American
Red Cross

W9-BVY-473

FIRST AID—
Responding to
Emergencies

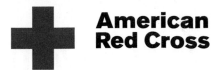

American Red Cross

FIRST AID—
Responding to Emergencies

Important certification information

American Red Cross certificates may be issued upon successful completion of a training program, which uses this textbook as an integral part of the course.
By itself, the text material does not constitute comprehensive Red Cross training. In order to issue American Red Cross certificates, your instructor must be authorized by the American Red Cross, and must follow prescribed policies and procedures. Make certain that you have attended a course authorized by the Red Cross. Ask your instructor about receiving American Red Cross certification, or contact your local chapter for more information.

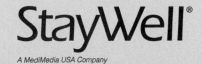

StayWell®

A MediMedia USA Company

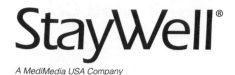

A MediMedia USA Company

Copyright © 2005 by The American National Red Cross. Revised edition 2007.

This participant's textbook is an integral part of the American Red Cross
First Aid—Responding to Emergencies course. By itself, it does not
constitute complete and comprehensive training for first aid. Please contact
your Red Cross chapter for further information on this course.

   The emergency care procedures outlined in this book reflect the standard
of knowledge and accepted emergency practices in the United States at the
time this book was published. It is the reader's responsibility to stay informed
of changes in emergency care procedures.

All rights reserved. No part of this publication may be reproduced, stored in
a retrieval system, or transmitted in any form or by any means, electronic,
mechanical, photocopying, recording, or otherwise, without prior written
permission from American Red Cross National Headquarters, Products and
Health and Safety Services.

The updates to this program are based on the 2005 Consensus on Science
for CPR and Emergency Cardiovascular Care (ECC) and meet the 2005
Guidelines for First Aid.

Printed in the United States of America

Composition by Graphic World
Printing/Binding by Banta Book Group

StayWell
780 Township Line Rd.
Yardley, PA 19067

Library of Congress cataloged the 4th edition as follows:

American Red Cross first aid : responding to emergencies.— 4th ed.
     p. ; cm.
   ISBN 978-1-58480-400-0
  1. First aid in illness and injury. 2. Medical emergencies.
[DNLM: 1. Emergencies—Programmed Instruction.
  2. First Aid—Programmed Instruction. WA 18.2 A512 2005]
  I. American Red Cross. II. American Red Cross first aid.

RC86.7.A477 2005
616.02'52—dc22

                                        2005002263

 09 10 / 9 8 7 6 5 4 3

Preface

This text is dedicated to the thousands of employees and volunteers of the American Red Cross who contribute their time and talent to supporting and teaching life-saving skills worldwide. And to the thousands of course participants and other readers who have decided to be prepared to take action when an emergency strikes.

*This Fourth Edition of the **First Aid—Responding To Emergencies** text has been updated with the latest science for First Aid, CPR and Emergency Cardiovascular Care (ECC 2005), and includes automated external defibrillation (AED) information and skills. The design has been significantly updated with a new format for skill sheets, key terms, sidebars and more. Skill sheets all now feature photos. Key content areas include a new Chapter 3, Before Giving Care, and Child and Adult AED content and skills being added to Chapter 7.*

This text is part of an integral training program with certification available from your local American Red Cross chapter. CPR and AED certifications are valid for 1 year while first aid certification is valid for 3 years. Contact your local American Red Cross at www.redcross.org for more information on how you can receive American Red Cross life-saving certification.

For more information about Red Cross training and services, visit www.redcross.org. For ordering information contact your local American Red Cross chapter or visit www.shopstaywell.com.

Acknowledgments

This textbook is the fourth edition of **American Red Cross First Aid—Responding to Emergencies**. *We have endeavored to improve and polish this text and course, which continue to meet the 2005 Consensus on Science for CPR and Emergency Cardiovascular Care (ECC) and meet 2005 Guidelines for First Aid. Many individuals shared in the development and revision process in various supportive, technical and creative ways. Each edition could not have been developed without the dedication and support of employees and volunteers.*

Fourth Edition—Pat Bonifer, Director; Mike Espino and Emilie Sparks Parker, Project Managers; John Beales, Ted T. Crites, CHES, Greg Stockton, Managers; C.P. Dail, Marc Madden and Connie Harvey, Senior Associates; Idabel Daly, Nancy J. Edmonds, Adreania McMillian, Mark Schraf and Stephan Widell, NREMT-P, Associates; Greta Petrilla, Marketing Manager; and Rhadames Avila and Betty Butler, Administrative Assistants.

The StayWell team for this fourth edition included: Nancy Monahan, Senior Vice President; Bill Winneberger, Senior Director of Manufacturing; Reed Klanderud, Marketing Director; Paula Batt, Sales Director; Shannon Bates, Managing Editor; Pam Billings, Product Manager; Carolyn Lemanski, Education Specialist/Higher Education; Jo Ann Emenecker, Editorial Project Manager; Bryan D. Elrod, Senior Developmental Editor; Louise Quinn, Publishing Coordinator; Stephanie Weidel, Senior Production Editor.

The American Red Cross and StayWell extend special thanks to Casey Berg, Katherine George and Vincent Knows.

Members of the American Red Cross Advisory Council on First Aid and Safety (ACFAS) also provided guidance and review—

Donald J. Gordon, PH.D., M.D.
Professor and Chairman, DEMT
University of Texas Health Science Center at
San Antonio
Chair, Advisory Council on First Aid and Safety
(ACFAS)
San Antonio, Texas

James A. Judge II, EMT-P, CEM
Executive Director, Lake-Sumter EMS, Inc.
Committee Member, Advisory Council on First
Aid and Safety (ACFAS)
Mount Dora, Florida

The American Red Cross thanks the following individuals for their reviews of this text or previous editions:

Stuart A. Balter, ATC, EMT-D
Hudson Valley Community College

Dayna S. Brown
Morehead State University

Kathleen C. Brown, MPH, BSN, CHES
University of Tennessee

Les Chatelain
University of Utah

Verallyn M. Cline
University of Wisconsin

Raymond A. Cranston
Farmington Hills Police Department

Susan T. Dempf, PhD
Canisius College

Dean W. Dimke
American Red Cross

Ann E. Graziadei
Gallaudet University

Arthur L. Grist, Sr.
University of Southern Illinois at Edwardsville

Susan J. Grosse
Milwaukee High School of the Arts

Kristen M. Haydon
American Red Cross Dallas Area Chapter

Joyce Holbrook Huner
Macomb Community College

Laird Hayes, EdD
American Red Cross Orange County Chapter

Richard C. Hunt, MD, FACEP
East Carolina University

Lisa Anne Johnson, EMT-P
Illinois State University

Constance S. LaBarbera, B.S., M.S., Ed.S., Ed.D.
Bossier Parish Community College

Louise Feasel Lindenmeyer
Shoreline Community College

Nancy S. Maylath, HSD
University of Toledo

Carol G. McKenzie, PhD
California State University

Tim McQuade, NYS EMT-P
Erie Community College

Marshall J. Meyer
American Red Cross Oregon Trail Chapter

Anthony Museulino
West Ontario County Chapter

Sean E. Page, MSN, CRNP, APRN-BC, CSN
American Red Cross York County Chapter

Deborah Radi
American Red Cross Greater Minneapolis Area Chapter

Catherine E. Rossilli
Westmont College

Tom Schmitz, NREMT
American Red Cross Greater Minneapolis Area Chapter

Barbara Ann Smink, RN, BSN
Boerne High School

Kemberley D. Wright
American Red Cross Rockingham County Chapter

The American Red Cross thanks the following organizations for their reviews of this text or previous editions:

American Camping Association

American College of Emergency Medicine

American College of Emergency Physicians

American Lyme Disease Foundation, Inc.

American Society of Poison Control Centers

Boy Scouts of America

Emergency Trauma Services Children's National Medical Center

Epilepsy Foundation for the National Capital Area

Girl Scouts of the USA

National Association of Emergency Medical Services Physicians

National Diabetes Information Clearinghouse

Practice Guidelines Wilderness Medical Society (WMS)

Shenandoah Mountain Rescue Group

Veterans Administration Medical Center

Contents

Detailed Table of Contents

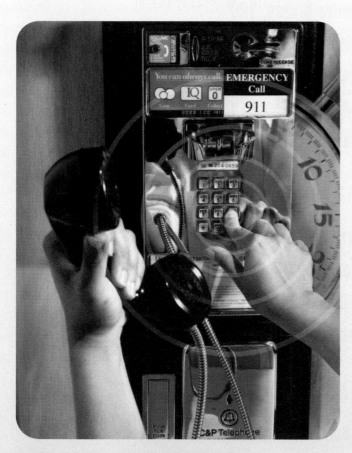

Chapter 2: Responding To An Emergency, 18

PART ONE: INTRODUCTION

Chapter 1: If Not You—Who?, 2

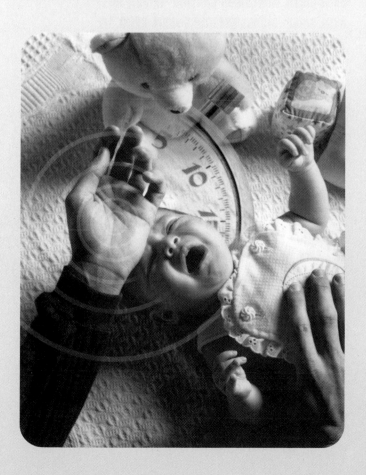

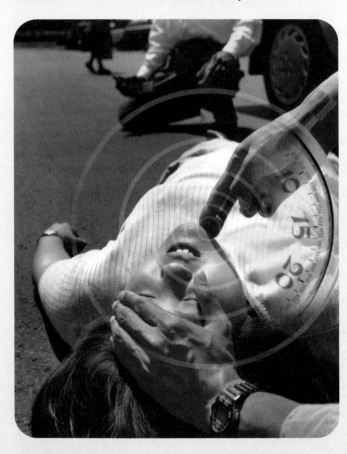

PART THREE: LIFE-THREATENING EMERGENCIES, 85

Chapter 6: Breathing Emergencies, 86

Chapter 7: Cardiac Emergencies and Unconscious Choking, 114

Chapter 8: Bleeding, 156

Chapter 9: Shock, 168

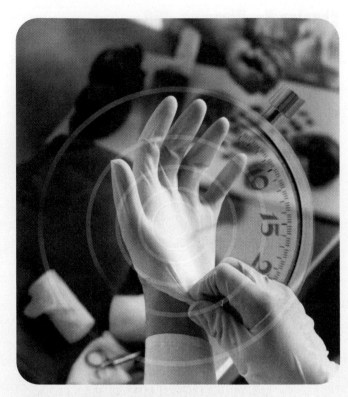

PART FOUR: INJURIES, 177

Chapter 10: Soft Tissue Injuries, 178

Chapter 11: Musculoskeletal Injuries, 204

Chapter 12: Injuries to the Extremities, 224

Chapter 13: Injuries to the Head, Neck and Back, 252

Chapter 14: Injuries to the Chest, Abdomen and Pelvis, 270

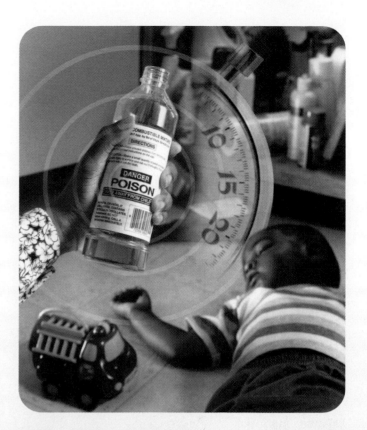

PART FIVE: MEDICAL EMERGENCIES, 283

Chapter 15: Sudden Illness, 284

Chapter 16: Poisoning, 302

Chapter 17: Bites and Stings, 318

Chapter 18: Substance Misuse and Abuse, 332

Chapter 19: Heat- and Cold-Related Emergencies, 350

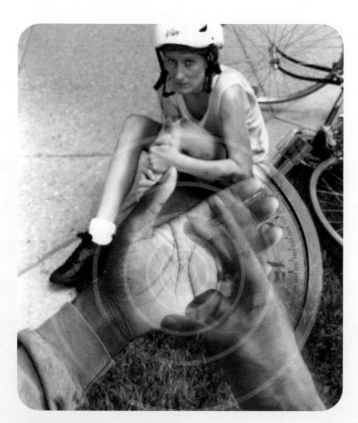

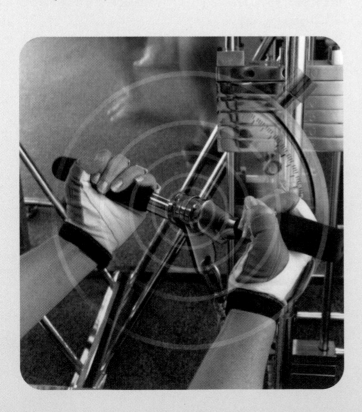

About This Course

WHY YOU SHOULD TAKE THIS COURSE

People need to know what to do in an emergency before medical help arrives. Since you, the citizen responder, are the person most likely to be first on the scene of an emergency, it is important that you know how to recognize emergencies and how to respond. This course will prepare you to make appropriate decisions regarding first aid care and to act on those decisions.

The first critical step in any emergency depends on the presence of someone who will take appropriate action. After completing this course, you should be able to—

* Recognize when an emergency has occurred.
* Follow the emergency action steps: **CHECK— CALL—CARE** for any emergency.
* Provide care for injury or sudden illness until professional medical help arrives.

This course clarifies when and how to call for emergency medical help, eliminating the confusion that is frequently a factor in any emergency. This course also emphasizes the importance of a safe, healthy lifestyle. The Healthy Lifestyles Awareness Inventory, which your instructor will provide, provides a means for you to evaluate your lifestyle, determine how you can improve it and help prevent lifestyle-related illness and injury.

HOW YOU WILL LEARN

Course content is presented in various ways. The textbook, which will be assigned reading, contains the information that will be discussed in class. Your instructor has the option to use video segments and power point display to support class discussions and other activities. These audiovisuals emphasize the key points that you will need to remember when making decisions in emergencies and will help you give appropriate care. They also present skills that you will practice in class. Participating in all class activities will increase your confidence in your ability to respond to emergencies.

The course design allows you to frequently evaluate your progress in terms of skills competency, knowledge and decision making. Certain chapters in the textbook include directions for skill practice sessions that are designed to help you learn specific first aid skills. Some of the practice sessions require practice on a manikin. Others give you the opportunity to practice with another person. This will give you a sense of what it would be like to care for a real person in an emergency situation and help reduce any concerns or fears you may have about giving care. Your ability to perform specific skills competently will be checked by your instructor during the practice sessions.

Your ability to make appropriate decisions when faced with an emergency will be enhanced as you participate in the class activities. Periodically, you will be given situations in the form of scenarios that provide you the opportunity to apply the knowledge and skills you have learned. These scenarios also provide an opportunity to discuss with your instructor the many different situations that you may encounter in any emergency.

REQUIREMENTS FOR COURSE COMPLETION CERTIFICATE

When this course is taught by a currently authorized American Red Cross instructor, you will be eligible for an American Red Cross course completion certificate. In order for you to receive an American Red Cross course completion certificate, you must—

- Correctly answer at least 80 percent or better in the appropriate sections on the final written exam(s).
- Participate in all skill sessions and scenarios.
- Demonstrate competency in all required skills.

The final written exam is designed to test your retention and understanding of the course material. You will take this exam at the end of the course. If you do not pass the written exam the first time, you may take a second exam.

If this course is taught at a college or university, there may be additional academic requirements, such as attendance and grading, that your instructor will explain to you.

TEXTBOOK

This textbook has been designed to facilitate your learning and understanding of the knowledge and skills required to effectively respond to emergency situations. The following pages graphically point out how to use this text to your best advantage.

Photographs, drawings, charts and graphs appear in all chapters, which illustrate skills, concepts and anatomical features.

Scenarios

Every chapter opener contains a brief scenario that presents an event involving some aspect of the chapter content. The story in the scenario will be used to answer the Application Questions in the chapter.

chapter 1

You and several friends are driving home after a softball game. It was a perfect afternoon for a game. You are discussing your team's prospects for making the play-offs when, several times, your attention is drawn to the car in front of you. It swerves across the double yellow line and veers back into its lane to avoid an oncoming car. You keep a safe distance behind the car. Suddenly, the car speeds up, runs a stop sign and smashes into a tree. You park your car a safe distance away from the accident scene and get out. As you approach the scene, you notice that the windshield is cracked in a star pattern, its edges red with blood. You see that the driver is motionless and bleeding from the forehead.

If Not You . . . Who?

Objectives

After reading this chapter, you should be able to—

- Describe two types of emergencies that require first aid.
- Describe your role in an emergency situation.
- Identify the most important action you can take in a non-life-threatening emergency.
- List five common barriers to action that may prevent people from responding to emergencies.
- Identify six ways bystanders can help at the scene of an emergency.

Objectives

At the beginning of each chapter is a bulleted list of objectives. Each item describes something you should know or be able to do after reading the chapter and participating in class activities. Read this list carefully, and refer back to it as you read the chapter. These objectives form the basis for test questions on the final exam.

Key Terms and Glossary Terms

A list of key terms with their definitions appears on the front page of each chapter in a purple box. You need to know these key terms and their meanings to understand the material in the chapters. These key terms are printed in **boldface italics** *the first time they are explained in the chapter and also appear, defined, in the Glossary. Some key terms are listed in more than one chapter because they are essential to your understanding of the material presented in each.*

Glossary terms are set in **bold** *in the text.*

---

4   PART ONE   INTRODUCTION

Introduction

An **emergency** is a situation demanding immediate action. An emergency can happen at any place (on the road, in your home, where you work), to anyone (a friend, relative, stranger) and at any time. This text provides you with basic *first aid* information and skills so that you will recognize and respond to any emergency appropriately. Your response may help save a life.

TYPES OF EMERGENCIES

There are two types of emergencies that require first aid: sudden illness or an injury. A *sudden illness* is a physical condition that requires immediate medical attention. Examples of sudden illness include a heart attack and a severe allergic reaction. An *in-*

jury is damage to the body from an external force, such as a broken bone from a fall. Emergencies can also be categorized as life-threatening and non-life-threatening. A *life-threatening emergency* is an illness or injury that impairs a victim's ability to circulate oxygenated blood to all the parts of his or her body. A *non-life-threatening emergency* is a situation that does not have an immediate impact on a victim's ability to circulate oxygenated blood, but still requires medical attention. You will learn more about caring for life-threatening and non-life-threatening emergencies as you progress through this text.

YOUR ROLE IN AN EMERGENCY

The *emergency medical services (EMS) system* is a network of community resources and medical personnel that provides emergency care to victims of life-threatening injury or sudden illness. Think of the EMS system as a chain made up of several links. Each link depends on the others for success. Without the involvement of *citizen responders* such as you, the EMS system cannot function effectively. As

KEY TERMS

Barriers to action: Reasons for not acting or for hesitating to act in an emergency situation.

Citizen responder: A layperson (someone who does not have special or advanced medical training or skill) who recognizes an emergency and decides to act.

Emergency: A situation requiring immediate action.

Emergency medical services (EMS) personnel: Trained and equipped community-based personnel who provide emergency care for ill or injured victims and who are often dispatched through a local emergency number.

Emergency medical services (EMS) system: A network of community resources and medical personnel that provides emergency care to victims of injury or sudden illness.

Emergency medical technician (EMT): A person who has successfully completed a state-approved emergency medical technician training program. The levels of EMTs are the EMT-Basic, EMT-Intermediate and EMT-Paramedic.

First aid: Immediate care given to a victim of injury or sudden illness until more advanced care can be obtained.

First responder: A person trained in emergency care that may be called on to give such care as a routine part of his or her job.

Good Samaritan laws: Laws that protect people who willingly give first aid without accepting anything in return.

Injury: Damage that occurs when the body is subjected to an external force, such as a blow, a fall, a collision, an electrical current or temperature extremes.

Life-threatening emergency: An illness or injury that impairs a victim's ability to circulate oxygenated blood to all the parts of his or her body.

Non-life-threatening emergency: A situation that does not have an immediate impact on a victim's ability to circulate oxygenated blood, but still requires medical attention.

Sudden illness: A physical condition requiring immediate medical attention.

SUMMARY

An emergency can happen at any place, and at any time. The emergency medical services (EMS) system is a network of community resources and medical personnel that provides emergency care to victims of injury or sudden illness. However, the EMS system cannot properly function without the actions of a trained citizen responder like you. By

CHAPTER 1   If Not You . . . Who?   15

learning to recognize an emergency and deciding to act (calling 9-1-1 or the local emergency number and giving care) you can help save the life of a victim of injury or sudden illness.

In the following chapters, you will learn how to manage different kinds of emergencies. You will learn emergency action steps that you can apply to any emergency situation and how to give care in both life-threatening and non-life-threatening situations.

Application Questions

Application Questions, designated with a blue heading in a pale gold box, challenge you to apply the information you have learned and build a solution. The questions are based on the scenario that appears on the chapter-opening page. These questions allow you to apply the information you have been learning to a real-life situation. Answers to the Application Questions are found in Appendix A of this text.

APPLICATION QUESTIONS

1. What immediate steps could you and your friends who witnessed the car crash take?

2. As you approach the victim of the car crash, you begin to feel faint and nauseated and are not sure you can proceed any farther. How can you still help?

3. The approximate time of the crash you witnessed was 4:50 p.m. The EMS personnel did not arrive until 5:25 p.m., and the victim did not arrive at the hospital until 6:30 p.m. What might have caused this delay in reaching the victim and getting him to the hospital?

Shock: The Domino Effect

- An injury causes severe bleeding.
- The heart attempts to compensate for the disruption of blood flow by beating faster.
- The victim first has a rapid pulse. More blood is lost. As blood volume drops, the pulse becomes weak or hard to find.
- The increased workload on the heart results in an increased oxygen demand. Therefore, breathing becomes faster.
- To maintain circulation of blood to the vital organs, blood vessels constrict in the arms, legs and skin. Therefore, the skin appears pale or ashen and feels cool.
- In response to the stress, the body perspires heavily and the skin feels moist.
- Because tissues of the arms and legs are now without oxygen, cells start to die.
- The brain now sends a signal to return blood to the arms and legs in an attempt to balance blood flow between these body parts and the vital organs.
- Vital organs now are not receiving adequate oxygen.
- The heart tries to compensate by beating even faster.

- More blood is lost and the victim's condition worsens.
- Without oxygen, the vital organs fail to function properly.
- As the brain is affected, the victim becomes restless, drowsy and eventually loses consciousness.
- As the heart is affected, it beats irregularly, resulting in an irregular pulse. The rhythm then becomes chaotic and the heart fails to circulate blood.
- There are no longer signs of circulation.
- When the heart stops, breathing stops.
- The body's continuous attempt to compensate for severe blood loss eventually results in death.

SUMMARY

Do not wait for shock to develop before giving care to a victim of injury or sudden illness. Always follow the general care steps for any emergency to minimize the progression of shock. Care for life-threatening conditions, such as breathing emergen-

cies or severe external bleeding, non-life-threatening conditions. key to managing shock effectively the local emergency number and as possible.

Sidebars

Feature articles called sidebars enhance the information presented in the main body of the text. They appear in most chapters and have a purple background. They present historical and current information and events that relate to the content of the chapter. You will not be tested on any information presented in these sidebars as part of the American Red Cross course completion requirements.

Tables

Tables, on a light gold background, are included in many chapters. They summarize key concepts and information and may aid in studying.

Table 4-1 Body Systems

SYSTEM	MAJOR STRUCTURES	HOW THE SYSTEM WORKS — PRIMARY FUNCTION	WITH OTHER BODY SYSTEMS
Respiratory	Airway and lungs	Supplies the body with oxygen and removes carbon dioxide through breathing	Works with the circulatory system to provide oxygen to cells; controlled by the nervous system
Circulatory	Heart, blood and blood vessels	Transports nutrients and oxygen to body cells and removes waste products	Works with the respiratory system to provide oxygen to cells; works in conjunction with the urinary and digestive systems to remove waste products; helps give skin color; controlled by the nervous system
Nervous	Brain, spinal cord and nerves	One of two primary regulatory systems in the body; transmits messages to and from the brain	Regulates all body systems through a network of nerves
Musculoskeletal	Bones, ligaments, muscles and tendons	Provides body's framework; protects internal organs and other underlying structures; allows movement; produces heat; manufactures blood components	Provides protection to organs and structures of other body systems; muscle action is controlled by the nervous system
Integumentary	Skin, hair and nails	An important part of the body's communication network; helps prevent infection and dehydration; assists with temperature regulation; aids in production of certain vitamins	Helps to protect the body from disease-producing organisms; together with the circulatory system, helps to regulate body temperature; under control of the nervous system; communicates sensation to the brain through the nerves
Endocrine	Glands	Secretes hormones and other substances into blood and onto skin	Together with the nervous system coordinates the activities of other systems
Digestive	Mouth, esophagus, stomach, intestines, pancreas, gallbladder and liver	Breaks down food into usable form to supply the rest of the body with energy	Works with the circulatory system to transport nutrients to the body
Genitourinary	Kidneys and bladder	Removes waste from the circulatory system and regulates water balance	
	Uterus and genitalia	Performs the process of sexual reproduction	

Boxes

Boxes contain information that may be useful or of interest to you. They appear throughout the textbook.

Child Safety

The following statements represent an awareness of child safety that can reduce the chances of injury to your child. Check each statement that reflects your lifestyle.

☐ I buckle my child into an approved automobile safety seat even when making short trips.

☐ I teach my child safety by behaving safely in my everyday activities.

☐ I supervise my child whenever he or she is around water and maintain fences and gates that act as barriers to water.

☐ I have checked my home for potential fire hazards and smoke detectors are installed and working.

☐ I have placed foods and small items that can choke my child out of his or her reach.

☐ I inspect my home, day-care center, school, babysitter's home or wherever my child spends time for potential safety and health hazards.

If you only checked one or two statements, you should consider making changes in your lifestyle now.

Home Safety

The following statements represent a safety-conscious lifestyle that can reduce your chances, and the chances of others, of injury in your home.

☐ The stairways and halls in my home are well lit.

☐ I have nonskid tread or securely fastened rugs on my stairs.

☐ I keep all medications out of reach of children and in a locked cabinet.

☐ I keep any poisonous materials out of the reach of children and in a locked cabinet.

☐ All rugs are firmly secured to the floor.

☐ I store all firearms, unloaded, in a locked place out of the reach of children, and ammunition is stored separately.

☐ I keep the handles of pots and pans on the stove turned inward when I am using them.

If you only checked one or two statements, you should consider making changes in your lifestyle now.

• Diving from a diving board should only occur if there is a safe diving envelope (the area of water in front of, below and to the sides of a diving board that is deep enough that a diver will not strike the bottom, regardless of the depth of the water or the design of the pool).

▸ Location of the nearest fire extinguisher and first aid kit

If you work in an environment where hazards exist, wear recommended safety equipment and follow safety procedures (**Fig. 24-5**). Both employers and employees must follow safety rules issued by

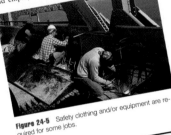

Figure 24-5 Safety clothing and/or equipment are required for some jobs.

STUDY QUESTIONS

1. Match each term with the correct definition.

   a. Carbohydrates
   b. Obesity
   c. Stress
   d. Cardiorespiratory endurance
   e. Aerobic exercise
   f. Saturated fat
   g. Calorie

   ———— A measure of the energy value of food.

   ———— A physiological or psychological response to real or imagined influences that alter an existing state of physical, mental or emotional balance.

   ———— The ability to take in, deliver and extract oxygen for physical work.

   ———— The fat in animal tissues and products.

   ———— Activities that require additional effort by the heart and lungs to meet the increased demand by the skeletal muscles for oxygen.

   ———— A condition characterized by excess of stored body fat.

   ———— Compounds that contain carbon, oxygen and hydrogen; the main source of energy for all body functions.

2. Fill in the blanks with the correct word or words.

   The leading cause of death in the United States is _____. The disease that is the leading cause of death is _____. The leading cause of death for people ages 1 to 39 is _____.

3. List three ways to reduce your risk of personal injury.

4. List two motor-vehicle safety guidelines.

5. List four guidelines for what to do in case the building you are in catches fire.

6. When Jake learned that his grandmother had fallen in the upstairs hall, he went to her house to see what he could do to make it safer for her. What hazards might he have discovered in the hall? What could he do to make the hall safer?

7. Your 2-year-old nephew is coming to visit. What can you do to make your kitchen safe?

Study Questions

At the end of each chapter are a series of Study Questions designed to test your retention and understanding of the chapter content and key terms. Completing these questions will help you determine how well you understand the material and also help you prepare for the final written exam. The answers to Study Questions are located in Appendix A of this text. Write the answers in your textbook and use additional paper, if necessary.

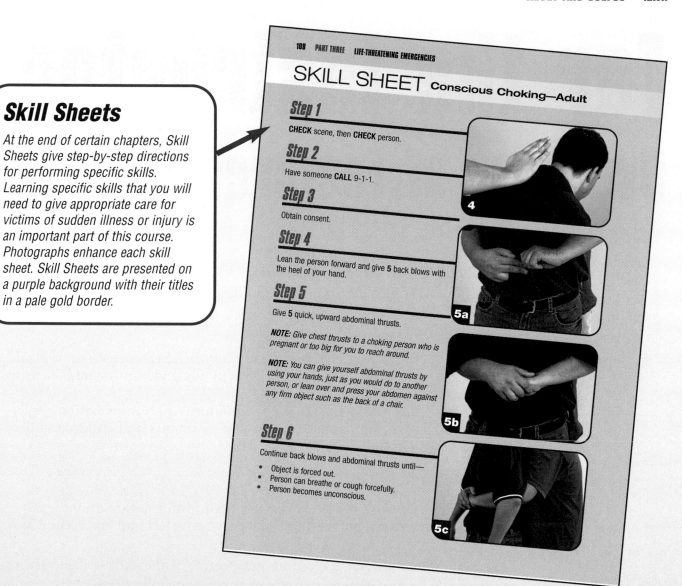

Skill Sheets

At the end of certain chapters, Skill Sheets give step-by-step directions for performing specific skills. Learning specific skills that you will need to give appropriate care for victims of sudden illness or injury is an important part of this course. Photographs enhance each skill sheet. Skill Sheets are presented on a purple background with their titles in a pale gold border.

108 PART THREE LIFE-THREATENING EMERGENCIES

SKILL SHEET Conscious Choking—Adult

Step 1

CHECK scene, then CHECK person.

Step 2

Have someone CALL 9-1-1.

Step 3

Obtain consent.

Step 4

Lean the person forward and give 5 back blows with the heel of your hand.

Step 5

Give 5 quick, upward abdominal thrusts.

NOTE: Give chest thrusts to a choking person who is pregnant or too big for you to reach around.

NOTE: You can give yourself abdominal thrusts by using your hands, just as you would do to another person, or lean over and press your abdomen against any firm object such as the back of a chair.

Step 6

Continue back blows and abdominal thrusts until—
- Object is forced out.
- Person can breathe or cough forcefully.
- Person becomes unconscious.

HOW TO USE THIS TEXTBOOK

You should complete the following five steps for each chapter to gain the most from this course:

1. Read the chapter objectives before reading the chapter.
2. As you read the chapter, keep the objectives in mind. When you finish, go back and review the objectives. Check to see that you can meet them without difficulty.
3. Review figures and illustrations. Read captions and labels.
4. Answer the Application Questions at the end of each chapter. Check your answers with those in Appendix A. If you cannot answer or do not understand the answers given, ask your instructor to help you with concepts or questions with which you are having difficulty.
5. Answer the Study Questions at the end of each chapter. Mark or write your answers in the text to facilitate your review or study. Answer as many questions as you can without referring to the chapter. Then review the information covering any questions you were unable to answer, and try them again. Check your responses to the questions with the answers in Appendix A. If you have not answered a question appropriately, reread that part of the chapter to ensure that you understand why the answer is correct. This exercise will help you gauge how much information you are retaining and which areas you need to review. If, after rereading that part of the chapter, you still do not understand, ask your instructor to help you.

For the Instructor
Overview of Features

The following provides a preview for instructors of new features and content in this fourth edition of Responding to Emergencies.

New Content:

- *Adult Automated External Defibrillator* (AED) focuses on typical AED equipment, using an AED safely for a victim of sudden cardiac arrest and working with EMS
- *Child Automated External Defibrillator* (AED) information, skills and recognizing cardiac emergencies in infants and children under 8 years old

New Chapter:

- *Before Giving Care* gives you important information about legal considerations, preventing disease transmission and emergency moves

New Skill Sheets provide a close-up perspective of the skill sequence being taught providing an easy-to-use reference to keep skills sharp

Streamlined CPR skills increase the ability of the student to remember skills when they are needed

Nationally recognized course completion certificate. American Red Cross First Aid, CPR and AED training is standardized and recognized by many national, state and local authorities

Courses developed by experts. American Red Cross materials are developed in collaboration with leading educational and medical authorities and reflect the most current information and techniques. Red Cross CPR and first aid courses are based on the 2005 Consensus on Science for CPR and Emergency Cardiovascular Care (ECC) and the 2005 Guidelines for First Aid.

Team Up with the American Red Cross—the Most Trusted Name in Health and Safety Training for More than 90 years.

For additional health and safety and disaster preparedness resources, visit *www.redcross.org* today or contact your local American Red Cross chapter.

Health Precautions

HEALTH PRECAUTIONS AND GUIDELINES DURING FIRST AID TRAINING

The American Red Cross has trained millions of people in first aid and CPR (cardiopulmonary resuscitation) using manikins as training aids.

The Red Cross follows widely accepted guidelines for cleaning and decontaminating training manikins. If these guidelines are adhered to, the risk of any kind of disease transmission during training is extremely low.

To help minimize the risk of disease transmission, you should follow some basic health precautions and guidelines while participating in training. You should take precautions if you have a condition that would increase your risk or other participants' risk of exposure to infections. Request a separate training manikin if you—

- Have an acute condition, such as a cold, a sore throat or cuts or sores on the hands or around your mouth.
- Know you are seropositive (have had a positive blood test) for hepatitis B surface antigen (HBsAg), indicating that you are currently infected with the hepatitis B virus.
- Know you have a chronic infection indicated by long-term seropositivity (long-term positive blood tests) for the hepatitis B surface antigen (HBsAg)* or a positive blood test for anti-HIV (that is, a positive test for antibodies to HIV, the virus that causes many severe infections including AIDS).
- Have had a positive blood test for hepatitis C (HCV).
- Have a type of condition that makes you unusually likely to get an infection.

To obtain information about testing for individual health status, go to: *www.cdc.gov/ncidod/diseases/hepatitis/c/faq.htm*

*A person with hepatitis B infection will test positive for the hepatitis B surface antigen (HBsAg). Most persons infected with hepatitis B will get better within a period of time. However, some hepatitis B infections will become chronic and will linger for much longer. These persons will continue to test positive for HBsAg. Their decision to participate in CPR training should be guided by their physician.

After a person has had an acute hepatitis B infection, he or she will no longer test positive for the surface antigen but will test positive for the hepatitis B antibody (anti-HBs). Persons who have been vaccinated for hepatitis B will also test positive for the hepatitis antibody. A positive test for the hepatitis B antibody (anti-HBs) should not be confused with a positive test for the hepatitis B surface antigen (HBsAg).

If you decide you should have your own manikin, ask your instructor if he or she can provide one for you to use. You will not be asked to explain why in your request. The manikin will not be used by anyone else until it has been cleaned according to the recommended end-of-class decontamination procedures. Because the number of manikins available for class use is limited, the more advance notice you give, the more likely it is that you can be provided a separate manikin.

GUIDELINES

In addition to taking the precautions regarding manikins, you can further protect yourself and other participants from infection by following these guidelines:
- Wash your hands thoroughly before participating in class activities.
- Do not eat, drink, use tobacco products or chew gum during classes when manikins are used.
- Clean the manikin properly before use.
  - For some manikins, this means vigorously wiping the manikin's face and the inside of its mouth with a clean gauze pad soaked with either a fresh solution of liquid chlorine bleach (¼ c sodium hypochlorite per gallon of tap water) or rubbing alcohol. The surfaces should remain wet for at least 1 minute before they are wiped dry with a second piece of clean, absorbent material.
  - For other manikins, it means changing the manikin's face. Your instructor will provide you with instructions for cleaning the type of manikin used in your class.
- Follow the guidelines provided by your instructor when practicing skills such as clearing a blocked airway with your finger.

PHYSICAL STRESS AND INJURY

Successful course completion requires full participation in classroom and skill sessions, as well as successful performance in skill and knowledge evaluations. Due to the nature of the skills in this course, you will be participating in strenuous activities, such as performing cardiopulmonary resuscitation (CPR) on the floor. If you have a medical condition or disability that will prevent you from taking part in the skills practice sessions, please let your instructor know so that accommodations can be made. If you are unable to participate fully in the course, you may "audit" the course and participate as much as you can or desire. In order to audit a course, you must let the instructor know before the training begins. Be aware that you will not be eligible to receive a course completion certificate.

Part ONE

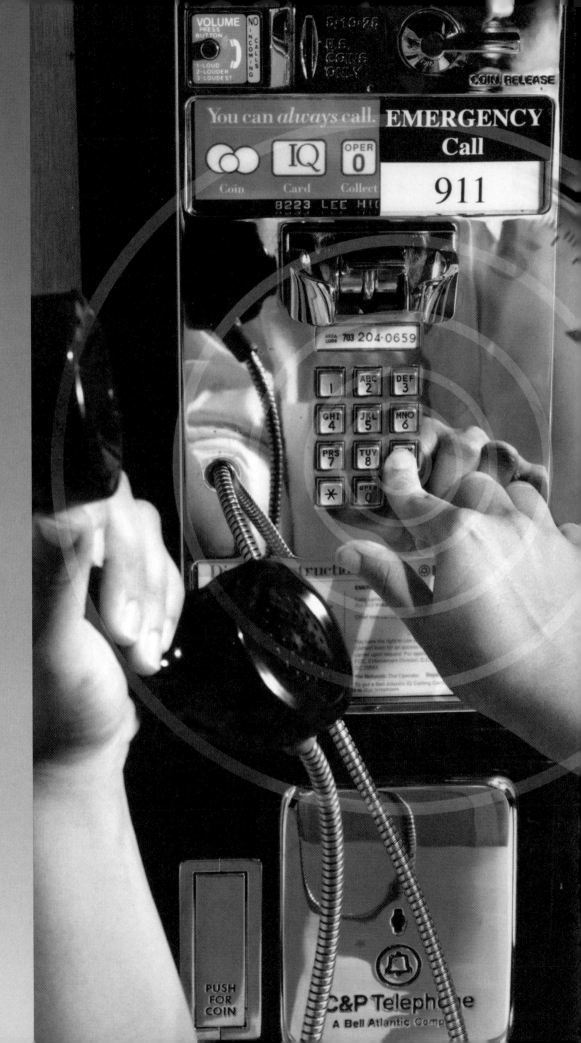

Introduction

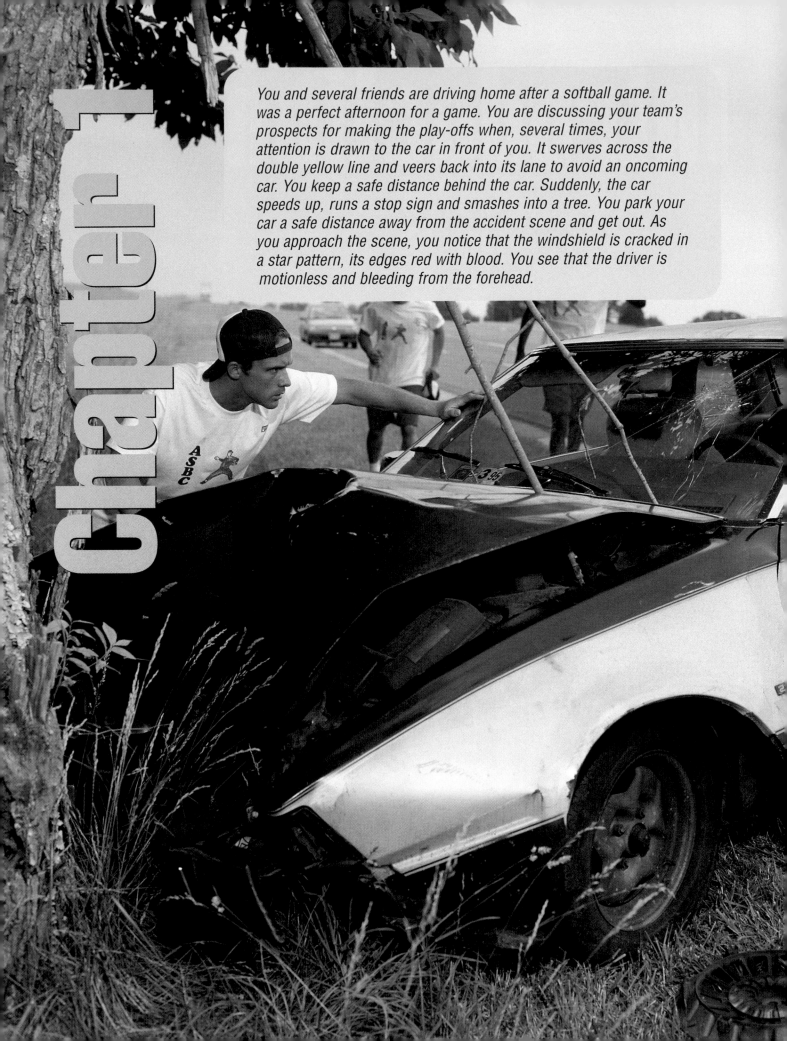

chapter 1

You and several friends are driving home after a softball game. It was a perfect afternoon for a game. You are discussing your team's prospects for making the play-offs when, several times, your attention is drawn to the car in front of you. It swerves across the double yellow line and veers back into its lane to avoid an oncoming car. You keep a safe distance behind the car. Suddenly, the car speeds up, runs a stop sign and smashes into a tree. You park your car a safe distance away from the accident scene and get out. As you approach the scene, you notice that the windshield is cracked in a star pattern, its edges red with blood. You see that the driver is motionless and bleeding from the forehead.

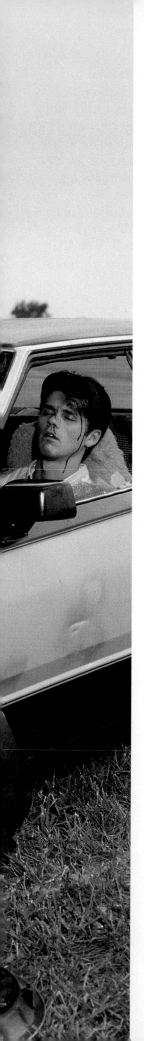

If Not You . . . Who?

Objectives

After reading this chapter, you should be able to—

■ *Describe two types of emergencies that require first aid.*

■ *Describe your role in an emergency situation.*

■ *Identify the most important action you can take in a non-life-threatening emergency.*

■ *List five common barriers to action that may prevent people from responding to emergencies.*

■ *Identify six ways bystanders can help at the scene of an emergency.*

Introduction

An **emergency** is a situation demanding immediate action. An emergency can happen at any place (on the road, in your home, where you work), to anyone (a friend, relative, stranger) and at any time. This text provides you with basic **first aid** information and skills so that you will recognize and respond to any emergency appropriately. Your response may help save a life.

TYPES OF EMERGENCIES

There are two types of emergencies that require first aid: sudden illness or an injury. A **sudden illness** is a physical condition that requires immediate medical attention. Examples of sudden illness include a heart attack and a severe allergic reaction. An **in-**

jury is damage to the body from an external force, such as a broken bone from a fall. Emergencies can also be categorized as life-threatening and non-life-threatening. A **life-threatening emergency** is an illness or injury that impairs a victim's ability to circulate oxygenated blood to all the parts of his or her body. A **non-life-threatening emergency** is a situation that does not have an immediate impact on a victim's ability to circulate oxygenated blood, but still requires medical attention. You will learn more about caring for life-threatening and non-life-threatening emergencies as you progress through this text.

YOUR ROLE IN AN EMERGENCY

The **emergency medical services (EMS) system** is a network of community resources and medical personnel that provides emergency care to victims of life-threatening injury or sudden illness. Think of the EMS system as a chain made up of several links. Each link depends on the others for success. Without the involvement of **citizen responders** such as you, the EMS system cannot function effectively. As

KEY TERMS

Barriers to action: Reasons for not acting or for hesitating to act in an emergency situation.

Citizen responder: A layperson (someone who does not have special or advanced medical training or skill) who recognizes an emergency and decides to act.

Emergency: A situation requiring immediate action.

Emergency medical services (EMS) personnel: Trained and equipped community-based personnel who provide emergency care for ill or injured victims and who are often dispatched through a local emergency number.

Emergency medical services (EMS) system: A network of community resources and medical personnel that provides emergency care to victims of injury or sudden illness.

Emergency medical technician (EMT): A person who has successfully completed a state-approved emergency medical technician training program. The levels of EMTs are the EMT-Basic, EMT-Intermediate and EMT-Paramedic.

First aid: Immediate care given to a victim of injury or sudden illness until more advanced care can be obtained.

First responder: A person trained in emergency care that may be called on to give such care as a routine part of his or her job.

Good Samaritan laws: Laws that protect people who willingly give first aid without accepting anything in return.

Injury: Damage that occurs when the body is subjected to an external force, such as a blow, a fall, a collision, an electrical current or temperature extremes.

Life-threatening emergency: An illness or injury that impairs a victim's ability to circulate oxygenated blood to all the parts of his or her body.

Non-life-threatening emergency: A situation that does not have an immediate impact on a victim's ability to circulate oxygenated blood, but still requires medical attention.

Sudden illness: A physical condition requiring immediate medical attention.

The EMS System

EMS CALL TAKER

EMS call takers work in emergency communications centers. When 9-1-1 is dialed, the call taker receives the call and quickly determines what help is needed. He or she then dispatches the appropriate *EMS personnel.* An increasing number of call takers are trained emergency medical dispatchers and can provide instructions on how to help until EMS personnel arrive.

FIRST RESPONDER

First responders are often the first people you turn to for help at the scene of an emergency. They may be firefighters, law enforcement officers, lifeguards, industrial safety officers or people with similar responsibility for the safety or well-being of the community. Because of the nature of their jobs, they are often close to the scene and have the necessary supplies and equipment to give care. First responders provide a critical transition between a citizen responder's basic level of care and the care provided by more advanced EMS personnel.

EMERGENCY MEDICAL TECHNICIANS

Emergency medical technicians (EMTs) are trained medical professionals who are dispatched to an emergency by the call taker. Once the emergency medical technicians arrive, they determine the victim's condition and give advanced care. There are three levels of training and certification—EMT-Basic, EMT-Intermediate and EMT-Paramedic.

Emergency Medical Technician-Basic (EMT-Basic)

In most of the United States, ambulance personnel are certified at least at the EMT-Basic level. The EMT-Basic is trained to assess a victim's condition and care for both life-threatening and non-life-threatening emergencies.

Emergency Medical Technician-Intermediate

An EMT-Intermediate has more advanced training that allows him or her to perform techniques such as administering medications and intravenous fluids.

EMT-Paramedics

EMT-Paramedics are highly specialized emergency medical technicians. In addition to performing basic life-support skills, paramedics can administer medications and intravenous fluids, provide advanced airway care and perform other advanced lifesaving techniques. They are trained to handle a wider range of conditions. Paramedics function at the highest level of out-of-hospital care.

a citizen responder, your primary role in an emergency includes—

▶ Recognizing that an emergency exists.
▶ Deciding to act.
▶ Taking action by calling 9-1-1 or the local emergency number.
▶ Giving care until medical help arrives.

In the first few minutes of an emergency, a citizen responder trained in first aid can provide help that can save a life or make the difference between a complete recovery and permanent **disability** (**Fig. 1-1,** *A-D*).

RECOGNIZING EMERGENCIES

The ability to recognize that an emergency has occurred is the first step toward taking appropriate action (**Table 1-1**). You may become aware of an emergency from certain indicators, including unusual noises, sights, odors, appearance or behavior (**Fig. 1-2,** *A-D*).

Unusual Noises

Unusual noises are often the first indicators that call your attention to an emergency. Some noises that may indicate an emergency include—

▶ Screaming, yelling, moaning or calling for help.
▶ Breaking glass, crashing metal or screeching tires.
▶ Sudden, loud or unidentifiable sounds.
▶ Unusual silence.

Unusual Sights

Unusual sights can also be a common indicator that an emergency has occurred. Sights that indicate a possible emergency include—

▶ A stopped vehicle on the roadside, especially in an unusual position.
▶ Broken glass.
▶ An overturned pot on the kitchen floor.

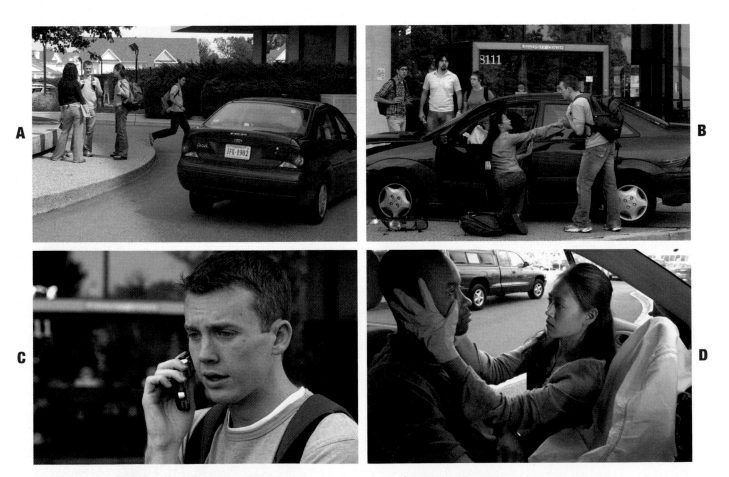

Figure 1-1 The role of the citizen responder includes **A,** recognizing an emergency, **B,** deciding to act, **C,** calling 9-1-1 or the local emergency number, and **D,** giving care until EMS personnel arrive.

▶ A spilled medicine container.
▶ Downed electrical wires.
▶ Sparks, smoke or fire.

Unusual Odors

Odors are part of our everyday lives, such as gasoline fumes at gas stations or smoke from a bonfire. However, when odors are stronger than usual, not easily identifiable or otherwise seem inappropriate, they may indicate an emergency. Always put your own safety first if you smell an unusual or very strong odor, because many fumes are poisonous. An unusual odor on a person's breath may also be a clue to an emergency situation. A person experiencing a diabetic emergency, for example, may have a breath odor that can be mistaken for the smell of alcohol. You will learn about diabetic emergencies in Chapter 15.

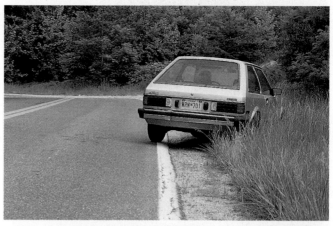

A

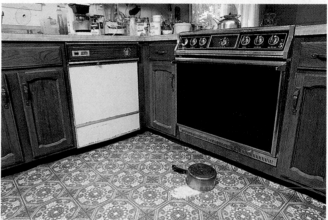

B

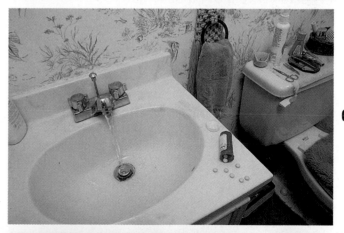

C

Table 1-1 Recognizing Emergencies

COMMON INDICATORS	EXAMPLES
Unusual noises	Screams, yells, moans or calls for help Breaking glass, crashing metal, screeching tires Sudden, loud or unidentifiable sounds Unusual silence
Unusual sights	Stopped vehicle on the roadside Broken glass Overturned pot in kitchen Spilled medicine container Downed electrical wires Sparks, smoke or fire
Unusual odors	Odors that are stronger than usual Unrecognizable odors Inappropriate odors
Unusual appearance or behavior	Unconsciousness Confused or unusual behavior Trouble breathing Clutching chest or throat Slurred, confused or hesitant speech Unexplainable confusion or drowsiness Sweating for no apparent reason Uncharacteristic skin color Inability to move a body part

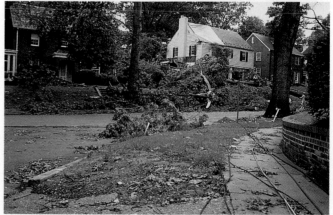

D

Figure 1-2   A-D, Unusual sights may indicate an emergency.

Unusual Appearance or Behavior

It may be difficult to tell if someone's appearance or behavior is unusual, particularly if he or she is a stranger. Certain behaviors or appearances could indicate an emergency (**Fig. 1-3**). If you see someone collapse to the floor, he or she obviously requires your immediate attention. You will not know if your help is needed until you approach the victim. He or she may merely have slipped and may not need your help. On the other hand, the person may be unconscious and need immediate medical assistance. Other behaviors and appearances that could indicate an emergency may be less obvious. They include—

▶ Unconsciousness.
▶ Confused or unusual behavior.
▶ Trouble breathing.
▶ Clutching the chest or throat.
▶ Slurred, confused or hesitant speech.
▶ Unexplainable confusion or drowsiness.
▶ Sweating for no apparent reason.
▶ Uncharacteristic skin color—pale, ashen, flushed or bluish skin.
▶ Inability to move a body part.

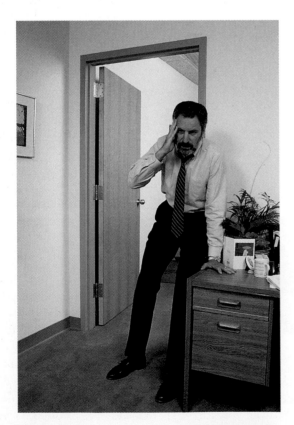

Figure 1-3 Unusual appearance may indicate an emergency.

These and other appearances and behaviors may occur alone or together. For example, a heart attack may be indicated by chest pain alone or may be accompanied by sweating and trouble breathing. You will learn more about the signals of a heart attack in Chapter 7.

DECIDING TO ACT

Once you recognize that an emergency has occurred, you must decide to act. Calling 9-1-1 or the local emergency number is the most important action you and other citizen responders can take. Early arrival of EMS personnel increases the victim's chances of surviving a life-threatening emergency.

Overcoming Barriers to Action

Sometimes people simply do not recognize that an emergency has occurred. At other times, people recognize an emergency but are reluctant to act. People have various reasons for hesitating or not acting. These reasons are called *barriers to action.* Common reasons people give for not acting include—

▶ The presence of bystanders.
▶ Uncertainty about the victim.
▶ The nature of the injury or illness.
▶ Fear of disease transmission.
▶ Fear of not knowing what to do or of doing something wrong.
▶ Being unsure of when to call 9-1-1.

Thinking about these barriers and mentally preparing yourself to overcome them will help you respond more confidently when an actual emergency occurs.

Presence of Bystanders

Bystanders can cause confusion at an emergency scene. It may not be easy to tell if anyone is giving first aid. In every emergency situation you should always ask if help is needed. Do not assume, just because a crowd has gathered, that someone is caring for the victim. You may feel embarrassed about coming forward in front of strangers. Do not let this feeling deter you from offering help when needed. You may be the only one at the scene who knows first aid. If someone else is already giving care, offer to help. Ensure that the crowd does not endanger it-

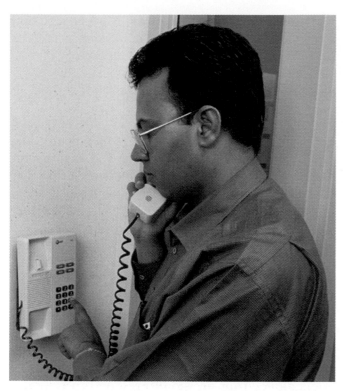

Figure 1-4   Bystanders can help you respond to emergencies.

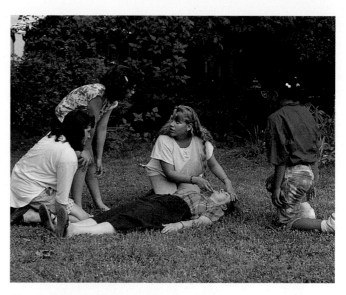

Figure 1-5   You may need to respond to an emergency involving someone whom you do not know.

self or the victim. Sometimes you may need to ask bystanders who are not helping to back away and give the victim and responders ample space.

Bystanders can be of great help in an emergency (**Fig. 1-4**). You can ask them to call for, meet and direct the ambulance; keep the area free of unnecessary traffic; or help you give first aid. You might send them for blankets or other supplies. Bystanders may have valuable information about what happened or may know the victim's medical history. Bystanders can also help comfort the victim and others at the scene.

Uncertainty About the Victim

Because most emergencies happen in or near the home, you are more likely to give care to a friend or family member than to a stranger (**Fig. 1-5**). However, this is not always the case. You may not know the victim and feel uncomfortable with the idea of touching a stranger. You may hesitate to act because the victim may be much older or younger than you, be of a different gender or race, not speak the same language or have a disabling condition. However, despite your reluctance, it is important to remember that the victim is a person in need of help and that

you can always take some type of action to help: call 9-1-1 or the local emergency number, volunteer to meet and guide EMS personnel to the scene or assist those who are giving care.

Sometimes victims of injury or sudden illness may act strangely or be uncooperative. The injury or illness, stress or other factors, such as the influence of alcohol or other substances, may make people act offensively. Do not take such behavior personally. Remember, an emergency can cause even the nicest person to act angry or unpleasant. If the victim's attitude or behavior keeps you from caring for him or her, you can still help. Call 9-1-1 or the local emergency number. Once the EMS system has been activated, manage bystanders and attempt to reassure the victim. If at any time the victim's behavior becomes a threat to you, you should withdraw from the immediate area.

Nature of the Injury or Illness

An injury or illness may sometimes be very unpleasant to handle. The presence of blood, vomit, unpleasant odors or torn or burned skin may disturb you. You cannot predict how you will respond to these and other factors in an emergency. Sometimes you may need to compose yourself before acting. If you must, turn away for a moment and take a few deep breaths, then give care. If you are still unable to give care, you can help in other ways, such as volunteering to call 9-1-1 or the local emergency number or managing other bystanders at the scene.

Fear of Disease Transmission

Today, many people worry about the possibility of being infected with a disease while providing first aid. Although diseases can be transmitted in a first aid situation, the actual risk is far less than you may think. In Chapter 3, you will learn how to take steps, such as hand washing and using protective barriers, to prevent disease transmission.

Fear of Doing Something Wrong

We all respond to emergencies in different ways. Whether trained or untrained, some people are afraid of doing the wrong thing and making the situation worse. Sometimes people worry that they might be sued. Do not be overly concerned about this. Lawsuits against those who give emergency care are highly unusual and rarely successful. All states have enacted *Good Samaritan laws* that protect people who willingly give first aid without accepting anything in return. See page 32 for more information on Good Samaritan laws.

It is not uncommon for people to have feelings that make them hesitate or fail to help. These barriers to action are personal and very real to the people who experience them. The decision to act is yours alone. Your decision to respond to emergencies should be guided by your own values, as well as by knowledge of the risks that may be present in various rescue situations.

TAKING ACTION

The Emergency Medical Services (EMS) System

The emergency medical services (EMS) system is a network of community resources and medical personnel that provides emergency care to victims of injury or sudden illness. As a citizen responder, you are responsible for activating this system by calling 9-1-1 or the local emergency number.

When You Call 9-1-1

When you call 9-1-1 or the local emergency number, your call will be automatically routed to the police, fire or EMS system (**Fig. 1-6, A**). When your call is answered, you will talk to an emergency call taker who has had special training in dealing with crises over the phone. The call taker will ask you for a phone number and address of the emergency and will ask other key questions to determine whether you need police, fire or EMS assistance (**Fig. 1-6, B**).

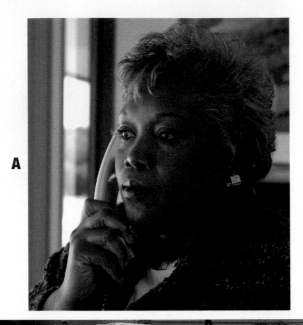

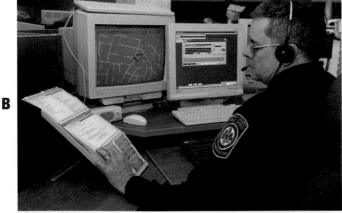

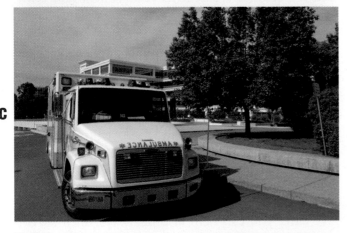

Figure 1-6 A-C, Many call takers give instructions to citizen responders for what to do before EMS personnel arrive.

It may seem that the call taker asks a lot of questions. The information you give helps the dispatcher to send the type of help needed, based on the severity of the emergency. Once the ambulance is on its way, the call taker may ask you to stay on the line and continue to talk to you (**Fig. 1-6, C**). Many dispatchers today are also trained to give instructions before EMS personnel arrive. These pre-arrival instructions, combined with your first aid training, help to ensure an effective emergency response.

When using a mobile phone to call 9-1-1, it is important to know that the system that identifies a

Wireless 9-1-1: Hundreds of Millions Served

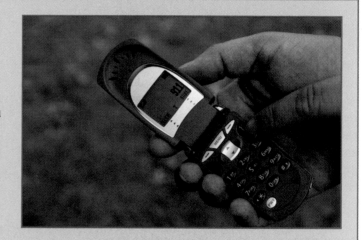

The 9-1-1 service was created in the United States in 1968 as a nationwide telephone number for the public to use to report emergencies and request emergency assistance. It gives the public direct access to an emergency communication center called a Public Service Answering Point, which is responsible for taking the appropriate action. The numbers 9-1-1 were chosen because they best fit the needs of the public and the telephone companies. They are easy to remember and dial, and they have never been used as an office, area or service code. Today, an estimated 200 million people call 9-1-1 each year. At least 99 percent of the population and 96 percent of the geographic United States is covered by some type of 9-1-1 service.

There are two types of 9-1-1 systems—Basic and Enhanced. A Basic 9-1-1 system automatically routes the emergency call to the Public Service Answering Point that handles the area where the phone is located. An Enhanced 9-1-1 system automatically displays the telephone number, address and name in which the phone is listed. If the caller is unable to remain on the line or is unable to speak or if the call is disconnected, the call taker can still obtain enough information to send help. Some 9-1-1 systems can reconnect a caller and transfer callers to other agencies or telephone numbers with a single button.

According to the Federal Communications Commissions (FCC) over 50 million people a year use wireless phones to call 9-1-1. That is more than double the number of people who used a wireless phone to activate the EMS in 1995. However, wireless phones are not associated with one fixed location or address, which can make it difficult to accurately determine the location of the caller or the emergency.

Current and future development of the 9-1-1 system includes initiatives to integrate the wireless technology more effectively. The FCC has adopted a variety of 9-1-1 rules aimed at improving the system's ability to locate wireless 9-1-1 callers. These rules apply to all cellular phone licensees, broadband Personal Communication Service and certain Special Mobile Radio licensees.

Because wireless 9-1-1 location information is not available everywhere it is important to remember the following tips when using a wireless phone to call 9-1-1:

▸ Tell the emergency operator the location of the emergency right away.
▸ Give the emergency operator your wireless phone number so that if the call gets disconnected, he or she can call you back.
▸ If your wireless phone is not "initialized" (i.e., you do not have a contract for service with a wireless service provider), and your emergency call gets disconnected, you must call the emergency operator back because he or she does not have your telephone number and cannot contact you.
▸ Learn to use the designated number in your state for highway accidents or other non-life-threatening incidents. Often states reserve specific numbers for these types of incidents. For example, "#77" is the number used for highway accidents in Virginia. The number to call for non-life-threatening incidents in your state can be located in the front of your phone book.
▸ Refrain from programming your phone to automatically dialing 9-1-1 when one button such as the "9" key is pressed. Unintentional wireless 9-1-1 calls, which often occur when auto-dial keys are inadvertently pressed, cause problems for emergency service call centers.
▸ If your wireless phone came pre-programmed with the auto-dial 9-1-1 feature already turned on, turn this feature off. Check your user manual to find out how.
▸ Lock your keypad when you are not using your wireless phone. This action also prevents accidental calls to 9-1-1.

SOURCES:
DISPATCH Monthly Magazine, www.911.dispatch.com. Accessed 6/24/04.
Federal Communications Commission, *www.fcc.gov/911/enhanced*. Accessed 6/24/04.
National Emergency Number Association, *www.nena.org*. Accessed 6/24/04.

caller's location and telephone is still in its infancy and is not available everywhere. Therefore, you should tell the call taker the location of the emergency and your mobile phone number in case you are disconnected.

Until Help Arrives

There are many actions you, other citizen responders or bystanders can take before EMS personnel arrive. Always follow the pre-arrival instructions provided by the call taker. These instructions may range from taking actions that make the scene safer and more accessible to EMS personnel (confining household pets, turning on extra lights, gathering the victim's medications) to giving more advanced care. You will learn to give more advanced care for an ill or injured person as you progress through this course.

PREPARING FOR EMERGENCIES

If you are prepared for emergencies, you can help ensure that care begins as soon as possible—for yourself, your family and your fellow citizens. Steps you can take in preparing for an emergency include becoming trained in first aid and making or purchasing a first aid kit.

First aid training provides you with both the knowledge and skills necessary to respond confidently to emergency situations. Your training will give you a basic plan of action to use in any emergency. You will be better able to manage your fears and overcome barriers to action by knowing what to do. Your training will enable you to respond more effectively in your role as a citizen responder.

You can be ready for most emergencies if you do the following things now:

▶ Keep important information about you and your family or household in a handy place, such as on the refrigerator door and in your automobile glove compartment (**Fig. 1-7**). Include your address, everyone's date of birth, medical conditions, allergies, and prescriptions and dosages. List everyone's physicians' names and phone numbers.

▶ Keep medical and insurance records up to date.

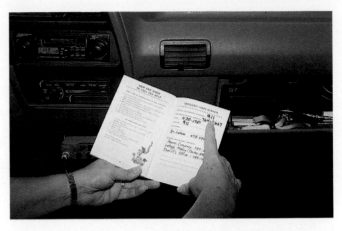

Figure 1-7 Keep important information in handy places, such as in your car's glove compartment.

▶ Find out if your community is served by the 9-1-1 system. If not, look up the local emergency number for police, fire, EMS services and poison control. These numbers are usually listed in the front of the telephone book.

▶ Teach children how to call for help as soon as they are old enough to use the telephone.

▶ Keep emergency telephone numbers listed in a handy place, such as by the telephone and in your first aid kit. Include the home and office phone numbers of family members, friends or neighbors who can help. Be sure to keep both the list and the telephone numbers current.

▶ Keep a first aid kit readily available in your home, automobile, workplace and recreation area (**Fig. 1-8**). Store each kit in a dry place and replace used contents regularly. A first aid kit should contain the following:

• 2 absorbent compress dressings (5 × 9 inches)
• 25 adhesive bandages (assorted sizes)
• 1 adhesive cloth tape (10 yards × 1 inch)
• 5 triple antibiotic ointment packets (approximately 1 gram each)
• 5 antiseptic wipe packets
• 2 packets of aspirin (81 mg each)
• 1 blanket (space blanket)
• 1 breathing barrier (with one-way valve)
• 1 instant cold compress
• 2 pairs of nonlatex gloves (size: large)
• 2 hydrocortisone ointment packets (approximately 1 gram each)

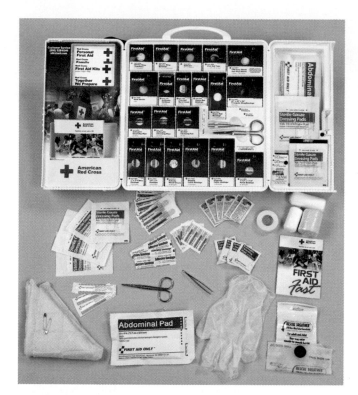

Figure 1-8 It is important to keep a well-stocked first aid kit in your home, automobile, workplace and recreation area.

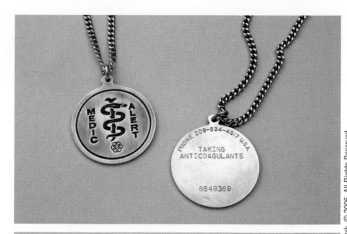

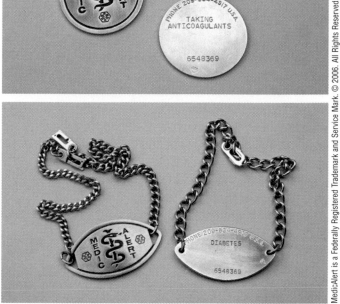

MedicAlert is a Federally Registered Trademark and Service Mark. © 2006. All Rights Reserved.

Figure 1-9 Medical ID tags and bracelets can provide important medical information about a victim.

- Scissors
- 1 roller bandage (3 inches wide)
- 1 roller bandage (4 inches wide)
- 5 sterile gauze pads (3 × 3 inches)
- 5 sterile gauze pads (4 × 4 inches)
- Oral thermometer (nonmercury/nonglass)
- 2 triangular bandages
- Tweezers
- First aid booklet

▶ Learn first aid and cardiopulmonary resuscitation (CPR) skills, and practice regularly.

▶ Make sure your house or apartment number is easy to read. Numerals are easier to read than spelled-out numbers. Report any downed or missing street signs to the proper authorities.

▶ Wear a medical ID bracelet if you have a potentially serious medical condition, such as epilepsy, diabetes, heart disease or allergies (**Fig. 1-9, A-B**).

SUMMARY

An emergency can happen at any place, to anyone and at any time. The emergency medical services (EMS) system is a network of community resources and medical personnel that provides emergency care to victims of injury or sudden illness. However, the EMS system cannot properly function without the actions of a trained citizen responder like you. By learning to recognize an emergency and deciding to act (calling 9-1-1 or the local emergency number and giving care) you can help save the life of a victim of injury or sudden illness.

In the following chapters, you will learn how to manage different kinds of emergencies. You will learn emergency action steps that you can apply to any emergency situation and how to give care in both life-threatening and non-life-threatening situations.

Honoring Our Heroes:

The Red Cross Certificate of Merit

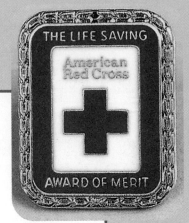

American Red Cross

CERTIFICATE *of* MERIT

awarded to

for selfless and humane action

Issued at Washington, D.C.

Honorary Chairman   *Chairman*

The Certificate of Merit is the highest honor that the American Red Cross awards to citizens. The Red Cross confers this certificate on individuals who are not part of the community's emergency medical system but who save or sustain a victim's life with skills learned in an American Red Cross Health and Safety course.

Although the survival of the victim is not a criterion for eligibility for the award, nominees for the award must have performed every possible lifesaving skill prior to the victim's receiving medical care. Sometimes team certificates are awarded. In such a case, each member of the team must contribute directly to the lifesaving act.

The Certificate of Merit program began in 1911 and was originally a cash award given annually to four railway workers who performed first aid. The next year, the Red Cross decided to recognize four individuals from the general public who demonstrated exemplary first aid skills. In 1915, water safety skills and rescues were included in the certificate criteria. From 1912 to 1925, the Red Cross gave cash awards to 66 individuals.

In 1928, the Red Cross reevaluated its cash award program. Because the cash awards could be given only to a few individuals a year and because the rescuers did not receive any lasting reminder of the award, the Red Cross decided to eliminate the cash award and institute the present-day Certificate of Merit. The certificate is signed by the President of the United States, who is also the honorary chairman of the American Red Cross (a tradition begun in 1913 by William Howard Taft), and often awarded in a local ceremony. Over 12,000 individuals have received a Certificate of Merit since 1911.

What kinds of people receive Certificates of Merit? A brief look at those individuals who were honored in previous years reveals that honorees come from all walks of life, are of all ages, from 4 to 76, and perform their life-saving skills in a variety of different places and situations. A 15-year-old gives rescue breathing to her father who suffers a stroke at home. A day-care worker gives abdominal thrusts to a 5-year-old who is choking on food during lunch. A woman controls bleeding, cares for shock, and checks breathing and signs of life for a victim of a stabbing at a gas station. During a water emergency, a man frees a companion from underneath an overturned canoe, splints the victim's broken leg, gives care for hypothermia and cares for shock.

Perhaps the one common element in all these cases is that the rescuer provided lifesaving skills in an emotionally charged situation. These individuals demonstrate that life-sustaining first aid care can be rendered even when the emergency threatens the life of a loved one, a child or a badly injured stranger. An American Red Cross training course can teach you the practical skills you need to help a person in danger and can equip you to handle an emergency even when you are frightened or feel panic.

APPLICATION QUESTIONS

1. What immediate steps could you and your friends who witnessed the car crash take?

2. As you approach the victim of the car crash, you begin to feel faint and nauseated and are not sure you can proceed any farther. How can you still help?

3. The approximate time of the crash you witnessed was 4:50 p.m. The EMS personnel did not arrive until 5:25 p.m., and the victim did not arrive at the hospital until 6:30 p.m. What might have caused this delay in reaching the victim and getting him to the hospital?

STUDY QUESTIONS

1. In each of the following three scenarios, circle the indicators of a potential emergency.

   a. I was fixing sandwiches and talking with my next-door neighbor, Mrs. Roberts, who had come by to borrow a book. My 3-year-old, Jenny, was in the next room playing with some puzzles. As Mrs. Roberts got up to leave, I heard a loud thump and a shriek from upstairs.
   b. I was on the bus headed for work. A man from the back of the bus came down the aisle, and I noticed that he was moving unsteadily. It was cold in the bus, but I noticed he was sweating and looked very pale. "I don't know where I am," I heard him mumble to himself.
   c. On my way into the grocery store from the parking lot, I heard the loud screech of tires and the crash of metal. I saw that a car had struck a telephone pole, causing the telephone pole to lean at an odd angle. Wires were hanging down from the pole. It was very frightening.

2. List five common barriers to taking action at the scene of an emergency.

3. How can a citizen responder overcome each of these barriers to action?

4. Match each term with the correct phrase.

a. First aid   d. Sudden illness
b. Citizen responder e. EMS system
c. Emergency   f. Barriers to action

___C___ A situation that requires immediate action.

___e___ A network of community resources and medical personnel that provides emergency care to victims of injury or sudden illness.

___a___ The immediate care given to a victim of injury or sudden illness until more advanced care can be obtained.

___d___ A physical condition, such as a heart attack, requiring immediate medical attention.

___b___ A layperson (someone who does not have special or advanced medical training or skill) who recognizes an emergency and decides to act.

___f___ Reasons for not acting or for hesitating to act in an emergency situation.

5. Identify six ways bystanders can help at the scene of an emergency.

Answers are listed in Appendix A.

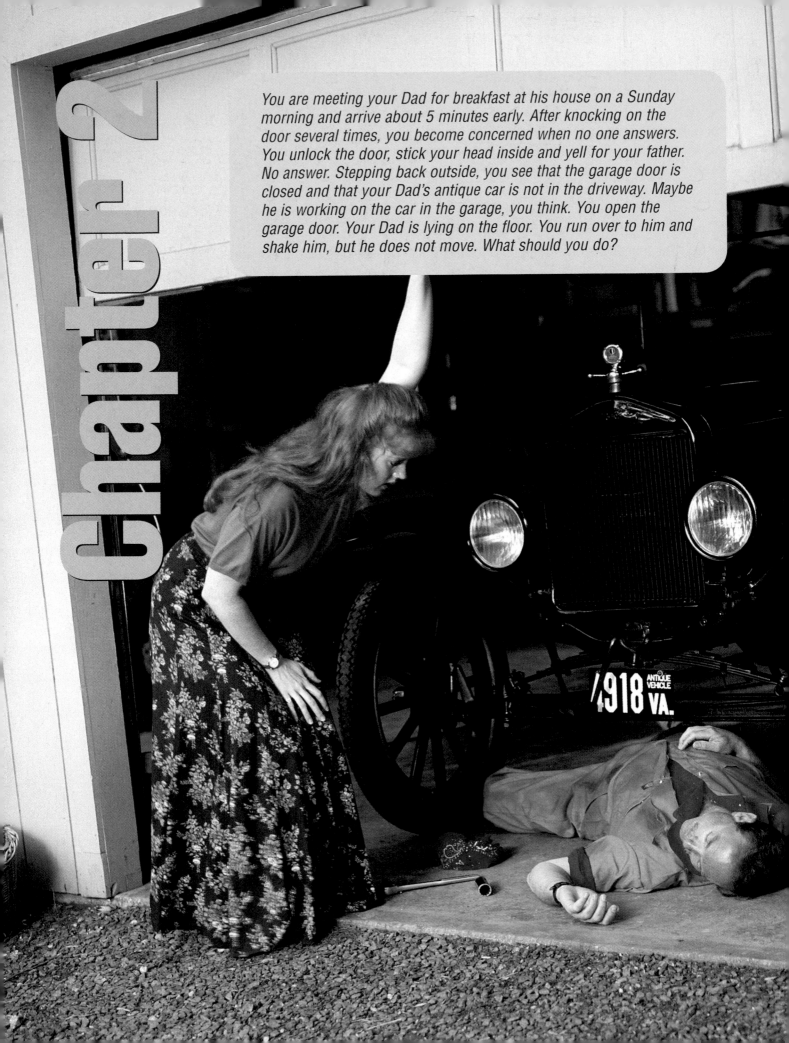

Chapter 2

You are meeting your Dad for breakfast at his house on a Sunday morning and arrive about 5 minutes early. After knocking on the door several times, you become concerned when no one answers. You unlock the door, stick your head inside and yell for your father. No answer. Stepping back outside, you see that the garage door is closed and that your Dad's antique car is not in the driveway. Maybe he is working on the car in the garage, you think. You open the garage door. Your Dad is lying on the floor. You run over to him and shake him, but he does not move. What should you do?

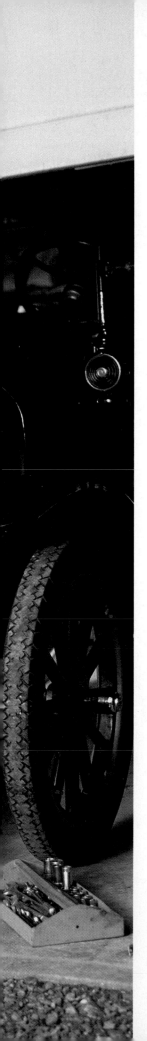

Responding to an Emergency

Objectives

After reading this chapter, you should be able to—

■ *Identify and describe the three emergency action steps.*

■ *List the four conditions considered life threatening in an emergency situation.*

■ *Explain when and how to call 9-1-1 or the local emergency number.*

Introduction

An emergency scene can be overwhelming. It poses questions that demand immediate answers. What should I do first? Where can I get help? What can I do to help the ill or injured person? By learning how to check an emergency scene and prioritize your actions, you will be able to respond effectively in any emergency situation.

EMERGENCY ACTION STEPS

The *emergency action steps* are three steps you should take in any emergency. These steps are—

▸ **CHECK** the scene and the victim.
▸ **CALL** 9-1-1 or the local emergency number.
▸ **CARE** for the victim.

Check

This emergency action step has two parts—checking the scene and checking the victim.

Checking the Scene

Before you can help the victim, you must make sure the scene is safe for you and any bystanders. Take time to check the scene and answer these questions:

▸ Is the scene safe?
▸ What happened?
▸ How many victims are there?
▸ Are bystanders available to help?

Look for anything that may threaten your safety and that of the victim and bystanders. Examples of dangers include downed power lines, falling rocks, traffic, a crime scene, a hostile crowd, violent behavior, fire, smoke, dangerous fumes, extreme weather and deep or swiftly moving water (**Fig. 2-1**). *Do not approach the victim if any of these dangers are present.* Go to a safe place and call 9-1-1 or the local emergency number. Do not risk becoming a victim yourself. Leave dangerous situations to professionals, such as firefighters and police officers, who have the training to deal with them. Once they make the scene safe, you can offer to help.

Find out what happened. Look around the scene for clues about what caused the emergency and the type and extent of the victim's injuries. You may discover a situation that requires your immediate attention. As you approach the victim, take in the whole picture. Nearby objects, such as shattered glass, a fallen ladder or a spilled bottle of medicine, might tell you what happened. If the victim is unconscious, checking the scene may be the only way to tell what happened (**Fig. 2-2**).

Look carefully for more than one victim. You may not spot everyone who needs help at first. For example, in a car crash, an open door may be a clue that a victim has left the car or was thrown from it. If one victim is bleeding or screaming loudly, you may overlook another victim who is unconscious. It is also easy in any emergency situation to overlook an infant or a small child. If you find more than one victim, ask yourself if there are any bystanders to help you. Even an untrained bystander can assist you by calling 9-1-1 or the local emergency number, retrieving first aid supplies and comforting and reassuring less seriously injured victims. A bystander who knows the victim may know whether he or she has any medical conditions or allergies.

As you move closer, continue to check the scene to see if it is still safe. At this point, you may see other dangers that were not obvious to you from a

K E Y   T E R M S

Consent: Permission to give care, given by the victim to the rescuer.

Emergency action steps: Three basic steps you should take in any emergency: **CHECK—CALL—CARE.**

Signs of life: Normal breathing or movement.

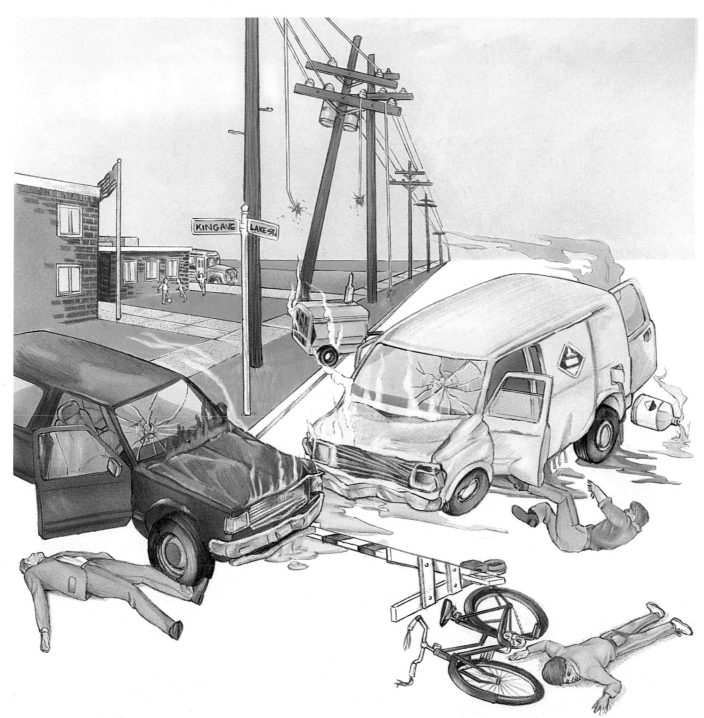

Figure 2-1   Check the scene for anything that may threaten your safety and that of the victims and bystanders. Can you identify the hazards shown above?

distance. You may also see clues to what happened or victims and bystanders you did not notice before.

Checking the Victim

Do not move a victim unless he or she is in immediate danger. If an immediate danger is present, such as rising flood water, try to move the victim as quickly and carefully as possible without making the situation worse. If no immediate danger exists,

tell the victim not to move. Also tell bystanders not to move the victim.

If you find that the victim has any life-threatening conditions, you must activate the EMS system as soon as possible (**Fig. 2-3**). Four of the conditions considered life threatening in an emergency situation are—

▸ Unconsciousness.
▸ Trouble breathing.

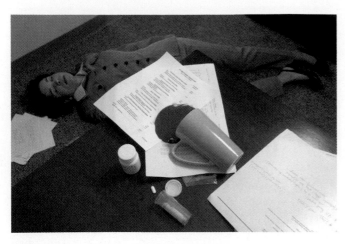

Figure 2-2 If the victim is unconscious, nearby objects may be your only clue to what has happened.

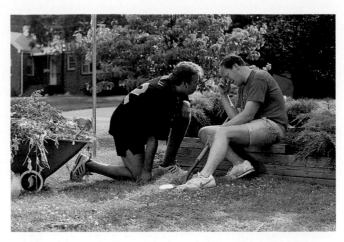

Figure 2-4 If the victim is conscious and has no life-threatening conditions, interview the victim and any bystanders.

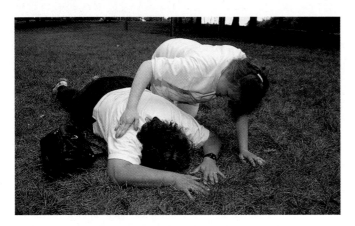

Figure 2-3 If the victim has life-threatening conditions, call 9-1-1 or the local emergency number immediately.

▶ No *signs of life* (normal breathing or movement) and, for children and infants, no pulse.
▶ Severe bleeding.

If the victim is conscious and appears to have no life-threatening conditions, introduce yourself and interview the victim and any bystanders to find out what happened (**Fig. 2-4**). You must get *consent* from a conscious adult victim before you begin to give care. Detailed information about checking a victim is described in Chapter 5.

Call

As a citizen responder, your top priority is to ensure that the victim receives more advanced care as soon as possible. The EMS system works more effectively if you can give information about the victim's condition when the call is placed. This information helps to ensure that the victim receives proper medical care as quickly as possible.

When to Call

At times, you may be unsure if EMS personnel are needed. Your first aid training will help you make the decision. As a general rule, call 9-1-1 or the local emergency number if the victim—

▶ Is unconscious or has an altered level of consciousness.
▶ Has trouble breathing or is breathing in a strange manner.
▶ Has chest discomfort, pain or pressure that persists for more than 3 to 5 minutes or goes away and comes back.
▶ Is bleeding severely.
▶ Has pressure or pain in the abdomen that does not go away.
▶ Is vomiting blood or passing blood.
▶ Has a seizure that lasts more than 5 minutes or has multiple seizures.
▶ Has a seizure and is pregnant.
▶ Has a seizure and is diabetic.
▶ Fails to regain consciousness after a seizure.
▶ Has a severe headache or slurred speech.
▶ Appears to be poisoned.
▶ Has injuries to the head, neck or back.
▶ Has possible broken bones.
▶ Has a severe (critical) burn.

You should also activate the EMS system if any of the following situations exist:

▶ Fire or explosion
▶ The presence of poisonous gas

▸ Downed electrical wires
▸ Swiftly moving or rapidly rising water
▸ Motor vehicle collisions
▸ Victims who cannot be moved easily

These conditions and situations do not comprise a complete list. Trust your instincts. If you think there is an emergency, there probably is. Do not hesitate to call EMS personnel if you are uncertain.

Making the Call

When calling 9-1-1 or the local emergency number, give the call taker the necessary information. Most EMS call takers will ask—

▸ The exact address or location and the name of the city or town. Be prepared to give the names of nearby intersecting streets (cross streets or roads); landmarks; and the name of the building, the floor and the room number.
▸ The telephone number and address from which the call is being made.
▸ The caller's name.
▸ What happened, for example, a motor vehicle collision, a fall, a fire, sudden onset of chest pain.
▸ The number of people involved.
▸ The condition of the victim(s), for example, unconsciousness, chest pain, trouble breathing, bleeding.
▸ The care being given.

Do not hang up until the call taker tells you to. Make sure the call taker has all the information needed to send the right help to the scene. Some EMS call takers may also be able to provide in-

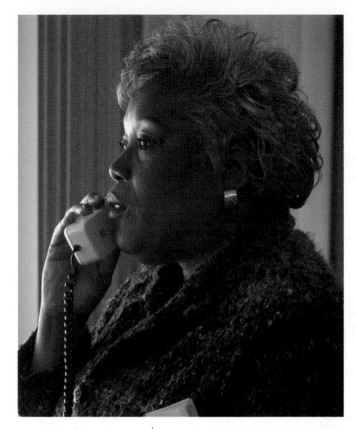

Figure 2-6 If possible, have a bystander call 9-1-1 or the local emergency number while you give care.

structions on how best to care for the victim until help arrives (**Fig. 2-5**).

If possible, ask a bystander to call 9-1-1 or the local emergency number for you (**Fig. 2-6**). Sending someone else to make the call allows you to stay with the victim. Tell the bystander the victim's condition and the care being given. Tell him or her to report to you after making the call and tell you what the call taker said.

If You Are Alone

If you are in a situation in which you are the only person other than the victim, you must make a decision to *Call First* or *Care First*. You should *Call First*, that is, call 9-1-1 or the local emergency number before giving care for—

▸ An unconscious adult victim or adolescent age 12 or older.
▸ A witnessed sudden collapse of a child or infant.
▸ An unconscious infant or child known to be at a high risk for heart problems.

Call First situations are likely to be cardiac emergencies, such as sudden cardiac arrest, where time is critical.

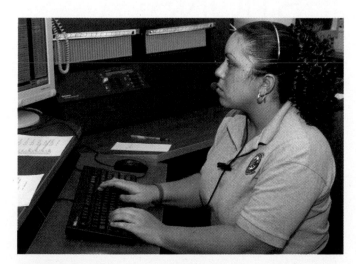

Figure 2-5 Some EMS call takers can provide instructions on how best to care for the victim until EMS personnel arrive.

Care First, that is, provide 2 minutes of care, then call 9-1-1 or the local emergency number for—

▶ An unconscious victim younger than age 12 when the collapse has not been witnessed.

▶ Any victim of a drowning.

Care First situations are likely to be related to breathing emergencies rather than sudden cardiac arrest. In these situations provide support for airway, breathing and circulation (ABCs) through rescue breaths and chest compressions, as appropriate.

Care for the Victim

Once you have checked the scene and the victim, you may need to give care. Always care for life-threatening conditions before those that are not life threatening. For example, a breathing emergency would take priority over an injured leg. While you are waiting for more advanced medical help, watch for changes in the victim's level of consciousness and breathing. A change in the victim's condition may be a signal of a serious illness or injury. A condition that may not appear serious at first may become serious with time. Help the victim rest comfortably, and keep him or her from getting chilled or overheated. Reassure the victim. You will learn more about how to care for an ill or injured person as you progress through this course.

SUMMARY

Emergency situations are often confusing and frightening. To take appropriate actions in any emergency, follow the three basic emergency action steps: **CHECK—CALL—CARE. CHECK** the scene and the victim, **CALL** 9-1-1 or the local emergency number to activate the EMS system and **CARE** for the victim until more advanced medical personnel arrive.

APPLICATION QUESTIONS

1. What dangers could exist in the garage?

2. What specific factors in the garage could influence your decision to move or not move your Dad?

3. After checking the scene in the garage, what would you do next? Why?

STUDY QUESTIONS

Answer the following questions based on the scenario below.

You are driving along the interstate. It is getting dark. Rain has been falling steadily, and is now beginning to freeze. Suddenly the tractor-trailer in front of you in your lane begins to sway and slide, then jackknifes and crashes onto its left side. Drivers put on their brakes and swerve, and by some miracle, everyone close by manages to avoid crashing into the fallen truck or each other. You pull onto the median and stop a safe distance behind the truck.

1. List the possible dangers to be aware of at the scene of this emergency.

2. Describe the actions you should take if you determine that the scene is unsafe.

You determined that the scene is safe and approach the tractor-trailer. You find the driver behind the wheel. You check the driver for life-threatening conditions.

3. List four life-threatening conditions that you may find.

You check the driver and discover that he is unconscious. You tell a bystander to call 9-1-1 or the local emergency number.

4. List the information that the bystander should have when calling EMS personnel.

5. Describe the actions you would take if no one else was available to help.

Answers are listed in Appendix A.

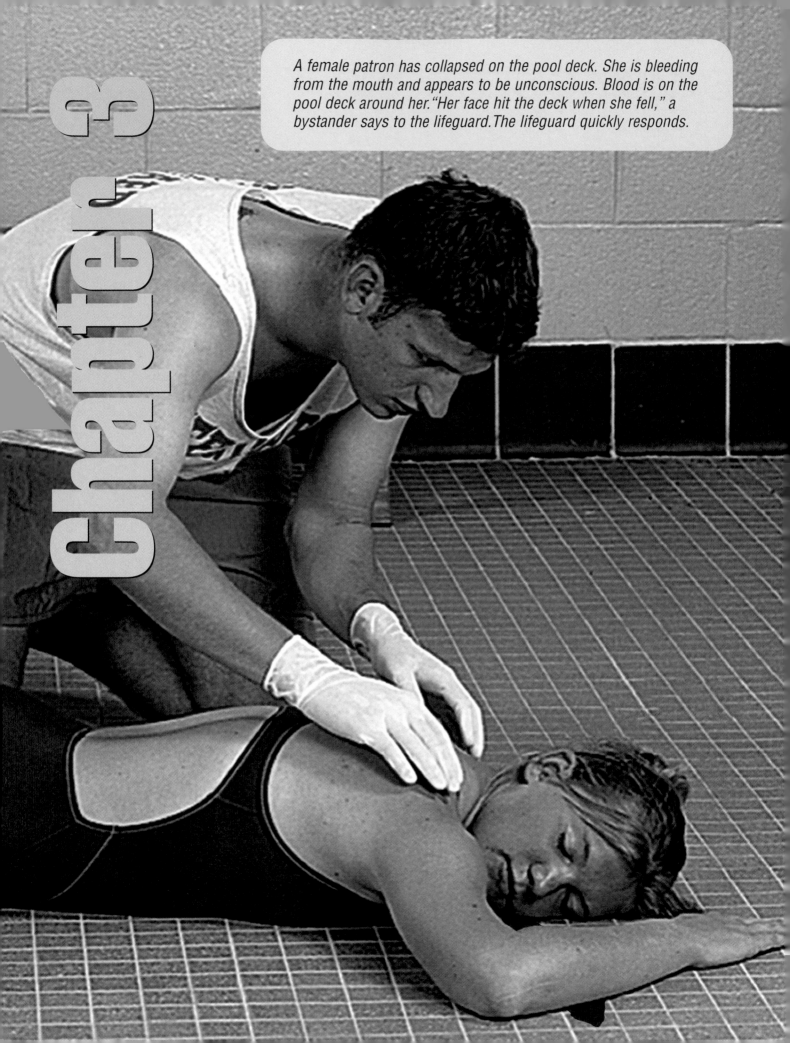

A female patron has collapsed on the pool deck. She is bleeding from the mouth and appears to be unconscious. Blood is on the pool deck around her. "Her face hit the deck when she fell," a bystander says to the lifeguard. The lifeguard quickly responds.

Before Giving Care

Objectives

After reading this chapter, you should be able to—

■ *List four conditions that must be present for disease transmission to occur.*

■ *Identify two ways in which a pathogen can enter the body.*

■ *Describe how to minimize the risk of disease transmission when giving care in a situation that involves visible blood.*

■ *Describe the difference between consent and implied consent.*

■ *Describe the purpose of Good Samaritan laws.*

■ *List six situations in which moving a victim is necessary.*

■ *List five limitations you should be aware of before you attempt to move someone.*

■ *Describe how to perform four emergency moves.*

After reading this chapter and completing the class activities, you should be able to—

■ *Demonstrate how to remove disposable gloves.*

Introduction

As a citizen responder, you have made an important decision to help an ill or injured person. However, in any emergency situation your top priority is to ensure your own safety. In this chapter, you will learn how to protect yourself from disease transmission and properly move a victim. In addition, this chapter provides you with some basic legal information you need to know before giving care.

PREVENTING DISEASE TRANSMISSION

To help protect against **disease transmission**, you first need to understand how infections occur, how diseases pass from one person to another and what you can do to protect yourself and others.

Infectious diseases are those you can catch from other people, animals, insects or things that have been in contact with the disease. Because some infectious diseases like hepatitis and human immunodeficiency virus (HIV) are very serious, you must learn how to protect yourself and others from disease transmission.

How Infections Occur

The disease process begins when a **pathogen** (germ) gets into the body. When pathogens enter the body, they can sometimes overpower the body's natural defense systems and cause illness. This type of illness is called an **infection**. Most infectious diseases are caused by **bacteria** and **viruses**.

Disease-Causing Agents

Bacteria are everywhere. They do not depend on other organisms for life and can live outside the human body. Most bacteria do not infect humans. Those that do may cause serious illness. Bacterial meningitis and **tetanus** are examples of diseases caused by bacteria. The body's ability to fight infection depends on its immune system. In a person with a healthy immune system, a bacterial infection is often avoided. However, another body may have difficulty fighting infection caused by bacteria. When an infection is present, physicians may prescribe antibiotics that either kill the bacteria or weaken them enough for the body to get rid of them. Commonly prescribed antibiotics include penicillin, erythromycin and tetracycline.

Unlike bacteria, viruses depend on other organisms to live and reproduce. Viruses can cause many diseases, including the common cold (caused by the rhinovirus). Once in the body, viruses may be difficult to eliminate because very few medications are effective against viral infections. Although there are some medications that kill or weaken viruses, the

KEY TERMS

Consent: Permission to give care, given by the victim to the rescuer.

Direct contact transmission: Occurs when infected blood or body fluids from one person enter another person's body at a correct entry site.

Disease transmission: The passage of a disease from one person to another.

Implied consent: Legal concept that assumes a person would consent to receive emergency care if he or she were physically able to do so.

Indirect contact transmission: Occurs when a person touches objects that have the blood or body fluid of an infected person, and that infected blood or body fluid enters the body through a correct entry site.

Personal protective equipment: The equipment and supplies that help prevent the rescuer from directly contacting infected materials.

Standard precautions: Safety measures taken to prevent exposure to blood and body fluids when giving care to ill or injured persons.

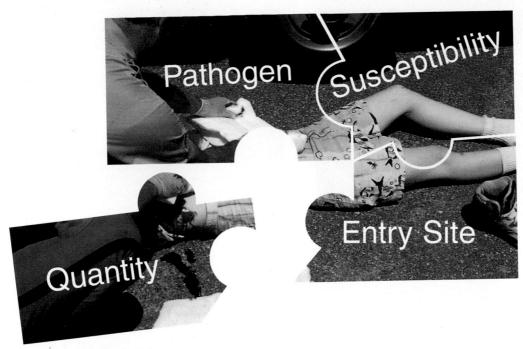

Figure 3-1   If any one of these conditions is missing, infection will not occur.

body's own immune system is the main defense against them.

How Bloodborne Pathogens Are Spread

For any diseases to be spread, including bloodborne diseases, all four of the following conditions must be met:

▶ A pathogen is present.
▶ There is enough of the pathogen present to cause disease.
▶ The pathogen passes through the correct entry site.
▶ A person is susceptible to the pathogen.

To understand how infections occur, think of these four conditions as pieces of a puzzle. All the pieces have to be in place for the picture to be complete. If any one of these conditions is missing, an infection cannot occur (**Fig. 3-1**).

Bloodborne pathogens such as hepatitis B virus (HBV), hepatitis C virus (HCV) and HIV can spread from person to person through *direct contact transmission* and *indirect contact transmission* with infected blood or other body fluids. HBV, HCV and HIV are not spread by food or water or by casual contact such as hugging or shaking hands. The highest risk of transmission is unprotected direct or indirect contact with infected blood.

Direct contact transmission occurs when the infected blood or body fluids from one person enter another person's body at a correct entry site. For example, direct transmission can occur through infected blood splashing in the eye or by directly touching body fluids from an infected person (**Fig. 3-2, A**).

Some bloodborne pathogens are also transmitted by indirect contact. Indirect contact transmission can occur when a person touches an object that contains the blood or another body fluid of an infected person, and that infected blood or other body fluid enters the body through a correct entry site. These objects include soiled dressings, equipment and work surfaces that are contaminated with an infected person's blood or other body fluids. For example, indirect contact can occur when a person picks up blood soaked bandages with a bare hand and the pathogens enter through a break in the skin on the hand (**Fig. 3-2, B**).

Standard Precautions When Giving Care

Standard precautions are safety measures taken to prevent exposure to blood and body fluids when giving care to ill or injured persons. This approach to infection control means that you should consider all body fluids and substances as infectious. These precautions and practices include personal hygiene,

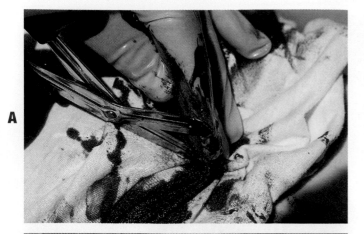

A

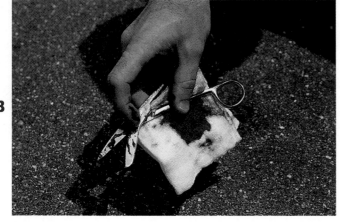

B

Figure 3-2 **A,** Direct contact transmission. **B,** Indirect contact transmission.

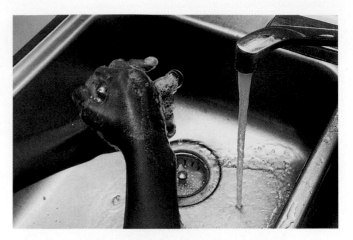

Figure 3-3 Thorough hand washing after giving care helps to protect you against disease.

using personal protective equipment and equipment for cleaning and disinfecting contaminated surfaces.

Personal Hygiene

Good personal hygiene habits, such as frequent hand washing, help to prevent disease transmission. You should always wash and scrub your hands after giving care, even if you never came into contact with a victim's blood or other body fluids (**Fig. 3-3**). To wash your hands correctly, you should—

▶ Wet your hands with water.
▶ Apply antimicrobial liquid soap to your hands.
▶ Rub your hands vigorously for at least 15 seconds, covering all surfaces of the hands and fingers.
   • Use soap and warm running water.
   • Scrub nails by rubbing them against the palms of your hands.
▶ Rinse hands with water.
▶ Dry your hands thoroughly with a paper towel.
▶ Turn off the faucet using the paper towel.

Personal Protective Equipment

Personal protective equipment is the equipment that helps keep you from directly contacting infected materials. This equipment includes disposable gloves (such as nitrile or vinyl) and breathing barriers used when performing rescue breaths. To reduce the risk of getting or transmitting an infectious disease, follow these guidelines for the use of protective equipment:

▶ Wear disposable (single-use) gloves whenever giving care, particularly if you may come in contact with blood or body fluids (**Fig. 3-4**).
▶ Remove jewelry, such as rings, bracelets and watches, before putting on disposable gloves.
▶ Cover any cuts, scrapes or sores prior to putting on protective equipment.

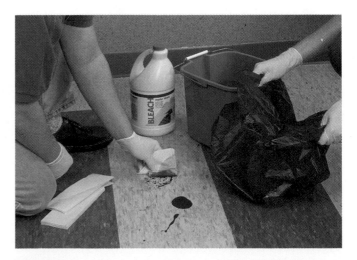

Figure 3-4 Personal protective equipment includes disposable gloves and protective barriers such as a face shield and resuscitation mask.

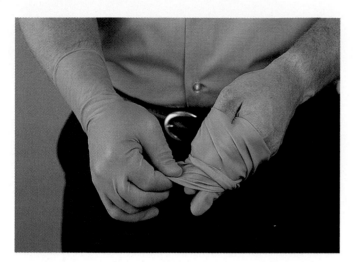

Figure 3-5   Remove disposable gloves without contacting the soiled part of the gloves, and dispose of them in a proper container.

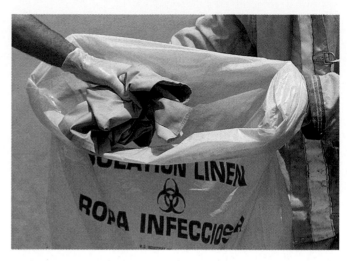

Figure 3-6   When cleaning up a blood spill, use protective equipment and place all contaminated materials in a labeled biohazard container.

- **Do not** use disposable gloves that are discolored, torn or punctured.
- **Do not** clean or reuse disposable gloves.
- Change gloves before you give care to a different victim.
- Wear protective coverings, such as a mask, eyewear or gown, whenever you are likely to come in contact with blood or other body fluids that may splash.
- Use breathing barriers, such as resuscitation masks or face shields, when giving rescue breaths.
- Remove disposable gloves without contacting the soiled part of the gloves, and dispose of them in a proper container (**Fig. 3-5**).

Cleaning Up a Blood Spill

If a blood spill occurs—

- Clean up the spill immediately or as soon as possible after the spill occurs.
- Use disposable gloves and other personal protective equipment when cleaning up spills.
- Wipe up the spill with paper towels or other absorbent materials.
- After the area has been wiped up, flood the area with a solution of approximately 1½ c liquid chlorine bleach to 1 gallon of fresh water (1 part bleach per 10 parts water). Let stand for at least 10 minutes.
- Dispose of the contaminated material used to clean up the spill in a labeled biohazard container (**Fig. 3-6**).

If You Are Exposed

If you are exposed to blood or other body fluid, wash the exposed area as quickly as possible. Be sure to notify a police officer or other professional on the scene, such as a firefighter or emergency medical technician, that you have been exposed. Seek medical attention.

LEGAL CONSIDERATIONS
Obtaining Consent

Before giving first aid to a conscious adult victim, you must get his or her permission to give care. This permission is referred to as *consent*. A conscious victim has the right to either refuse or accept care. To get consent you must tell the victim—

1. Who you are.
2. Your level of training.
3. The care you would like to give.

Only then can a conscious victim give you consent. Do not give care to a conscious victim who refuses it. Even if a victim does not give consent, you should still call 9-1-1. If the conscious victim is an infant or child, get permission to give care from the parent or guardian.

If the victim is unconscious or unable to respond due to the illness or injury, consent is implied. *Implied consent* means you can assume that if the person could respond, he or she would agree to be cared for. Consent is also implied for an infant or child if a parent or guardian is not present or immediately available.

Good Samaritan Laws

All states have enacted **Good Samaritan laws**. These laws give legal protection to people who willingly provide emergency care to ill or injured persons without accepting anything in return.

When a citizen responds to an emergency and acts as a reasonable and prudent person would under the same conditions, Good Samaritan immunity generally prevails. This legal immunity protects you, as a citizen responder, from being sued and found financially responsible for the victim's injury. For example, a reasonable and prudent citizen responder would—

▸ Move a victim only if his or her life was endangered.
▸ Check the victim for life-threatening emergencies before giving further care.
▸ Call 9-1-1 or the local emergency number.
▸ Ask a conscious victim for permission before giving care.
▸ Give care only to the level of his or her training.
▸ Continue to give care until more highly trained personnel arrive.

Good Samaritan laws were enacted to encourage people to help others in emergency situations. They require that the "good Samaritan" responder use common sense and a reasonable level of skill, not to exceed the scope of the individual's training in emergency situations. They assume that each person would do his or her best to save a life or prevent further injury.

People are rarely sued for helping in an emergency. However, the existence of Good Samaritan laws does not mean that someone cannot sue. In rare cases, courts have ruled that these laws do not apply when an individual responder's response was grossly or willfully negligent or reckless or when the responder abandoned the victim after initiating care.

Good Samaritan laws vary from state to state. If you are interested in finding out about your state's Good Samaritan laws, contact a legal professional or your state attorney general's office, or check with your local library.

REACHING AND MOVING VICTIMS

Usually, when you give first aid, you will not face hazards that require moving the victim immediately. In most cases, you can follow the emergency action steps by **CHECKING** the scene and the victim, **CALLING** 9-1-1 or the local emergency number and **CARING** for the victim where you find him or her. Moving a victim needlessly can lead to further injury. For example, if the victim has a fracture of the leg, movement could result in the end of the bone tearing the skin. Soft tissue damage, damage to nerves, blood loss and infection all could result unnecessarily.

You should move a victim only when you can do so safely and when there is immediate danger such as—

▸ Fire.
▸ Presence of toxic gas.
▸ Risk of drowning.
▸ Risk of explosion.
▸ A collapsing structure (**Fig. 3-7**).
▸ Uncontrollable traffic hazards.

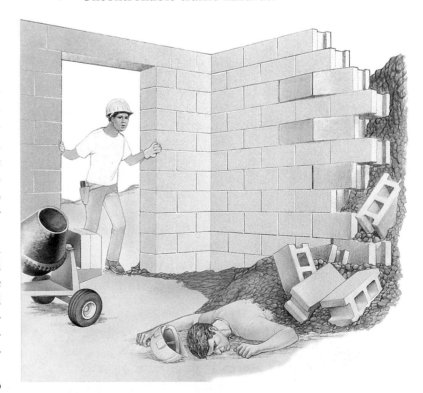

Figure 3-7 You should move a victim only if he or she is in immediate danger.

Before you act, consider the following limitations to moving one or more victims quickly and safely:

▶ Dangerous conditions at the scene
▶ The size of the victim
▶ Your physical ability
▶ Whether others can help you
▶ The victim's condition

Considering these limitations will help you decide how to proceed. For example, if you are injured, you may be unable to move the victim and will only risk making the situation worse. If you become part of the problem, EMS personnel will have one more victim to rescue.

To protect yourself and the victim, follow these guidelines when moving a victim:

▶ Only attempt to move a person you are sure you can comfortably handle.
▶ Bend your body at the knees and hips.
▶ Lift with your legs, not your back.
▶ Walk carefully, using short steps.
▶ When possible, move forward rather than backward.
▶ Always look where you are going.
▶ Support the victim's head, neck and back, if necessary.
▶ Avoid bending or twisting a victim with a possible head, neck or back injury.

Gaining Access

Sometimes you cannot give care because the victim is inaccessible. One example is a situation in which someone is able to call 9-1-1 or the local emergency number for help but is unable to unlock the door of the home or office. Victims may also be inaccessible in motor vehicle collisions. Vehicle doors are sometimes locked or crushed, windows may be rolled up or the vehicle may be unstable. Fire, water or other obstacles may prevent you from safely reaching the victim.

You must immediately begin to think of how to safely gain access to the victim. If you cannot reach the victim, you cannot check him or her or give care. But remember, when attempting to reach a victim, your safety is the most important consideration. Protect yourself and the victim by doing only what you are trained to do and by using equipment appropriate for the situation. In traffic, items such

as reflective markers or flares and flashlights may help keep you safe by alerting other drivers.

Emergency Moves

You can move a person to safety in many different ways, but no one way is best for every situation. The objective is to move a person to safety without injuring yourself or causing further injury to the victim. The following are four common types of emergency moves:

▶ Walking assist
▶ Pack-strap carry
▶ Two-person seat carry
▶ Clothes drag

All of these emergency moves can be done by one or two people and without any equipment.

Walking Assist

The most basic emergency move is the walking assist. Either one or two responders can use this method with a conscious victim. To perform a walking assist, place the victim's arm across your shoulders and hold it in place with one hand. Support the victim with your other hand around the victim's waist. In this way, your body acts as a crutch, supporting the victim's weight while you both walk (**Fig. 3-8, _A_**). A second rescuer, if present, can support the victim in the same way on the other side (**Fig. 3-8, _B_**). This assist is not appropriate to use if you suspect that the victim has a head, neck or back injury.

Pack-Strap Carry

The pack-strap carry can be used with both conscious and unconscious victims. To use it with an unconscious victim requires a second person to help position the victim on your back. To perform the pack-strap carry, have the victim stand or have a second person support the victim. Position yourself with your back to the victim, back straight, knees bent, so that your shoulders fit into the victim's armpits. Cross the victim's arms in front of you and grasp the victim's wrists (**Fig. 3-9, _A_**). Lean forward slightly and pull the victim up and onto your back (**Fig. 3-9, _B_**). Stand up and walk to safety. Depending on the size of the victim, you may be able to hold both of the victim's wrists with one hand, leav-

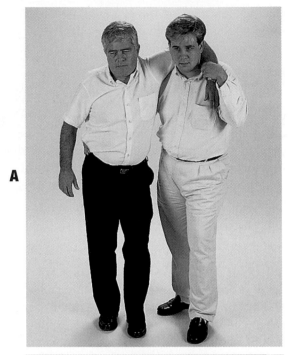

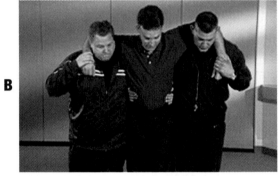

Figure 3-8 The most basic emergency move is the walking assist. **A**, The rescuer's body supports the victim's weight. **B**, A second rescuer can support the victim from the other side.

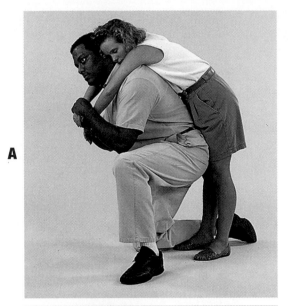

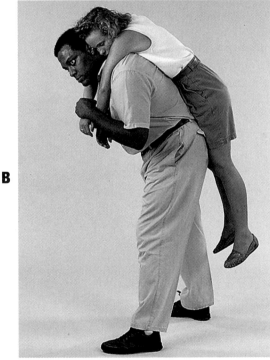

Figure 3-9 **A**, To perform the pack strap-carry, position yourself with your back to the victim. Cross the victim's arms in front of you and grasp the victim's wrists. **B**, Lean forward slightly and pull the victim onto your back.

ing your other hand free to help maintain balance, open doors and remove obstructions. This assist is not appropriate to use if you suspect that the victim has a head, neck or back injury.

Two-Person Seat Carry

The two-person seat carry requires a second responder. This carry can be used for any victim who is conscious and not seriously injured. Put one arm behind the victim's thighs and the other across the victim's back. Interlock your arms with those of a second rescuer behind the victim's legs and across the victim's back (**Fig. 3-10, *A***). Lift the victim in the "seat" formed by the rescuers' arms (**Fig. 3-10, *B***).

Clothes Drag

The clothes drag can be used to move a conscious or unconscious victim suspected of having a head, neck or back injury (**Fig. 3-11**). This move helps keep the victim's head and neck stabilized. Grasp the victim's clothing behind the neck, gathering enough to secure a firm grip. Using the clothing, pull the victim (head-first) to safety.

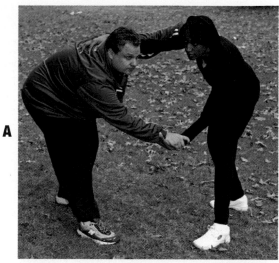

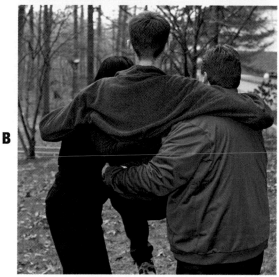

Figure 3-10   The two-person seat carry can be used for anyone who is conscious or not seriously injured. **A.** Lock arms under the victim's legs and across the victim's back. **B,** Lift the victim in the seat formed by the rescuer's arms.

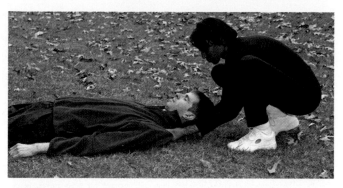

Figure 3-11   Use the clothes drag to move a person suspected of having a head, neck or back injury.

During the move, the victim's head is cradled by both clothing and the responder's arms. This emergency move is exhausting and may cause back strain for the rescuer, even when done properly.

SUMMARY

In any emergency situation, your top priority is to ensure your own safety. Protect yourself from disease transmission by wearing personal protective equipment, such as disposable gloves and breathing barriers and following good personal hygiene practices, such as hand washing. Always check the scene for safety before you approach a victim, and be sure to obtain consent from an adult victim who is conscious and alert. Never move a victim unless the scene is or becomes unsafe. If you must move a victim, be sure to do so in a manner that is safe for you and will not cause the victim any further harm. By thinking before you give care, you will not only be ensuring the safety of the victim but also your own.

APPLICATION QUESTIONS

1. What steps should the lifeguard take before giving care?

2. What steps to prevent disease transmission?

STUDY QUESTIONS

For Questions 1-5, circle the letter of the correct answer.

1. Disease transmission from a victim to a rescuer requires four conditions to be present. Which of the following is **NOT** one of these four?

   a. The victim may or may not be infected with the disease.
   b. The responder must be exposed to the infected victim's body substance.
   c. There must be enough of the pathogen present to cause infection.
   d. The pathogen passes through a correct entry site.

2. You are providing first aid to a child who has fallen off her bike. An untrained bystander picks up the gauze with blood on it. He is not wearing gloves. His action is an example of exposure through—

   a. Direct contact.
   b. Bacterial contact.
   c. Viral contact.
   d. Indirect contact.

3. Safety measures you can use to prevent disease transmission include—

   a. Calling 9-1-1 or the local emergency number.
   b. Using personal protective equipment such as disposable gloves.
   c. Wiping up a blood spill with a paper towel and placing the paper towel in the nearest wastebasket.
   d. Monitoring the victim until EMS personnel arrive.

4. To obtain a victim's consent to give care, you must tell the victim—

   a. Your level of training.
   b. Your age.
   c. What you think is wrong.
   d. Your job.

5. Which would you use to move a victim with a suspected head, neck or back injury?

   a. Pack-strap carry
   b. Walking assist
   c. Clothes drag
   d. Two-victim seat carry

6. List four situations in which it may be necessary to move a victim.

7. List four limitations you should consider before attempting to move a victim.

8. List four guidelines to follow when moving a victim.

9. Name four common types of emergency moves.

Answers are listed in Appendix A.

SKILL SHEET Removing Disposable Gloves

Step 1

Partially remove the first glove.

- Pinch the glove at the wrist, being careful to touch only the glove's outside surface.

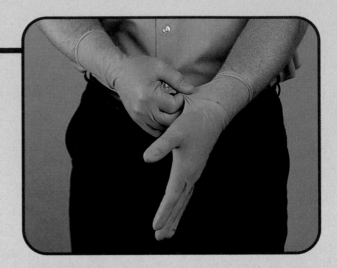

- Pull the glove toward the fingertips without completely removing it.
- The glove is now partly inside out.

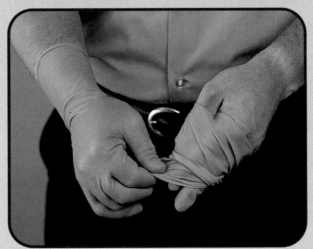

Step 2

Remove the second glove.

- With your partially gloved hand, pinch the outside surface of the second glove.
- Pull the second glove toward the fingertips until it is inside out, and then remove it completely.

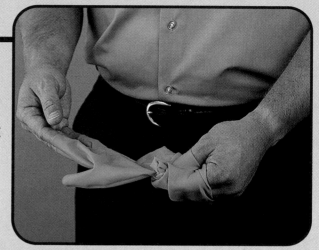

Step 3

Finish removing both gloves.

- Grasp both gloves with your free hand.
- Touch only the clean interior surface of the glove.

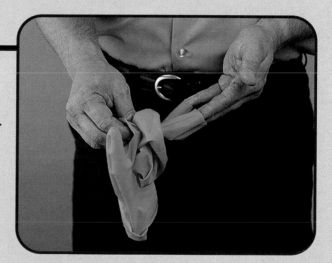

Step 4

After removing both gloves—

- Discard gloves in an appropriate container.
- Wash your hands thoroughly.

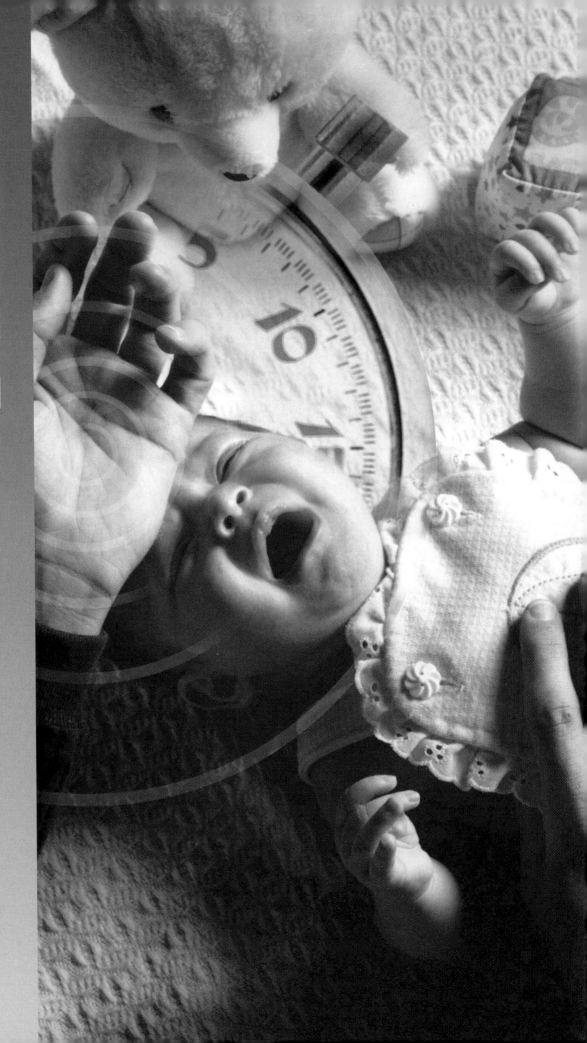

Part

TWO

Assessment

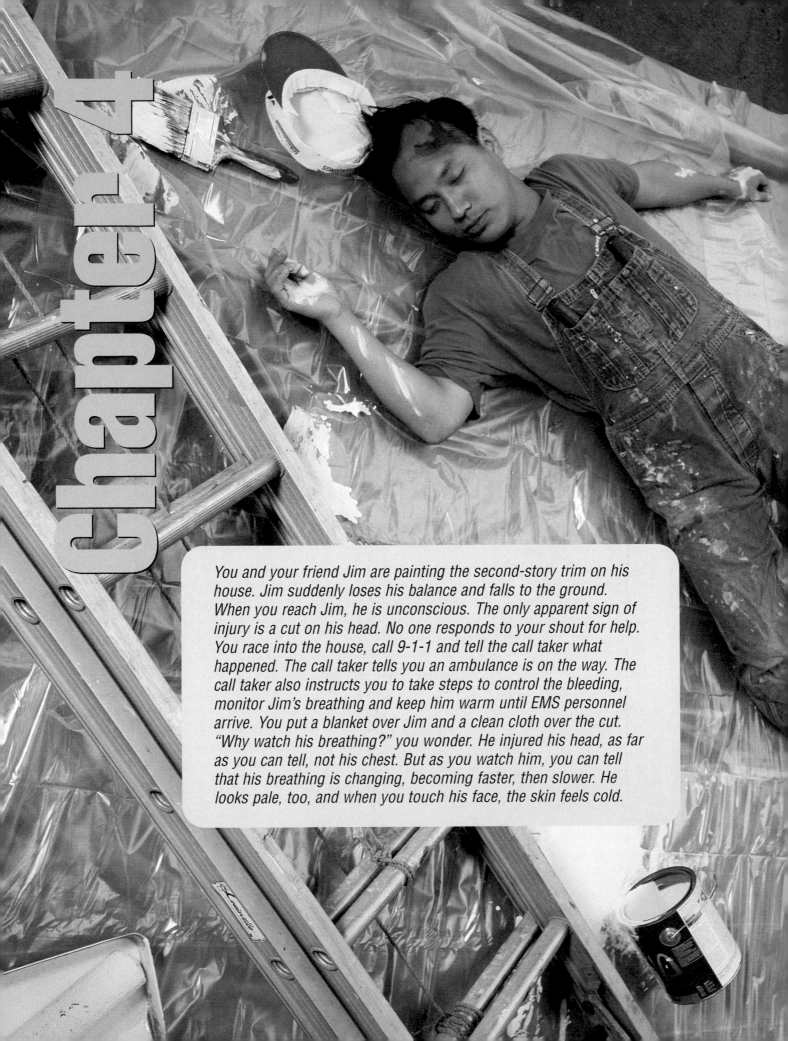

chapter 4

You and your friend Jim are painting the second-story trim on his house. Jim suddenly loses his balance and falls to the ground. When you reach Jim, he is unconscious. The only apparent sign of injury is a cut on his head. No one responds to your shout for help. You race into the house, call 9-1-1 and tell the call taker what happened. The call taker tells you an ambulance is on the way. The call taker also instructs you to take steps to control the bleeding, monitor Jim's breathing and keep him warm until EMS personnel arrive. You put a blanket over Jim and a clean cloth over the cut. "Why watch his breathing?" you wonder. He injured his head, as far as you can tell, not his chest. But as you watch him, you can tell that his breathing is changing, becoming faster, then slower. He looks pale, too, and when you touch his face, the skin feels cold.

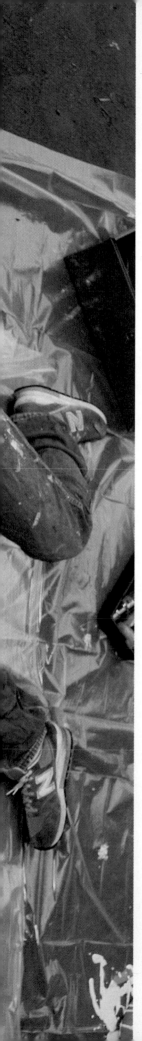

Body Systems

Objectives

After reading this chapter, you should be able to—

■ *Identify the five body cavities and the major structures in each cavity.*

■ *Identify the eight body systems and the major structures in each system.*

■ *Describe the primary functions of each of the eight body systems.*

■ *Give one example of how the body systems work together.*

■ *Describe conditions within each body system that require emergency care.*

Introduction

The human body is a miraculous machine. It performs many complex functions, each of which helps us live. You do not need to be an expert in human body structure and function to give effective care. Neither should you need a medical dictionary to effectively describe an injury. By knowing a few key structures, their functions and their locations, you can recognize a serious illness or injury and accurately communicate with EMS personnel about a victim's condition.

To remember the locations of the body structures, it helps to learn to visualize the structures that lie beneath the skin. The structures you can see or feel are reference points for locating the internal structures you cannot see or feel. For example, to locate the pulse on either side of the neck, you can use the Adam's apple on the front of the neck as a reference point. Using reference points will help you describe the location of injuries and other problems you may find. This chapter provides you with an overview of

important reference points, terminology and the structure and functions of eight body systems. Understanding the body systems and how they interact and depend on each other to keep the body functioning will help you give appropriate care to an ill or injured person.

BODY CAVITIES

A body cavity is a space in the body that contains organs, such as the heart, lungs and liver. The five major cavities, illustrated in **Figure 4-1**, are the—

▶ **Cranial cavity,** located in the head. It contains the brain and is protected by the skull.
▶ **Spinal cavity,** extending from the bottom of the skull to the lower back. It contains the spinal cord and is protected by the bones of the spine (vertebrae).
▶ **Thoracic cavity,** located in the **trunk.** It contains the heart, lungs and other important structures. It is protected by the **rib cage** and the upper spine.
▶ **Abdominal cavity,** located in the trunk between the **diaphragm** and the pelvis. It contains many organs, including the liver, gallbladder, pancreas, intestines, stomach, kidneys and spleen. Because most of the abdominal cavity is not protected by any bones, the

KEY TERMS

Airway: The pathway for air from the mouth and nose to the lungs.
Arteries: Large blood vessels that carry oxygenated blood away from the heart to the rest of the body.
Body system: A group of organs and other structures that work together to carry out specific functions.
Bone: A dense, hard tissue that forms the skeleton.
Brain: The center of the nervous system; controls all body functions.
Cells: The basic units of all living tissue.
Heart: A muscular organ that circulates blood throughout the body.
Lungs: A pair of light, spongy organs in the chest that provide the mechanism for taking oxygen in and removing carbon dioxide during breathing.

Muscle: A fibrous tissue that is able to contract, allowing and causing movement of organs and body parts.
Nerve: A part of the nervous system that sends impulses to and from the brain and all body parts.
Organ: A collection of similar tissues acting together to perform specific body functions.
Pulse: The beat you feel with each heart contraction.
Skin: The tough, supple membrane that covers the surface of the body.
Spinal cord: A bundle of nerves extending from the brain at the base of the skull to the lower back; protected by the spinal column.
Tissue: A collection of similar cells that act together to perform specific body functions.
Veins: Blood vessels that carry oxygenated blood from all parts of the body to the heart.

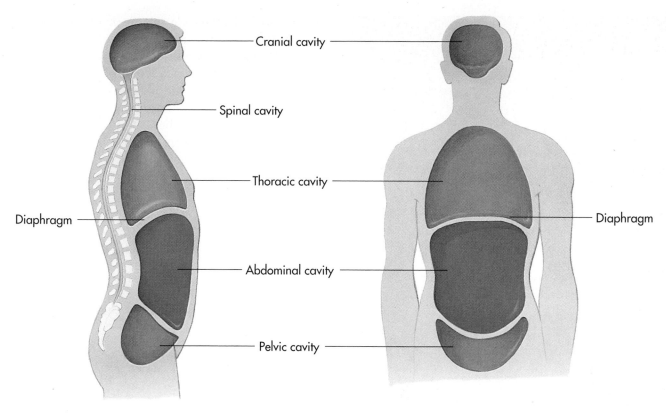

Figure 4-1   The five major cavities of the body.

organs within it are especially vulnerable to injury.

▶ **Pelvic cavity,** located in the pelvis, the lowest part of the trunk. It contains the bladder, rectum and reproductive organs. It is protected by the pelvic bones and the lower portion of the spine.

Knowing the general location and relative size of major organs in each cavity will help you assess a victim's injury or illness. The major organs and their functions are more fully described in the next section of this chapter and in later chapters.

BODY SYSTEMS

The body is made up of billions of microscopic *cells,* the basic units of all living tissue. There are many different types of cells. Each type contributes in a specific way to keep the body functioning normally. Collections of similar cells form *tissues,* which form organs **(Fig. 4-2).** An *organ* is a collection of similar tissues acting together to perform specific body functions. **Vital organs** perform functions that are essential for life. They include the brain, heart and lungs.

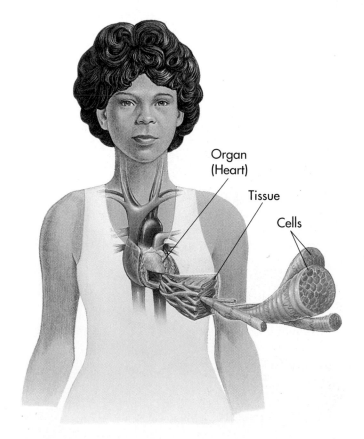

Figure 4-2   Cells and tissues make up organs.

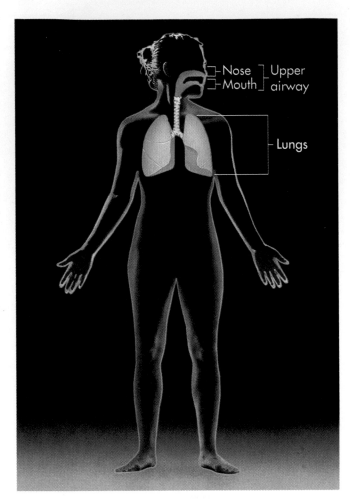

Figure 4-3 The respiratory system.

A *body system* is a group of organs and other structures that are especially adapted to perform specific body functions. They work together to carry out a function needed for life. For example, the heart, blood and blood vessels make up the circulatory system. The **circulatory system** keeps all parts of the body supplied with oxygen-rich blood. For the body to work properly, all of the following systems must work well together:

▸ Respiratory
▸ Circulatory
▸ Nervous
▸ Musculoskeletal
▸ Integumentary
▸ Endocrine
▸ Digestive
▸ Genitourinary

The Respiratory System

The body must have a constant supply of oxygen to stay alive. The **respiratory system** supplies the body with oxygen through breathing. When you **inhale**, air fills the lungs and the **oxygen** in the air is transferred to the blood. The blood carries oxygen to all parts of the body. This same system removes **carbon dioxide**, a waste gas. Carbon dioxide is transferred from the blood to the lungs. When you **exhale**, air is forced from the lungs, expelling carbon dioxide and other waste gases. This breathing process is called **respiration**.

Structure and Function

The respiratory system includes the airway and lungs. **Figure 4-3** shows the parts of the respiratory system. The *airway*, the passage through which air travels to the lungs, begins at the nose and mouth. Air passes through the nose and mouth, through the **pharynx** (the throat), **larynx** (the voice box) and **trachea** (the windpipe), on its way to the lungs (**Fig. 4-4**). The *lungs* are a pair of light, spongy organs in the chest that provide the mechanism for taking oxygen in and removing carbon dioxide during breathing. Behind the trachea is the esophagus. The **esophagus** is a tube that carries food and liquids from the mouth to the stomach. A small flap of tissue, the **epiglottis**, covers the trachea when you swallow to keep food and liquids out of the lungs.

Air reaches the lungs through two tubes called **bronchi**. The bronchi branch into increasingly smaller tubes called **bronchioles** (**Fig. 4-5, A**). These

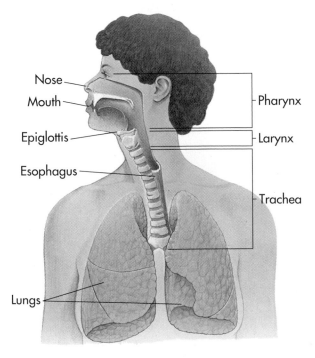

Figure 4-4 The respiratory system includes the pharynx, larynx and trachea.

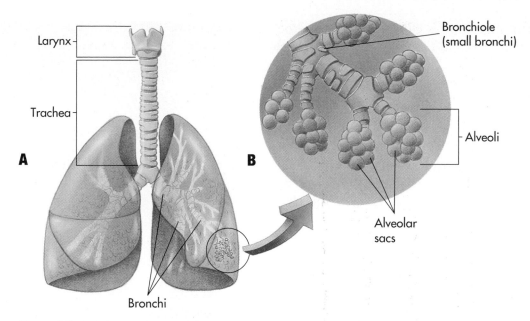

Figure 4-5   **A,** The bronchi branch into many small tubes. **B,** Oxygen and carbon dioxide pass into and out of blood through the walls of the alveoli and the capillaries.

tubes eventually end in millions of microscopic air sacs called alveoli. Oxygen and carbon dioxide pass into and out of the blood through the thin cell walls of the **alveoli** and microscopic blood vessels called **capillaries** (**Fig. 4-5,** *B*).

Air enters the lungs when you inhale and leaves the lungs when you exhale. When the diaphragm and the chest muscles contract, you inhale. The chest expands, drawing air into the lungs. When the chest muscles and diaphragm relax, pushing air from the lungs, the chest cavity becomes smaller and you exhale (**Fig. 4-6**). (The average adult breathes about 12 to 20 times per minute, and a child or infant, depending on age, breathes between 20 to 40 times per minute.) This ongoing breathing process is involuntary—meaning you do not have to think about it—and is controlled by the brain.

Conditions That Require Emergency Care

Because of the body's constant need for oxygen, it is important to recognize trouble breathing and to provide emergency care immediately. Some causes of trouble breathing include airway obstructions, asthma, allergies and injuries to the chest. Trouble breathing is referred to as **respiratory distress**.

If a victim has respiratory distress, you may hear or see noisy breathing or gasping. The victim may be conscious or unconscious. The conscious victim may be anxious or excited or may say that he or she feels short of breath. The victim's skin, particularly the lips and under the nails, may have a

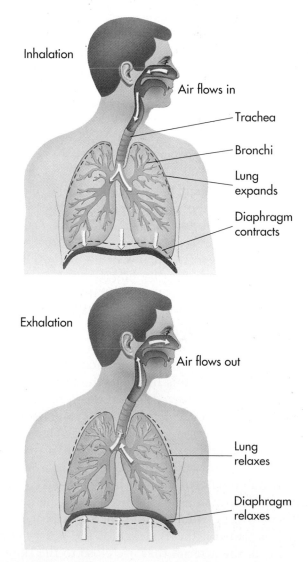

Figure 4-6   The chest muscles and the diaphragm contract as you inhale and relax as you exhale.

blue tint. This condition is called **cyanosis** and oc-curs when the blood and tissues do not get enough oxygen.

A victim who stops breathing has **respiratory arrest**. Respiratory arrest is a life-threatening emer-gency. Without the oxygen obtained from breath-ing, other body systems cannot function. For exam-ple, without oxygen, the heart muscle stops functioning. The circulatory system will fail.

Respiratory problems require immediate at-tention. Making sure the airway is open and clear is critical. You may have to breathe for a non-breathing victim or give care to someone who is choking. Breathing for the victim is called **rescue breathing**. These skills are discussed in detail in Chapter 6.

The Circulatory System

The **circulatory system** works with the respiratory system to carry oxygen-rich blood to every body cell. It also carries other nutrients throughout the body, removes waste and returns oxygen-poor blood to the lungs. The circulatory system includes the heart, blood and blood vessels. **Figure 4-7** shows this system.

Structure and Function

The heart is a muscular organ located behind the **sternum**, or breastbone. The *heart* circulates blood throughout the body through veins and arteries. *Arteries* are large blood vessels that carry blood away from the heart to the rest of the body. The ar-teries subdivide into smaller blood vessels and ulti-mately become microscopic capillaries. The capil-laries transport blood to all the cells of the body and nourish them with oxygen.

After the oxygen in the blood is transferred to the cells, *veins* carry the blood back to the heart. The heart circulates this blood to the lungs to pick up more oxygen before circulating it to other parts of the body. This cycle is called the **circulatory cy-cle**. The cross section of the heart in **Figure 4-8** shows how blood moves through the heart to com-plete the circulatory cycle.

The pumping action of the heart is called a **con-traction**. Contractions are controlled by the heart's electrical system, which makes the heart beat regu-larly. You can feel the evidence of the heart's con-tractions in the arteries that are close to the skin—for instance, at the neck or the wrist. The beat you feel with each contraction is called the *pulse*. The

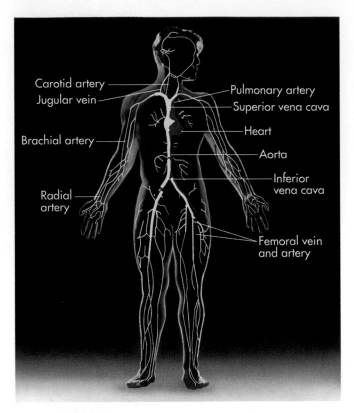

Figure 4-7   The circulatory system.

heart must beat regularly to deliver oxygen to body cells to keep the body functioning properly.

Conditions That Require Emergency Care

The following circulatory problems threaten the de-livery of oxygen to body cells:

▸ Blood loss caused by severe bleeding, such as a severed artery
▸ Impaired circulation, such as a blood clot
▸ Failure of the heart to pump adequately, such as a heart attack

Body tissues die when they do not receive oxy-gen. For example, when an artery supplying the brain with blood is blocked, brain tissue dies. When an artery supplying the heart with blood is blocked, heart muscle tissue dies. This damage of heart muscle is a life-threatening emergency—a heart attack.

When a person has a heart attack, the heart func-tions irregularly and may stop. If the heart stops, breathing will also stop. When the heart stops beat-ing or beats too weakly to pump blood effectively, it is called **cardiac arrest**. Victims of either heart attack or cardiac arrest need immediate emergency care. Cardiac arrest victims need to have circula-

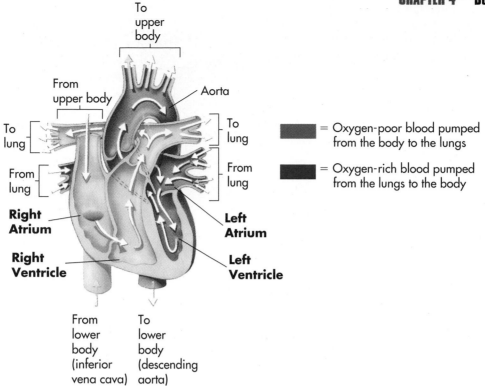

To
upper
body

From
upper body

Aorta

To
lung

To
lung

From
lung

From
lung

**Right
Atrium**

**Left
Atrium**

**Right
Ventricle**

**Left
Ventricle**

From
lower
body
(inferior
vena cava)

To
lower
body
(descending
aorta)

= Oxygen-poor blood pumped
from the body to the lungs

= Oxygen-rich blood pumped
from the lungs to the body

Figure 4-8   The heart is a two-sided pump made up of four chambers. A system of one-way valves keeps blood moving in the proper direction to complete the circulatory cycle.

tion maintained artificially by receiving chest compressions and rescue breathing. This combination of compressions and breaths is called **cardiopulmonary resuscitation** or **CPR.** You will learn more about the heart and how to perform CPR in Chapter 7.

The Nervous System

The **nervous system,** the most complex and delicate of all body systems, is one of the body's two major regulating and coordinating systems. (The other is the endocrine system, discussed later in this chapter.) The nervous system depends on a number of different sensory organs in the body to provide information about internal and external conditions that permit it to regulate and coordinate the body's activities.

Structure and Function

The *brain,* the center of the nervous system, is the master organ of the body. It regulates all body functions, including the respiratory and circulatory systems. The primary functions of the brain are the sensory, motor and integrated functions of consciousness, memory, emotions and use of language.

The brain transmits and receives information through a network of nerves. **Figure 4-9** shows the nervous system. The *spinal cord,* a large bundle of nerves, extends from the brain through a canal in the **spine,** or backbone. *Nerves* extend from the brain and spinal cord to every part of the body.

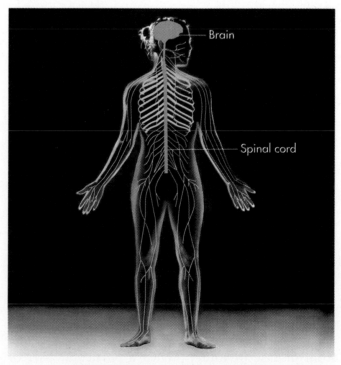

Brain

Spinal cord

Figure 4-9   The nervous system.

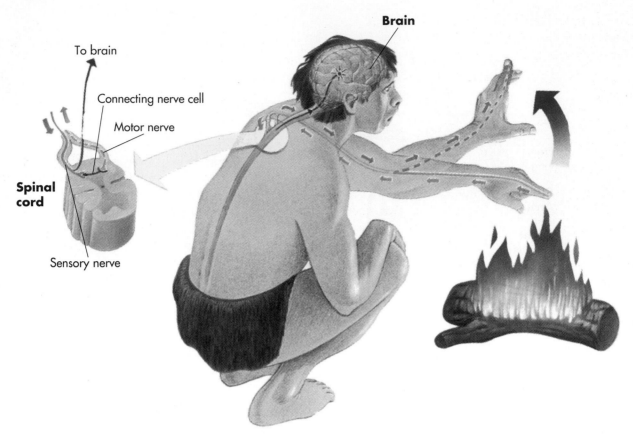

Figure 4-10 Messages are sent to and from the brain by way of the nerves.

Nerves transmit information as electrical impulses from one area of the body to another. Some nerves conduct impulses from the body to the brain, allowing you to see, hear, smell, taste and feel. These functions are the sensory functions. Other nerves conduct impulses from the brain to the muscles to control motor functions or movement (**Fig. 4-10**).

The integrated functions of the brain are more complex. One of these functions is **consciousness.** Normally, when you are awake, you are fully conscious. In most cases, being conscious means that you know who you are, where you are, the approximate date and time and what is happening around you. Your consciousness level can vary. For example, you can be highly aware in certain situations and less aware during periods of relaxation, sleep, illness or injury.

Conditions That Require Emergency Care

Brain cells, unlike other body cells, cannot regenerate or grow back. Once brain cells die or are damaged, they are not replaced. Brain cells may die from disease or injury. When a particular part of

the brain is diseased or injured, a person may lose the body functions controlled by that area of the brain. For example, if the part of the brain that regulates breathing is damaged, the person may stop breathing.

Illness or injury may change a person's level of consciousness. Consciousness may be affected by emotions, in which case the victim may be intensely aware of what is going on. At other times, the victim's mind may seem to be dull or cloudy. Illness or injury affecting the brain can also alter memory, emotions and the ability to use language.

A head injury can cause a temporary loss of consciousness. Any head injury causing a loss of consciousness can also cause brain injury and must be considered serious. These injuries require evaluation by medical professionals because injury to the brain can cause blood to form pools in the skull. Pooling blood puts pressure on the brain and limits the supply of oxygen to the brain cells.

Injury to the spinal cord or a nerve can result in a permanent loss of feeling and movement below the injury. This condition is called **paralysis.** For example, a lower back injury can result in paralysis of the legs; a neck injury can result in paralysis of all four limbs. A broken bone or a deep wound can also cause nerve damage, resulting in a loss of sensation or movement. In Chapter 13, you will learn about techniques for caring for head, neck and back injuries.

The Musculoskeletal System

The **musculoskeletal system** is made up of the bones, ligaments, muscles and tendons and comprises most of the body's weight. Together, these structures are primarily responsible for posture, locomotion and other body movements, but they are also responsible for many other functions that are not as obvious.

Structure and Function

The musculoskeletal system performs each of the following functions: supporting the body, protecting internal organs, allowing movement, storing minerals, producing blood cells and producing heat.

Bones and Ligaments

The body has over 200 bones. *Bone* is dense, hard tissue that forms the skeleton. The skeleton forms the framework that supports the body (**Fig. 4-11**). Where two or more bones join, they form a **joint**. **Figure 4-12** shows a typical joint. Bones are usually held together at joints by fibrous bands of tissue called **ligaments**. Bones vary in size and shape, allowing them to perform specific functions.

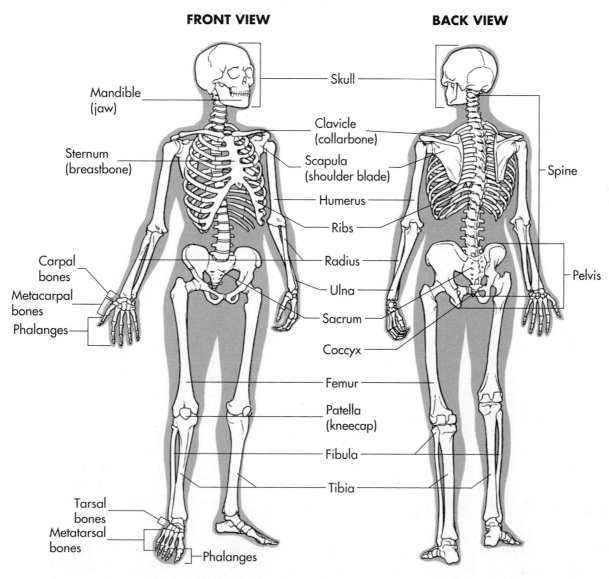

FRONT VIEW   **BACK VIEW**

Mandible (jaw) — Skull
Sternum (breastbone) — Clavicle (collarbone)
Scapula (shoulder blade)
Humerus
Ribs
Spine
Carpal bones — Radius
Metacarpal bones — Ulna
Phalanges — Sacrum
Pelvis
Coccyx
Femur
Patella (kneecap)
Fibula
Tibia
Tarsal bones
Metatarsal bones
Phalanges

Figure 4-11   Major bones of the body.

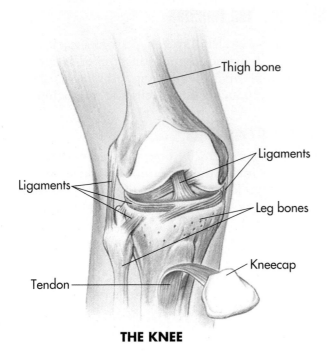

THE KNEE

Figure 4-12   A typical joint.

The bones of the skull protect the brain. The spine is made of bones called **vertebrae** that protect the spinal cord. The **ribs** are bones that attach to the spine and to the breastbone, forming a protective shell for vital organs, such as the heart and lungs.

In addition to supporting and protecting the body, bones aid movement. The bones of the arms and legs work like a system of levers and pulleys to position the hands and feet so that they can function. Bones of the wrist, hand and fingers are progressively smaller to allow for fine movements like writing. The small bones of the feet enable you to walk smoothly. Together, the bones of the foot work as shock absorbers when you walk, run or jump. Bones also store minerals and produce certain blood cells.

Muscles and Tendons

Muscles are made of special tissue that can contract and relax, resulting in movement. **Figure 4-13** shows the major muscles of the body. **Tendons** are

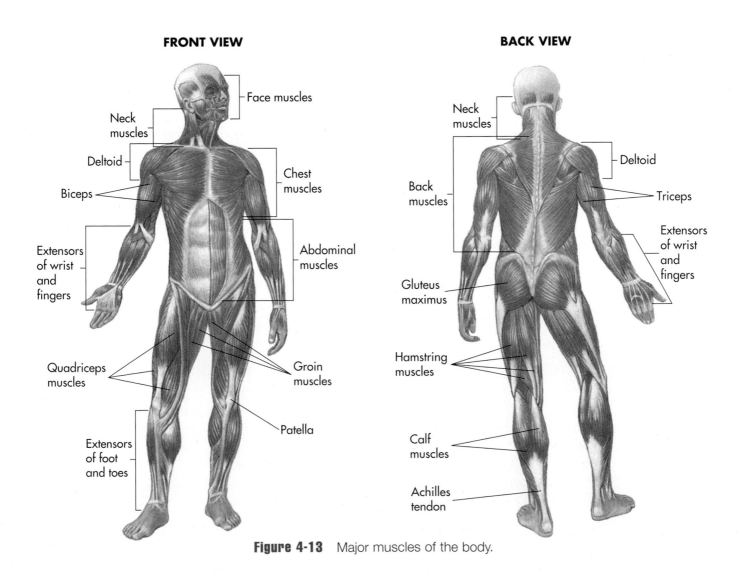

Figure 4-13   Major muscles of the body.

tissues that attach muscles to bones. Muscles band together to form muscle groups. Muscles work together in groups to produce movement (**Fig. 4-14**). Working muscles produce heat. Muscles also protect underlying structures, such as bones, nerves and blood vessels. Muscle action is controlled by the nervous system. Nerves carry information from the muscles to the brain. The brain processes this information and directs the muscles through the nerves (**Fig. 4-15**).

Muscle actions are either voluntary or involuntary. Involuntary muscles, such as the heart, are automatically controlled by the brain. You do not have to think about involuntary muscles to make them work. Voluntary muscles, such as leg and arm muscles, are most often under your conscious control but often work automatically. You are sometimes aware of telling them to move, but you do not think about walking, for example, you just do it.

Conditions That Require Emergency Care

Injuries to bones and muscles include fractures, dislocations, strains and sprains. A **fracture** is a broken bone. Dislocations occur when bones of a joint are

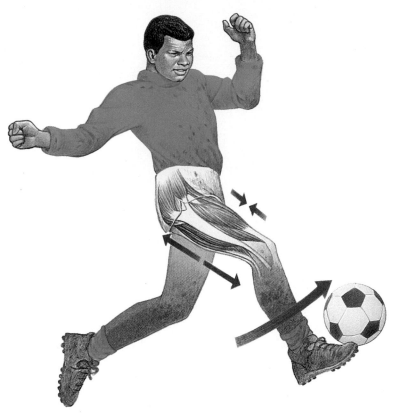

Figure 4-14   Muscle groups work together to produce movement.

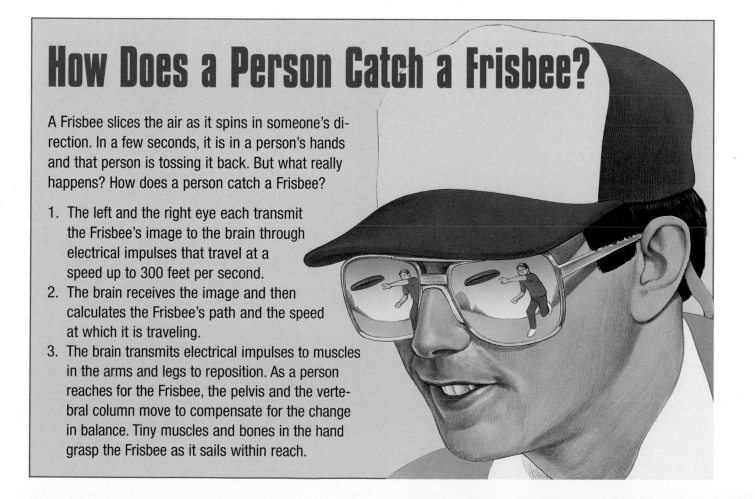

How Does a Person Catch a Frisbee?

A Frisbee slices the air as it spins in someone's direction. In a few seconds, it is in a person's hands and that person is tossing it back. But what really happens? How does a person catch a Frisbee?

1. The left and the right eye each transmit the Frisbee's image to the brain through electrical impulses that travel at a speed up to 300 feet per second.
2. The brain receives the image and then calculates the Frisbee's path and the speed at which it is traveling.
3. The brain transmits electrical impulses to muscles in the arms and legs to reposition. As a person reaches for the Frisbee, the pelvis and the vertebral column move to compensate for the change in balance. Tiny muscles and bones in the hand grasp the Frisbee as it sails within reach.

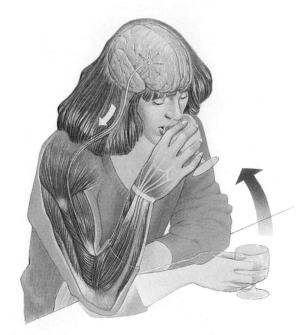

Figure 4-15   The brain controls muscle movement.

moved out of place, which is usually caused by physical trauma. **Strains** are injuries to muscles and tendons; **sprains** are injuries to ligaments. Although injuries to bones and muscles may not look serious, nearby nerves, blood vessels and other organs may be damaged. Regardless of how they appear, these injuries may cause lifelong disabilities or become

life-threatening emergencies. For example, torn ligaments in the knee can limit activity, and broken ribs can puncture the lungs and cause trouble breathing.

When you provide emergency care, remember that injuries to muscles and bones often result in additional injuries. You will learn more about musculoskeletal injuries and how to care for them in later chapters.

The Integumentary System

The **integumentary system** consists of the skin, hair and nails (**Fig. 4-16**). Most important among these structures is the skin. The skin protects the body and helps keep fluids within the body. It prevents **infection** by keeping out disease-producing **microorganisms**, or **pathogens**.

Structure and Function

The *skin* is made of tough, elastic fibers that stretch without easily tearing, protecting the skin from injury. The skin also helps make vitamin D and stores minerals.

The outer surface of the skin consists of dead cells that are continually rubbed away and replaced by new cells. The skin contains the hair roots, oil glands and sweat glands. Oil glands help to keep

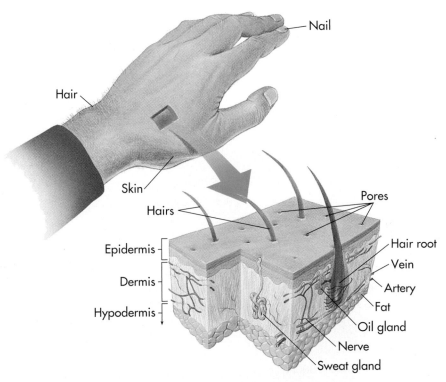

Figure 4-16   The skin, hair and nails make up the integumentary system.

the skin soft, supple and waterproof. Sweat glands and pores help regulate body temperature by releasing sweat. The nervous system monitors blood temperature and causes you to sweat if blood temperature rises even slightly. Although you may not see or feel it, sweat is released to the skin's surface.

Blood supplies the skin with nutrients and helps provide its color. When blood vessels dilate (become wider), the blood circulates close to the skin's surface. This dilation can make some people's skin appear flushed or red and makes the skin feel warm. The reddening may not appear with darker skin. When blood vessels constrict (become narrower), not as much blood is close to the skin's surface, causing the skin to look pale or ashen and feel cool. In people with darker skin, color changes may be most easily seen in the nail beds and the **mucous membranes** inside the mouth and inside the lower eyelids.

Nerves in the skin make it very sensitive to sensations such as touch, pain and temperature. Therefore, the skin is also an important part of the body's communication network and is a type of sensory organ.

Conditions That Require Emergency Care

Although the skin is tough, it can be injured. Sharp objects may puncture, cut or tear the skin. Rough objects can scrape it, and extreme heat or cold may burn or freeze it. Burns and skin injuries that cause bleeding may result in the loss of vital fluids. Germs may enter the body through breaks in the skin, causing infection that can become serious. In later chapters, you will learn how to care for skin injuries, such as burns and cuts.

The Endocrine System

The **endocrine system** is the second of the two regulatory systems in the body. Together with the nervous system, it coordinates the activities of other body systems.

Structure and Function

The endocrine system consists of several glands (**Fig. 4-17**). **Glands** are organs that release substances into the blood or onto the skin. Some glands produce **hormones**, substances that enter the bloodstream and influence tissue activity in various parts of the body. For example, the thyroid gland makes a hormone that controls **metabolism**, the process by

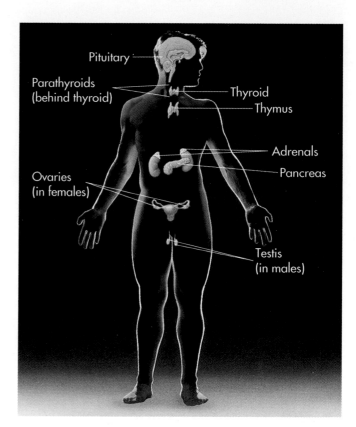

Figure 4-17   The endocrine system.

which all cells convert nutrients to energy. Other glands include the sweat and oil glands in the skin.

Conditions That Require Emergency Care

You do not need to know all the glands in the endocrine system or the hormones they produce. Problems in the endocrine system usually develop slowly and seldom become emergencies. Knowing how hormones work in general, however, helps you understand how some illnesses seem to develop suddenly.

For example, an emergency occurs when too much or too little of a hormone called insulin is secreted into the blood. Normally, insulin is secreted by small glands embedded in the pancreas. Without insulin, cells cannot use the sugar they need from food. Too much insulin forces blood sugar rapidly into the cells, lowering blood sugar levels and depriving the brain of the blood sugar it needs to function normally. Too little insulin results in too high a level of sugar in the blood. The condition in which the body does not produce enough insulin and blood sugar is abnormally high is called **diabetes**. Blood sugar levels that rise or fall abnormally can make a person ill, sometimes severely so. You will learn more about this kind of emergency in Chapter 15.

The Digestive System

The **digestive system**, also called the gastrointestinal system, consists of organs that work together to take in and break down food and eliminate waste. This digestive process provides the body with water, **electrolytes** and other nutrients.

Structure and Function

The major structures of the digestive system include the mouth, esophagus, stomach, intestines, pancreas, gallbladder and liver (**Fig. 4-18**). Food entering the system is broken down into a form the body can use. As food passes through the system, the body absorbs nutrients that can be converted to energy to be used by the cells. The unabsorbed portion continues through the system and is eliminated as waste.

Conditions That Require Emergency Care

Because most digestive system organs are in the unprotected abdominal cavity, they are very vulnerable to injury. Such an injury can occur, for example, if a body strikes a car's steering wheel in a collision.

These organs can also be damaged by a penetrating injury, such as a stab or gunshot wound. Damaged organs may bleed internally, causing severe loss of blood, or may spill waste products into the abdominal cavity. Such a spill can result in severe infection. Chapter 14 discusses in more detail how to recognize and care for abdominal injuries.

The Genitourinary System

The **genitourinary system** is made up of two systems: the urinary system and the reproductive system. Although relatively close together in the body, they have very different functions. The urinary system plays a major role in managing body fluid and eliminating waste products. The reproductive system's primary purpose is to reproduce human life.

Structure and Function

The **urinary system** consists of organs that eliminate waste products filtered from the blood (**Fig. 4-19**). The primary organs are the kidneys and the bladder. The **kidneys** are located behind the abdominal cavity just beneath the chest, one on each side. They filter wastes from the circulating blood to form urine.

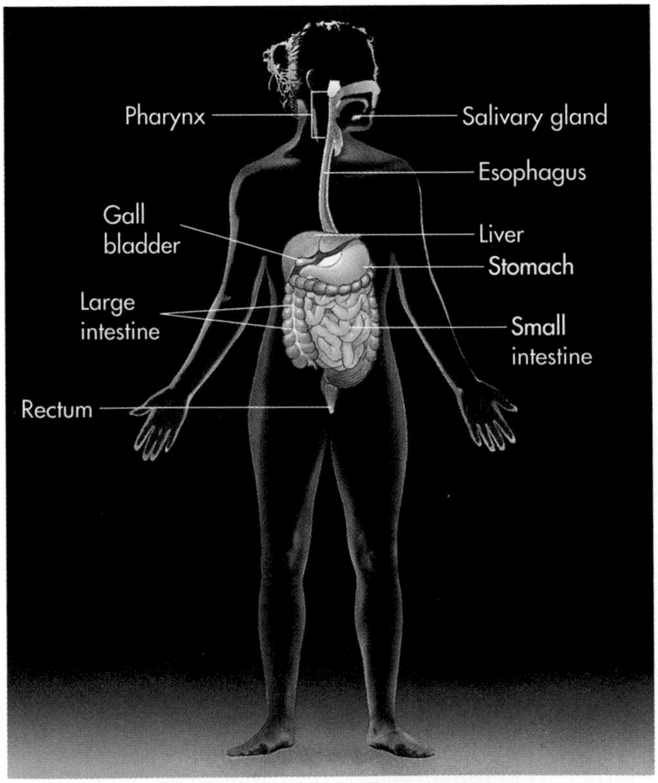

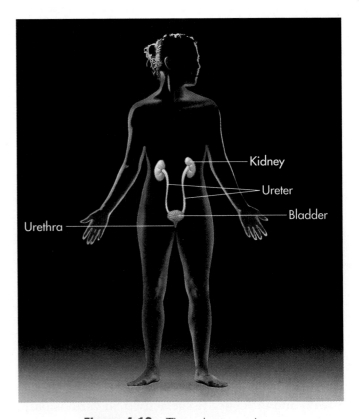

Figure 4-18 The digestive system.

Figure 4-19 The urinary system.

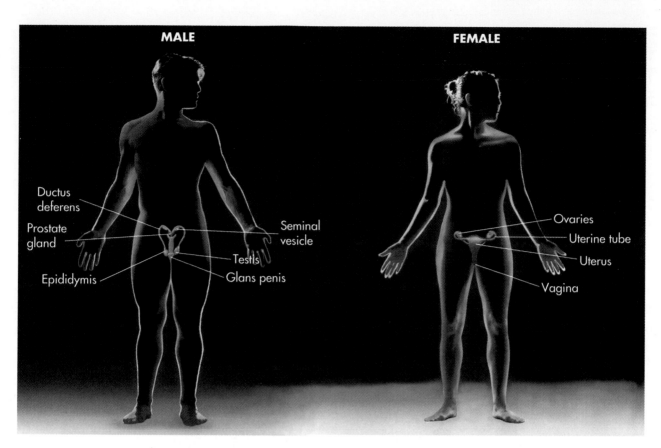

Figure 4-20 The male and female reproductive systems.

Urine is then stored in the **bladder**, a small muscular sac. The bladder stretches as it fills and then shrinks back after the urine is released.

The female and male **reproductive systems** include the organs for sexual reproduction (**Fig. 4-20**). Injuries to the abdominal or pelvic area can damage organs in either system.

The female reproductive organs are smaller than many major organs and are protected by the pelvic bones. The soft tissue external structures are more susceptible to injury, although such injury is uncommon. The male reproductive organs are located outside of the pelvis and are more vulnerable to injury.

Conditions That Require Emergency Care

The frequency of injuries to the organs of the urinary system depends on their vulnerability. Unlike the abdominal organs, the kidneys are partially protected by the lower ribs, making them less vulnerable to injury. But the kidneys may be damaged by a significant blow to the back just below the rib cage or by a penetrating wound, such as a stab or gun-

shot wound. Anyone with an injury to the back below the rib cage may have injured one or both kidneys. Because of the kidney's rich blood supply, such an injury often causes severe internal bleeding, often manifested by blood in the urine.

The bladder is injured less frequently than the kidneys, but injuries to the abdomen can rupture the bladder, particularly when it is full. Bone fragments from a fracture of the pelvis can also pierce the bladder or intestines.

Injuries to urinary system organs may not be obvious but should be suspected if there are significant injuries to the back just below the rib cage or to the abdomen. Chapter 14 discusses signals to watch for and how to give care for such injuries.

The external reproductive organs, called **genitalia**, have a rich supply of blood and nerves. Injuries to these organs may cause bleeding but are rarely life threatening. Injuries to the genitalia are usually caused by a blow to the pelvic area but may result from sexual assault or rape. Although such injuries are rarely life threatening, they almost always cause the victim extreme distress. Such a victim may refuse care.

Table 4-1 Body Systems

SYSTEM	MAJOR STRUCTURES	PRIMARY FUNCTION	HOW THE SYSTEM WORKS WITH OTHER BODY SYSTEMS
Respiratory	Airway and lungs	Supplies the body with oxygen and removes carbon dioxide through breathing	Works with the circulatory system to provide oxygen to cells; controlled by the nervous system
Circulatory	Heart, blood and blood vessels	Transports nutrients and oxygen to body cells and removes waste products	Works with the respiratory system to provide oxygen to cells; works in conjunction with the urinary and digestive systems to remove waste products; helps give skin color; controlled by the nervous system
Nervous	Brain, spinal cord and nerves	One of two primary regulatory systems in the body; transmits messages to and from the brain	Regulates all body systems through a network of nerves
Musculoskeletal	Bones, ligaments, muscles and tendons	Provides body's framework; protects internal organs and other underlying structures; allows movement; produces heat; manufactures blood components	Provides protection to organs and structures of other body systems; muscle action is controlled by the nervous system
Integumentary	Skin, hair and nails	An important part of the body's communication network; helps prevent infection and dehydration; assists with temperature regulation; aids in production of certain vitamins	Helps to protect the body from disease-producing organisms; together with the circulatory system, helps to regulate body temperature; under control of the nervous system; communicates sensation to the brain through the nerves
Endocrine	Glands	Secretes hormones and other substances into blood and onto skin	Together with the nervous system coordinates the activities of other systems
Digestive	Mouth, esophagus, stomach, intestines, pancreas, gallbladder and liver	Breaks down food into usable form to supply the rest of the body with energy	Works with the circulatory system to transport nutrients to the body
Genitourinary	Kidneys and bladder	Removes waste from the circulatory system and regulates water balance	
	Uterus and genitalia	Performs the process of sexual reproduction	

INTERRELATIONSHIPS OF BODY SYSTEMS

Each body system plays a vital role in survival (**Table 4-1**). Body systems work together to help the body maintain a constant healthy state. When the environment changes, body systems adapt to the new conditions. For example, because your musculoskeletal system works harder when you exercise, your respiratory and circulatory systems must also work harder to meet your body's increased oxygen demands. Your body systems also react to the stresses caused by illness or injury.

Body systems do not work independently of each other. The impact of an injury or illness is rarely restricted to one body system. For example, a stroke may result in brain damage that will impair movement and feeling. Injuries to the ribs can make breathing difficult. If the heart stops beating for any reason, breathing will also stop.

In any significant illness or injury, body systems may be seriously affected. The condition that results from a progressive failure of a body system or systems is called **shock**. Shock is the inability of the circulatory system to provide adequate oxygen to all parts of the body, especially the cells of the vital organs. You will learn more about shock in Chapter 9.

Generally, the more body systems involved in an emergency, the more serious the emergency. Body systems depend on each other for survival. In serious injury or illness, the body may not be able to keep functioning. In these cases, regardless of your best efforts, the victim may die.

SUMMARY

The body includes a number of systems, all of which must work together for the body to function properly. The brain, the center of the nervous system, controls all body functions including those of the other body systems. Knowing a few key structures, their functions and their locations helps you to understand more about these body systems and how they relate to injuries and sudden illnesses. Injury or illness that affects one body system can have a serious impact on other systems. Fortunately, basic care is usually all you need to give until EMS personnel arrive. By learning the basic principles of care described in later chapters, you may be able to make the difference between life and death.

APPLICATION QUESTIONS

1. Why did the call taker tell you to watch Jim's breathing?

2. Which body systems appear to have been affected by Jim's fall?

STUDY QUESTIONS

1. Complete the table with the correct system, structures or function(s).

Systems	Structures	Function
		Supplies the body with the oxygen it needs through breathing
	Heart, blood and blood vessels	
Integumentary		
Musculoskeletal		
		Regulates all body functions; a communication network

2. Match each term with the correct definition.

a. Arteries	e. Tissue
b. Organ	f. Spinal cord
c. Cell	g. Respiration
d. Endocrine system	h. Veins

_____ The process of breathing.

_____ A large bundle of nerves extending from the brain through the spine.

_____ A collection of similar cells that perform a specific function.

_____ A body system that regulates and coordinates the activities of other body systems by producing chemicals that influence the activity of tissues.

_____ The basic unit of living tissue.

_____ Blood vessels that carry oxygenated blood from the heart to the body.

_____ Blood vessels that carry blood to the heart.

_____ A collection of similar tissues acting together to perform a specific body function.

In questions 3 through 9, circle the letter of the correct answer.

3. Which structure is not located in or part of the thoracic cavity?

a. The liver
b. The rib cage
c. The heart
d. The lungs

4. The two body systems that work together to provide oxygen to the body cells are—

   a. Musculoskeletal and integumentary.
   b. Circulatory and musculoskeletal.
   c. Respiratory and circulatory.
   d. Endocrine and nervous.

5. One of the main functions of the integumentary system is to—

   a. Transmit information to the brain.
   b. Produce blood cells.
   c. Prevent infection.
   d. Secrete hormones.

6. The function of the digestive system is to—

   a. Perform the process of reproduction.
   b. Transport nutrients and oxygen to body cells.
   c. Break down food into a form the body can use for energy.
   d. All of the above.

7. Which structure in the airway prevents food and liquid from entering the lungs?

   a. The trachea
   b. The epiglottis
   c. The esophagus
   d. The bronchi

8. If a person's use of language suddenly becomes impaired, which body system might be injured?

   a. The musculoskeletal system
   b. The nervous system
   c. The integumentary system
   d. The circulatory system

9. Which two body systems will react initially to alert a victim to a severe cut?

   a. Circulatory, respiratory
   b. Respiratory, musculoskeletal
   c. Nervous, respiratory
   d. Circulatory, nervous

Answers are listed in Appendix A.

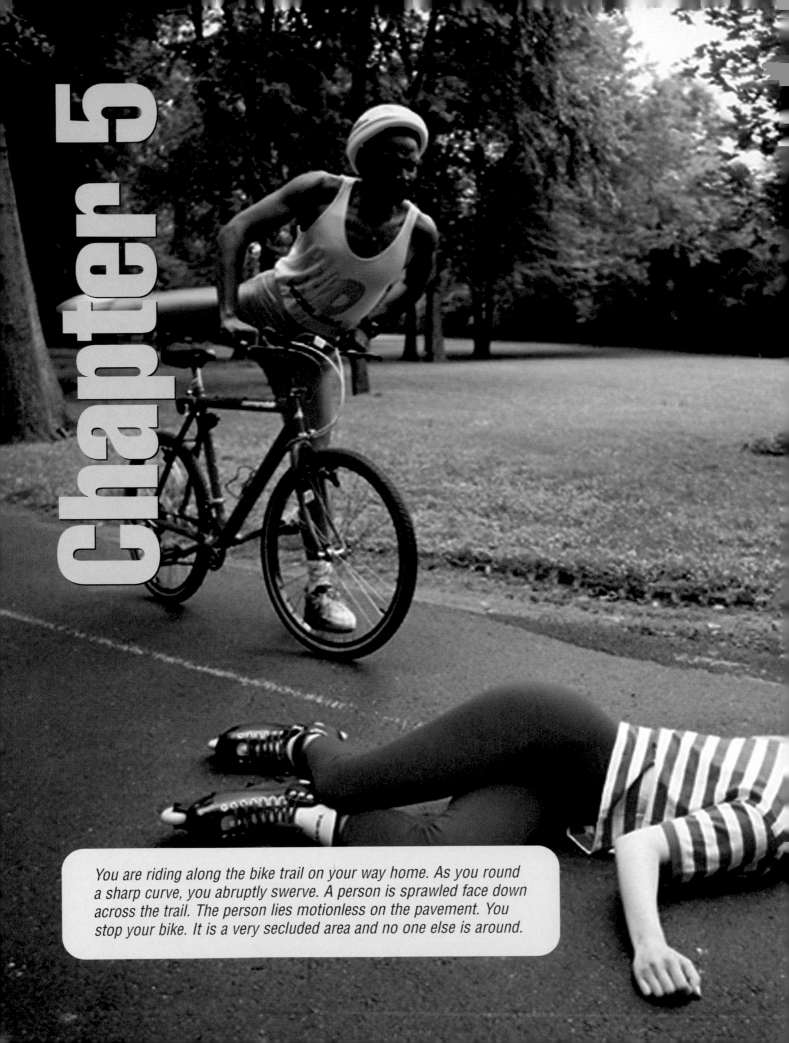

Chapter 5

You are riding along the bike trail on your way home. As you round a sharp curve, you abruptly swerve. A person is sprawled face down across the trail. The person lies motionless on the pavement. You stop your bike. It is a very secluded area and no one else is around.

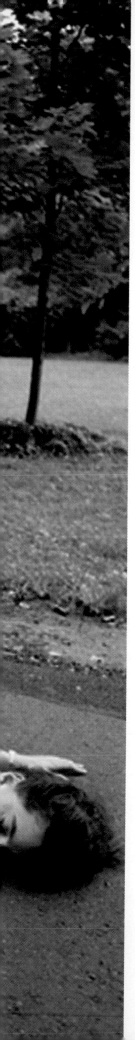

Checking the Victim

Objectives

After reading this chapter, you should be able to—

- Describe how to check for life-threatening conditions for an adult, child or infant.

- Identify and explain at least three questions you should ask the victim or bystanders in an interview.

- Describe how to check for non-life-threatening conditions for an adult, child or infant.

After reading this chapter and completing the class activities, you should be able to—

- Demonstrate how to check an unconscious adult, child or infant.

- Demonstrate how to check a conscious adult, child or infant.

Introduction

In earlier chapters, you learned that as a citizen responder trained in first aid, you can make a difference in an emergency—you may even save a life. You learned how to recognize an emergency and to follow the emergency action steps: CHECK—CALL—CARE. More importantly, you learned that your decision to act can have a significant impact on the victim's chance of survival. You can always do something to help.

In this chapter, you will learn how to check an injured or ill person for life-threatening conditions. You will also learn how to interview a conscious victim and any bystanders, check for non-life-threatening conditions and give basic care in any emergency until EMS personnel arrive.

CHECKING FOR LIFE-THREATENING CONDITIONS

After checking the scene, you should check the victim first for life-threatening conditions. Life-threatening conditions include—

▶ Unconsciousness.
▶ Trouble breathing.
▶ No *signs of life* (normal breathing or movement) and, for children and infants, no pulse.
▶ Severe bleeding.

The actions you will take depend on the conditions you find.

Shock

When someone becomes suddenly ill or is injured, normal body functions may be interrupted. In cases of minor injury or illness, the interruption is brief and the body is able to compensate quickly. With more severe injuries or illness, however, the body is unable to meet its demand for oxygen. The condition in which the body fails to circulate oxygen-rich blood to all the parts of the body is known as shock. If left untreated, shock can lead to death. Always look for the signals of shock whenever you are giving care. You will learn how to recognize and treat a victim for shock in Chapter 9.

Checking for Consciousness

First, determine if the victim is conscious. Tap him or her on the shoulder and shout, "Are you okay?" For an infant, gently tap the infant's shoulder or flick the foot. Do not jostle or move the victim.

If the victim is conscious and alert, introduce yourself, get the victim's consent to give care and attempt to find out what happened. Look for signals of injury or illness, ask the victim to describe what he or she is experiencing, for example, dizziness or pain. Perhaps a bystander is available to help answer questions and to call 9-1-1 or the local emergency number if necessary.

If the victim is unconscious, the situation is different. Unconsciousness is always a life-threatening condition. Call 9-1-1 or the local emergency number immediately. Ideally, someone will be available to make the call while you care for the victim.

Remember that if you are in a situation in which you are the only person other than the victim, you should—

Call First, that is, call 9-1-1 or the local emergency number before giving care for—

▶ An unconscious adult victim or adolescent age 12 or older.

KEY TERMS

Head-tilt/chin-lift technique: Technique used to open a victim's airway by pushing down on the forehead while pulling up on the bony part of the jaw.

Signs of life: Normal breathing or movement.

▶ An unconscious infant or child known to be at a high risk for heart problems.

▶ A witnessed sudden collapse of a child or infant.

Care First, that is, give 2 minutes of care, then call 9-1-1 or the local emergency number for—

▶ An unwitnessed collapse of an unconscious person younger than 12 years old.

▶ Any victim of a drowning.

If you must leave the scene to call 9-1-1 or the local emergency number, carefully position an unconscious victim on one side in case he or she vomits while you are gone. This position is called a **recovery position** (**Fig. 5-1**). Roll the victim onto his or her side, and bend the top leg and move it forward. Position the head and neck so that the face is angled toward the ground. Avoid twisting the neck and back as you roll the victim onto his or her side. If you suspect a head, neck or back injury and a clear, open airway can be maintained, do not move the victim unnecessarily. If a clear, open airway **cannot** be maintained or if you must leave the victim to get help, move the victim onto his or her side while keeping the head, neck and back in a straight line by placing the victim in a modified High Arm In Endangered Spine (H.A.IN.E.S.) recovery position.

If the victim is conscious, tell him or her that you are going to get help. Make the victim as comfortable as possible.

After calling 9-1-1 or the local emergency number, return to the victim, complete the check and give care until EMS personnel arrive.

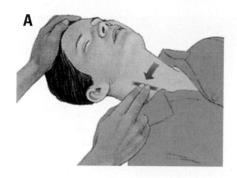

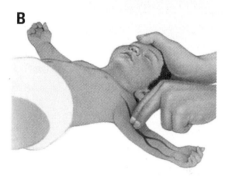

Figure 5-2, A-B   Check for a pulse on a **A,** child or **B,** infant.

Checking for a Pulse—Child and Infant

To find out if the heart is beating, check for a pulse (**Fig. 5-2, A-B**) for no more than 10 seconds. To check for signs of life, look for normal breathing or movement, then check for a pulse for no more than 10 seconds for children and infants if no breathing or movement is found.

CHECKING AN UNCONSCIOUS PERSON

If you find that the person is unconscious and 9-1-1 or the local emergency number has been called, find out if there are other conditions that threaten the person's life. Always check to see if an unconscious person—

▶ Has an open airway.

▶ Shows signs of life (movement or breathing).

▶ Is bleeding severely.

An easy way to remember what you need to check is to think of ABC, which stands for—

▶ Airway—open the airway.

▶ Breathing—check for movement or breathing.

▶ Circulation—check for signs of life (including a pulse for a child or infant) and severe bleeding.

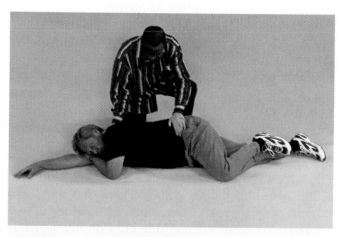

Figure 5-1   If you are alone and must leave an unconscious victim, position the person on one side in case he or she vomits while you are gone.

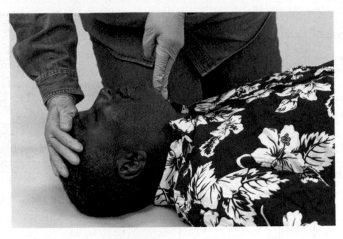

Figure 5-3 Open an unconscious person's airway using the head-tilt/chin-lift technique.

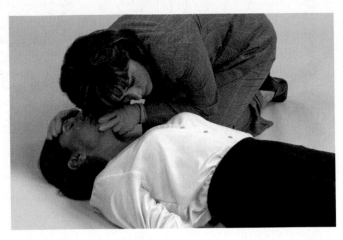

Figure 5-4 Look, listen and feel for movement and breathing for no more than 10 seconds.

Airway

Once you or someone else has called 9-1-1 or the local emergency number, you must check to see if the person has an open airway and is breathing. An open airway allows air to enter the lungs for the person to breathe. If the airway is blocked, the person cannot breathe. This is a life-threatening condition.

When someone is unconscious and lying on his or her back, the tongue may fall to the back of the throat and block the airway. To open an unconscious person's airway, push down on his or her forehead while pulling up on the bony part of the jaw with two or three fingers of your other hand to lift the chin (**Fig. 5-3**). This procedure, known as the *head-tilt/chin-lift technique,* moves the tongue away from the back of the throat, allowing air to enter the lungs.

Breathing

After opening the airway, you must check an unconscious person carefully for signals of breathing. Look, listen and feel for these signals. Position yourself so that you can hear and feel air as it escapes from the nose and mouth. At the same time, look to see if the victim's chest clearly rises and falls. Look, listen and feel for movement and breathing for no more than 10 seconds (**Fig. 5-4**). If the person is not breathing, give 2 rescue breaths with each breath lasting about 1 second (**Fig. 5-5**). If the air goes in (chest clearly rises), check for a

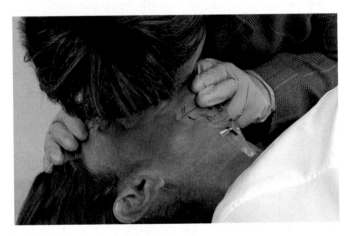

Figure 5-5 Keep the airway open and give 2 rescue breaths.

pulse for children and infants. In an unconscious adult, you may detect an irregular, gasping or shallow breath. This is known as an agonal breath. Do not confuse this for normal breathing. You should begin CPR immediately. Agonal breaths do not occur frequently in children.

Sometimes food, liquid or other objects will block the person's airway. When this happens, you will need to remove whatever is blocking the airway.

If air does go in but the child or infant is not breathing, you may need to perform rescue breathing. Rescue breathing is a technique used to provide a non-breathing victim with oxygen. You will learn how to perform rescue breathing in Chapter 6.

If the person is breathing, his or her heart is beating and is circulating blood. In this case, maintain an open airway by using the head-tilt/chin-lift

Checking for a Pulse— Child and Infant

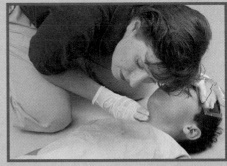

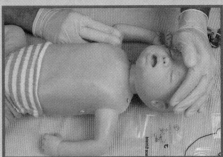

For a child, feel for the pulse at either of the **carotid arteries** located in the neck. To find the carotid pulse, feel for the Adam's apple and slide your fingers into the groove at the side of the neck. Sometimes the pulse may be difficult to find, because it may be slow or weak. If at first you do not find a pulse, find the Adam's apple and again slide your fingers into place. When you think you are in the right spot, take no more than 10 seconds to feel for the pulse. Feel for the pulse on the side of the child's neck closer to you.

For an infant, feel for the **brachial pulse** in the upper arm.

technique as you continue to look for other life-threatening conditions.

Circulation

It is very important to recognize breathing emergencies in children and infants and to act before the heart stops beating. Adults' hearts frequently stop beating because they are diseased. Infants' and children's hearts, however, are usually healthy. When an infant's or child's heart stops, it is usually the result of a breathing emergency.

If an adult is not breathing and you have given him or her 2 rescue breaths, you must then assume the problem is a cardiac emergency and begin CPR immediately.

If a child or infant shows no signs of life (movement or breathing), you will have to check for a pulse for no more than 10 seconds. If you find a pulse but no breathing, give rescue breathing. If the child or infant does not show signs of life or a pulse, the heart is not beating properly.

You must keep blood circulating in the person's body until emergency medical help arrives. To do this, you will have to perform cardiopulmonary resuscitation (CPR). Rescue breathing for infants and children is discussed in Chapter 6. CPR is discussed in Chapter 7.

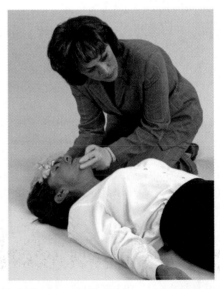

Figure 5-6   Check for severe bleeding by scanning from head to toe.

Severe Bleeding

After checking for signs of life, quickly check for severe bleeding. Bleeding is severe when blood spurts from the wound or cannot be easily controlled. Look over the victim's body from head to toe for signals of bleeding, such as blood-soaked clothing or blood pooling around the victim (**Fig. 5-6**).

Bleeding usually looks more serious than it is. A small amount of blood on a slick surface or mixed with water almost always looks like a great deal of blood. Severe bleeding is not always easy to recognize. You must make a decision based on your best judgment. Severe bleeding must be controlled as soon as possible. Make sure you protect yourself against disease transmission by keeping a barrier between you and the victim's blood. You will learn more about severe bleeding in Chapter 8.

CHECKING A CONSCIOUS VICTIM

Once you have determined that a victim is conscious and has no immediate life-threatening conditions, you can begin to check for other conditions that may need care. Checking a conscious victim with no immediate life-threatening conditions involves two basic steps:

1. Interview the victim and bystanders.
2. Check the victim from head to toe.

Interviewing the Victim and Bystanders

Ask the victim and bystanders simple questions to learn more about what happened and to learn about the victim's condition. These interviews should not take much time. Remember to first identify yourself and to get the victim's consent to give care. Begin by asking the victim's name. Using the victim's name will make him or her feel more comfortable. Gather additional information by asking the victim the following questions:

▸ What happened?
▸ Do you feel pain or discomfort anywhere?
▸ Do you have any allergies?
▸ Do you have any medical conditions, or are you taking any medication?

If the victim feels pain, ask him or her where the pain is located and to describe it. You can often expect to get descriptions such as burning, crushing, throbbing, aching or sharp pain. Ask when the pain started and what he or she was doing when it began. Ask the victim to rate his or her pain on a scale of 1-10 (1 being mild and 10 being severe).

Sometimes a victim may not be able to provide you with the proper information. Infants or children may be frightened, or the victim may not speak your language. Ask family members, friends

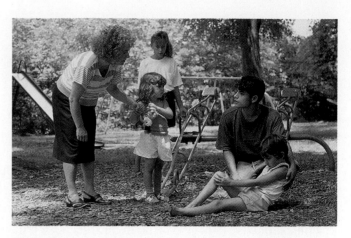

Figure 5-7 Parents or other adults may be able to give you helpful information or help you communicate with a sick or injured child.

or bystanders what happened. They may be able to give you helpful information or help you communicate with the victim (**Fig. 5-7**). You will learn more about communicating with people with special needs in Chapter 21.

Write down the information you learn during the interview. If possible, have someone else write down the information or help you remember it. This information can be given to EMS personnel when they arrive. Providing this information may help EMS personnel to determine the type of medical care the victim should receive. Information might include what medications the victim is taking and any allergies he or she has.

Checking the Victim from Head to Toe

Before you begin to check the victim, tell him or her what you are going to do. Have the victim tell you if any areas hurt. Avoid touching any painful area or having the victim move any area that is painful. Use your senses—sight, sound, touch and smell—to detect anything abnormal. Think about how the body normally looks. Be alert for any signals of injuries—anything that looks or sounds unusual. If you are uncertain, compare the injured side to the other side of the body. Watch for facial expressions, and listen for a tone of voice that may reveal pain. Look for a medical ID tag or bracelet. This tag may tell you what might be wrong, who to call for help and what care to give (**Fig. 5-8**).

Begin your check at the victim's head, examining the scalp, face, ears, eyes, nose and mouth.

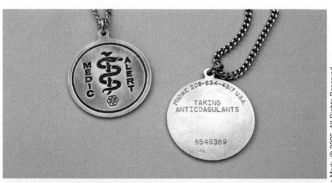

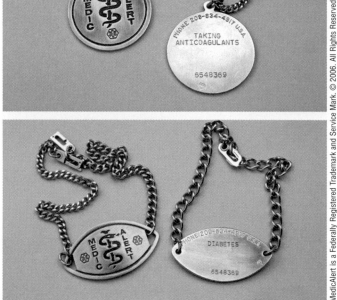

MedicAlert is a Federally Registered Trademark and Service Mark. © 2006. All Rights Reserved.

Figure 5-8 Medical ID tags and bracelets can provide important information about the victim.

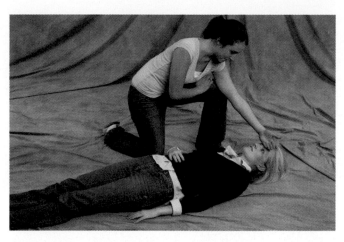

Figure 5-9 Feel the skin with the back of your hand to determine the skin's temperature.

Look for cuts, bumps, bruises and depressions. Look for signals that may indicate a serious problem. Watch for changes in consciousness. Notice if the victim is drowsy, not alert or confused. Look for changes in or any trouble breathing. A healthy person breathes regularly, quietly and easily. Abnormal breathing includes noisy breathing, such as gasping for air or making gurgling or whistling sounds; breathing that is unusually fast or slow; and breathing that is painful.

The skin's appearance and temperature often indicate something about the victim's condition. Notice how the skin looks and feels. A victim with a flushed, pale or ashen (gray) face may be ill. Note if the skin is reddish, bluish, pale or ashen. Darker skin looks ashen instead of pale. Determine the temperature of the skin by feeling it with the back of your hand (**Fig. 5-9**). Skin that is cool, moist, warm or dry to the touch may indicate a medical problem. In later chapters, you will learn more about what these changes may mean and what first aid to give.

If the victim becomes unconscious and the call has not already been made, stop your check and call 9-1-1 or the local emergency number immediately. Return to the victim and continuously check him or her for any life-threatening conditions that may appear. Remain at the victim's head,

where it is easiest to check for breathing and signs of life.

If you do not suspect an injury to the head, neck or back, determine if the victim has any specific injuries by asking him or her to try to move each body part in which he or she feels no pain or discomfort. To check the neck, ask the injured person if he or she has neck pain. If he or she does not, ask the person to slowly move his or her head from side to side (**Fig. 5-10**). Check the shoulders by asking the person to shrug them (**Fig. 5-11**). Check the chest and abdomen by asking the person to try to take a deep breath and then blow the air out (**Fig. 5-12**). Ask if he or she is experiencing pain during breathing. Check each arm by first asking the person if he or

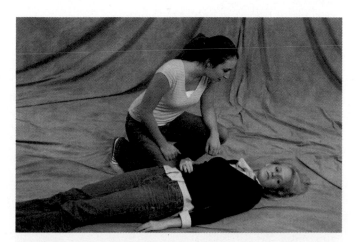

Figure 5-10 Ask the victim to gently move his or her head from side to side to check the neck.

she can move the fingers and the hand. Next, ask if he or she can bend the arm (**Fig. 5-13**). In the same way, check the hips and legs by first asking if he or she can move the toes, foot and ankle. Then determine if the victim can bend the leg (**Fig. 5-14**). Check one extremity at a time.

If the victim can move all the body parts without pain or discomfort and has no other apparent signals of injury or illness, have him or her attempt to rest for a few minutes in a sitting position (**Fig. 5-15**). Help the victim slowly stand when he or she is ready (**Fig. 5-16**).

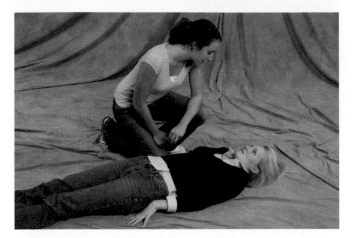

Figure 5-11   Ask the victim to shrug his or her shoulders to check the shoulders.

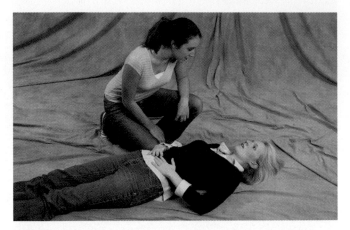

Figure 5-12   To check the chest and abdomen, ask the victim to breathe deeply and then blow the air out. Ask if he or she is experiencing pain.

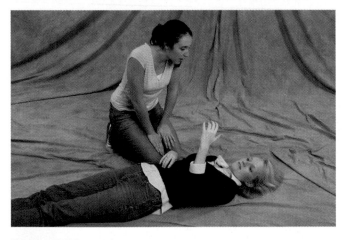

Figure 5-13   Check the arms by asking the victim to bend his or her arms one at a time.

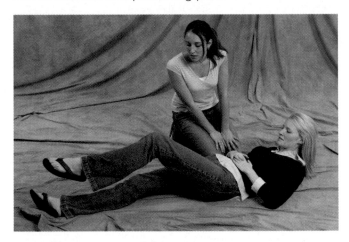

Figure 5-14   Check the legs by asking the victim to bend his or her legs one at a time.

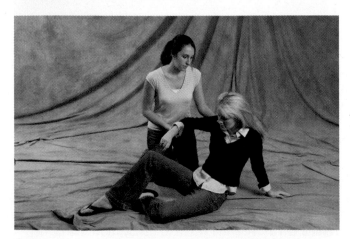

Figure 5-15   If there are no signals of obvious injuries, help the victim into a sitting position.

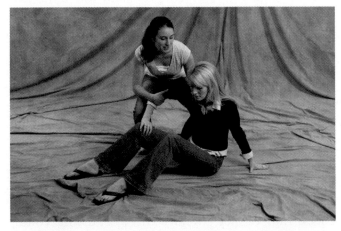

Figure 5-16   Help the victim slowly stand when he or she is ready.

From Horses to Helicopters—*A History of Emergency Care*

Emergency care originated during the French emperor Napoleon's campaigns in the late 1700s. The surgeon-in-chief for the Grand Army, Dominique Jean Larrey, became the first physician to try to save the wounded during battles instead of waiting until the fighting was over (Major R). Using horse-drawn litters, Larrey and his men dashed onto the battlefield in what became known as "flying ambulances."

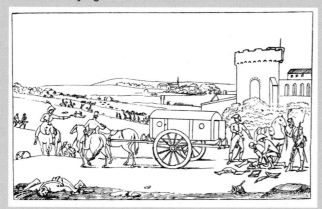

By the 1860s, the wartime principles of emergency care were applied to emergencies in some U.S. cities. In 1878, a writer for *Harper's New Monthly Magazine* explained how accidents were reported to the police, who then notified a local hospital by a telegraph signal. He described an early hospital ambulance ride in New York City (Rideing WH). "A well-kept horse was quickly harnessed to the ambulance; and as the surgeon took his seat behind, having first put on a jaunty uniform cap with gold lettering, the driver sprang to the box . . . and with a sharp crack of the whip we rolled off the smooth asphalt of the courtyard and into the street. . . . As we swept around corners and dashed over crossings, both doctor and driver kept up a sharp cry of warning to pedestrians" (Rideing WH). While booming industrial cities developed emergency transport systems, rural populations had only rudimentary services. In most small towns, the mortician had the only vehicle large enough to handle the litters, so emergency victims were just as likely to ride in a hearse to the hospital as in an ambulance (Division of Medical Sciences).

Cars gave Americans a faster system of transport, but over the next 50 years, car collisions also created the need for more emergency vehicles. In 1966, a major report questioned the quality of emergency services (Division of Medical Sciences). Dismayed at the rising death toll on the nation's highways, the U.S. Congress passed laws in 1966 and 1973 ordering the improved training of ambulance workers and emergency department staffs, an improved communication network and the development of regional units with specialized care.

Today, the telegraph signal has been replaced by the telephone and mobile phone. Today more than 99 percent of the U. S. population has access to basic 9-1-1 services. In some areas, a computer connected to the enhanced 9-1-1 system displays the caller's name, address and phone number, even if the caller cannot speak. Ambulance workers have changed from coachmen to trained medical professionals who can provide life-saving care at the scene. Horses have been replaced by ambulances and helicopters equipped to provide the most advanced pre-hospital care available.

The EMS system has expanded in sheer numbers and in services. Today, there are more than 800,000 EMS providers delivering care. In addition, many organizations, such as hospitals, have become more integrated with the EMS system to ensure quality care. Physicians and nurses continue the patient's care after they arrive at the hospital.

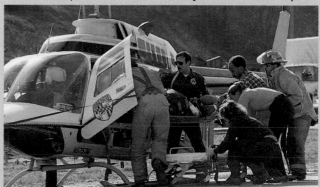

If patients suffer from critical conditions, such as heart attacks, burns, spinal cord injuries or other traumatic injuries or if the patients are children, the EMS system now has developed regional centers where specialists and specialized equipment are always available. In two centuries, the EMS system has evolved from horses to helicopters. As technology continues to advance, it is difficult to imagine what changes the future will bring.

SOURCES

Division of Medical Sciences, National Academy of Sciences. National Research Council: *Accidental death and disability: the neglected disease of modern society,* Washington, D.C., September 1966.

Major R, M.D.: *A History of Medicine,* Springfield, Ill. Charles C. Thomas, 1954.

National Registry of Emergency Medical Technicians Web site. *www.nremt.org/about/ems_learn.asp.* Accessed 7/22/04.

National Emergency Number Association. *www.nena.org.* Accessed 6/24/04.

Rideing WH: Hospital Life in New York, *Harper's New Monthly Magazine* 57 (171), 1878.

If the person feels dizzy, is unable to move a body part or is experiencing pain with movement, help him or her rest in the most comfortable position. Keep the person from getting chilled or overheated, and reassure him or her. Determine what additional care is needed and whether to call 9-1-1 or the local emergency number.

Giving Care

Once you complete the head-to-toe examination, give care for any specific injuries you find. To give care for the victim until EMS personnel arrive, follow these general guidelines:

▶ Do no further harm.
▶ Monitor breathing and consciousness.
▶ Help the victim rest in the most comfortable position.
▶ Keep the victim from getting chilled or overheated.
▶ Reassure the victim.
▶ Give any specific care needed.

Deciding Whether to Transport the Victim

Whether you transport an injured victim or wait for EMS personnel depends on many factors, including the availability of advanced medical care, the severity of the injury or illness, and your judgment. If you do decide to transport the victim yourself, ask someone else to come with you to help keep the victim comfortable. Be sure you know the quickest route to the nearest medical facility with emergency-care capabilities. Pay close attention to the victim and watch for any changes in his or her condition.

Do not transport a victim—

▶ When the trip may aggravate the injury or illness or cause additional injury.
▶ When the victim has or may develop a life-threatening condition.
▶ If you are unsure of the nature of the injury or illness.

With a life-threatening condition or if there is a possibility of further injury, call 9-1-1 or the local emergency number and wait for help.

Discourage a victim from driving himself or herself to the hospital. An injury may restrict movement, or the victim may become groggy or faint. A sudden onset of pain may be distracting. Any of these conditions can make driving dangerous for the victim, passengers, other drivers and pedestrians.

SPECIAL CONSIDERATIONS
Checking Infants and Children

Infants (age 0 to 1) and children (age 1 to 12) receive care that is slightly different from that provided for adult victims.

When checking a child or infant for life-threatening conditions, follow the same steps as for an adult. However, if you are alone and find an unconscious child or infant who is not breathing, but does have a pulse, give rescue breathing for about 2 minutes before calling 9-1-1 or the local emergency number. Providing 2 minutes of rescue breathing will get oxygen into the child or infant and may prevent the heart from stopping.

When checking a child for non-life-threatening conditions, observe the child before touching him or her. Look for signals that indicate changes in consciousness, any trouble breathing, and any apparent injuries or conditions. All signals may change as soon as you touch the child because he or she may become anxious or upset. If a parent or guardian is present, ask him or her to help calm the infant or child. Parents can also tell you if the child has a medical condition that you should be aware of (**Fig. 5-17**).

Communicate clearly with the parent or guardian and the child. Explain what you are going to do. Get at eye level with the child. Talk slowly and in a friendly manner. Use simple words. Ask questions that the child can answer easily. Often a parent or guardian will be holding a crying child. Check the child while the parent or guardian holds him or her. When you begin the examination, begin at the toes instead of the head. Checking in this order gives the child the opportunity to get used to the process and allows him or her to see what is going on.

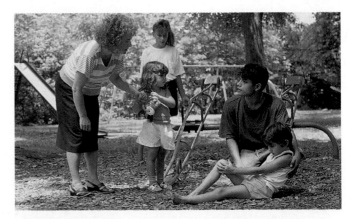

Figure 5-17   Parents or other adults may be able to give you helpful information or help you communicate with a sick or injured child.

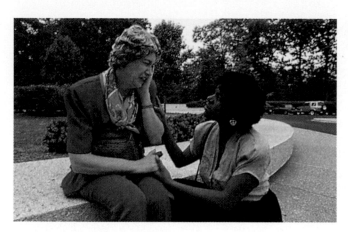

Figure 5-18 Speak to an elderly victim at eye level so that he or she can see or hear you more clearly.

Checking Older Adults

When checking an older adult (over 65), attempt to learn the victim's name and use it when you speak to him or her. Consider using Mrs., Mr. or Ms. as a sign of respect. Get at the victim's eye level so that he or she can see and hear you more clearly (**Fig. 5-18**). If the victim seems confused, it may be the result of vision or hearing loss. Someone who needs glasses to see is likely to be very anxious without them. If he or she usually wears eyeglasses and cannot find them, try to locate them. Notice if he or she has a hearing aid. Speak a little more slowly and clearly and look at the victim's face while you talk. If the victim is truly confused, try to find out if the confusion is the result of the injury or a condition he or she already has. Information from family members or bystanders is frequently helpful. The victim may be afraid of falling, so if he or she is standing, offer an arm or hand. Remember that an older victim may need to move very slowly.

Try to find out what medications the person is taking and if he or she has any medical conditions so that you can tell EMS personnel. Look for a medical ID bracelet or necklace, which often provides you with the victim's name and address and information about any specific condition the victim has. Be aware that an elderly person may not recognize the signals of a serious condition. An elderly person may also minimize any signals for fear of losing his or her independence or being placed in a nursing home. You will learn more about communicating with older adults in Chapter 21.

SUMMARY

Many variables affect dealing with emergencies. By following the emergency action steps: **CHECK—CALL—CARE,** you can ensure that the victim receives the best possible care. If possible, check victim in position found.

Determine if the victim has any life-threatening conditions. Life-threatening conditions include unconsciousness, trouble breathing, no signs of life and severe bleeding. Call 9-1-1 or the local emergency number if a victim appears to have any of these signals.

If you find no life-threatening conditions, interview the victim and any bystanders and perform a head-to-toe examination (toe-to-head for a child or infant) to find and care for any other injuries. If you do not give care, these conditions could become life threatening.

APPLICATION QUESTIONS

1. What might you do to make the scene safe for you to check the victim?

2. What kinds of injuries or other conditions might the victim on the bike trail have?

3. If the victim on the bike trail does not respond when you tap on his or her shoulder, what would your next step be?

4. If you find that the victim on the trail is conscious, is breathing and has no severe bleeding, what should you do next?

STUDY QUESTIONS

1. Match each emergency action step with the actions it includes.

   a. Check the scene.
   b. Check the victim for life-threatening emergencies.
   c. Call 9-1-1 or the local emergency number.
   d. Care for the victim.

   _____ Open the airway.

   _____ Look for bystanders who can help.

   _____ Interview the victim and bystanders.

   _____ Check for movement and breathing.

   _____ Do a head-to-toe examination.

   _____ Call 9-1-1 or the local emergency number.

   _____ Look for victims.

   _____ Check for severe bleeding.

   _____ Look for dangers.

   _____ Check for pulse (child or infant).

   _____ Look for clues to determine what happened.

   _____ Obtain the victim's consent.

2. List four life-threatening conditions.

Use the following scenario to answer questions 3 and 4.

Several people are clustered in the middle of a street. A car is stopped in the right lane. As you approach the group, you can see a mangled bicycle lying on the pavement. You see your neighbor sitting next to it. No one seems to be doing anything. You approach your neighbor and kneel next to him.

3. What type of dangers could be present at the scene? What could you do to make the scene safer?

4. You determine that your neighbor has no life-threatening emergencies. What should you do next?

Use the following scenario to answer question 5.

You walk into your boss's office for a meeting. You see a cup of coffee spilled on the desk. You find him lying on the floor, motionless. What should you do?

5. Based on the scenario above number the following actions in order:

___4___ Open the airway.

___1___ Check the scene.

___5___ Check for signs of life and severe bleeding.

___2___ Check for consciousness.

___3___ Call 9-1-1 or the local emergency number.

In questions 6 through 9, circle the letter of the correct answer.

6. What is the purpose of your initial check of the victim?

    a. To check for minor injuries
    b. To determine if any life-threatening conditions need immediate care
    c. To get consent from the victim before giving care
    d. To ask for information about the cause of the injury or illness

7. Once you determine the victim has no life-threatening conditions, you should—

    a. Call 9-1-1 or the local emergency number.
    b. Transport the victim to the nearest hospital.
    c. Check for other injuries or conditions that could become life threatening if not cared for.
    d. Check for consciousness.

8. Before beginning a check for life-threatening conditions, you should first—

    a. Position the victim so that you can open the airway.
    b. Check the scene.
    c. Check for bystanders.
    d. Call 9-1-1 or the local emergency number.

9. After checking for consciousness, you determine that the victim is unconscious. What should you do next?

    a. Call 9-1-1 or the local emergency number.
    b. Give 2 rescue breaths.
    c. Check for signs of life and severe bleeding.
    d. Begin a check for non-life-threatening conditions.

Answers are listed in Appendix A.

SKILL SHEET Checking an Unconscious Adult (Age 12 or Older)

Check the scene and the victim. *Remember: Always follow standard precautions to prevent disease transmission. Use protective equipment (disposable gloves and breathing barriers). Wash your hands thoroughly after giving care.*

CHECK scene, then **CHECK** person.

Step 1

Tap shoulder and shout, "Are you okay?"

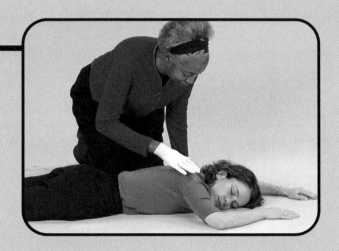

Step 2

No response, **CALL** 9-1-1.

NOTE: If an unconscious person is face-down—roll face-up supporting head, neck and back.

Step 3

Open airway (tilt head, lift chin).

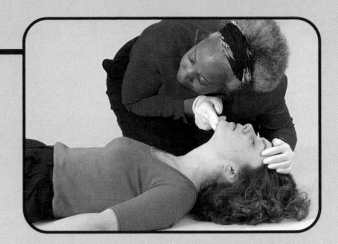

Step 4

CHECK for signs of life (movement and breathing) for no more than 10 seconds. If no signs of life, give **2** rescue breaths.

NOTE: Irregular, gasping or shallow breathing is NOT normal breathing.

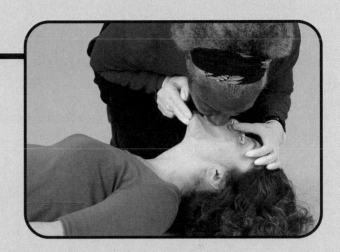

Step 5

If there is normal breathing, place the person in recovery position and monitor Airway, Breathing and Circulation (ABCs).

Step 6

If breaths go in—quickly scan the body for severe bleeding and get into position to perform CPR or use an AED (if AED is immediately available).

SKILL SHEET Checking an Unconscious Child
(Ages 1 to 12)

Check the scene and the victim. *Remember: Always follow standard precautions to prevent disease transmission. Use protective equipment (disposable gloves and breathing barriers). Wash your hands thoroughly after giving care.*

Step 1

CHECK scene, then **CHECK** child.

Step 2

Obtain consent from parent or guardian, if present.

Step 3

Tap shoulder and shout, "Are you okay?"

Step 4

No response, **CALL** 9-1-1.
If alone—

- Give about **2** minutes of **CARE**.
- Then **CALL** 9-1-1.

NOTE: If an unconscious child is face-down—roll face-up supporting head, neck and back.

Step 5

Open airway (tilt head, lift chin), **CHECK** for signs of life (movement and breathing) for no more than **10** seconds.

Step 6

If no breathing, give **2** rescue breaths.

Step 7

If breaths go in, **CHECK** for pulse (and severe bleeding).

Step 8

If breathing normally, place in recovery position and monitor Airway, Breathing and Circulation (ABCs).

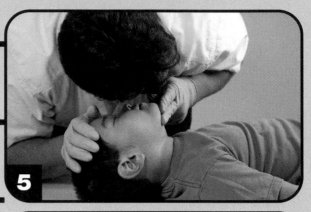

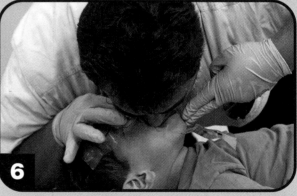

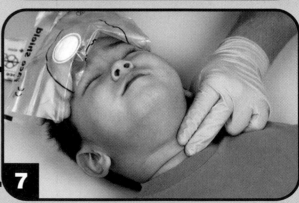

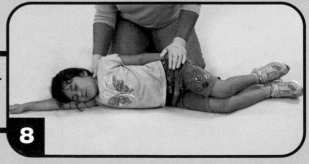

SKILL SHEET Checking an Unconscious Infant
(Under Age 1)

Check the scene and the victim. *Remember: Always follow standard precautions to prevent disease transmission. Use protective equipment (disposable gloves and breathing barriers). Wash your hands thoroughly after giving care.*

Step 1

CHECK scene, then CHECK infant.

Step 2

Obtain consent from parent or guardian, if present.

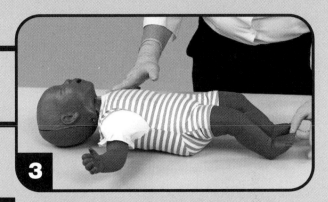

Step 3

Flick foot or tap shoulder and shout, "Are you okay?"

Step 4

No response, CALL 9-1-1.
If alone—

- Give about **2** minutes of CARE.
- Then CALL 9-1-1.

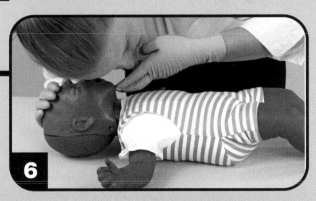

Step 5

If an unconscious infant is face-down—
roll face-up supporting head, neck and back.

Step 6

Open airway (tilt head, lift chin), CHECK for signs of life (movement and breathing) for no more than **10** seconds.

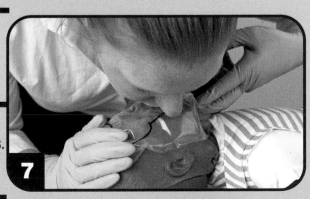

Step 7

If no breathing, give **2** rescue breaths.

Step 8

If breaths go in, CHECK for pulse (and severe bleeding).

Step 9

If breathing normally, place in recovery position and monitor Airway, Breathing and Circulation (ABCs).

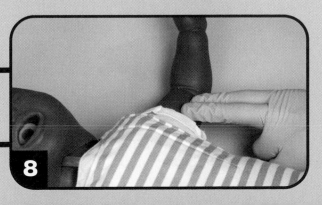

SKILL SHEET Checking a Conscious Victim

Check the scene and the victim. *Remember: Always follow standard precautions to prevent disease transmission. Use protective equipment (disposable gloves and breathing barriers). Wash your hands immediately after giving care.*

Step 1

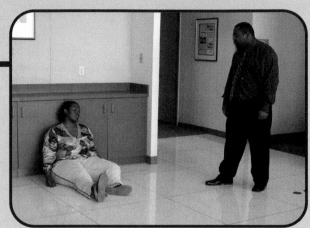

Interview the person.

- Introduce yourself, tell him or her your level of training, and get permission to give care.

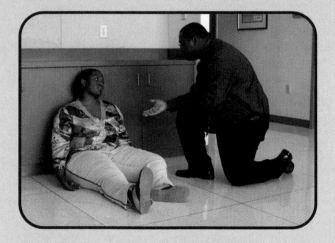

- Ask—
  - What is your name?
  - What happened?
  - Do you feel pain or discomfort anywhere?
  - Do you have any allergies?
  - Do you have any medical conditions, or are you taking any medication?

Note: Send someone to CALL 9-1-1 or the local emergency number any time a life-threatening emergency becomes apparent.

Step 2

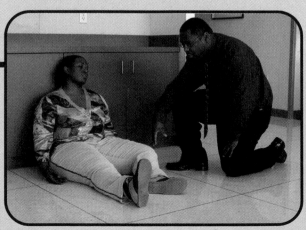

Check head to toe.

- Visually inspect the body.
- Before you begin, tell the person what you are going to do.
- Look carefully for bleeding, cuts, bruises and obvious deformities.
- Look for a medical ID bracelet or necklace.

Note: Do not ask the person to move any areas in which he or she has discomfort or pain or if you suspect injury to the head, neck or back.

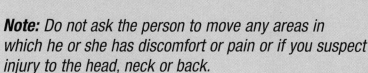

Step 3

Check the head.

- Look at the scalp, face, ears, eyes, nose and mouth for cuts, bumps, bruises and depressions.
- Notice if the victim is drowsy, not alert or confused.

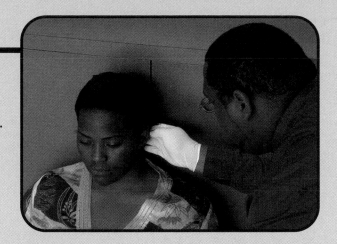

Step 4

Check skin appearance and temperature.

- Feel the person's forehead with the back of your hand.
- Look at the person's face and lips.
- Ask yourself, is the skin—
    - Cold or hot?
    - Unusually wet or dry?
    - Pale, bluish or flushed?

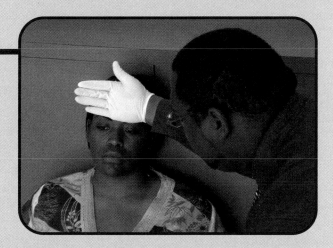

Step 5

Check the neck.

- If there is no discomfort and no suspected injury to the neck, ask the person to move the head slowly from side to side.
- Note pain, discomfort or inability to move.

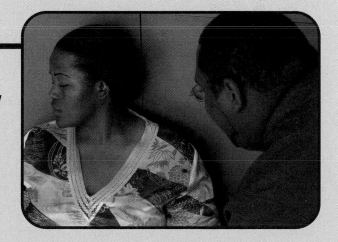

SKILL SHEET **Checking a Conscious Victim**

Step 6

Check the shoulders.

- Ask the person to shrug his or her shoulders.

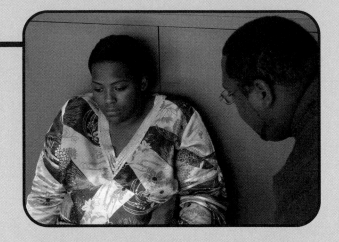

Step 7

Check the chest and abdomen.

- Ask the person to take a deep breath and blow air out.
- Ask if he or she is experiencing pain during breathing.

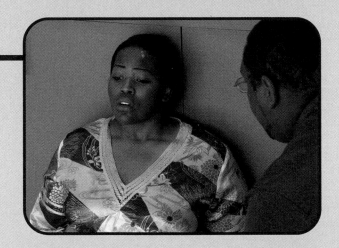

Step 8

Check the arms.

- Check one arm at a time.
- Ask the person to—
  - Move hands and fingers.
  - Bend the arm.

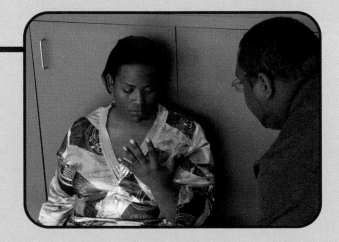

Step 9

Check the hips and legs.

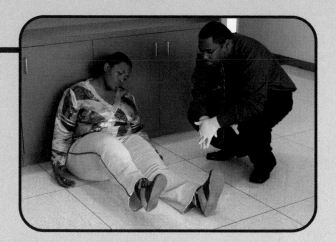

Step 10

CARE for any conditions you find.

If the person can move all body parts without pain or discomfort and has no other apparent signals of injury or illness—

- *Have him or her rest for a few minutes in a sitting position.*
- *Help the person slowly stand when he or she is ready, if no further difficulty develops.*

If the person is unable to move a body part or is experiencing pain on movement or dizziness—

- *Help him or her rest in the most comfortable position.*
- *Keep the person from getting chilled or overheated.*
- *Reassure him or her.*
- *Determine whether to call 9-1-1 or the local emergency number.*

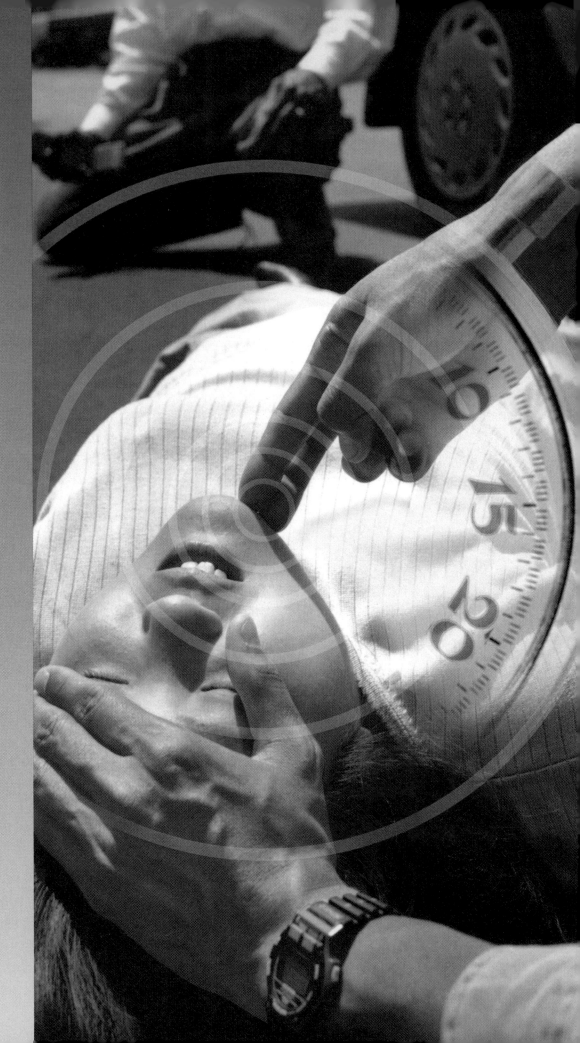

Part

THREE

Life-Threatening Emergencies

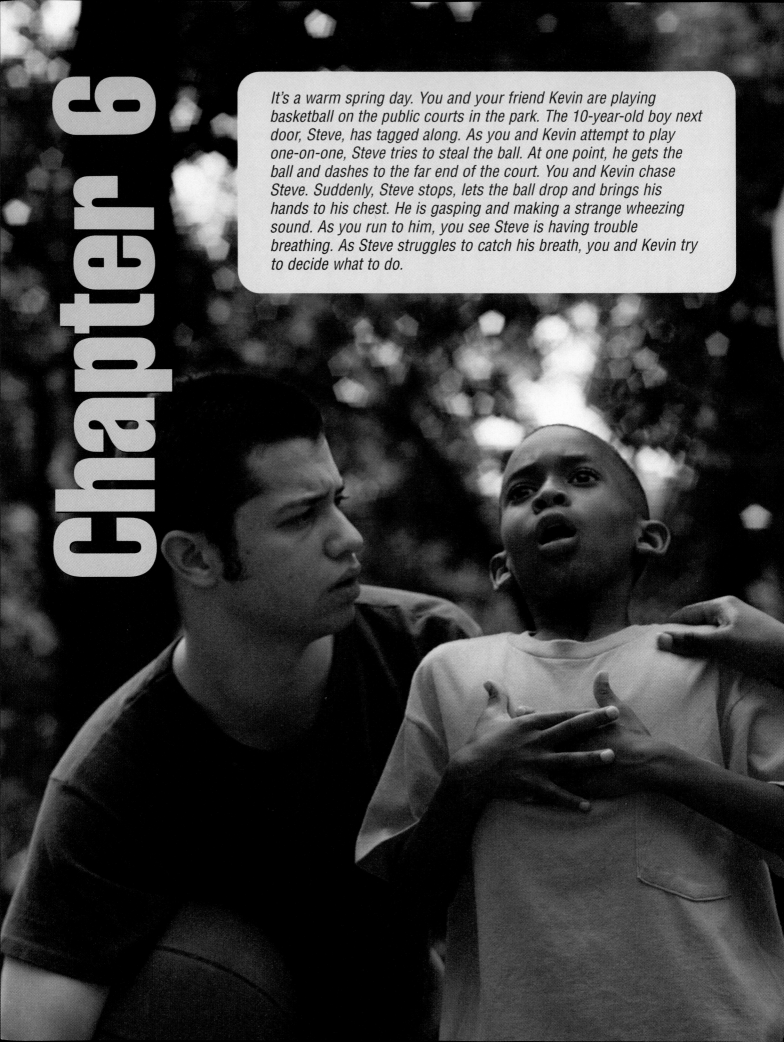

Chapter 6

It's a warm spring day. You and your friend Kevin are playing basketball on the public courts in the park. The 10-year-old boy next door, Steve, has tagged along. As you and Kevin attempt to play one-on-one, Steve tries to steal the ball. At one point, he gets the ball and dashes to the far end of the court. You and Kevin chase Steve. Suddenly, Steve stops, lets the ball drop and brings his hands to his chest. He is gasping and making a strange wheezing sound. As you run to him, you see Steve is having trouble breathing. As Steve struggles to catch his breath, you and Kevin try to decide what to do.

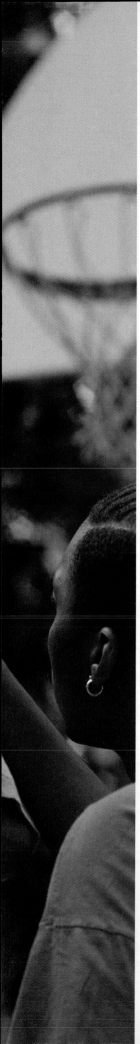

Breathing Emergencies

Objectives

After reading this chapter, you should be able to—

- Identify the causes of breathing emergencies.
- Identify signals of respiratory distress.
- Identify conditions that cause respiratory distress.
- Identify common causes of choking for adults, children and infants.
- Describe the care for a conscious choking adult, child and infant.
- Describe the care for a victim experiencing respiratory distress.
- Describe the care for a victim in respiratory arrest.
- Describe when and how to use breathing barriers.

After reading this chapter and completing the class activities, you should be able to—

- Demonstrate how to provide rescue breathing for a child or infant.
- Demonstrate how to provide care for a conscious choking adult, child and infant.
- Demonstrate how to give care for a victim in respiratory distress.

Introduction

In this chapter, you will learn how to care for someone who is having trouble breathing or who has stopped breathing. As you read in Chapter 5, you should follow the emergency action steps: CHECK—CALL—CARE in any emergency situation. Check to see if the scene is safe and if the victim has any life-threatening conditions. If the victim appears to have a life-threatening condition, send someone to immediately call 9-1-1 or the local emergency number. Finally, care for any conditions you may find.

THE BREATHING PROCESS

As you read in Chapter 4, the human body requires a constant supply of oxygen for survival. When you breathe air into your lungs, the oxygen in the air is transferred to the blood. The blood transports the oxygen to the brain, other organs, muscles and other parts of the body. Without oxygen, brain cells can begin to die in 4 to 6 minutes (**Fig. 6-1**). Some tissues, such as the brain, are very sensitive to oxygen deprivation. Unless the brain receives oxygen within minutes, permanent brain damage or death will result.

BREATHING EMERGENCIES

There are two types of **breathing emergencies**: respiratory distress and respiratory arrest. Respiratory distress is a condition in which breathing becomes difficult. Respiratory arrest occurs when breathing stops. Both of these emergencies are considered life threatening.

Respiratory Distress

Respiratory distress is the most common breathing emergency. Respiratory distress can be caused by a variety of conditions including—

▶ A partially obstructed airway.
▶ Illness.
▶ Chronic conditions, such as emphysema or asthma.
▶ Electrocution.
▶ Heart attack.
▶ Injury to the head, chest, lungs or abdomen.
▶ Allergic reactions.
▶ Drugs.
▶ Poisoning.
▶ Emotional distress.

Respiratory distress can lead to respiratory arrest.

Signals of Respiratory Distress

A victim of respiratory distress may show various signals. Victims may look as if they cannot catch their breath, or they may gasp for air. They may

KEY TERMS

Airway obstruction: Complete or partial blockage of the airway, which prevents air from reaching a person's lungs; the most common cause of respiratory emergencies.

Anatomical airway obstruction: Complete or partial blockage of the airway by the tongue or swollen tissues of the mouth and throat.

Aspirate: Inhalation of blood, vomit or other foreign material into the lungs.

Cyanotic: Bluish discoloration of the skin around the mouth or the fingertips resulting from a lack of oxygen in the blood.

Mechanical airway obstruction: Complete or partial blockage of the airway by a foreign object, such as a piece of food or a small toy, or by fluids such as vomit or blood.

Rescue breathing: A technique of breathing for a non-breathing child or infant.

Respiratory arrest: A condition in which breathing has stopped.

Respiratory distress: A condition in which breathing is difficult.

Stoma: An opening in the front of the neck through which a person whose larynx has been removed breathes.

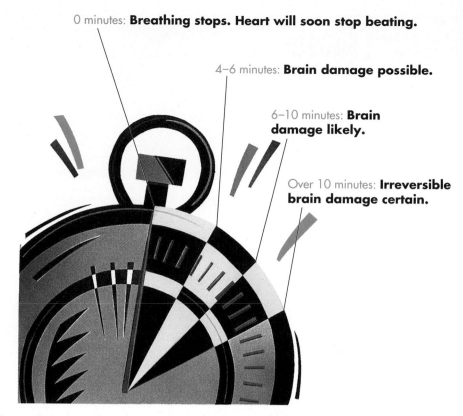

0 minutes: **Breathing stops. Heart will soon stop beating.**

4–6 minutes: **Brain damage possible.**

6–10 minutes: **Brain damage likely.**

Over 10 minutes: **Irreversible brain damage certain.**

Figure 6-1 Time is critical in life-threatening emergencies. Unless the brain gets oxygen within minutes of when breathing stops, brain damage or death will occur.

appear to breathe faster or slower than normal. Breaths may be unusually deep or shallow. They may make unusual noises, such as wheezing, gurgling or high-pitched sounds like crowing.

The victim's skin appearance and temperature can also indicate respiratory distress. At first, the victim's skin may be unusually moist and appear flushed. Later, it may appear pale, ashen or *cyanotic* and feel cool as the oxygen level in the blood falls. Victims may say they feel dizzy or light-headed. They may feel pain in the chest or tingling in the hands, feet or lips. Understandably, the victim may be apprehensive or fearful. Any of these signals is a clue that the victim may be in respiratory distress.

Conditions That Cause Respiratory Distress

Asthma

Asthma is a condition that narrows the air passages and makes breathing difficult. During an asthma attack, the air passages become constricted, or narrowed, as a result of a spasm of the muscles lining the bronchi (the air passages that lead from the trachea to the alveoli) or swelling of the bronchi themselves.

The Centers for Disease Control and Prevention (CDC) estimated that in the year 2001, 20.3 million Americans were affected by asthma. Asthma is more common in children and young adults than in older adults, but its frequency and severity is increasing in all age groups in the United States. Asthma is the third-ranking cause of hospitalization among those younger than age 15.

Asthma attacks may be triggered by an allergic reaction to food, pollen, a drug, an insect sting or emotional stress. For some people, cold air or physical activity may induce asthma. **Wheezing,** a common signal of asthma, is the hoarse whistling sound made when exhaling. Wheezing occurs because air becomes trapped in the lungs. Usually, people diagnosed with asthma control attacks with medication. These medications stop the muscle spasm, opening the airway, which makes breathing easier.

Emphysema

Emphysema is a disease in which the lungs and alveoli lose their ability to exchange carbon dioxide and oxygen effectively. Emphysema is a chronic (long-lasting or frequently recurring) disease and

Signals of Respiratory Distress

▸ Trouble breathing.
  • Breathing is slow or rapid.
  • Breaths are unusually deep or shallow.
  • Victim is gasping for breath.
  • Victim is wheezing, gurgling or making high-pitched noises.
▸ Victim's skin is unusually moist or cool.
▸ Victim's skin has a flushed, pale, ashen or bluish appearance.
▸ Victim feels short of breath.
▸ Victim feels dizzy or light-headed.
▸ Victim feels pain in the chest or tingling in hands, feet or lips.
▸ Victim feels apprehensive or fearful.

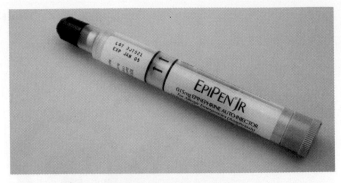
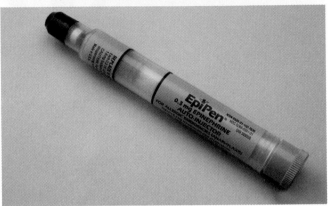

Figure 6-2   People who know they are allergic to certain substances or bee stings may carry an **anaphylaxis kit** with medication that reverses the allergic reaction.

will worsen over time. The most common signal of emphysema is shortness of breath. Exhaling is extremely difficult. In advanced cases, the victim may feel restless, confused and weak, and may even go into respiratory or cardiac arrest.

Bronchitis

Bronchitis is a condition resulting in inflammation of the lining of the trachea, bronchi and bronchioles. This inflammation causes a buildup of mucus that obstructs the passage of air and air exchange in the lungs. Chronic bronchitis is most commonly caused by long-term smoking; however, exposure to environmental irritants and pollutants may also lead to bronchitis. A person with bronchitis will typically have a persistent cough and may feel tightness in the chest and have trouble breathing. As with emphysema, the person may also feel restless, confused and weak, and may even go into respiratory or cardiac arrest.

Anaphylactic Shock

Anaphylactic shock, also known as **anaphylaxis,** is a severe allergic reaction. Air passages may swell and restrict a person's breathing. Anaphy-

laxis may be caused by insect stings, food, other **allergens** or certain medications. Signals of anaphylaxis include a rash; a feeling of tightness in the chest and throat; and swelling of the face, neck and tongue. The person may also feel dizzy or confused. If not recognized early and cared for quickly, an anaphylactic shock can become a life-threatening emergency. Some people know that they are allergic to certain substances or to bee stings. They may have learned to avoid these substances or bees and may carry medication to reverse the allergic reaction (**Fig. 6-2**). People who have severe allergic reactions may wear a medical ID bracelet or necklace.

Hyperventilation

Hyperventilation occurs when breathing is faster than normal. This rapid breathing can upset the body's balance of oxygen and carbon dioxide. Hyperventilation often results from fear or anxiety and is likely to occur in people who are tense and nervous. It can also be caused by head injuries; severe bleeding; or illnesses such as high fever, heart failure, lung disease or diabetic emergencies. It can also be triggered by asthma or exercise. A characteristic signal of hyperventilation is deep, rapid breathing. Despite their efforts to breathe, people who are hyperventilating feel that they cannot get enough air or that they are suffocating. Therefore, they are often fearful and apprehensive, or they may appear confused. They may say that they feel dizzy or that their fingers and toes or lips feel numb or tingly.

If the victim's breathing is rapid and he or she shows signals of an injury or an underlying illness or condition, call 9-1-1 or the local emergency number immediately. This person needs advanced care right away. If, however, the victim's breathing is rapid and you are sure that it is caused by emotion, such as excitement, tell him or her to relax and breathe slowly. Reassurance is often enough to correct hyperventilation. If the breathing still does not slow down, the person could have a serious problem. When breathing is too fast, slow, noisy or painful, call 9-1-1 or the local emergency number immediately.

Care for Respiratory Distress

Recognizing the signals of respiratory distress and quickly giving care is a key step to preventing other life-threatening conditions, such as respiratory arrest. You do not need to know the specific cause of a victim's respiratory distress to effectively give care. To care for a victim of respiratory distress, you should—

▶ **CHECK** the scene to ensure your safety before you approach a victim. The victim's condition may have been caused by an unsafe environmental condition, such as the presence of toxic fumes.
▶ **CHECK** the victim for consciousness. If the victim is conscious, you know that he or she is breathing and that his or her heart is beating.
▶ **CALL 9-1-1 or the local emergency number.** Even though the victim is conscious, respiratory distress is a life-threatening emergency and requires immediate care from EMS personnel. Send someone to call 9-1-1 or the local emergency number. Continue to check for other life-threatening conditions, such as severe bleeding.
▶ **CARE** for the conditions you find:
  • Help the victim rest in a comfortable position. In most cases, it is easier for the victim to breathe in a sitting position (**Fig. 6-3**).

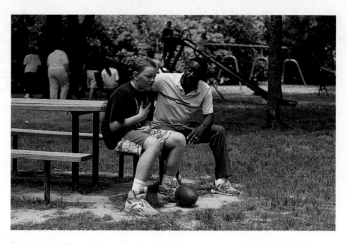

Figure 6-3 A person who is having trouble breathing may breathe more easily in a sitting position.

  • Loosen any tight clothing, especially around the neck and abdomen.
  • Open a door or window to provide fresh air. You may also move the victim to fresh air if it is safe to do so and will not cause further harm.
  • Make sure someone has called 9-1-1 or the local emergency number for help.
  • If the victim is conscious, check for other life-threatening conditions, such as severe bleeding.
  • Interview the victim and any bystanders. As you check the victim, remember that a person who has trouble breathing may have trouble talking. Therefore, talk to any bystanders who may know about the victim's condition. The victim can confirm answers or answer yes-or-no questions by nodding. The victim can also write down his or her answers.
  • Continue to monitor the victim's ABCs (airway, breathing and circulation). Watch for additional signals of respiratory distress.
  • Calm and reassure the victim. Help maintain normal body temperature by preventing chilling on a cool day or by providing shade on a hot day.
  • Assist the victim in taking his or her prescribed medication for the condition if trained and state or local regulations allow. Medications may include oxygen, an inhalant (bronchial dilator) or epinephrine.

Special Considerations

Children and Respiratory Distress

Infections of the respiratory system are more common in children and infants than in adults. These can range from minor infections, such as the common cold, to life-threatening infections that block the airway. Signals of respiratory distress in children include—

▶ Agitation.
▶ Unusually fast or slow breathing.
▶ Drowsiness.
▶ Noisy breathing.
▶ Pale, ashen, flushed or bluish skin color.
▶ Breathing trouble increases.
▶ Altered level of consciousness.
▶ Increased heart rate.

A common childhood illness that causes respiratory distress is croup. **Croup** is a viral infection that causes swelling of the tissues around the vocal cords. Besides the basic signals of respiratory distress and a cough that sounds like the bark of a seal, croup is often preceded by 1 or 2 days of illness, sometimes with a fever. Croup occurs more often in the winter months, and its signals are more evident in the evening. Croup is not generally life threatening but can be very frightening for the child and the parents or guardian.

Another childhood illness is **epiglottitis,** a bacterial infection that causes a severe inflammation of the epiglottis. You may recall from Chapter 4 that the epiglottis is a flap of tissue above the vocal cords

that seals off the airway during swallowing. When the epiglottis becomes infected, it can swell and completely block the airway. A child with epiglottitis will appear ill and have a high fever and a sore throat. He or she will often be sitting up and straining to breathe. The child will be very frightened, so be sure to keep the child calm. Saliva will often be dripping from the mouth because swelling of the epiglottis prevents the child from swallowing.

You do not need to distinguish between croup and epiglottitis, because the care you give will be the same. First aid for a child in respiratory distress includes allowing him or her to remain in the most comfortable position for breathing. If the child's breathing does not appear to improve, or at the first signal that the child's condition is worsening, call 9-1-1 or the local emergency number. Do not attempt to place any object in the child's mouth. Be aware that a child's airway may become completely blocked as a result of epiglottitis. A child with a blocked airway has a life-threatening emergency and needs immediate medical help.

AIRWAY OBSTRUCTION— CONSCIOUS VICTIM

Airway obstruction is the most common cause of respiratory emergencies. The two types of airway obstruction are anatomical and mechanical. A person suffering from an anatomical or mechanical airway obstruction is choking.

An *anatomical airway obstruction* occurs if the airway is blocked by the tongue or swollen tissues of the mouth and throat. This type of obstruction may result from injury to the neck or a medical emergency, such as anaphylaxis.

A *mechanical airway obstruction* occurs when the airway is partially or completely blocked by a foreign object, such as a piece of food or a small toy, or by fluids, such as vomit or blood.

Causes

Common causes of choking include—

▶ Trying to swallow large pieces of poorly chewed food.
▶ Drinking alcohol before or during meals. Alcohol dulls the nerves that aid swallowing, making choking on food more likely.

Care for Respiratory Distress

▶ Check for life-threatening conditions.
▶ Call 9-1-1 or the local emergency number.
▶ Help the victim rest comfortably.
▶ Check for non-life-threatening conditions.
▶ Reassure the victim.
▶ Assist with medication.
▶ Keep the victim from getting chilled or overheated.
▶ Monitor ABCs.

▶ Wearing dentures. Dentures make it difficult for the wearer to sense whether food is fully chewed before swallowing.

▶ Eating while talking excitedly or laughing or eating too fast.

▶ Walking, playing or running with food or objects in the mouth.

Signals

A person with an obstructed airway can quickly stop breathing, lose consciousness and die. You must be able to recognize that the airway is obstructed and immediately give care. A person who is choking may have either a complete or partial airway obstruction.

Partial Airway Obstruction

A victim with a partial airway obstruction can still move air to and from the lungs. This air allows the victim to cough in an attempt to dislodge the object. The victim may also be able to move air past the vocal cords to speak. The victim may clutch at his or her throat with one or both hands as a natural reaction to choking. This action is the universal distress signal for choking (**Fig. 6-4**). If the victim is coughing forcefully or wheezing, do not interfere with attempts to cough

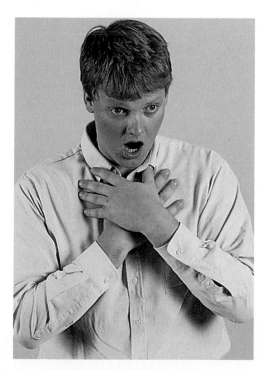

Figure 6-4 Clutching the throat with one or both hands is universally recognized as a distress signal for choking.

up the object. A victim who is getting enough air to cough or speak also has enough air entering the lungs to breathe. Stay with the victim and encourage him or her to continue coughing to clear the obstruction. If coughing persists, call for help.

Complete Airway Obstruction

A partial airway obstruction can quickly become a complete airway obstruction. A person with a completely blocked airway is choking and is unable to cough, speak or breathe. Sometimes the victim may cough weakly and ineffectively or make high-pitched noises. All of these signals tell you the victim is not getting enough air to sustain life. Act immediately! If a bystander is available, have him or her call 9-1-1 or the local emergency number while you begin to give care.

Care for an Airway Obstruction

A combination of 5 **back blows** followed by 5 **abdominal thrusts** provides an effective way to clear the airway obstruction in an adult or child. Back blows are helpful in dislodging the object that is in the airway (**Fig. 6-5**). Abdominal thrusts compress the abdomen and create pressure that forces the diaphragm higher into the thoracic cavity, thus increasing pressure within the lungs and airway. This pressure simulates a cough, forcing air trapped in the lungs to push the object out of the airway, like a cork from a bottle of champagne. Continue to provide 5 back blows and 5 abdominal thrusts until the person can cough forcefully, speak or breathe, or becomes unconscious.

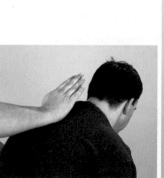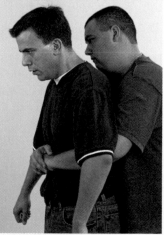

Figure 6-5 Provide 5 back blows and 5 abdominal thrusts until the person can cough forcefully, speak or breathe, or becomes unconscious.

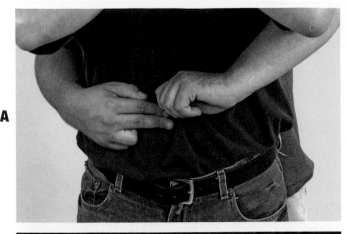

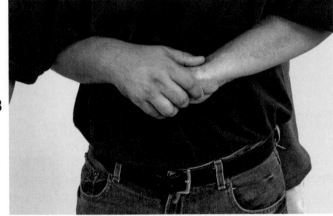

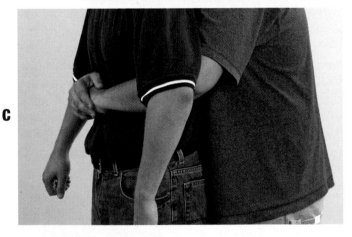

Figure 6-6   Abdominal thrusts: **A,** Place the thumb side of your fist against the middle of the victim's abdomen. **B,** Grab your fist with your other hand. **C,** Give quick, upward thrusts into the abdomen.

Conscious Adult or Child

A combination of 5 back blows followed by 5 abdominal thrusts is an effective way to clear an airway obstruction. To give back blows—
▸ Position yourself slightly behind the person.
▸ Provide support by placing one arm diagonally across the chest and lean the person forward.

▸ Firmly strike the person between the shoulder blades with the heel of your other hand.
If the back blows do not clear the obstruction, give abdominal thrusts.

To give abdominal thrusts to a conscious choking adult or child, stand or kneel behind the victim and wrap your arms around his or her waist. Make a fist with one hand and place the thumb side against the middle of the victim's abdomen, just above the navel and well below the lower tip of the breastbone (**Fig. 6-6, A-B**). Grab your fist with your other hand and give quick, upward thrusts into the abdomen (**Fig. 6-6, C**). Each thrust is a separate and distinct attempt to dislodge the obstruction. The skill sheets at the end of this chapter show this technique in detail.

Conscious Infant

An infant can easily swallow small objects, such as pebbles, coins, beads and parts of toys, which can then block the airway. Infants also often choke because their eating skills develop slowly. Therefore, they can easily choke on foods such as nuts, hot dogs, grapes and popcorn, which are often the perfect size to block their smaller airways.

If you determine that a conscious infant cannot cough, cry or breathe, perform 5 back blows followed by 5 chest thrusts. Position the infant face-up on your forearm. Place your other hand on top of the infant, using your thumb and fingers to hold the infant's jaw while sandwiching the infant between your forearms. Turn the infant over so that he or she is face-down on your forearm (**Fig. 6-7, A**). Lower your arm onto your thigh so that the infant's head is lower than his or her chest, then give 5 firm back blows with the heel of your hand between the infant's shoulder blades (**Fig. 6-7, B**). Maintain support of the infant's head and neck by firmly holding the jaw between your thumb and forefinger. Each blow should be a separate and distinct attempt to dislodge the object.

To give chest thrusts, you will need to place the infant in a face-up position. Start by placing your free hand and forearm along the infant's head and back so that the infant is sandwiched between your two hands and forearms (**Fig. 6-8, A**). Continue to support the infant's head between your thumb and finger from the front while you cradle the back of the head with your other hand. Turn the infant onto his or her back. Lower your arm that is supporting the infant's back onto your opposite thigh. The infant's head should be lower than his or her chest,

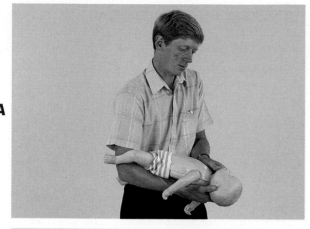

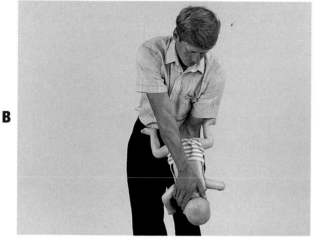

Figure 6-7 **A,** To give back blows, sandwich the infant between your forearms. Support the infant's head and neck by holding the jaw between your thumb and forefinger. **B,** Turn the infant over so that he or she is facedown on your forearm. Give 5 firm back blows with the heel of your hand while supporting the arm that is holding the infant on your thigh.

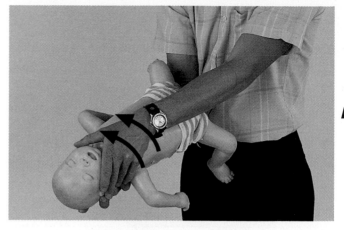

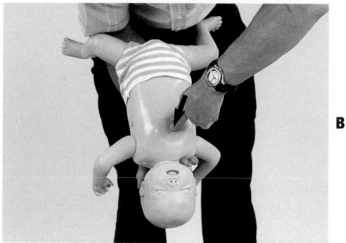

Figure 6-8 To give chest thrusts, sandwich the infant between your forearms. Continue to support the infant's head. **A,** Turn the infant onto his or her back and support your arm on your thigh. The infant's head should be lower than the chest. **B,** Give 5 chest thrusts.

which will assist in dislodging the object. Give 5 chest thrusts.

To locate the correct place to give chest thrusts, imagine a line running across the infant's chest between the nipples. Place the pads of two or three of your fingers just under this imaginary line. If you feel the notch at the end of the infant's breastbone, move your fingers up toward the nipple line (**Fig. 6-8, *B***).

Use the pads of the index and middle fingers to compress the breastbone. Compress the breastbone ½ to 1 inch; let the breastbone return to its normal position. Keep your fingers in contact with the infant's breastbone. You can give back blows and chest thrusts effectively whether you stand or sit, as long as the infant is supported on your

thigh. If the infant is large or your hands are too small to adequately support the infant, you may prefer to sit. The infant's head must be lower than his or her chest. Continue back blows and chest thrusts until the object is forced out, the infant begins to breathe on his or her own or the infant becomes unconscious.

Special Considerations

Chest Thrusts

In some instances, abdominal thrusts are not the best method of care for a conscious choking adult or child. For example, if you cannot reach far enough

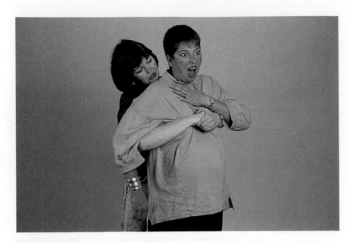

Figure 6-9 Give chest thrusts if you cannot reach around the victim to give abdominal thrusts, or if the victim is noticeably pregnant.

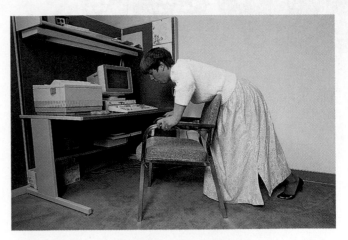

Figure 6-10 To give abdominal thrusts to yourself, press your abdomen onto a firm object, such as the back of a chair.

around the victim to give effective abdominal thrusts, you should give chest thrusts. You should also give chest thrusts instead of abdominal thrusts to choking victims who are obviously pregnant or known to be pregnant.

To give chest thrusts to a conscious victim, stand behind the victim and place your arms under the victim's armpits and around the chest. As with abdominal thrusts, make a fist with one hand and place the thumb side against the center of the victim's breastbone. Be sure that your fist is centered on the breastbone, not on the ribs. Also make sure that your fist is not near the lower tip of the breastbone. Grab your fist with your other hand and thrust inward. Repeat these thrusts until the victim can cough, speak or breathe or until the victim becomes unconscious (**Fig. 6-9**).

If You Are Alone

If you are alone and choking and no one is around who can help, you can give yourself abdominal thrusts in one of two ways. Make a fist with one hand and place the thumb side on the middle of your abdomen slightly above your navel and well below the tip of your breastbone. Grasp your fist with your other hand and give quick, upward thrusts. You can also lean forward and press your abdomen over any firm object, such as the back of a chair, a railing or a sink. Be careful not to lean over anything with a sharp edge or a corner that might injure you (**Fig. 6-10**).

Conscious Choking Adult or Child Who Becomes Unconscious

While giving abdominal thrusts to a conscious choking adult or child, you should anticipate that the victim will become unconscious if the obstruction is not removed. If the victim becomes unconscious, carefully lower him or her to the floor. Call 9-1-1 or the local emergency number if someone has not already called.

Open the victim's airway using the head-tilt/chin-lift technique and attempt 2 rescue breaths. Often the throat muscles relax enough after a person becomes unconscious to allow air past the obstruction and into the lungs. You will know air has made it successfully into the lungs if the victim's chest rises and falls with each rescue breath. If air does not go into the lungs and the chest does not rise, perform chest compressions. You will learn more about performing chest compressions and providing care for an unconscious choking adult or child in Chapter 7.

Conscious Choking Infant Who Becomes Unconscious

If a conscious choking infant becomes unconscious, lower the infant to a table or the floor and open his or her airway. Call 9-1-1 or the local emergency number if someone has not already done so. Open the infant's airway. Then attempt 2 rescue breaths. If air still does not go in, position the infant for chest compressions. Give 30 chest compressions followed by a visual check for an object. If you see an object, try to remove it with your little finger (**Fig. 6-11**). If you do not see an object, or after your attempt to remove an object with your little finger, give 2 rescue breaths. Continue the sequence of providing 30 chest compressions followed by an attempt to remove an object if you see it, followed by attempting 2 rescue breaths, until you are able to get air in or EMS personnel arrive and take over (**Fig. 6-12, *A-B***). If you are able to get air into the infant, check for signs of life and a pulse. You will learn more about caring for an infant with no signs of life in Chapter 7.

RESPIRATORY ARREST

In *respiratory arrest*, breathing stops. The person gets no oxygen. The body can function without oxygen for only a few minutes before body systems begin to fail. Without oxygen, the heart muscle stops functioning, causing the circulatory system to fail. When the heart stops, other body systems start to fail. However, you can keep the person's respiratory system functioning artificially by giving rescue breathing.

Signals for Respiratory Arrest

Signals for a victim in respiratory arrest include—

▶ Absence of breathing.
▶ Skin color (ashen or cyanotic).

Care for Respiratory Arrest

Rescue breaths are a way of breathing air into a victim's lungs to supply that person with the oxygen he or she needs to survive. Rescue breaths are given as a part of CPR and to infants and children who are not breathing but still have a pulse.

Rescue breaths work because the air you breathe into the victim contains more than enough oxygen to keep that person alive. The air you take

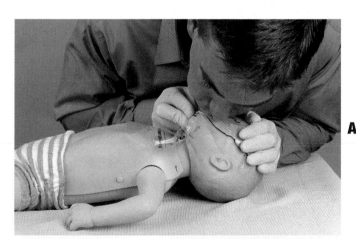
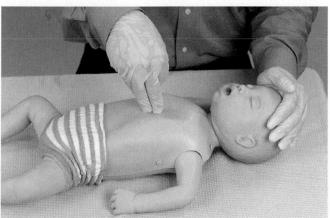

Figure 6-12 **A,** If the breaths do not go in, reposition the airway and give breaths again. **B,** If air still does not go in, position the infant for chest compressions.

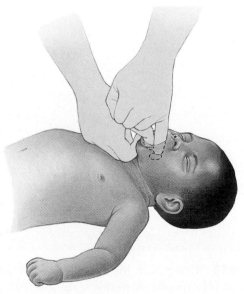

Figure 6-11 Lift the jaw upward. If you see an object, try to remove it with your little finger.

in with every breath contains about 21 percent oxygen, but your body uses only 5 percent of that oxygen. The air you breathe out of your lungs and into the victim's lungs contains about 16 percent oxygen, enough to keep someone alive.

Rescue Breathing for Infants and Children

If you discover that a child or infant is unconscious, not breathing and has a pulse and no one is available to call 9-1-1 or the local emergency number, give 2 minutes of care and then make the call yourself. Rescue breathing for a child or an infant is performed in much the same way as a rescue breath for an adult. However, there are some minor variations. These variations take into account the anatomical and physiological differences between an adult and a child or infant.

Rescue Breathing for a Child

To provide rescue breathing for a child, use less air in each breath and deliver breaths at a slightly faster rate. You do not need to tilt a child's head as far back as an adult's to open the airway. (Tilt the head gently back only far enough to allow your breaths to go in (**Fig. 6-13**). Use the fingers and not the thumb to lift the lower jaw at the chin up and outward. Keep your fingers on the bony part of the jaw.) Tipping the child's head back too far may obstruct the airway. Take a normal breath, not a deep breath, and give 1 breath every 3 seconds for a child or infant. Each breath should last about 1 second.

Rescue Breathing for an Infant

When giving rescue breathing to an infant, it is easier to cover both the nose and mouth with your mouth than to pinch the nose (**Fig. 6-14**). Take a normal breath, not a deep breath, and give 1 breath every 3 seconds for an infant. Each breath should last about 1 second. Be careful not to over-inflate an infant's lungs. Breathe only until you see the chest clearly rise. After 2 minutes of rescue breathing (about 40 breaths), recheck for signs of life and a pulse for no more than 10 seconds. If the child or infant has a pulse but is not breathing, continue rescue breathing. Recheck for signs of life and a pulse and breathing about every 2 minutes.

Breathing Barriers

You may not feel comfortable with the thought of giving rescue breaths, especially to someone you do not know. Disease transmission is an understandable concern, even though the chances of contracting a disease from providing rescue breaths are extremely low. CPR breathing barriers, such as resuscitation masks and face shields, create a barrier between your mouth and nose and the victim's. This barrier can help protect you from contact with blood and other body fluids. Many barriers are small enough to fit in a pocket, first aid kit or in the glove compartment of a car (**Fig. 6-15, A-B**). When using a CPR breathing barrier during rescue breathing, follow the same procedures already described. Depend-

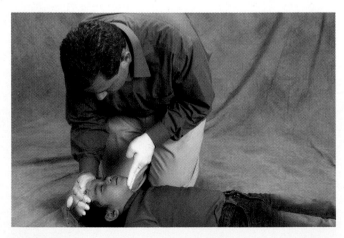

Figure 6-13 Tilt the head and lift the chin to open the airway.

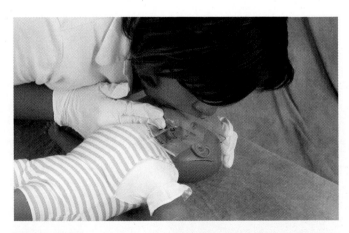

Figure 6-14 Cover both the nose and mouth of the infant with your mouth when giving rescue breathing to an infant.

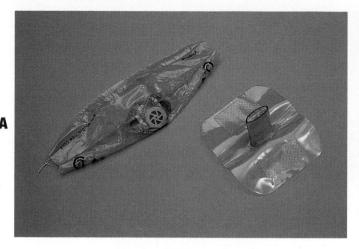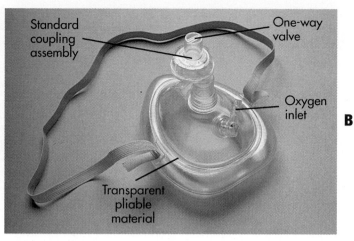

Figure 6-15   A, A face shield or, **B,** a mask, when placed between your mouth and nose and the victim's, can help prevent you from contacting a person's saliva or other body fluids.

ing on the barrier, you may have to modify how you open the airway and maintain the correct airway position. While the use of CPR breathing barriers is preferred to mouth-to-mouth contact, you should not delay rescue breathing while searching for a breathing barrier or learning how to use one.

When to Stop Care

Do not stop rescue breathing unless one of the following situations occurs:

▶ The scene becomes unsafe.
▶ The victim begins to breathe on his or her own.
▶ Another trained person takes over for you.
▶ EMS personnel arrive on the scene and take over.
▶ You are too exhausted to continue.

Special Considerations

Rescue breathing is a very simple skill to perform. However, several situations exist that may require special attention. Being familiar with these situations will help you give care for a person in respiratory arrest.

Air in the Stomach

The most common complication of rescue breathing is air in the stomach. Air in the stomach can cause **gastric distention**. Gastric distention can be serious because it can make the victim vomit. If an unconscious person vomits, he or she may *aspirate* stomach contents or other material, such as saliva or blood, which can hamper rescue breathing.

Common causes of gastric distention include—

▶ Breathing into the victim with too much force. This situation often occurs when the victim's head is not tilted back far enough and the airway is not completely open.
▶ Breathing too quickly. This increases pressure in the airway, causing air to enter the stomach.
▶ Breathing into the victim longer than 1 second in duration.

To avoid forcing air into the stomach, be sure to keep the victim's head tilted correctly for his or her size and age. Breathe into the victim only enough to make the chest clearly rise. Breaths should not be given too quickly or too hard. Pause between breaths long enough for the victim's lungs to empty and for you to take another breath.

Laryngectomies: A Breath of Fresh Air

Years ago a person diagnosed with cancer of the larynx had a small chance of survival. Today, advances in drugs, surgical techniques and radiation therapy have led to increased survival rates. Laryngeal cancer is now one of the most curable cancers.

Cancer of the larynx may involve the vocal cords and surrounding tissue, giving rise to signals such as voice changes or trouble breathing or swallowing. Surgical removal of the larynx, known as a total laryngectomy, is a common procedure for treating laryngeal cancer. The person who has this procedure is a laryngectomee. When the entire larynx is removed, a connection no longer exists between the mouth, the nose and the windpipe. A surgical opening, called a stoma, is made in the front of the neck, and the windpipe is attached to it. The patient breathes only through the stoma and not through the mouth or nose. This person is called a "total neck breather."

Some people have a condition that hinders the effectiveness of their airway, such as growths or vocal cord paralysis. They can be assured of an adequate air supply by having an opening made from the outside of the neck into the windpipe. A tube is inserted to prevent the opening from growing together again. This opening is also called a stoma. Because these individuals still have a larynx, they may be able to breathe to some degree through the nose and mouth. They are called "partial neck breathers."

Although someone who has had a total laryngectomy no longer has vocal cords, that person is still able to speak. The only aspect of speech they no longer have is the ability to generate sound. Many laryngectomees communicate using an instrument called an artificial larynx, which generates sound electronically. The head of the instrument is held against the neck and the sound vibrates through the neck and into the mouth. The person shapes the word just as if the sound came from the vocal cords. Sometimes the resulting sound from neck placement is not satisfactory, in which case a cap with a small straw-like tube is put on the head of the instrument, and the tube is placed into the corner of the mouth. In this way, the sound is delivered directly into the mouth, and the person uses more normal pronunciation to shape the sound into speech.

Another way a laryngectomee makes sound is by using the same sound source we all use when we burp. The location of the sound is the upper end of the food tube, or esophagus. The laryngectomee learns to move the air into the esophagus and make controlled sound, as the air comes back out. With practice, the sound becomes refined and very effective for speech. This is known as esophageal speech. A variation of this form of communication is known as tracheoesophageal speech. A small surgical opening is created between the windpipe and esophagus. A valved tube is put in the opening. The tube allows air from the lungs to enter the esophagus, and the individual produces esophageal speech by exhaling rather than by injecting air into the esophagus.

The International Association of Laryngectomees (IAL) was formed in 1952 as an organization dedicated to supporting laryngectomees and their families. There are nearly 300 member clubs located throughout the United States and in several foreign countries. Supported by the American Cancer Society, the IAL is also a conduit for public information and education regarding laryngectomees. The IAL has been dedicated to helping educate emergency and public workers on the special needs of neck breathers in certain emergency situations, such as respiratory arrest. Through their efforts, many lives have been saved.

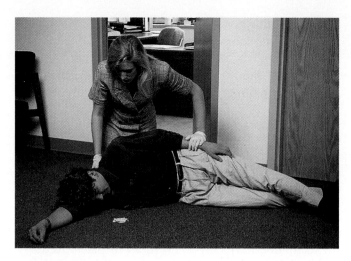

Figure 6-16   If the victim vomits, roll the victim on the side and clear the mouth of any objects.

Vomiting

When you give rescue breaths, the victim may vomit, whether or not gastric distention occurs. If the victim vomits, roll him or her onto one side (**Fig. 6-16**). If the person vomits and is unconscious and lying down, position the person on his or her side. Avoid twisting the neck and back. This positioning helps to prevent vomit from entering the lungs. Quickly wipe the victim's mouth clean, reposition the victim on his or her back, reopen the airway and continue with rescue breathing.

Mouth-to-Nose Breathing

Sometimes you may not be able to make an adequate seal over a victim's mouth to perform a rescue breath. The victim's jaw or mouth may be injured or your mouth may be too small to cover the victim's. If so, provide mouth-to-nose rescue breaths as follows:

▸   Maintain the head-tilt position with one hand on the forehead. Use your other hand to close the victim's mouth, making sure to push on the chin and not on the throat.
▸   Open your mouth wide, take a deep breath, seal your mouth tightly around the victim's nose and breathe into the victim's nose (**Fig. 6-17**). Open the victim's mouth between breaths, if possible, to let air out.

Mouth-to-Stoma Breathing

Some people have had an operation to remove all or part of the upper end of their airway. They breathe through an opening called a *stoma* in the front of the neck (**Fig. 6-18**). Air passes directly into the airway through the stoma instead of through the mouth and nose.

Most people with a stoma wear a medical ID tag or carry a card identifying this condition. You may not see the stoma immediately. You will probably notice the opening in the neck as you tilt the head back to check for breathing or move clothing.

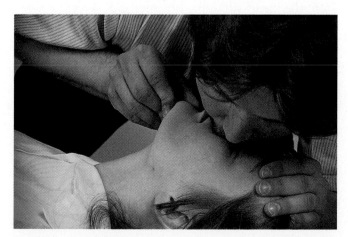

Figure 6-17   For mouth-to-nose breathing, keep the head tilted back, close the victim's mouth and seal your mouth around the victim's nose.

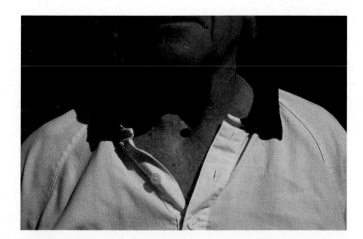

Figure 6-18   You may need to give rescue breaths to a victim with a stoma, which is an opening in the front of the neck.

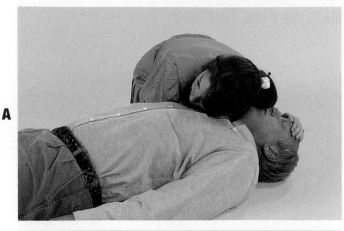

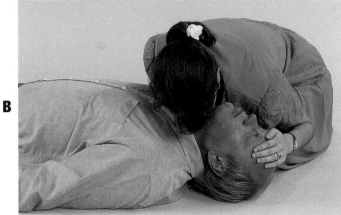

Figure 6-19 **A,** To check for breathing, look, listen and feel for breaths with your ear over the stoma. **B,** To give rescue breaths, seal your mouth around the stoma and breathe into the victim.

A stoma may be obscured by clothing, such as a turtleneck, sweater or a scarf.

To give rescue breaths to someone with a stoma, you must give breaths through the stoma instead of the mouth or nose. Follow the same basic steps as in mouth-to-mouth breathing, except—

1. Look, listen and feel for breathing with your ear over the stoma (**Fig. 6-19, A**).
2. Give breaths into the stoma, breathing at the same rate as for mouth-to-mouth breathing (**Fig. 6-19, B**).
3. Remove your mouth from the stoma between breaths to let air flow back out.

If the chest does not clearly rise when you give rescue breaths, suspect that the victim may have had only part of the larynx removed. Some air thus continues to flow through the larynx to the lungs during normal breathing. When giving mouth-to-stoma breathing, air may leak through the nose and mouth, diminishing the amount of your rescue breaths that reaches the lungs. If this occurs, you need to seal the nose and mouth with your hand to prevent air from escaping during rescue breaths.

Victims with Dentures

If you know or see that the victim is wearing dentures, do not automatically remove them. Dentures help you give rescue breaths by supporting the victim's mouth and cheeks during mouth-to-mouth breathing. If the dentures are loose, the head-tilt/chin-lift technique may help keep them in place. Remove the dentures only if they become so loose that they block the airway or make it difficult for you to give breaths.

Victims with Suspected Head, Neck or Back Injuries

You should suspect a head, neck or back injury if the person—

▶ Was involved in a motor vehicle crash.
▶ Was injured as a result of a fall from a height greater than the victim's standing height. Complains of neck or back pain.
▶ Has tingling or weakness in extremities.
▶ Is not fully alert.
▶ Appears intoxicated.
▶ Appears to be frail or over 65 years of age.

If you suspect the victim may have a head, neck or back injury, you should try to minimize movement of the head and neck when opening the airway with the head-tilt chin-lift method. Victims who have a suspected spinal injury should not be moved. But if an open airway cannot be maintained or the responder must leave the victim to get help, place the victim in a modified High Arm In Endangered Spine (H.A.IN.E.S.) recovery position.

You will learn more about caring for head, neck and back injuries in Chapter 13.

SUMMARY

Breathing emergencies are life-threatening conditions. There are two types of breathing emergencies: respiratory distress and respiratory arrest. Respiratory distress is a condition in which breathing becomes difficult. Respiratory arrest occurs when breathing stops. As a citizen responder, your role is to recognize the signals of a breathing emergency, call 9-1-1 or the local emergency number and give appropriate care. By knowing how to care for breathing emergencies, you are now better prepared to care for cardiac and other emergencies. You will learn about cardiac emergencies in Chapter 7.

APPLICATION QUESTIONS

1. What signals was Steve exhibiting and experiencing in the opening scenario?

2. Would knowing the cause of Steve's problem change the care you give? Why or why not?

3. Could the cause of Steve's respiratory distress lead to respiratory arrest? Why or why not?

4. If Steve went into respiratory arrest, what would you do?

5. Is it possible that Steve's condition may lead to an anatomical airway obstruction? Why?

STUDY QUESTIONS

1. Match each term with the correct definition.

a. Airway obstruction
b. Head-tilt/chin-lift
c. Aspiration
d. Rescue breathing
e. Epiglottitis
f. Respiratory arrest
g. Anatomical airway obstruction
h. Respiratory distress

_____ Inhaling blood, vomit or other foreign material into the lungs.

_____ Technique of breathing for a non-breathing child or infant.

_____ Blockage of the airway that prevents air from reaching the victim's lungs.

_____ Condition in which breathing stops.

_____ Condition in which breathing becomes difficult.

_____ Technique for opening the airway.

_____ Occurs if the airway is blocked by the tongue or swollen tissues of the mouth and throat.

_____ Condition in which the epiglottis swells.

2. Circle four signals associated with respiratory distress that you find in the following scenario.

When Rita walked into Mr. Boyd's office, she found him collapsed across his desk. His eyes were closed but she could hear him breathing, making a high whistling noise. He was flushed, sweating and seemed to be trembling uncontrollably. When he heard Rita, he raised his head a little, "My chest hurts," he gasped, "and I feel dizzy and can't seem to catch my breath." He looked frightened.

3. List three causes of choking.

4. Match each type of care with its purpose.

    a. Back blows and abdominal thrusts
    b. Recognizing and caring for respiratory distress
    c. Giving rescue breaths

    _____ Supply oxygen to the lungs when someone has stopped breathing.

    _____ Force a foreign object out of the airway.

    _____ May prevent respiratory arrest from occurring.

In questions 5 through 16, circle the letter of the correct answer.

5. Which of the following is a signal of respiratory distress?

    a. Gasping for air
    b. Breathing that is slower than normal
    c. Wheezing
    d. All of the above

6. How are asthma, hyperventilation and anaphylactic shock alike?

    a. They require rescue breathing.
    b. They are forms of respiratory distress.
    c. They are always life threatening.
    d. They occur only in children and infants.

7. Care for victims of respiratory distress always includes which of the following?

    a. Helping the victim rest in a comfortable position
    b. Giving the victim water to drink
    c. Giving rescue breathing
    d. Delivering abdominal thrusts

8. Which of the following statements about rescue breathing is true?

    a. It supplies the body with oxygen necessary for survival.
    b. It always requires clearing the airway of foreign objects.
    c. It is given to children and infants who are not breathing but do have a pulse.
    d. It is given only when two rescuers are present.

9. For which condition would a child or infant need rescue breathing?

    a. Unconsciousness
    b. Unconsciousness and respiratory distress
    c. Unconsciousness, respiratory arrest, with pulse.
    d. Unconsciousness, respiratory distress, with no pulse.

10. When you give rescue breaths, how much air should you breathe into the victim?

    a. Enough to make the stomach clearly rise
    b. Enough to make the chest clearly rise
    c. Enough to feel resistance
    d. Enough to fill the victim's cheeks

11. Which action is a part of the care for an unconscious adult victim with an obstructed airway?

    a. Giving 2 rescue breaths
    b. Giving chest compressions
    c. Calling 9-1-1 or the local emergency number
    d. All of the above

12. What should you do for a conscious infant who is choking and cannot cry, cough or breathe?

    a. Give back blows and chest thrusts.
    b. Give 1 rescue breath.
    c. Give abdominal thrusts.
    d. Lower the infant to the floor and open the airway.

13. After giving 2 rescue breaths to an adult victim with an obstructed airway who becomes unconscious, what should you do next?

    a. Give chest compressions if the chest does not rise.
    b. Look for an object in the back of the throat and attempt to remove it if it is visible.
    c. Check for signs of life, give 2 rescue breaths and look for and remove an object if it is visible at the back of the throat.
    d. Check for and remove an object if it is visible at the back of the throat and then check for signs of life.

14. After 2 minutes of rescue breathing, you check a child for signs of life including a pulse. The child has a pulse but still is not breathing. What should you do?

    a. Continue rescue breathing by giving 2 breaths.
    b. Continue rescue breathing by giving 1 breath every 3 seconds.
    c. Stop rescue breathing for 2 minutes.
    d. Reposition the airway.

15. While eating dinner, a friend suddenly starts to cough weakly and makes high-pitched noises. What should you do?

    a. Lower him to the floor, check for and remove an object if it is visible at the back of the throat, give 2 breaths and up to 5 abdominal thrusts.
    b. Give back blows and abdominal thrusts until the object is dislodged or he becomes unconscious.
    c. Encourage him to continue coughing to try to dislodge the object.
    d. Open the airway using the head-tilt/chin-lift technique.

16. A woman is choking on a piece of candy but is conscious and coughing forcefully. What should you do?

    a. Slap her on the back until she coughs up the object.
    b. Give abdominal thrusts.
    c. Encourage her to continue coughing.
    d. Perform a check at the back of the throat.

17. Number in order the following actions for performing rescue breathing, starting from the time you discover that an unconscious child victim is not breathing.

    _____ Check for signs of life including a pulse and severe bleeding.

    _____ Give 1 breath about every 3 seconds.

    _____ Give 2 breaths.

    _____ Recheck for signs of life and a pulse after 2 minutes.

Answers are listed in Appendix A.

SKILL SHEET **Conscious Choking—Adult**
(If person cannot cough, speak or breathe)

Step 1

CHECK scene, then **CHECK** person.

Step 2

Have someone **CALL** 9-1-1.

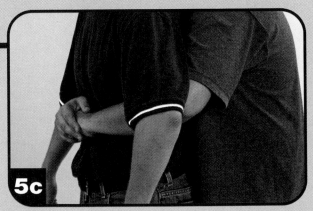

Step 3

Obtain consent.

Step 4

Lean the person forward and give **5** back blows with the heel of your hand.

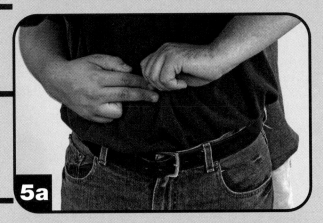

Step 5

Give **5** quick, upward abdominal thrusts.

NOTE: *Give chest thrusts to a choking person who is pregnant or too big for you to reach around.*

NOTE: *You can give yourself abdominal thrusts by using your hands, just as you would do to another person, or lean over and press your abdomen against any firm object such as the back of a chair.*

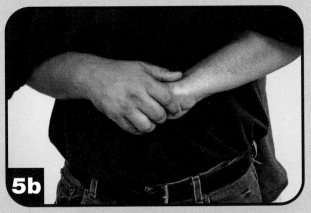

Step 6

Continue back blows and abdominal thrusts until—

- Object is forced out.
- Person can breathe or cough forcefully.
- Person becomes unconscious.
- If adult becomes unconscious, follow steps on pp. 142-143.

SKILL SHEET Conscious Choking—Child
(If child cannot cough, speak or breathe)

Step 1

CHECK scene, then CHECK child.

Step 2

Have someone CALL 9-1-1.

Step 3

Obtain consent from parent or guardian, if present.

Step 4

Lean the child forward and give 5 back blows with the heel of your hand.

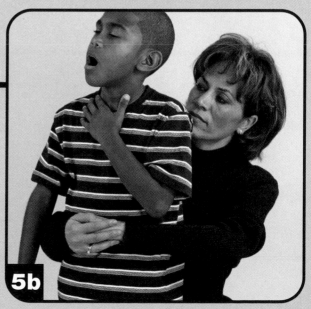

Step 5

Give 5 quick, upward abdominal thrusts.

NOTE: *For a child, stand or kneel behind the child, depending on his or her size.*

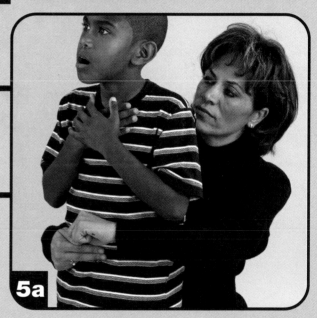

Step 6

Continue back blows and abdominal thrusts until—

- Object is forced out.
- Child can breathe or cough forcefully.
- Child becomes unconscious.
- If child becomes unconscious, follow steps on pp. 146-147.

SKILL SHEET Conscious Choking—Infant

Check the scene and the infant. *Remember: Always follow standard precautions to prevent disease transmission.*

Step 1

Obtain permission to provide care (if parent or guardian is present).

Step 2

If the infant cannot cough, cry or breathe, have someone else call 9-1-1 or the local emergency number.

Step 3

Carefully position the infant face-down on your forearm.

- Support the infant's head and neck with your hand.
- Lower the infant onto your thigh, keeping the infant's head lower than his or her chest.

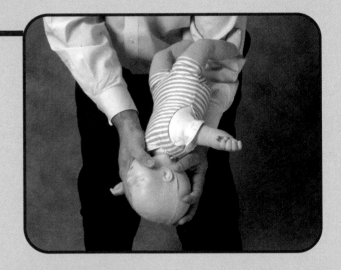

Step 4

Give **5** firm back blows between the infant's shoulder blades with the heel of your hand.

- Each blow should be a separate and distinct attempt to dislodge the object.

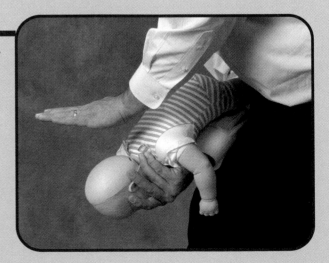

Step 5

Carefully position the infant face-up on your forearm.

- Support the infant's head and neck with your hand.
- Lower the infant onto your thigh, keeping the infant's head lower than his or her chest.

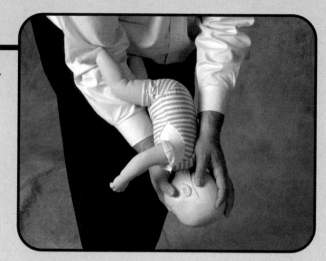

Step 6

Give **5** chest thrusts.

- Place two or three fingers on the center of the infant's chest, about 1 finger width below an imaginary line between the nipples.
- Compress the breastbone $\frac{1}{2}$ to 1 inch, 5 times.

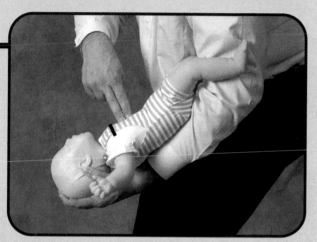

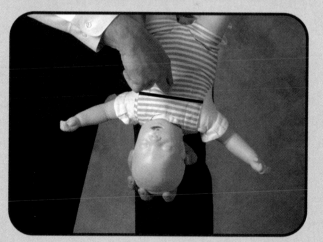

Step 7

Repeat cycles of back blows and chest thrusts until—

- The object is expelled.
- The infant starts to breathe, cry or cough forcefully.
- The infant becomes unconscious.

If the infant becomes unconscious, follow the steps on pp. 150-151.

SKILL SHEET   Rescue Breathing for a Child

Complete *"Checking an Unconscious Child (Ages 1-12)"* Steps 1-7 in Chapter 5, page 78.
Remember: Always follow standard precautions to prevent disease transmission.

If a child is not breathing but has a pulse—

Step 8

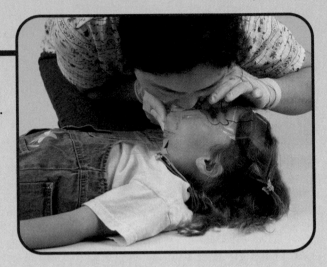

Give **1** rescue breath about every **3** seconds.

- Continue for about 2 minutes—about 40 breaths.

Step 9

Recheck for signs of life and a pulse about every
2 minutes.

- Continue rescue breathing as long as a pulse
  is present but the child is not breathing.

SKILL SHEET Rescue Breathing for an Infant

Complete *"Checking an Unconscious Infant (Under Age 1)"* Steps 1-8 in Chapter 5, page 79.
Remember: Always follow standard precautions to prevent disease transmission.

If an infant is not breathing but has a pulse—

Step 9

Give **1** rescue breath about every **3** seconds.

- Continue for 2 minutes—about 40 breaths.

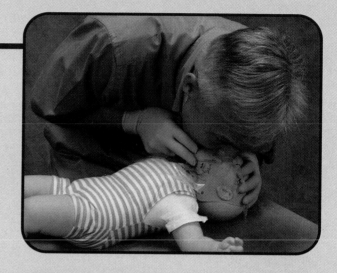

Step 10

Recheck for signs of life and a pulse about every **2** minutes.

- Continue rescue breathing as long as a pulse is present but the infant is not breathing.

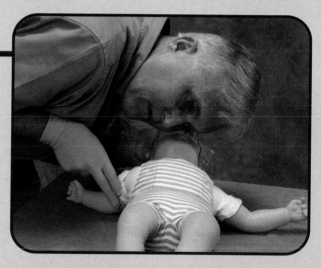

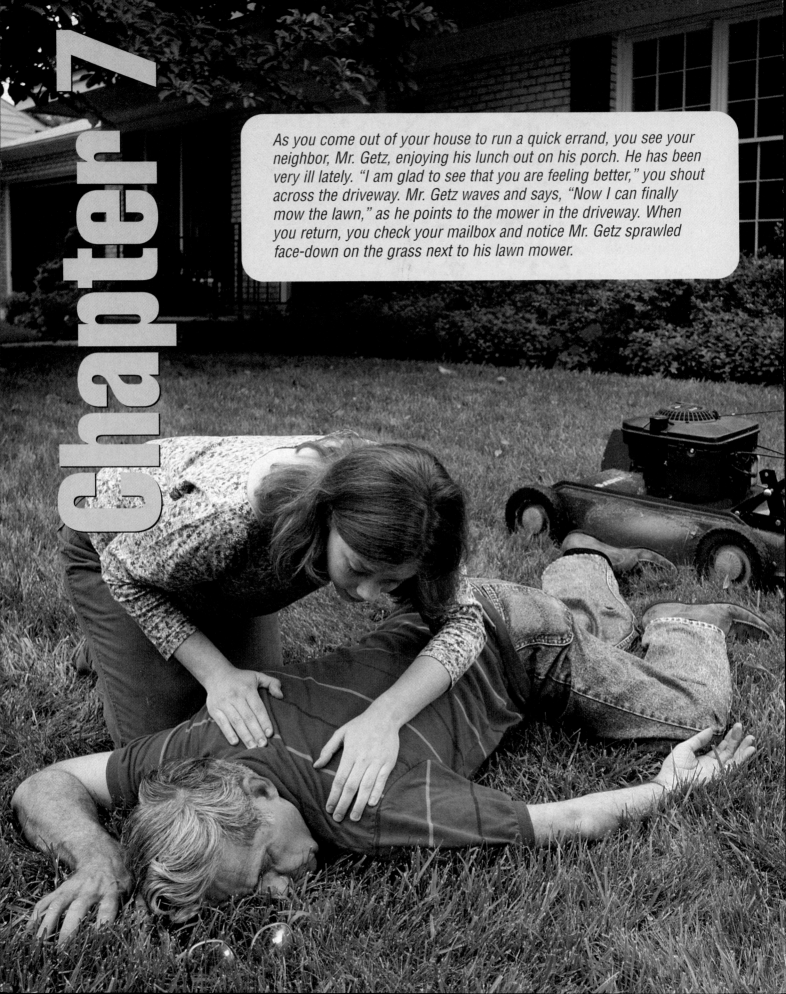

Chapter 7

As you come out of your house to run a quick errand, you see your neighbor, Mr. Getz, enjoying his lunch out on his porch. He has been very ill lately. "I am glad to see that you are feeling better," you shout across the driveway. Mr. Getz waves and says, "Now I can finally mow the lawn," as he points to the mower in the driveway. When you return, you check your mailbox and notice Mr. Getz sprawled face-down on the grass next to his lawn mower.

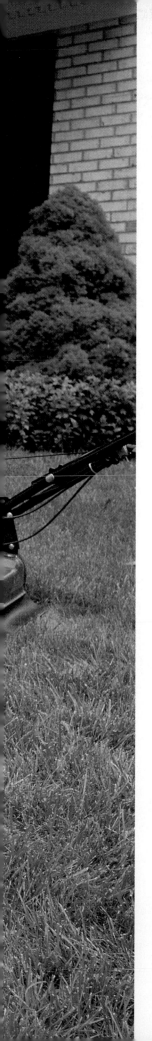

Cardiac Emergencies and Unconscious Choking

Objectives

After reading this chapter, you should be able to—

- Identify the links in the Cardiac Chain of Survival.
- List the signals of a heart attack for both men and women.
- Describe the care for a victim of a heart attack.
- Describe the role of CPR in cardiac arrest.
- Describe defibrillation and how it works.
- Describe the general steps for the use of an automated external defibrillator (AED).
- List the precautions for the use of an AED.

After reading this chapter and completing the appropriate class activities, you should be able to demonstrate—

- How to perform CPR for an adult, child and infant.
- How to care for an unconscious choking adult, child and infant.
- How to use an AED to care for an adult or child in cardiac arrest.

Introduction

In this chapter, you will learn how to recognize and give care for a victim of a cardiac emergency. This chapter also discusses risk factors of cardiovascular disease—the leading cause of cardiac emergencies—and what you can do to control those risks. Finally, you will learn what to do if an unconscious victim is not breathing and the rescue breaths you give do not go in (unconscious choking).

CARDIOVASCULAR DISEASE

Cardiovascular disease—abnormal conditions that affect the heart and blood vessels—is the leading cause of death for men and women in the United States. An estimated 61 million Americans suffer from some form of cardiovascular disease. About 950,000 Americans die of cardiovascular disease each year. The principal components of cardiovascular disease—coronary heart disease and stroke—account for more than 40 percent of all deaths in the United States.

Cardiovascular disease develops slowly. Fatty deposits of **cholesterol** and other material gradually build up on the inner walls of the arteries. This condition, called **atherosclerosis**, causes a progressive narrowing of blood vessels. Because atherosclerosis develops gradually, it can remain undetected for many years. Most people with atherosclerosis are unaware of it. Fortunately, atherosclerosis can be slowed or stopped by adopting a healthy lifestyle. You will learn more about maintaining a healthy lifestyle in Chapter 24 of this text.

The most common type of cardiovascular disease is *coronary heart disease* (also called coronary artery disease). Coronary heart disease occurs when the arteries that supply oxygen-rich blood to the heart muscle (*coronary arteries*) harden or narrow from the build-up of fatty deposits (atherosclerosis). As a result, the flow of oxygen-rich blood to the heart decreases. If the heart muscle is deprived of this blood, it dies. If enough of the heart muscle dies, the heart cannot circulate the blood effectively to other parts of the body (**Fig. 7-1**).

K E Y   T E R M S

Angina pectoris: Chest pain that comes and goes at different times; commonly associated with cardiovascular disease.

Asystole: A condition where the heart has stopped generating electrical activity.

Atherosclerosis: A condition in which fatty deposits build up on the walls of the arteries.

Cardiac arrest: A condition in which the heart has stopped beating or beats too ineffectively to generate a pulse.

Cardiopulmonary resuscitation (CPR): A technique that combines chest compressions and rescue breathing for a victim whose heart and breathing have stopped.

Cardiovascular disease: Disease of the heart and blood vessels.

Cholesterol: A fatty substance made by the body and found in certain foods; too much in the blood can cause fatty deposits on artery walls that may restrict or block blood flow.

Coronary arteries: Blood vessels that supply the heart muscle with oxygen-rich blood.

Coronary heart disease (also called coronary artery disease): Occurs when the coronary arteries that supply oxygen-rich blood to the heart muscle become hardened or narrowed from the build-up of fatty deposits.

Defibrillation: An electrical shock that disrupts the electrical activity of the heart long enough to allow the heart to spontaneously develop an effective rhythm on its own.

Heart attack: A sudden illness involving the death of heart muscle tissue when it does not receive oxygen-rich blood; also known as myocardial infarction.

Risk factors: Conditions or behaviors that increase the chance that a person will develop a disease.

Ventricular fibrillation (V-fib): An abnormal heart rhythm characterized by disorganized electrical activity, which results in the quivering of the ventricles.

Ventricular tachycardia (V-tach): An abnormal heart rhythm characterized by rapid contractions of the ventricles.

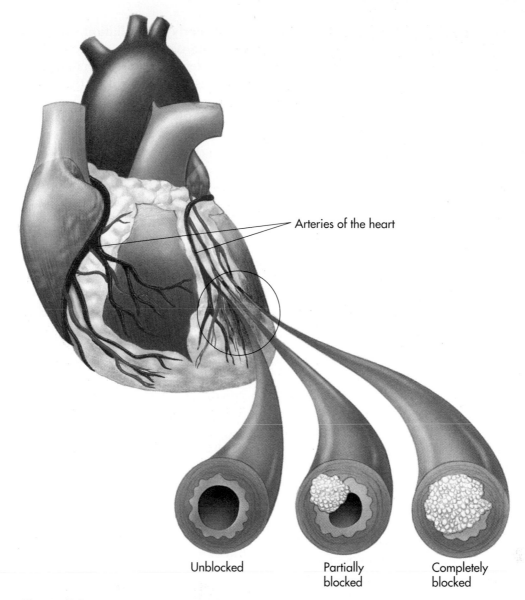

Arteries of the heart

Unblocked   Partially   Completely
                   blocked   blocked

Figure 7-1   Buildup of fatty materials on the inner walls of the arteries reduces blood flow to the heart muscle and may cause a heart attack.

CARDIAC EMERGENCIES

Two common cardiac emergencies are a heart attack (also known as myocardial infarction) and cardiac arrest. A **heart attack** refers to a condition in which the blood flow to some part of the heart muscle is compromised and the heart begins to die. If enough of the muscle dies, the heart cannot circulate blood effectively. The term **cardiac arrest** refers to a condition in which the heart stops beating.

The Cardiac Chain of Survival

A victim who has no signs of life is said to be **clinically dead** (**Fig. 7-2**). However, the cells of the brain and other vital organs will continue to live for a short period of time until oxygen is depleted. This victim needs **cardiopulmonary resuscitation** (CPR), which is a combination of chest compressions and rescue breathing. (The term "cardio" refers to the heart, and "pulmonary" refers to the lungs.) Performed together, rescue breaths and chest compressions artificially take over the functions of the lungs and heart, increasing the victim's chance of survival by keeping the brain supplied with oxygen until advanced medical care can be given.

However, even under the best of conditions, CPR only generates about one-third of the normal blood flow to the brain. Therefore, CPR alone is not enough to help someone survive cardiac arrest. Early CPR given by bystanders, combined with early **defibrillation** and **advanced cardiac life sup-**

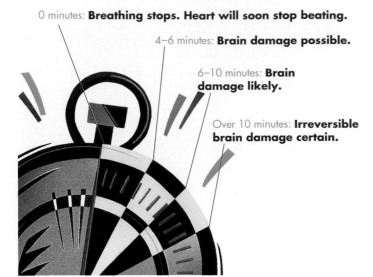

0 minutes: **Breathing stops. Heart will soon stop beating.**

4–6 minutes: **Brain damage possible.**

6–10 minutes: **Brain damage likely.**

Over 10 minutes: **Irreversible brain damage certain.**

Figure 7-2   Clinical death is a condition in which the heart and breathing stop. Without resuscitation, clinical death will result in biological death. Biological death is the irreversible death of brain cells.

port by EMS personnel, give the victim of cardiac arrest the best chance for survival. This concept is known as the Cardiac Chain of Survival.

The greatest chance of survival from cardiac arrest occurs when the following sequence of events—the Cardiac Chain of Survival—happens as rapidly as possible (**Fig. 7-3**):

1. **Early recognition and early access.** The sooner 9-1-1 or the local emergency number is called the sooner early advanced medical care arrives.
2. **Early CPR.** Early CPR helps circulate blood that contains oxygen to the vital organs until an AED is ready to use or advanced medical personnel arrive.

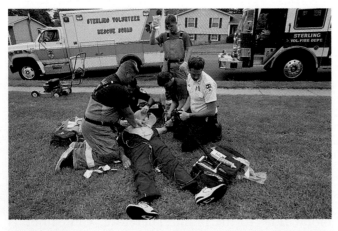

Figure 7-3   Use of a **defibrillator** and other advanced measures may restore a heartbeat in a victim of cardiac arrest.

3. **Early defibrillation.** Most victims of sudden cardiac arrest need an electric shock called defibrillation. Each minute that defibrillation is delayed reduces the chance of survival by about 10 percent.
4. **Early advanced medical care.** This is given by trained medical personnel, who provide further care and transport to hospital facilities.

HEART ATTACK

Heart attacks are caused by obstructions in the **coronary arteries**. Most people who die from a heart attack do so within 1 to 2 hours after the first signals appear. Because the obstruction may be a clot, early treatment with medication that dissolves clots can help in minimizing damage to the heart. Many lives might have been saved if bystanders or the victim had been aware of the signals of a heart attack and acted promptly.

Signals of a Heart Attack

The most prominent signal of a heart attack is persistent chest pain or discomfort. The pain can range from discomfort to an unbearable crushing sensation in the chest. The victim may describe it as an uncomfortable pressure, squeezing, tightness, aching or constricting, or a heavy sensation in the chest. Often, the pain is felt in the center of the chest behind the sternum. The pain may spread to the shoulder, arm, neck or jaw (**Fig. 7-4**). The pain is constant and usually not relieved by resting, changing position or taking medication. Any severe chest pain that lasts longer than 3 to 5 minutes or chest pain that is accompanied by other signals of a heart attack should receive emergency medical care immediately.

Another prominent indicator of a heart attack is trouble breathing. The victim may be breathing faster than normal because the body is trying to get much-needed oxygen to the heart. The victim's pulse may be faster or slower than normal, or irregular. The victim's skin may be pale, ashen or bluish, particularly around the face. The skin may also be moist from perspiration. The victim may feel nauseous and may vomit. These signals result from the stress the body experiences when the heart does not work effectively.

Nearly half of all deaths from heart attack are women. As with men, the most common signal for

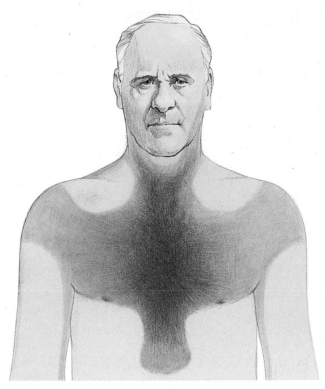

Figure 7-4 Heart attack pain is most often felt in the center of the chest, behind the breastbone. It may spread to the shoulder, arm, neck or jaw.

a heart attack in a woman is chest pain or discomfort. But women are somewhat more likely than men to experience some other common signals, particularly shortness of breath, nausea or vomiting and arm, back, neck, jaw or stomach pain.

Many heart attack victims delay seeking care. Nearly half of all heart attack victims wait 2 or more hours before going to the hospital. Victims often deny that they are having a heart attack. Some heart attack victims can have relatively mild signals and often mistake the signals for indigestion.

Care for a Heart Attack

The most important first aid measure is to be able to recognize the signals of a heart attack and take action. A heart attack victim may deny the seriousness of the signals he or she is experiencing. Do not let this denial influence you. If you think that the victim might be having a heart attack, you must act. Make sure you follow the emergency action steps: **CHECK—CALL—CARE.**

1. Send someone to call 9-1-1 or the local emergency number.

Aspirin Can Lessen Heart Attack Damage

You may be able to help a conscious person who is showing early signals of a heart attack by offering him or her an appropriate dose of aspirin when the signals first begin. However, you should never delay calling 9-1-1 or the local emergency number to do this. Always call 9-1-1 or the local emergency number as soon as you recognize the signals, and then help the person to be comfortable before you give the aspirin.

Then, if the person is able to take medicine by mouth, ask if he or she—

▶ Is allergic to aspirin.

▶ Has a stomach ulcer or stomach disease.

▶ Is taking any blood thinners, such as Coumadin™ or Warfarin™.

▶ Has been told by a doctor not to take aspirin.

If the person answers no to all of these questions, you may offer him or her two chewable (162 mg) baby aspirins, or up to one 5-grain (325 mg) adult aspirin tablet with a small amount of water. Be sure that you only use aspirin and not Tylenol, acetaminophen, Motrin, Advil or ibuprofen, which are painkillers. Likewise, do not use coated aspirin products or products meant for multiple uses such as cold, fever and headache.

You may also offer these doses of aspirin if you have cared for the person and he or she has regained consciousness and is able to take the aspirin by mouth.

2. Have the victim stop what he or she is doing and rest comfortably. Having the victim rest eases the heart's need for oxygen. Many victims find it easier to breathe while sitting (**Fig. 7-5**).

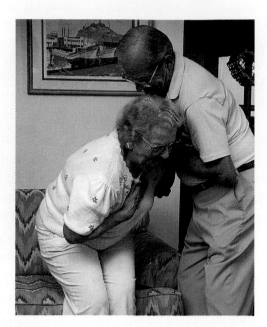

Figure 7-5 Tell a victim with severe chest pain to stop and rest. Many victims find breathing easier while sitting.

3. Loosen any restrictive clothing.
4. Monitor the victim closely until EMS personnel arrive. Note any changes in appearance or behavior.
5. Be prepared to perform CPR or use an AED if the victim stops breathing and has no other signs of life.

Talk to bystanders and the victim to get more information. Ask the victim if he or she has a history of heart disease. Some victims who have heart disease take prescribed medications for chest pain. You can help by getting the medication for the victim. Keep a calm and reassuring manner. Comforting the victim helps reduce anxiety and eases some of the discomfort. Do not try to drive the victim to the hospital yourself. The victim's condition could quickly deteriorate while you are en route.

Angina Pectoris

Some people with narrowed arteries may experience chest pain or pressure that comes and goes at different times. This type of pain is called *angina pectoris*, a medical term for pain in the chest. Angina pectoris, often referred to simply as angina, develops when the heart needs more oxygen than it gets. When the coronary arteries are narrow and the heart needs more oxygen, such as during physical activity or emotional stress, heart muscle tissues may not get enough oxygen. This lack of oxygen can cause a constricting chest pain that may spread

Signals of a Heart Attack

Persistent chest pain or discomfort that lasts longer than 3 to 5 minutes, or goes away and comes back.

▸ Chest pain spreading to the shoulders, neck, jaw, stomach, back or arms.

▸ Shortness of breath or trouble breathing.

▸ Nausea or vomiting.

▸ Dizziness, light-headedness or fainting.

▸ Pale, ashen (grayish) or bluish skin.

▸ Sweating.

▸ Denial.

In addition to persistent chest pain, women are somewhat more likely to experience some of the other warning signals, particularly—

• Shortness of breath.

• Nausea or vomiting.

• Back or jaw pain.

to the neck, jaw and arms. Pain associated with angina seldom lasts longer than 3 to 5 minutes.

A victim who knows that he or she has a history of angina may tell you he or she has prescribed medication that will temporarily widen the arteries and therefore help relieve the pain. A medication often prescribed is nitroglycerin. **Nitroglycerin** is commonly prescribed as a small tablet that dissolves under the tongue. It is also available in a spray. Sometimes nitroglycerin patches are placed on the chest. Once absorbed into the body, nitroglycerin dilates the blood vessels to make it easier for blood to reach heart muscle tissue, thus relieving the chest pain. Most angina patients are advised by their doctors to take three nitroglycerin doses over a 10-minute period. If there is no relief after 10 minutes, they are instructed to call for help.

CARDIAC ARREST

Cardiac arrest occurs when the heart stops beating or beats too ineffectively to generate a pulse and blood cannot be circulated to the brain and other vital organs. Cardiac arrest is a life-threatening

Care for a Heart Attack

‣ Recognize the signals of a heart attack.
‣ Call 9-1-1 or the local emergency number.
‣ Help the victim rest comfortably.
‣ Loosen any restrictive clothing.
‣ Assist the victim with any prescribed medication.
‣ Monitor breathing and other signs of life.
‣ Be prepared to perform CPR or use an AED if the victim's heart stops beating.

emergency because the body's vital organs are no longer receiving oxygen-rich blood.

Causes

Cardiovascular disease is the most common cause of cardiac arrest. Drowning, suffocation and certain drugs can cause breathing to stop, which will soon lead to cardiac arrest. Severe injuries to the chest or severe blood loss can also cause the heart to stop beating. Electrocution disrupts the heart's electrical activity and can cause the heart to stop. Stroke or other types of brain damage can also stop the heart. In some cases a victim of cardiac arrest may not have shown any warning signals. This condition is called **sudden death.**

Signals of Cardiac Arrest

A victim in cardiac arrest is unconscious and shows no signs of life. The absence of signs of life is the primary signal of cardiac arrest. Signs of life include—normal breathing, movement, a pulse (children and infants). The victim's skin may be pale, ashen or bluish, particularly around the face. The skin may also be moist from perspiration.

CPR FOR AN ADULT

Follow the emergency action steps: **CHECK— CALL—CARE** to determine if an unconscious adult needs CPR.

1. **CHECK** the scene and the victim.
2. If the victim is unconscious, send someone or **CALL** 9-1-1 or the local emergency number.
3. **CHECK** for signs of life for no more than 10 seconds. If the person is not breathing, give 2 rescue breaths.
4. If there are no signs of life (movement or breathing), provide **CARE** by giving CPR. Begin CPR with chest compressions at a rate of 100 compressions per minute. CPR can help circulate blood containing oxygen through a combination of chest compressions and rescue breaths.

Chest Compressions

Chest compressions are a method of making the blood flow when the heart is not beating. Chest compressions create pressure within the chest cavity that moves blood through the circulatory system. For chest compressions to be the most effective, the victim should be on his or her back on a firm, flat surface. The victim's head should be on the same level as the heart or lower. CPR is not effective if the victim is on a soft surface, like a sofa or mattress, or is sitting up in a chair.

Locate Proper Hand Position

It is important to locate the correct hand position while performing chest compressions. The correct hand position allows you to give the most effective compressions without further injuring the victim.

To locate the correct hand position on an adult victim—

1. Place the heel of one hand on the victim's sternum (breastbone), at the center of his or her chest.
2. Place your other hand directly on top of the first hand.
3. Use the heel of your hand to apply pressure on the sternum. Try to keep your fingers off the chest by interlacing them or holding them upward. Applying pressure with your fingers can lead to inefficient chest compressions or unnecessary damage to the chest (**Fig. 7-6**).

If you have arthritis or a similar condition, you may use an alternate hand position, grasping the wrist of the hand on the chest with your other hand (**Fig. 7-7**). You will find the correct hand position in the same way.

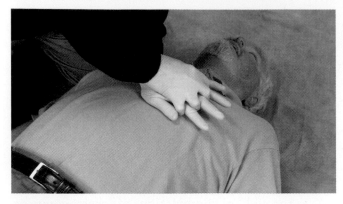

Figure 7-6 Place the heel of your hand on the sternum. Place your other hand directly on top of the first hand. Interlace your fingers and use the heel of your bottom hand to apply pressure on the sternum.

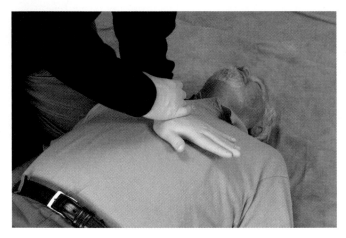

Figure 7-7 Grasping the wrist of the hand positioned on the chest is an alternate hand position for giving chest compressions.

In most cases, the victim's clothing will not interfere with your ability to correctly position your hands on his or her chest. Sometimes a layer of thin clothing will help keep your hands from slipping, because the victim's chest may be moist with sweat. If you cannot find the correct hand position, bare the victim's chest. You should not be overly concerned that you may not be able to find the correct hand position if the victim is obese, because fat does not accumulate as much over the sternum as it does elsewhere.

Position of the Rescuer

Your body position is important when providing chest compressions. Compressing the victim's chest straight down provides the best blood flow. The correct body position is also less tiring for you.

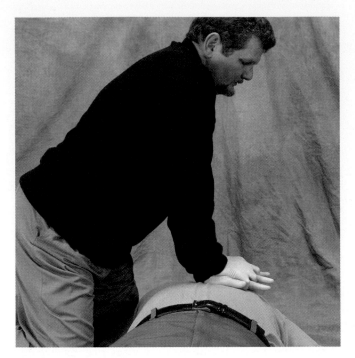

Figure 7-8 With your hands in place, position yourself so that your shoulders are directly over your hands, arms straight and elbows locked.

Kneel beside the victim with your hands in the correct position. Straighten your arms and lock your elbows so that your shoulders are directly over your hands (**Fig. 7-8**). When you press down in this position, you will be pushing straight down onto the sternum. Locking your elbows keeps your arms straight and prevents you from tiring quickly.

Compressing the chest requires less effort in this position. When you press down, the weight of your upper body creates the force needed to compress the chest. Push with the weight of your upper body, not with your arm muscles. Push straight down. Do not rock back and forth. Rocking results in less effective compressions and wastes much needed energy. If your arms and shoulders tire quickly, you are not using the correct body position. After each compression, release the pressure on the chest without removing your hands or changing hand position and allow the chest to return to its normal position before starting the next compression (**Fig. 7-9**).

Compression Technique

Each compression should push the sternum down from 1½ to 2 inches. The downward and upward movement should be smooth, not jerky. Maintain a

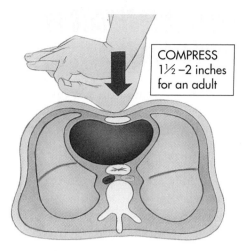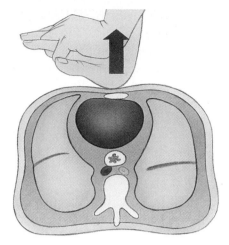

COMPRESS
1½ –2 inches
for an adult

Figure 7-9 Push straight down with the weight of your body, then release, allowing the chest to return to the normal position.

steady down-and-up rhythm, and do not pause between compressions. Spend half of the time pushing down and half of the time coming up. When you press down, the walls of the heart squeeze together, forcing the blood to empty out of the heart. When you come up, release all pressure on the chest. This release lets the chambers of the heart fill with blood between compressions. Keep your hands in their correct position on the sternum. If your hands slip, find the notch as you did before, and

reposition your hands correctly before continuing compressions.

Give compressions at the rate of about 100 per minute. As you do compressions, count aloud, "One and two and three and four and five and six and . . ." up to 30. Counting aloud will help you pace yourself. Push down as you say the number and come up as you say "and." You should be able to do the 30 compressions in about 18 seconds. Even though you are compressing the chest at a rate of about 100 times per minute, you will not actually perform 100 compressions in a minute, because you must stop compressions and give 2 breaths between each set of 30 compressions.

Compression/Breathing Cycles

When you perform CPR, give cycles of 30 compressions and 2 breaths. For each cycle, give 30 chest compressions, then open the airway with the head-tilt/chin-lift technique and give 2 rescue breaths (**Fig. 7-10**). For each new cycle of compressions and breaths, find the correct hand position in the middle of the chest.

Special Considerations

Multiple Responders

If two responders trained in CPR are at the scene, you should both identify yourselves as CPR-trained responders. One of you should call 9-1-1 or the lo-

Figure 7-10 Give 30 compressions, then 2 breaths.

cal emergency number for help, if this has not been done, while the other provides CPR. If the first responder is tired and needs help, the first responder should tell the second responder to take over. The second responder should immediately begin CPR, starting with chest compressions.

When to Stop CPR

Once you begin CPR, you should try not to interrupt the blood flow being created by your compressions. However, you can stop CPR if—

▸ The scene becomes unsafe.
▸ The victim shows obvious signs of life.
▸ An AED becomes available and is ready to use.
▸ Another trained rescuer arrives and takes over.
▸ You are too exhausted to continue.

If the victim shows an obvious sign of life, keep the airway open and monitor ABCs closely until EMS personnel arrive.

CARDIAC EMERGENCIES IN CHILDREN AND INFANTS

Unlike adults, children do not often initially suffer a cardiac emergency. In general, a child or infant suffers a respiratory emergency; then a cardiac emergency develops. Motor vehicle crashes, drowning, smoke inhalation, poisoning, airway obstruction, firearm injuries and falls are all common causes of respiratory emergencies that can develop into a cardiac emergency. A cardiac emergency can also result from an acute respiratory condition, such as an asthma attack and severe epiglottitis. If you recognize that an infant or child is in respiratory distress or respiratory arrest, give the care you learned in Chapter 6.

CPR FOR CHILDREN AND INFANTS

As with an adult, for an infant or child, use the emergency action steps: **CHECK—CALL—CARE** to determine if you need to perform CPR. Because

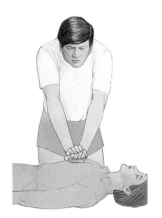
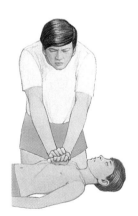
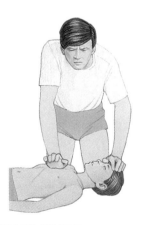
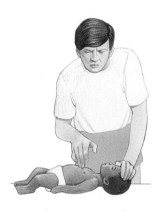

CPR SKILL COMPARISON CHART

Skill Components	Adult	Child	Infant
HAND POSITION:	Two hands in center of chest (on lower half of sternum)	One or two hands in center of chest (on lower half of sternum)	Two or three fingers on lower half of chest (one finger width below nipple line)
COMPRESS:	1½ to 2 inches	1 to 1½ inches	½ to 1 inch
BREATHE:	Until the chest rises (about 1 second per breath)	Until the chest rises (about 1 second per breath)	Until the chest rises (about 1 second per breath)
CYCLE:	30 compressions 2 breaths	30 compressions 2 breaths	30 compressions 2 breaths
RATE:	30 compressions in about 18 seconds (100 compressions per minute)	30 compressions in about 18 seconds (100 compressions per minute)	30 compressions in about 18 seconds (100 compressions per minute)

Figure 7-11   The technique for CPR differs slightly for adults, children and infants.

infants and children have smaller bodies and faster breathing and heart rates, the CPR techniques you use will be different. You must adjust your hand position, the rate of compressions and the number of compressions and breaths in each cycle. **Figure 7-11** compares CPR techniques for adults, children and infants.

CPR for a Child

To find out if an unconscious child needs CPR, begin by checking for life-threatening conditions. If you find that the child shows no signs of life (movement and breathing) and no pulse, begin CPR by performing chest compressions. To perform chest compressions—

▸ Locate the proper hand position on the middle of the chest as you would for an adult.
▸ Alternately, you can use a one-handed technique by placing one hand on the child's chest and the other hand on the forehead to maintain an open airway.
▸ Place the shoulder(s) over the hand(s).
▸ Compress the chest smoothly to a depth of about 1½ inches using the heel of the hand (**Fig. 7-12**).
  • Lift up, allowing the chest to fully return to its normal position, but keep contact with the chest.
  • Repeat compressions, performing 30 compressions in about 18 seconds.

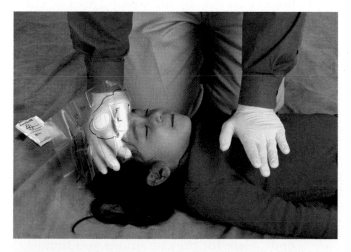

Figure 7-12 Alternate 1-handed technique: Place one hand on the child's chest and the other hand on the forehead to maintain an open airway.

After giving 30 compressions, remove your compression hand(s) from the chest, lift the chin and give 2 rescue breaths. The breaths should last about 1 second. Use the head-tilt/chin-lift technique to ensure that the child's airway is open. After giving the breath, place your hand(s) in the same position as before and continue compressions.

Keep repeating the cycles of 30 compressions and 2 rescue breaths. Continue CPR until an AED becomes available and ready, EMS or another trained responder arrives and takes over or the child shows obvious signs of life.

CPR for an Infant

To find out if an infant needs CPR, begin by checking for life-threatening conditions. Start by checking the infant's signs of life. If the infant shows no signs of life (movement and breathing) and no pulse, begin CPR by performing chest compressions. Position the infant face-up on a firm, flat surface. The infant's head must be on the same level as the heart or lower. Stand or kneel facing the infant from the side. *Bare the infant's chest.* Keep the hand on the infant's head to maintain an open airway. Use the fingers of your other hand to give compressions.

To find the correct location for compressions—

▸ Think of an imaginary line running across the chest between the nipples (**Fig. 7-13, A**).
▸ Place the pads of two or three fingers just below the imaginary line on the sternum. If you feel the notch at the end of the infant's sternum, move your fingers up a bit (**Fig. 7-13, B**).
▸ Use the pads of two or three fingers to compress the chest. Compress the chest ½ to 1 inch. Push straight down. Your compressions should be smooth, not jerky (**Fig. 7-13, C**).
▸ Keep a steady rhythm. Do not pause between compressions except to give breaths. When your fingers are coming up, release pressure on the infant's chest completely, but do not let your fingers lose contact with the chest. Compress at a rate of *about* 100 compressions per minute. That rate is slightly faster than the rate of compressions for a child.

When you complete 30 compressions, give 2 rescue breaths, covering the infant's nose and mouth with your mouth. The breath should take about 1 second. Keep repeating cycles of 30 compressions and 2 breaths.

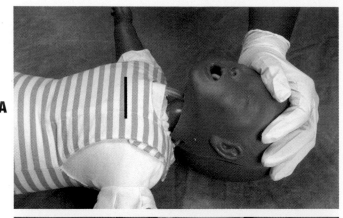

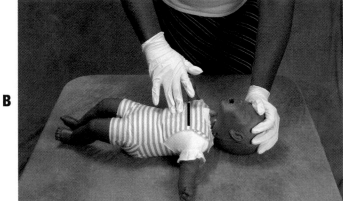

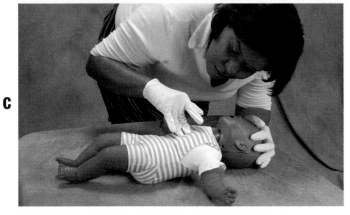

Figure 7-13   To locate compression position: **A,** imagine a line running across the chest between the infant's nipples. **B,** Place the pads of two or three fingers in the middle of the chest. **C,** Use the pads of the fingers to compress the chest.

Continue CPR until EMS or another trained responder arrives and takes over or the child shows obvious signs of life.

UNCONSCIOUS CHOKING—
ADULT OR CHILD

During your check for life-threatening conditions, you may discover that an unconscious victim is not breathing and the 2 rescue breaths you give do not go in. In this case, reposition the victim's airway and give 2 breaths again. You may not have tilted the victim's head far enough back the first time. If the breaths still will not go in, assume that the victim's airway is obstructed. To care for a unconscious adult or child with an airway obstruction—

1. Locate the correct hand position for chest compressions. Use the same techniques that you learned in CPR.
2. Remove breathing barrier when giving chest compressions. Perform chest compressions. Compress an adult's chest to a depth of about 2 inches 30 times in about 18 seconds. Compress a child's chest to a depth of about 1½ inches 30 times in about 18 seconds (**Fig 7-14, A**).
3. Look for a foreign object. Open the victim's mouth. Look inside the victim's mouth for a foreign object. If you see an object, remove it with your finger (**Fig. 7-14, B**).
4. Give 2 rescue breaths (**Fig. 7-14, C**). If the breaths do not go in, repeat cycles of chest compressions, foreign object check and 2 rescue breaths until—
   • The scene becomes unsafe.
   • The object is removed and the chest clearly rises with rescue breaths.
   • The victim starts to breathe on his or her own.
   • EMS personnel or another trained responder arrives and takes over.
   • You are too exhausted to continue.
5. If the breaths go in and the chest clearly rises, check for signs of life (including a pulse for children) for no more than 10 seconds. Care for the conditions you find.

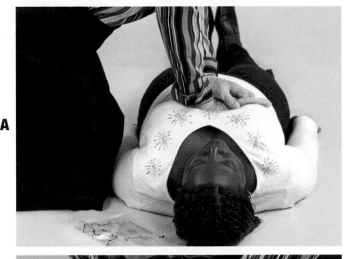

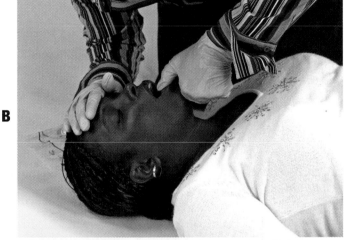

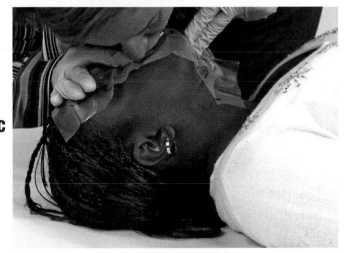

Figure 7-14   A, Compress an adult's chest about 2 inches 30 times in about 18 seconds. Compress a child's chest about 1½ inches 30 times in about 18 seconds. **B,** Look for a foreign object. If you see an object, remove it with your finger. **C,** Give 2 rescue breaths.

UNCONSCIOUS CHOKING—INFANT

If you determine an infant is unconscious, not breathing and you cannot get air into the lungs, reposition the airway by retilting the head and give 2 more rescue breaths. If you still cannot get air into the infant, assume that the airway is obstructed. To care for a unconscious infant with an airway obstruction—

1. Locate the correct hand position for chest compressions (**Fig. 7-15, A**). Use the same techniques that you learned in CPR.
2. Remove breathing barrier when giving chest compressions. Give 30 chest compressions (**Fig. 7-15, B**). Each compression should be about ½ to 1 inch deep.
3. Look for a foreign object. If the object is seen, remove it using your little finger (**Fig 7-15, C**).
4. Give 2 rescue breaths. If the breaths do not go in, repeat cycles of chest compressions, foreign object check and 2 rescue breaths until—
   - The scene becomes unsafe.
   - The object is removed and the chest clearly rises with rescue breaths.
   - The infant starts to breathe on his or her own.
   - EMS personnel or another trained responder arrives and takes over.
   - You are too exhausted to continue.
5. If the breath goes in and the chest clearly rises, check for signs of life (including a pulse) for no more than 10 seconds. Care for the conditions you find.

AUTOMATED EXTERNAL DEFIBRILLATORS (AED)

As stated earlier, most victims of sudden cardiac arrest need an electric shock called **defibrillation.** Each minute that defibrillation is delayed reduces the chance of survival by about 10 percent. Therefore, the sooner the shock is administered, the greater the likelihood of the victim's survival. By learning how to use an **automated external de-**

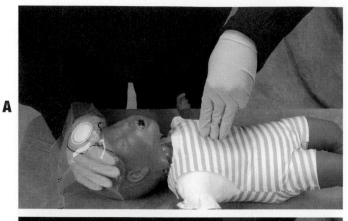

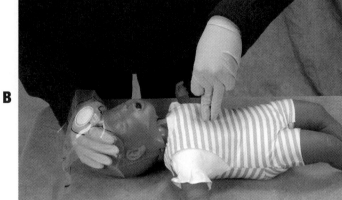

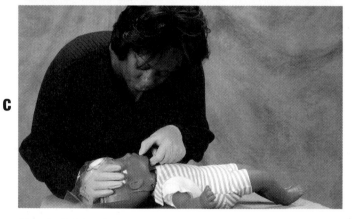

Figure 7-15 To care for an unconscious choking infant, **A,** find the correct position for chest compressions. **B,** Compress the chest 30 times about ½ to 1 inch deep. **C,** Look for an object in the mouth by lifting the jaw. If you see an object, remove it with your little finger.

fibrillator (AED), you can make a difference before EMS personnel arrive.

The Heart's Electrical System

The heart's electrical system controls its pumping action. In normal conditions, specialized cells of the heart initiate and transmit electrical impulses. These

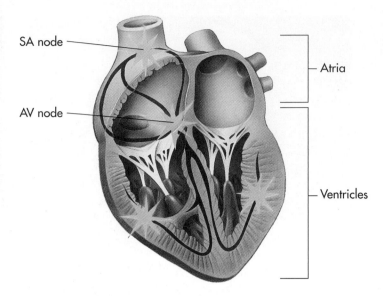

Figure 7-16 The heart's electrical system.

cells make up the conduction system. Electrical impulses travel through the upper chambers of the heart, called the atria, to the lower chambers of the heart, called the ventricles (**Fig. 7-16**).

The normal point of origin of the electrical impulse is the sinoatrial (SA) node above the atria. This impulse travels to a point midway between the atria and ventricles. This point is called the atrioventricular (AV) node. The pathway divides after the AV node into two branches, the right and left ventricles. These right and left branches become a network of fibers, called Purkinje fibers, which spread electrical impulses across the heart. Under normal conditions, this impulse reaches the muscular walls of the ventricles and causes the ventricles to contract. This contraction forces blood out of the heart to circulate through the body. The contraction of the left ventricle results in a pulse. The pauses between the pulse beats are the periods between contractions. When the heart muscles contract, blood is forced out of the heart. When they relax, blood refills the chambers.

Electrical activity of the heart can be evaluated with a cardiac monitor or electrocardiograph. Electrodes attached to an electrocardiograph pick up electrical impulses and transmit them to a monitor. This graphic record is referred to as an electrocardiogram (ECG). Heart rhythms appear on an ECG as a series of peaks and valleys.

When the Heart Fails

Any damage to the heart from disease or injury can disrupt the heart's electrical system. This disruption can result in an abnormal heart rhythm that can stop circulation. The two most common abnormal rhythms that initially present in sudden cardiac arrest victims are *ventricular fibrillation (V-fib)* and *ventricular tachycardia (V-tach)*. V-fib is a state of totally disorganized electrical activity in the heart. It results in fibrillation, or quivering, of the ventricles. In this state, the ventricles cannot pump blood and there are no signs of life, including no pulse for a child or infant. V-tach refers to a very rapid contraction of the ventricles. Although there is electrical activity resulting in a regular rhythm, the rate is often so fast that the heart is unable to pump blood properly. As with V-fib, there are no signs of life, including no pulse.

The Amazing Heart

Too often, we take our hearts for granted. The heart beats about 70 times each minute or more than 100,000 times a day. During an average lifetime, the heart will beat nearly 3 billion times. The heart circulates about a gallon of blood per minute or about 40 million gallons in an average lifetime. The heart circulates blood through about 60,000 miles of blood vessels.

Defibrillation

In many cases, V-fib and V-tach rhythms can be corrected by early defibrillation. Delivering an electrical shock with an AED disrupts the electrical activity of V-fib and V-tach long enough to allow the heart to spontaneously develop an effective rhythm on its own. If V-fib or V-tach is not interrupted, all electrical activity will eventually cease, a condition called *asystole*. Asystole cannot be corrected by defibrillation. Remember that you cannot tell what rhythm, if any, the heart has by checking for signs of life. CPR, started immediately and continued until defibrillation, helps maintain a low level of circulation in the body until the abnormal rhythm can be corrected by defibrillation.

USING AN AED—ADULT

With cardiac arrest, an AED should be used as soon as it is available and safe to do so. Be sure to call 9-1-1 or the local emergency number. CPR in progress is stopped only when the AED is ready to use. Most AEDs can be operated by following these simple steps:

1. Turn on the AED (**Fig. 7-17, A**).
2. Wipe the victim's chest dry. Apply the pads to the victim's bare chest (**Fig. 7-17, B**). Place one pad on the victim's upper right chest and the other pad on the victim's lower left side. Plug the connector into the AED.
3. Let the AED analyze the heart rhythm (**Fig. 7-17, C**) (or push the button marked "analyze," if indicated and prompted by the AED). Advise all responders and bystanders to "Stand clear." Do not touch the victim. If the AED tells you "No shock advised," begin CPR.
4. Deliver a shock by pushing the button if indicated and prompted by the AED (**Fig. 7-17, D**). Ensure that no one, including you, is touching the victim and that there are no hazards present.

In some cases, defibrillation is not required and the AED will not prompt you to deliver a shock. If no shock is indicated, give CPR. Leave the AED attached to the victim. The skill sheets at the end of this chapter provide step-by-step practice of using an AED.

AED Precautions

When operating an AED, you should avoid certain actions and situations that could harm you, other responders or bystanders and the victim. The

A Matter of Choice

Instructions that describe a person's wishes about medical treatment are called advance directives. These instructions are used when a person can no longer make his or her own health-care decisions. If a person is able to make decisions about medical treatment, advance directives do not interfere with his or her right to do so.

The Patient Self-Determination Act of 1990 provides that adults who are admitted to a hospital or a health-care facility or who receive assistance from certain organizations that receive funds from Medicare or Medicaid have the right to make fundamental choices about their own care. They must be told about their right to make decisions and about the level of life support that would be provided in an emergency situation. They should be of-

fered the opportunity to make these choices at the time of admission.

Conversations with relatives, friends or physicians, while the patient is still capable of making decisions, are the most common form of advance directives. However, because conversations may not be recalled accurately, the courts consider written directives more credible.

Two examples of written advance directives are living wills and durable powers of attorney for health care. The types of health-care decisions covered by these documents vary depending on the state where you live. Talking with a legal professional can help determine which advance directive options are recognized in your state and what they do and do not cover.

The instructions that are permitted in a living will vary from state to state. A living will generally allows a person to refuse only medical care that "merely prolongs the process of dying," as in the case of a terminal illness.

A person uses a durable power of attorney for health care to authorize someone to make medical decisions for him or her in any situation in which he or she can no longer make them. This authorized person is called a health-care surrogate or proxy. This surrogate, with the information given by the patient's physician, may consent to or refuse medical treatment on the patient's behalf. In this case, he or she would support the patient's needs and wishes around the health-care decisions and the advance directives.

"Do not resuscitate" (DNR) orders mean that if a person has determined that if his or her heartbeat or breathing stops, he or she should not be resuscitated. The choice of DNR orders may be covered in a living will or in the durable power of attorney for health care.

Appointing someone to act as a health-care surrogate, along with writing down your instructions, is the best way to formalize your wishes about medical care. Some of these documents can be obtained through a personal physician, an attorney or various state and health-care organizations.

A lawyer is not always needed to execute advance directives. However, if you have any questions concerning advance directives, it is wise to obtain legal advice.

Copies of your advance directives should be provided to all personal physicians, family members and the person chosen as your health-care surrogate. Tell them what documents have been prepared and where the original and copies are located. Discuss the document with all parties so that they understand the intent of all the requests. Keep these documents updated.

Keep in mind that advance directives are not limited to elderly persons or people with terminal illnesses. Advance directives should be considered by anyone who has decided on the care he or she would like to have provided. An unexpected illness or injury could create a need for decisions at any time.

Knowing about living wills, durable powers of attorney for health care and DNR orders can help you and your loved ones prepare for difficult decisions. If you are interested in learning more about your rights and the options available to you in your state, contact a legal professional.

SOURCES

Hospital Shared Services of Colorado, Stockard Inventory Program: *Your right to make health care decisions,* Denver, 1991.2.

Title 42 United States Code, Section 1395 cc(a)(1)(Q)(A) Patient Self-Determination Act.

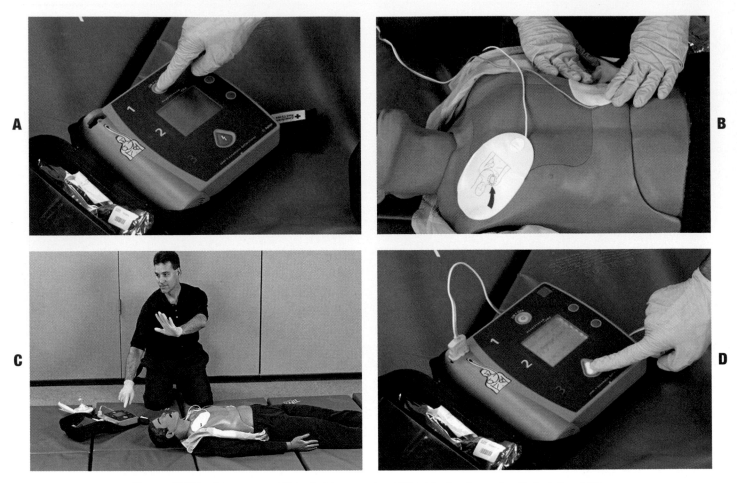

Figure 7-17   To use an AED: **A,** Turn on the AED. **B,** Apply pads. **C,** Let the AED analyze the heart rhythm. **D,** Deliver a shock if indicated.

following precautions should be taken when operating an AED:

▶ Do not touch the victim while the AED is analyzing. Touching or moving the victim may affect analysis.

▶ Do not touch the victim while the AED is defibrillating. You or others could be shocked.

▶ Do not use alcohol to wipe the victim's chest dry. Alcohol is flammable.

▶ Do not defibrillate someone around flammable or combustible materials, such as gasoline or free-flowing oxygen.

▶ Do not use an AED in a moving vehicle. Movement may affect the analysis.

▶ Do not use an AED on a victim in contact with water. Move the victim away from puddles of water or swimming pools, or out of the rain before defibrillating.

▶ Do not use an AED and/or electrode pads designed for adult victims on a child younger than age 8 or weighing less than 55 pounds unless pediatric pads specific to the device are not available. Local protocols may differ on this and should be followed.

▶ Do not use an AED on a victim wearing a nitroglycerin patch or other patch on the chest. With a gloved hand, remove any patches from the chest before attaching the device.

▶ Do not use a mobile phone or conduct radio transmissions within 6 feet of the AED. This may interrupt analysis.

Special Resuscitation Situations

Some situations require you to pay special attention when using an AED. Be familiar with these situations and know how to respond appropriately.

Always use common sense when using an AED and follow the manufacturer's recommendations.

AEDs Around Water

If a victim has been removed from water, remove wet clothing, if possible. Dry the victim's chest and attach the AED. The victim should not be in a puddle of water, nor should the rescuer be kneeling in a puddle of water when operating an AED.

If it is raining, take steps to ensure that the victim is as dry as possible and sheltered from the rain. Ensure that the victim's chest is wiped dry. Minimize delaying defibrillation, though, when taking steps to provide for a dry environment. The electrical current of an AED is very directional between the electrode pads. AEDs are very safe, even in rain and snow, when all precautions and manufacturer's operating instructions are followed.

AEDs and Implantable Devices

Some people whose hearts are weak and not able to generate electrical impulse may have had a pacemaker implanted. These small implantable devices may sometimes be located in the area below the right collarbone. There may be a small lump that can be felt under the skin. Sometimes the pacemaker is placed somewhere else. Other individuals may have an implantable cardioverter-defibrillator (ICD), a miniature version of an AED, which acts to automatically recognize and restore abnormal heart rhythms. If visible or you know that the victim has an implanted device, do not place the defibrillation pads directly over the implanted device. This may interfere with the delivery of the shock. Adjust pad placement if necessary, and continue to follow the established protocol. If you are not sure, use the AED if needed. It will not harm the victim or rescuer.

AEDs and Nitroglycerin Patches

People with a history of cardiac problems may use nitroglycerin patches (**Fig. 7-18**). These patches are usually placed on the chest. If you encounter a victim with a patch on his or her chest, remove it with a gloved hand. Nitroglycerin patches pose a possible absorption risk for rescuers, not an explosion hazard. Nitroglycerin patches look very similar to nicotine patches that people use to stop smoking.

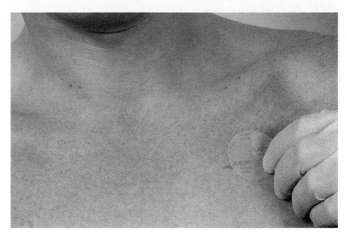

Figure 7-18   Look for medication patches.

Although these patches do not interfere with defibrillation, time may be wasted attempting to identify the type of patch. Therefore, any medication patches that are on the victim's chest should be removed.

Hypothermia

Victims of hypothermia have been resuscitated successfully even after prolonged exposure. It will take longer to do your check, or assessment, of the victim since you may have to check for signs of life and/or a pulse for up to 30 to 45 seconds. If you do not feel a pulse, begin CPR until an AED becomes readily available. If the victim is wet, dry his or her chest and attach the AED. If a shock is indicated, deliver a shock. If there is still no pulse, continue CPR. Follow local protocols as to whether additional shocks should be delivered. Continue CPR and protect the victim from further heat loss. CPR or defibrillation should not be withheld to rewarm the victim. Rescuers should take care not to shake a hypothermia victim unnecessarily as this could result in ventricular fibrillation.

Trauma and AEDs

If a person is in cardiac arrest resulting from traumatic injuries, an AED may still be used. Defibrillation should be administered according to local protocols.

AED Maintenance

For defibrillators to perform optimally, they must be maintained like any other machine. The AEDs that are available today require minimal maintenance. These devices have various self-testing features. However, it is important that operators are familiar with any visual or audible warning prompts the AED may have to warn of malfunction or a low battery. It is important that you read the operator's manual thoroughly and check with the manufacturer to obtain all necessary information regarding maintenance.

In most instances, if the machine detects any malfunction, you should contact the manufacturer. The device may need to be returned to the manufacturer for service. While AEDs require minimal maintenance, it is important to remember the following:

▸ Follow the manufacturer's specific recommendations for periodic equipment checks.

▸ Make sure that the batteries have enough energy for one complete rescue. (A fully charged backup battery should be readily available.)

▸ Make sure that the correct defibrillator pads are in the package and are properly sealed.

▸ Check any expiration dates on defibrillation pads and batteries and replace as necessary.

▸ After use, make sure that all accessories are replaced and that the machine is in proper working order.

▸ If at any time the machine fails to work properly or warning indicators are recognized, discontinue use and contact the manufacturer immediately.

USING AN AED—CHILD

Most cardiac arrest in children is not sudden. The most common causes of cardiac arrest in children are—airway problems, breathing problems, trauma or an accident (such as automobile accident, drowning, electrocution or poisoning), a hard blow to the chest (such as *Commotio Cordis*), congenital heart disease or sudden infant death syndrome (SIDS). AEDs equipped with pediatric AED pads are capable of delivering lower levels of energy to a victim between 1 and 8 years of age or weighing less than 55 pounds. Use the same general steps and precautions that you would when using an AED on an adult victim.

1. Turn on the AED.
2. Apply the pads to the child's chest.
   - Make sure that you are using pediatric AED pads.
   - Wipe the child's chest dry.
   - Place one pad on the child's upper right chest and the other pad on the child's lower left side (**Fig. 7-19, A**).
   - Make sure the pads are not touching. If the pads are at risk of touching each other, place one pad on the child's chest

A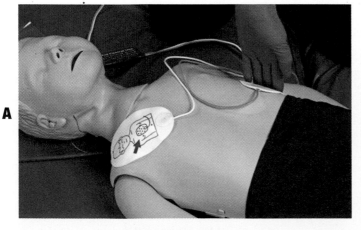

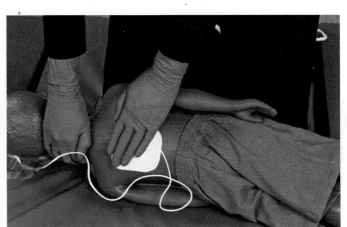 B

Figure 7-19 **A,** Place one pad on the child's upper right chest and the other pad on the child lower left side, or **B,** place one pad on the child's chest and the other pad on the child's back.

and the other pad on the child's back (**Fig. 7-19, *B***).

3. Plug the connector into the AED.

4. Let the AED analyze the heart rhythm (or push the "analyze" button if indicated and prompted by the AED).
   - Advise all responders and bystanders to "stand clear." Do not touch the child.

5. Deliver a shock by pushing the "shock" button if indicated and prompted by the AED. Ensure that no one is touching the child, including you, and that there are no hazards present (such as standing puddles of water).

- If the AED tells you "No shock advised," give 5 cycles (or about 2 minutes) of CPR.

SUMMARY

Cardiac emergencies present a major health threat to our communities. By learning to recognize the signals of cardiac emergencies and how to give care, you can make a difference.

APPLICATION QUESTIONS

1. Could atherosclerosis have led to Mr. Getz's collapse?

2. If Mr. Getz had experienced chest pain, how might stopping and resting have prevented his collapse?

3. Is it possible that Mr. Getz may have suffered a cardiac arrest? Why or why not?

4. Why is it important to know if Mr. Getz may be suffering cardiac arrest?

5. If Mr. Getz is in cardiac arrest, why will CPR alone not sustain his life?

STUDY QUESTIONS

1. Match each term with the correct definition.

   a. Cardiac arrest
   b. Cardiopulmonary
      resuscitation (CPR)
   c. Cholesterol
   d. Coronary arteries

   e. Heart
   f. Heart attack
   g. Cardiovascular disease
   h. Angina pectoris

   _____ A muscular organ that circulates blood throughout the body.

   _____ A fatty substance that builds up on the inner walls of arteries.

   _____ The leading cause of death for men and women in the United States.

   _____ Temporary chest pain caused by a lack of oxygen to the heart.

   _____ Blood vessels that supply the heart with oxygen-rich blood.

   _____ A combination of chest compressions and rescue breaths.

   _____ Condition that results when the heart stops beating or beats too ineffectively to circulate blood.

   _____ A sudden illness involving the death of heart muscle tissue caused by insufficient oxygen-rich blood reaching the cells.

2. Identify the signals of cardiac arrest.

3. List the situations in which a citizen responder may stop CPR.

4. Describe the conditions that most often cause cardiac arrest in children and infants.

In questions 5 through 12, circle the letter of the correct answer.

5. Which is the most common signal of a heart attack?

   a. Profuse sweating
   b. Persistent chest pain
   c. Pale skin
   d. Trouble breathing

6. Which of the following best describes the chest pain associated with heart attack?

   a. An uncomfortable pressure
   b. Persistent pain that may spread to the shoulder, arm, neck or jaw
   c. Throbbing pain in the legs
   d. a and b

7. What may happen as a result of a heart attack?

   a. The heart functions inadequately.
   b. The heart may stop.
   c. Some heart muscle tissue may die from lack of oxygen.
   d. All of the above.

8. Which should you do first to care effectively for a person having a heart attack?

   a. Position the victim for CPR.
   b. Begin rescue breathing.
   c. Call 9-1-1 or the local emergency number immediately.
   d. Call the person's physician.

9. How can you know if a person's heart is beating?

   a. The person is breathing.
   b. The person shows another sign of life.
   c. The person is conscious.
   d. Any or all of the above.

10. When is CPR needed for an adult?

   a. When the victim is conscious
   b. For every heart attack victim
   c. When the victim shows no signs of life
   d. When the heart attack victim loses consciousness

11. Which is the purpose of CPR?

   a. To keep a victim's airway open
   b. To identify any immediate threats to life
   c. To supply the vital organs with blood containing oxygen
   d. All of the above

12. CPR artificially takes over the functions of which two body systems?

   a. Nervous and respiratory systems
   b. Respiratory and circulatory systems
   c. Circulatory and nervous systems
   d. Circulatory and musculoskeletal systems

Use the following scenario to answer questions 13 and 14:

It is Saturday afternoon; you and your mother are at home watching a tennis match on television. At the commercial break, your mother mumbles something about indigestion and heads to the medicine cabinet to get an antacid. Twenty minutes later, you notice that your mom does not respond to a great play made by her favorite player. You ask what is wrong, and she complains that the antacid has not worked. She states that her chest and shoulder hurt. She is sweating heavily. You notice that she is breathing fast and she looks ill.

13. List the signals of a heart attack that you find in the scenario.

While waiting for EMS personnel to arrive, your mother loses consciousness.

14. Number in order the following actions you would now take.

_____ Open the airway and check for signs of life. *(There are none.)*

_____ Give 2 rescue breaths.

_____ Check for responsiveness.

_____ Correctly position your hands.

_____ Give cycles of 30 compressions and 2 breaths.

15. Number in order the following actions for giving care to an unconscious choking infant, starting from the time you first realize your breaths will not go in.

___5___ Give 30 chest compressions.

___1___ Check for an object.

___4/3___ Repeat 2 rescue breaths.

___6/2___ Reposition the infant's airway.

___2___ Remove an object if you see one.

Answers are listed in Appendix A.

SKILL SHEET CPR—Adult

Complete *"Checking an Unconscious Adult (Age 12 or Older)"* Steps 1-5 in Chapter 5, pages 76-77. *Remember: Always follow standard precautions to prevent disease transmission. Use protective equipment (disposable gloves and breathing barriers). Wash your hands immediately after giving care.*

Step 6

If the victim shows no signs of life—

Place the heel of one hand on the victim's sternum (breastbone) in the middle of the chest and place your other hand directly on top of the first hand.

Step 7

Position the shoulders over the hands.

- Compress the chest smoothly to a depth of about 2 inches—**30** times at a rate of about 100 compressions per minute.

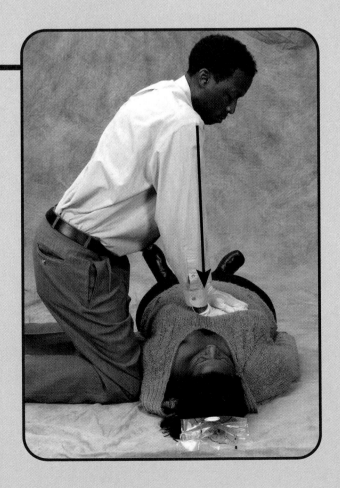

Step 8

Give **2** rescue breaths.

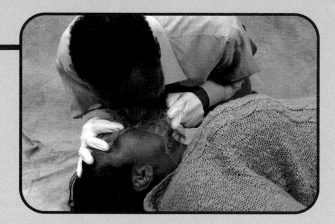

Step 9

Continue CPR.

Note: Continue CPR until—

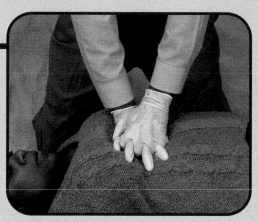

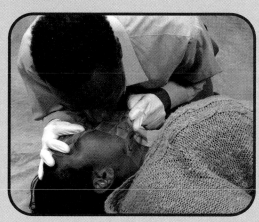

- The scene becomes unsafe.
- The victim shows an obvious sign of life.
- An AED becomes readily available and is ready to use.
- You are too exhausted to continue.
- EMS personnel arrive and take over.
- Another trained responder arrives and takes over.

If there are signs of life—
Keep the airway open and monitor the victim until EMS arrives and takes over.

SKILL SHEET   Unconscious Choking—Adult

Complete *"Checking an Unconscious Adult (Ages 12 or Older)"* Steps 1-5 in Chapter 5, pages 76-77. *Remember: Always follow standard precautions to prevent disease transmission. Use protective equipment (disposable gloves and breathing barriers). Wash your hands immediately after giving care.*

Step 6

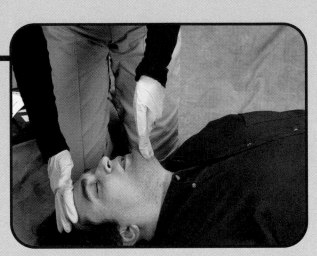

If the rescue breaths do not go in—

Reposition the victim's airway by tilting the head farther back and try 2 rescue breaths again.

If breaths still do not go in—

Step 7

Find the hand position in the middle of the chest.

Step 8

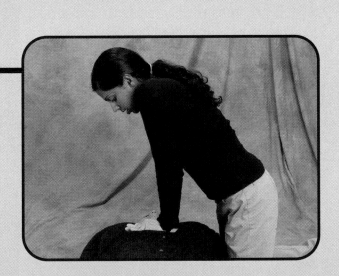

Position the shoulders over the hands.

• Compress the chest **30** times to a depth of about 2 inches.

Note: Remove any breathing barriers when giving chest compressions.

Step 9

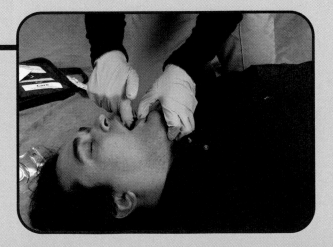

Lift the jaw and tongue and look inside the mouth.

• If you see an object, remove it with a finger.

Step 10

Try **2** rescue breaths.

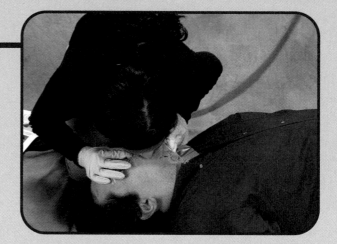

If the breaths still do not go in—

Step 11

Continue cycles of chest compressions, foreign object check and rescue breaths until—

* The scene becomes unsafe.
* The object is removed and the chest clearly rises with rescue breaths.
* The victim starts to breathe on his or her own.
* EMS personnel or another trained responder arrives and takes over.
* You are too exhausted to continue.

If breaths go in—

Step 12

Check for signs of life for no more than 10 seconds.

Step 13

If there are no signs of life—
Give CPR.

SKILL SHEET CPR—Child

Complete *"Checking an Unconscious Child (Ages 1 to 12)"* Steps 1-7 in Chapter 5, page 78. *Remember: Always follow standard precautions to prevent disease transmission. Use protective equipment (disposable gloves and breathing barriers). Wash your hands immediately after giving care.*

Step 8

If the child shows no signs of life and no pulse—
Find the hand position in the middle of the chest.

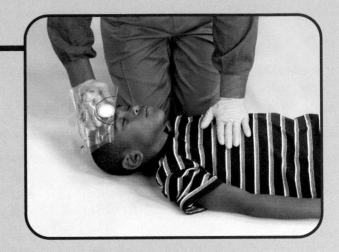

Step 9

Position the shoulders over the hands.

- Compress the chest **30** times smoothly to a depth of about 1½ inches.

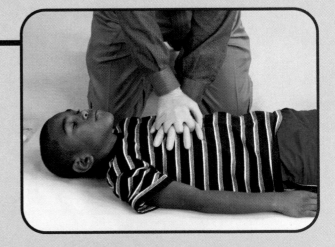

Step 10

Give **2** rescue breaths.

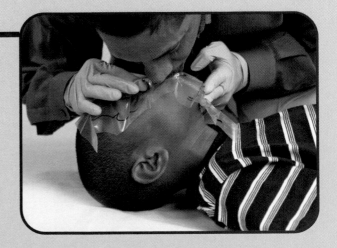

Step 11

Continue CPR.

Note: Continue CPR until—

- The scene becomes unsafe.
- The child shows obvious signs of life.
- An AED becomes readily available and is ready to use.
- You are too exhausted to continue.
- EMS personnel arrive and take over.
- Another trained responder arrives and takes over.

SKILL SHEET   Unconscious Choking—Child

Complete *"Checking an Unconscious Child (Ages 1 to 12)"* Steps 1-6 in Chapter 5, page 78.
Remember: Always follow standard precautions to prevent disease transmission. Use protective equipment (disposable gloves and breathing barriers). Wash your hands immediately after giving care.

Step 7

If the rescue breaths do not go in, reposition the child's airway. Place the child's head back into the neutral position, then attempt the head-tilt/chin-lift again.

• Try **2** rescue breaths again.

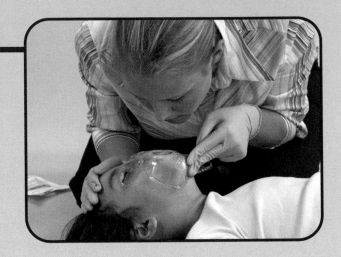

If breaths still do not go in—

Step 8

Find the hand position in the middle of the chest.

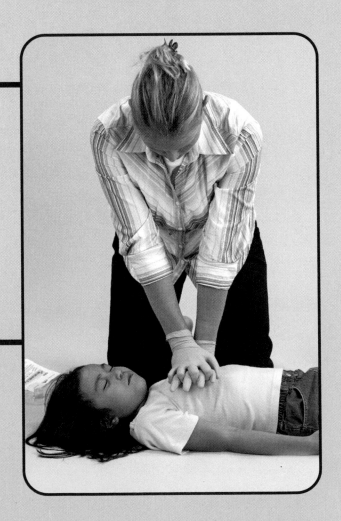

Step 9

Position your shoulders over the hands.

• Compress the chest **30** times to a depth of about 1½ inches—at a rate of about 100 compressions per minute.

Note: Remove any breathing barrier when giving chest compressions.

Step 10

Lift the jaw and tongue and look inside the mouth.

- If you see an object, remove it with a finger.

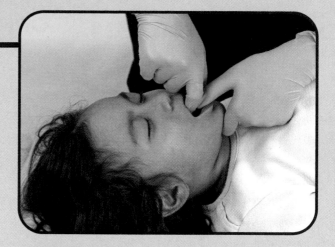

Step 11

Try **2** rescue breaths.

If the breaths still do not go in—

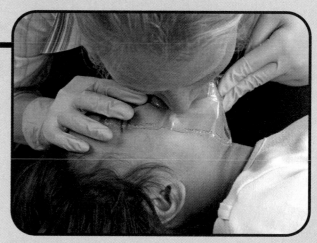

Step 12

Continue cycles of chest compressions, foreign object check and rescue breaths until—

- The scene becomes unsafe.
- The object is removed and the chest clearly rises with rescue breaths.
- The child starts to breathe on his or her own.
- EMS personnel or another trained responder arrives and takes over.
- You are too exhausted to continue.

If breaths go in—

Step 13

Check for signs of life and a pulse for no more than 10 seconds.

Step 14

If there is a pulse, but no breathing—
Give rescue breathing.

If there is no pulse—
Give CPR.

SKILL SHEET   CPR—Infant

Complete *"Checking an Unconscious Infant (Under Age 1),"* Steps 1-8 in Chapter 5, page 79.
Remember: Always follow standard precautions to prevent disease transmission. Use protective equipment (disposable gloves and breathing barriers). Wash your hands immediately after giving care.

Step 9

If the infant shows no signs of life and no pulse—
Find the finger position in the center of the chest over the breastbone.

- Place the other hand on the forehead to maintain an open airway.
- Place the pads of two or three fingers just below an imaginary line between the nipples.
- Place the pads of the two fingers next to your index finger on the sternum.

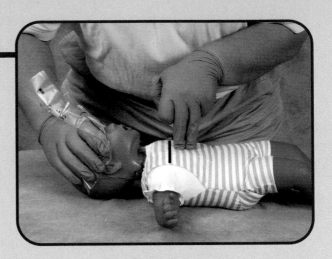

Step 10

Compress the chest smoothly to a depth of about ½ to 1 inch—**30** times at a rate of about 100 compressions per minute.

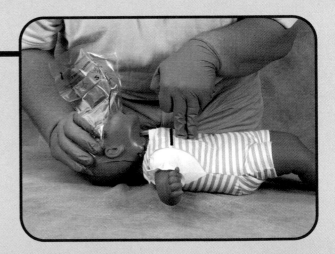

Step 11

Give **2** rescue breaths.

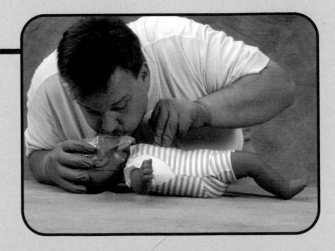

Step 12

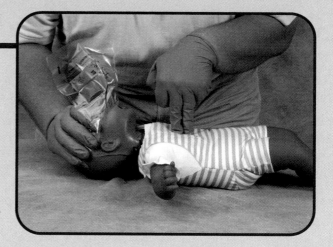

Continue CPR.

Note: Continue CPR until—
- The scene becomes unsafe.
- The infant shows obvious signs of life.
- You are too exhausted to continue.
- EMS personnel arrive and take over.
- Another trained responder arrives and takes over.

SKILL SHEET Unconscious Choking—Infant

Complete *"Checking an Unconscious Infant (Under Age 1)"* Steps 1-7 in Chapter 5, page 79.
Remember: Always follow standard precautions to prevent disease transmission. Use protective equipment (disposable gloves and breathing barriers). Wash your hands immediately after giving care.

Step 8

If the rescue breaths do not go in, reposition the infant's airway by placing the infant's head back into the neutral position, then attempting the head-tilt/chin-lift again. Try 2 rescue breaths again.

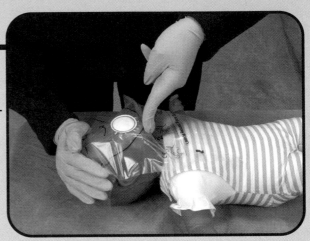

If breaths still do not go in—

Step 9

Find the finger position in the center of the chest over the breastbone.

- Place the pads of two or three fingers just below an imaginary line between the nipples.
- Place the pads of these fingers next to your index finger on the middle of the chest (sternum).
- Place the other hand on the forehead to maintain an open airway.

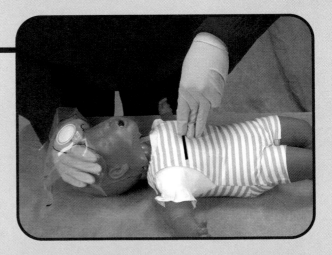

Step 10

Compress the chest smoothly to a depth of about ½ to 1 inch—**30** times at a rate of about 100 compressions per minute.

Note: Remove any breathing barrier when giving chest compressions.

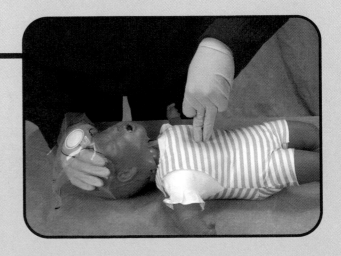

Step 11

Lift the jaw and tongue and look inside the mouth.

- If you see an object, remove it with your little finger.

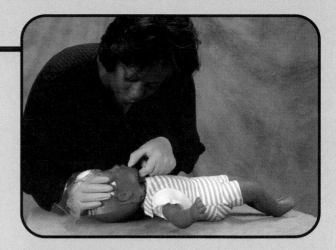

Step 12

Try **2** rescue breaths.

If the breaths still do not go in—

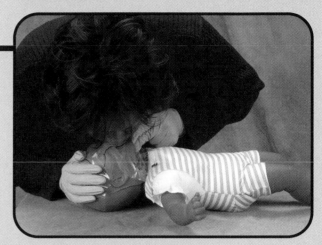

Step 13

Continue cycles of chest compressions, foreign object check and rescue breaths until—

- The scene becomes unsafe.
- The object is removed and the chest clearly rises with rescue breaths.
- The infant starts to breathe on his or her own.
- EMS personnel or another trained responder arrives and takes over.
- You are too exhausted to continue.

If the breaths go in—

Step 14

Check for signs of life and a pulse for no more than 10 seconds.

Step 15

If there is a pulse, but no breathing—
Give rescue breathing.

If there is no pulse—
Give CPR.

SKILL SHEET

Using an AED—Adult (over age 8 or more than 55 pounds)

Complete *"Checking an Unconscious Adult"* Steps 1-5 in Chapter 5, pages 76-77. *Remember: Always follow standard precautions to prevent disease transmission. Use protective equipment (disposable gloves and breathing barriers). Wash your hands immediately after giving care.*

If the victim shows no signs of life—

Step 6

Turn on the AED and prepare it for use.

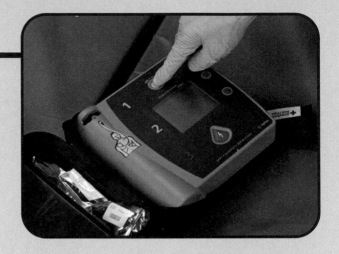

Step 7

Wipe the victim's chest dry.

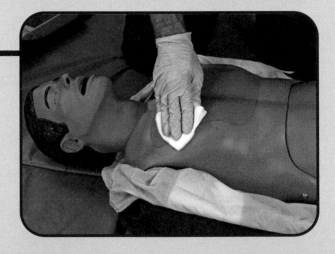

Step 8

Attach the AED pads to the victim.

- Peel the backing off one pad at a time and, following the diagram, press the pad firmly to the victim's bare skin.
- Place one pad on the victim's upper right chest and other pad on the lower left side.
- Plug in connector, if necessary.

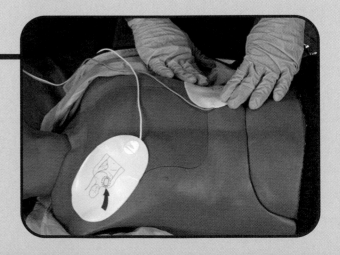

Step 9

Make sure no one, including you, is touching the victim.

• Say, "EVERYONE, STAND CLEAR!"

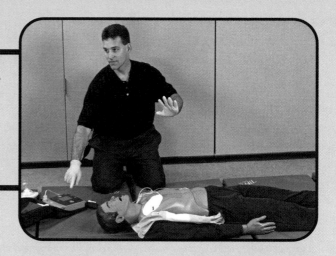

Step 10

Allow the AED to analyze the heart's rhythm.

Step 11

Make sure no one, including you, is touching the victim.

Say, "EVERYONE, STAND CLEAR!"

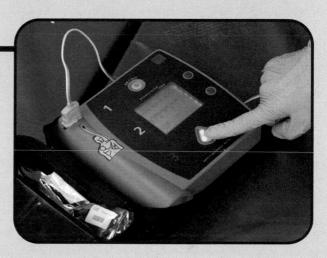

• Deliver a shock if prompted by pushing the "shock" button.

• Give **5** cycles, or about **2** minutes of CPR unless there are obvious signs of life. Let AED reanalyze. If no shock advised, give 5 cycles or about 2 minutes of CPR.

Note: When there are no signs of life and an AED is on the way, give CPR until the AED is ready to use. When the AED arrives, turn it on and follow Steps 6 through 11.

SKILL SHEET

Using an AED—Child (child ages 1-8 or less than 55 pounds)

Complete *"Checking an Unconscious Child"* Steps 1-7 in Chapter 5, page 78. *Remember: Always follow standard precautions to prevent disease transmission. Use protective equipment (disposable gloves and breathing barriers). Wash your hands immediately after giving care.*

If the child shows no signs of life and no pulse—

Step 8

Turn on the AED and prepare it for use.

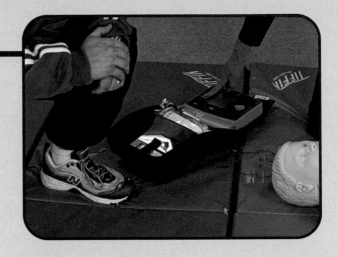

Step 9

Wipe the child's chest dry.

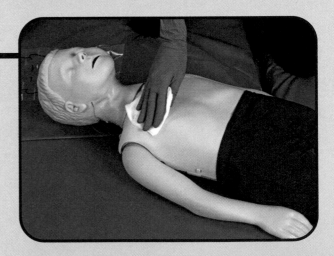

Step 10

Attach the pediatric AED pads to the child.

- Check to be certain that you are using pediatric pads.
- Peel the backing off one pad at a time and, following the diagram, press the pad firmly to the child's bare skin.

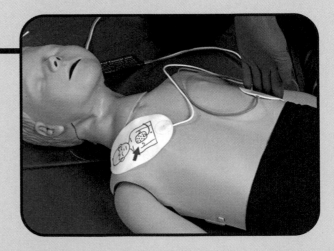

- Place one pad on the child's upper right chest and other pad on the lower left side.
  Note: *If the pads risk touching each other, place one pad on child's chest and other on child's back.*
- Plug in connector, if necessary.

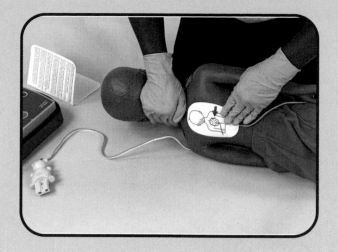

Step 11

Make sure no one, including you, is touching the child.

- Say, "EVERYONE, STAND CLEAR!"

Step 12

Allow the AED to analyze the heart's rhythm.

Step 13

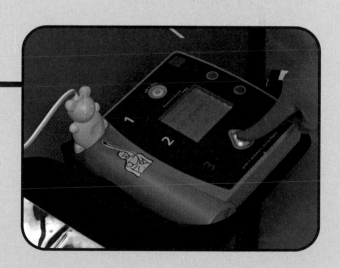

Make sure no one, including you, is touching the child.

Say, "EVERYONE, STAND CLEAR!"

- Deliver a shock if prompted by pushing the "shock" button.

- Give **5** cycles, or about **2** minutes of CPR unless there are obvious signs of life. Let AED reanalyze. If no shock advised, give 5 cycles or about 2 minutes of CPR.

Note: When there are no signs of life and an AED is on the way, give CPR until the AED is ready to use. When the AED arrives, turn it on and follow Steps 8 through 13.

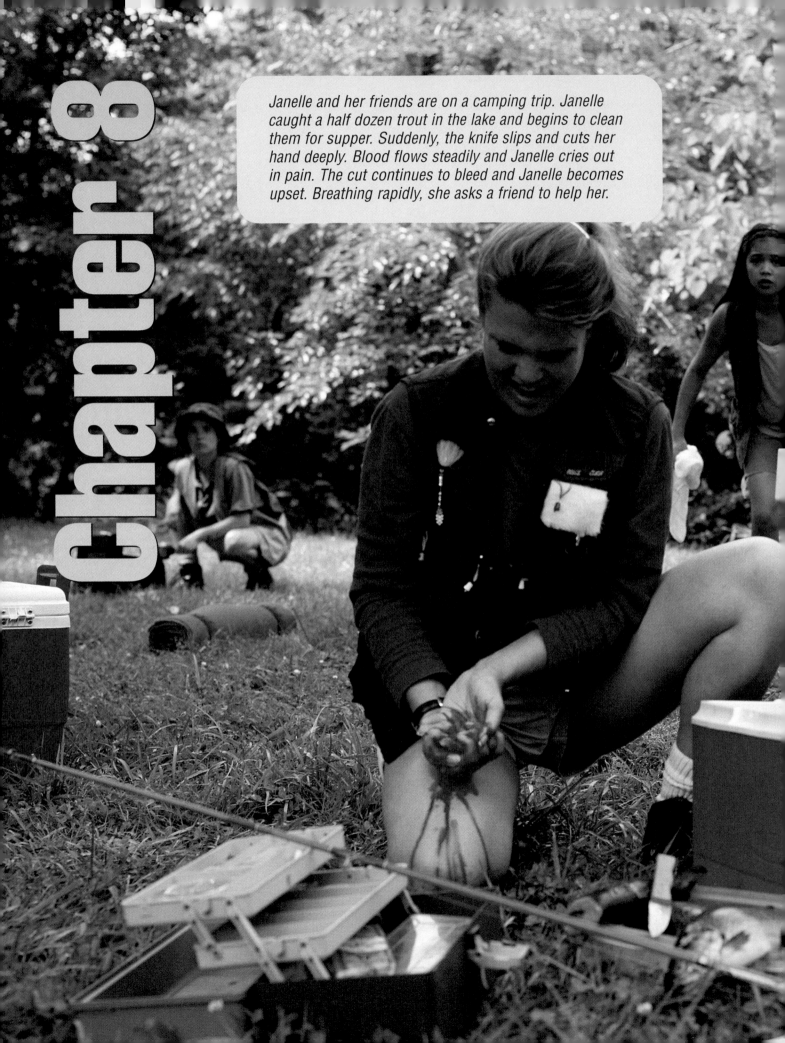

chapter 8

Janelle and her friends are on a camping trip. Janelle caught a half dozen trout in the lake and begins to clean them for supper. Suddenly, the knife slips and cuts her hand deeply. Blood flows steadily and Janelle cries out in pain. The cut continues to bleed and Janelle becomes upset. Breathing rapidly, she asks a friend to help her.

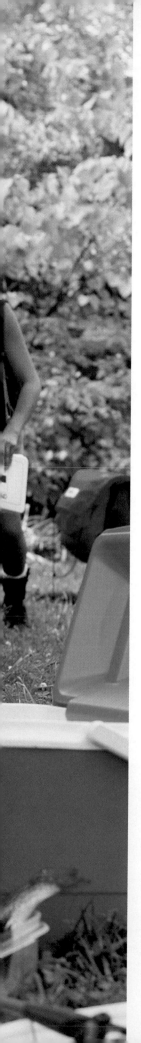

Bleeding

Objectives

After reading this chapter, you should be able to—

- ■ *Explain why severe bleeding must be controlled immediately.*

- ■ *Identify two signals of life-threatening external bleeding.*

- ■ *Describe the care for external bleeding.*

- ■ *Describe how to minimize the risk of disease transmission when giving care in a situation that involves visible blood.*

- ■ *Identify the signals of internal bleeding.*

- ■ *Describe the care for internal bleeding.*

After reading this chapter and completing the class activities, you should be able to demonstrate—

- ■ *How to control external bleeding.*

Introduction

*Bleeding is the escape of blood from arteries, capillaries or veins. A large amount of bleeding occurring in a short amount of time is called a **hemorrhage**. Bleeding is either external or internal. External bleeding, bleeding you can see coming from a wound, is usually obvious because it is visible (Fig. 8-1, A). Internal bleeding, bleeding inside the body, is often difficult to recognize (Fig. 8-1, B). Uncontrolled bleeding, whether external or internal, is a life-threatening emergency. As you learned in previous chapters, severe bleeding can result in death. In this chapter, you will learn how to recognize and give care for both internal and external bleeding.*

BLOOD AND BLOOD VESSELS

What is Blood?

Blood consists of liquid and solid components and comprises approximately 7 percent of the body's total weight. The average adult has a blood volume of between 10 and 12 pints. The liquid part of the blood is called **plasma**. The solid components include red and white blood cells and cell fragments called **platelets**.

Plasma makes up about half the total *blood volume*. Composed mostly of water, plasma maintains the blood volume needed for normal function of the circulatory system. Plasma also contains nutrients essential for energy production, growth and cell maintenance; carries waste products for elimination; and transports the other blood components.

White blood cells are a key disease-fighting part of the immune system. They defend the body against invading microorganisms, or pathogens. They also aid in producing antibodies that help the body resist infection.

Red blood cells account for most of the solid components of the blood. They are produced in the marrow in the hollow center of large bones, such as the long bones of the arm (humerus) and the thigh (femur). Red blood cells number nearly 260 million in each drop of blood. The red blood cells transport oxygen from the lungs to the body cells and carbon dioxide from the cells to the lungs. Red blood cells outnumber white blood cells about 1000 to 1.

Platelets are disk-shaped structures in the blood that are made up of cell fragments. Platelets are an essential part of the blood's clotting mechanism because of their tendency to bind together. Platelets help stop bleeding by forming blood clots at wound sites. Until blood clots form, bleeding must be controlled artificially.

Blood has three major functions:

▸ Transporting oxygen, nutrients and wastes.
▸ Protecting against disease by producing antibodies and defending against pathogens.

KEY TERMS

Arteries: Large blood vessels that carry oxygenated blood from the heart to the rest of the body.

Blood volume: The total amount of blood circulating within the body.

Capillaries: Microscopic blood vessels linking arteries and veins; they transfer oxygen and other nutrients from the blood to all body cells and remove waste products.

Clotting: The process by which blood thickens at a wound site to seal a hole or tear in a blood vessel and stops bleeding.

Direct pressure: The pressure applied on a wound to control bleeding, for example, by one's gloved hand.

External bleeding: Bleeding that can be seen coming from a wound.

Internal bleeding: Bleeding inside the body.

Pressure bandage: A bandage applied snugly to create pressure on a wound to aid in controlling bleeding.

Veins: Blood vessels that carry oxygenated blood from all parts of the body to the heart.

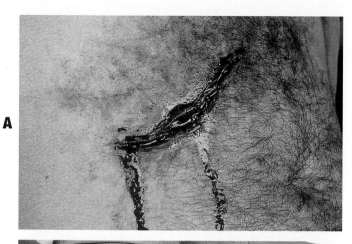

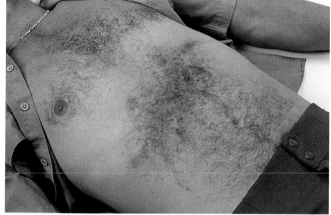

Figure 8-1   A, External bleeding is more easily recognized than **B,** internal bleeding.

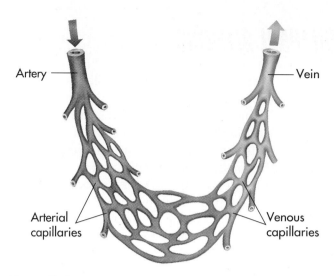

Figure 8-2   Blood flows through the three major types of blood vessels: arteries, capillaries and veins.

▶ Maintaining body temperature by circulating throughout the body.

Blood Vessels

Blood is channeled through blood vessels. The three major types of blood vessels are **arteries, capillaries** and **veins** (**Fig. 8-2**). Arteries carry blood away from the heart. Arteries vary in size. The smallest ones carry blood to the capillaries. Capillaries are microscopic blood vessels linking arteries and veins. They transfer oxygen and other nutrients from the blood into the cells. Capillaries pick up waste products, such as carbon dioxide, from the cells and move them into the veins. The veins carry blood back to the heart. The veins also carry waste products from the cells to the kidneys, intestines and lungs, where waste products are eliminated.

Because the blood in the arteries is closer to the pumping action of the heart, blood in the arteries travels faster and under greater pressure than blood in the capillaries or veins. Blood flow in the arteries pulses with the heartbeat; blood in the veins flows more slowly and evenly.

WHEN BLEEDING OCCURS

When bleeding occurs, a complex chain of events is triggered in the body. The brain, heart and lungs immediately attempt to compensate for blood loss to maintain the flow of oxygen-rich blood to the body tissues, particularly to the vital organs. The brain, recognizing a blood shortage, signals the heart to circulate more blood and to constrict blood vessels in the extremities. The brain signals the lungs to work harder, providing more oxygen.

Other important reactions to bleeding occur on a microscopic level. Platelets collect at the wound site in an effort to stop blood loss through clotting. White blood cells prevent infection by attacking microorganisms that enter through breaks in the skin. Over time, the body manufactures extra red blood cells to help transport more oxygen to the cells.

Blood volume is also affected by bleeding. Normally, excess fluid is absorbed from the bloodstream by the kidneys, lungs, intestines and skin. However, when bleeding occurs, this excess fluid is reabsorbed into the bloodstream as plasma. This reabsorption helps to maintain the critical balance of fluids needed by the body to keep blood volume constant. Bleeding that is severe enough to critically reduce the blood volume is life threatening because tissues will die from lack of oxygen. Life-threatening bleeding can be either external or internal.

EXTERNAL BLEEDING

External bleeding occurs when a blood vessel is opened externally, such as through a tear in the skin. Each type of blood vessel bleeds differently. Arterial bleeding (bleeding from an artery) is often rapid and severe. It is life threatening. Because arterial blood is under more pressure, it usually spurts from the wound, making it difficult for clots to form. Because clots do not form as rapidly, arterial bleeding is harder to control. The high concentration of oxygen gives arterial blood a bright red color.

Venous bleeding (bleeding from the veins) is generally easier to control than arterial bleeding. Veins are damaged more often because they are closer to the skin's surface. Venous blood is under less pressure than arterial blood and flows steadily from the wound without spurting. Only damage to veins deep in the body, such as those in the trunk or thigh, produces severe bleeding that is difficult to control. Because it is oxygen poor, venous blood is dark red or maroon.

Capillary bleeding, the most common type of bleeding, is usually slow because the vessels are small and the blood is under low pressure. It is often described as oozing from the wound. Clotting occurs easily with capillary bleeding. The blood is usually a paler red than arterial blood.

Most external bleeding you will encounter will be minor. You will be able to control it easily with pressure, and it usually stops by itself within 10 minutes. Sometimes, however, the damaged blood vessel is too large or the blood is under too much pressure for effective clotting to occur. In these cases, bleeding can be life threatening, and you will need to recognize and control it promptly when you check for life-threatening conditions.

Care for External Bleeding

External bleeding is usually easy to control. Generally, the pressure created by placing a sterile dressing and then a gloved hand, or even a gloved hand by itself, on a wound can control external bleeding. This technique is called applying *direct pressure*. Pressure placed on a wound restricts the blood flow through the wound and allows normal *clotting* to occur. Pressure on a wound can be maintained by applying a bandage snugly to the injured area. A bandage applied snugly to control bleeding is called a *pressure bandage*.

In some cases, direct pressure may not immediately control bleeding. This is an indication of severe external bleeding. Signals of severe external bleeding include—

▶ Blood spurting from the wound.
▶ Bleeding that fails to stop after all measures have been taken to control it.

A tourniquet, a tight band placed around an arm or leg to help constrict blood flow to a wound, is no longer generally recommended for use by laypersons because it too often does more harm than good. A tourniquet can cut off the blood supply to the limb below it and can damage skin, nerves and muscle by crushing the underlying tissue.

To give first aid for external bleeding, follow these general steps:

1. **CHECK** scene, then **CHECK** person.
2. Obtain consent.
3. Cover with a sterile dressing.
4. Apply direct pressure until bleeding stops.
5. Cover dressing with bandage.
6. If bleeding does not stop—
   • Apply additional dressings and bandages and continue to apply pressure.
   • Take steps to minimize shock, monitor the ABCs.
   • **CALL** 9-1-1 if not already done.

▶ Place direct pressure on the wound with a sterile gauze pad or any clean cloth, such as a washcloth, towel or handkerchief. Press hard. Using a pad or cloth will help keep the wound free from germs and aid clotting. Place your gloved hand over the pad and apply firm pressure (**Fig. 8-3, A**). If you do not have disposable gloves or an appropriate barrier, have the injured person apply pressure with his or her hand.

▶ Apply a pressure bandage to hold the gauze pads or cloth in place (**Fig. 8-3, B**).

▶ If blood soaks through the bandage, add more pads and bandages to help absorb the blood. Continue to apply pressure. Do not remove any blood-soaked pads. This can interfere with clotting.

▶ Make sure to call 9-1-1 or the local emergency number.

▶ Continue to monitor the victim's airway, breathing and circulation. Observe the victim closely for signals that may indicate that his or her condition is worsening, such as faster or slower breathing rates, changes in skin appearance and restlessness. Give additional care as needed.

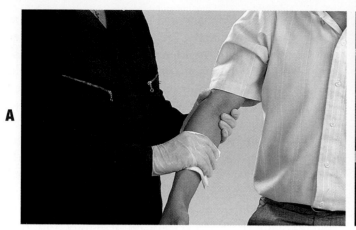 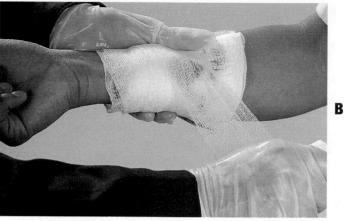

Figure 8-3   A, Apply direct pressure to the wound using a sterile gauze pad or clean cloth. **B,** Apply a pressure bandage. The victim may be able to help you.

INTERNAL BLEEDING

Internal bleeding is the escape of blood from arteries, capillaries or veins into spaces in the body. Severe internal bleeding can occur from injuries caused by a blunt force, such as a driver being thrown against the steering wheel in a car crash, or a chronic medical condition, such as an ulcer. Internal bleeding may also occur when an object, such as a knife or bullet, penetrates the skin and damages internal structures. A fractured bone, such as a rib, could penetrate and damage vital organs. In any traumatic injury, you should always suspect internal bleeding. For example, if a motorcycle rider is thrown from a bike, you may not see any serious external bleeding; however, you should consider that the impact may have caused internal injuries.

Signals of Severe Internal Bleeding

Severe internal bleeding is often difficult to recognize because its signals are not obvious and may take time to appear. These signals include—

▶ Soft tissues, such as those in the abdomen, that are tender, swollen or hard.
▶ Swelling, tenderness or rigidity in the injured area.
▶ Anxiety or restlessness.
▶ Rapid, weak pulse.
▶ Rapid breathing, shortness of breath.
▶ Skin that feels cool or moist or looks pale, ashen or bluish.
▶ Bruising in the injured area.

▶ Nausea, vomiting or coughing up blood.
▶ Abdominal pain.
▶ Excessive thirst.
▶ Decreased level of consciousness.
▶ Severe headache.

Many of these signals can also indicate a condition called shock. Shock is a progressive condition in which the circulatory system fails to circulate oxygen-rich blood to all parts of the body. You will learn more about shock in Chapter 9.

Care for Internal Bleeding

First aid for controlling internal bleeding depends on the severity and site of the bleeding. For minor internal bleeding, such as a bruise on an arm, apply an ice pack or a chemical cold pack to the injured area to help reduce pain and swelling. Always remember to place something, such as a gauze pad or a towel, between the source of cold and the skin to prevent damage to the skin.

If you suspect internal bleeding caused by serious injury, call 9-1-1 or the local emergency number. You can do little to control serious internal bleeding effectively. Activating the EMS system is the best help that you can give. EMS personnel must rapidly transport the victim to the hospital. Usually, the victim needs immediate surgery. While waiting for EMS personnel to arrive, follow the general care steps for any emergency.

▶ Do no further harm.
▶ Monitor breathing and consciousness.

▸ Help the victim rest in the most comfortable position.

▸ Keep the victim from getting chilled or overheated.

▸ Reassure the victim.

▸ Give any specific care needed.

SUMMARY

One of the most important things you can do in any emergency is to recognize and control life-threatening bleeding. Check for severe bleeding while checking for life-threatening conditions. External bleeding is easily recognized and should be cared for immediately by using direct pressure. Avoid contact with the injured person's blood by using standard precautions such as using disposable gloves and washing your hands with soap and water immediately or as soon as possible after giving care.

Although internal bleeding is less obvious, it can also be life threatening. Recognize when a serious injury has occurred, and suspect internal bleeding. You may not identify internal bleeding until you check for non-life-threatening conditions. When you identify or suspect life-threatening bleeding, activate the EMS system immediately and give care until EMS personnel arrive and take over.

APPLICATION QUESTIONS

1. From the description, would you suspect that Janelle's bleeding is a result of an injury to an artery, a vein or capillaries? Why?

2. How could Janelle's situation become life threatening?

3. What steps should Janelle's friend take to try to control Janelle's bleeding?

4. What precautions should Janelle's friend use to minimize the risk of disease transmission while giving care?

STUDY QUESTIONS

1. Match each term with the correct definition.

   a. External bleeding
   b. Direct pressure
   c. Pressure bandage
   d. Internal bleeding
   e. Arteries
   f. Veins

   _____ Using your gloved hand to apply pressure on the wound to control bleeding

   _____ Bleeding that can be seen coming from a wound

   _____ The escape of blood from an artery, vein or capillary into spaces inside the body

   _____ Blood vessels that carry blood from all parts of the body to the heart

   _____ Vessels that transport blood to the capillaries for distribution to the cells

   _____ A bandage applied snugly to maintain pressure on the wound to control bleeding

2. List two signals of life-threatening external bleeding.

3. Describe how to control external bleeding.

4. List five signals of internal bleeding.

5. Describe how to control minor internal bleeding.

Use the following scenario to answer questions 6 and 7:

The usual Saturday morning baseball game is in progress. A few spectators are standing around on the sidelines. As Milo takes a swing at a curve ball, he loses his grip on the bat, which flies several feet, hitting Chris hard on the thigh. Chris drops to the ground, clutching his leg. The skin where the leg was struck immediately becomes red and begins to swell.

6. What type of bleeding do you suspect Chris has?

7. What steps would you take to care for Chris?

Circle the letter of the correct answer.

8. A child has a deep cut on his arm. His face is moist and very pale. What would you do first?

   a. Have someone call 9-1-1 or the local emergency number.
   b. Apply direct pressure to the wound with a dressing.
   c. Place an ice pack on the affected arm.
   d. Apply pressure at the closest pressure point.

Answers are listed in Appendix A.

SKILL SHEET   Controlling External Bleeding

CHECK the scene for safety. **CHECK** the victim, following standard precautions. **CALL** 9-1-1 or the local emergency number if necessary. To **CARE** for a victim who is bleeding—

Step 1

Cover the wound with a dressing and press firmly against the wound with a gloved hand until bleeding stops.

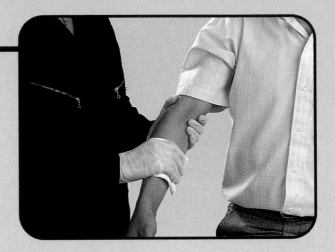

Step 2

Cover the dressing with a pressure bandage.

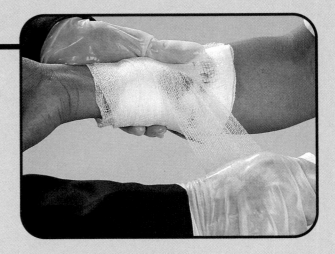

Step 3

If bleeding does not stop—

- Apply additional dressings and bandages.
- Take steps to minimize the effects of shock.
- Call 9-1-1 if not already done.

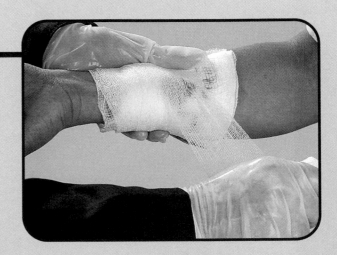

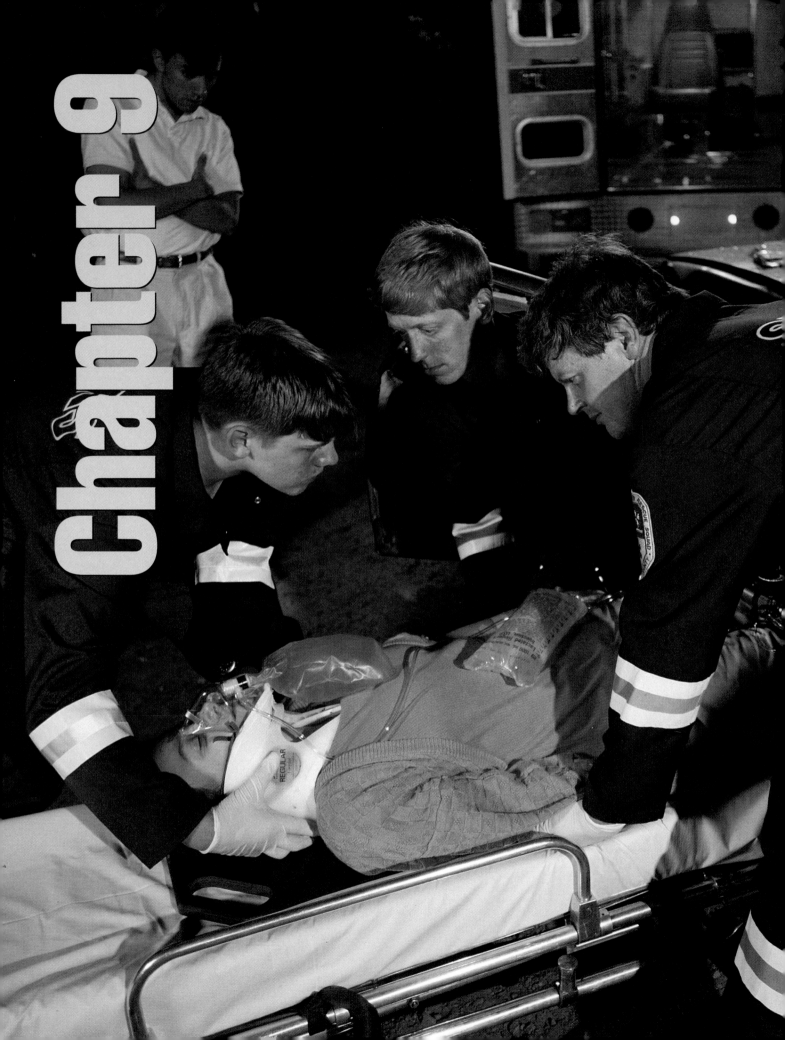

Chapter 9

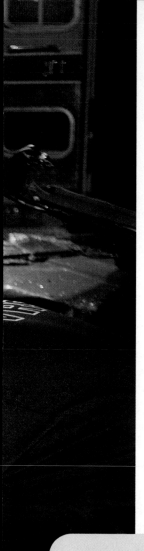

Shock

Objectives

After reading this chapter, you should be able to—

- List two conditions that can result in shock.

- Identify five types of shock and the conditions that cause each of them.

- List at least seven signals of shock.

- Explain what care can be given to minimize shock.

10:55 p.m. *On an isolated road, a large deer leaps into the path of an oncoming car traveling 55 mph. The driver, a 21-year-old college track star, cannot avoid the collision. In the crash, both of her legs are crushed and pinned in the wreckage.*

11:15 p.m. *Another car finally approaches. Seeing the crashed car, the driver stops and comes forward to help. He finds the woman conscious but restless and in obvious pain. He says he will go to call an ambulance at the nearest house, about a mile down the road. He assures her that he will return.*

11:25 p.m. *When the driver returns, he sees that the woman's condition has changed. She is now breathing faster, looks pale and appears drowsy. He holds her hand to comfort her and notices that her skin feels cold and moist.*

11:30 p.m. *The rescue squad arrives 10 minutes after receiving the phone call. The man explains that the woman became drowsy and is no longer conscious. Her breathing has become very irregular. The EMS personnel immediately go to work.*

Introduction

The driver in the scenario on the previous page was a victim of a progressively deteriorating life-threatening condition called shock. When the body experiences an injury or sudden illness, the body triggers a series of responses to compensate for any negative effects. When the body's attempts to compensate fail, the victim can progress into shock. Shock is a life-threatening condition. In this chapter, you will learn to recognize and give care to minimize shock.

SHOCK

When the body is healthy, three conditions are needed to maintain adequate blood flow:

▶ The heart must be working well.
▶ An adequate amount of oxygen-rich blood must be circulating in the body.
▶ The blood vessels must be intact and able to adjust blood flow.

Shock is a progressive condition in which the circulatory system fails to circulate oxygen-rich blood to all parts of the body. When *vital organs*, such as the brain, heart and lungs, do not receive oxygen-rich blood, they fail to function properly. When vital organs do not function properly, a series of responses is triggered in an attempt to keep them from failing.

When someone is injured or becomes suddenly ill, these normal body functions may be interrupted. In cases of minor injury or illness, this interruption is brief because the body is able to compensate quickly. With more severe injuries or illnesses, however, the body may be unable to ad-

just. When the body is unable to meet its demand for oxygen because blood fails to circulate adequately, shock occurs.

The Body's Responses

You learned in Chapter 4 that the heart circulates blood by contracting and relaxing in a consistent rhythmic pattern. The heart adjusts its speed and the force of its contractions to meet the body's changing demand for oxygen. For instance, when a person exercises, the heart beats faster and more forcefully to move more oxygen-rich blood to meet the working muscles' demand for more oxygen (**Fig. 9-1**).

Similarly, when someone suffers a severe injury or sudden illness that affects the flow of blood, the heart beats faster and stronger at first to adjust to the increased demand for oxygen. Because the heart is beating faster, breathing must also speed up to meet the body's increased demand for oxygen. You can detect these changes by observing and listening to the victim's appearance and breathing when you check for non-life-threatening conditions.

For the heart to do its job properly, an adequate amount of blood must circulate within the body. The body can compensate for some decrease in *blood volume*. Consider what happens when you donate blood. An adult can lose 1 pint of blood over a 10- to 15-minute period without any significant stress to the body. (This amount is smaller for children and infants.) Fluid is reabsorbed from the kidneys, lungs and intestines to replace lost blood volume. In addition, the body immediately begins to manufacture the blood's solid components. However, with severe injuries involving greater or more rapid blood loss, the body may not be able to adjust adequately. Body cells do not receive enough oxygen, and shock occurs. Any significant fluid loss from the body, such as from severe bleeding or burns or even from diarrhea or vomiting, can lead to shock.

KEY TERMS

Blood volume: The total amount of blood circulating within the body.
Shock: The failure of the circulatory system to provide adequate oxygen-rich blood to all parts of the body.

Vital organs: Organs whose functions are essential to life, including the brain, heart and lungs.

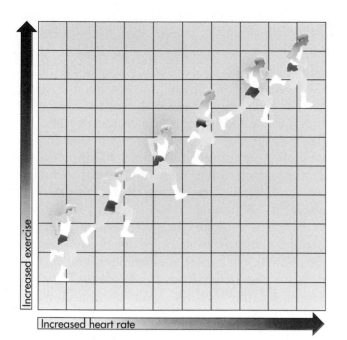

Figure 9-1   When a person exercises, the heart adjusts its speed to meet the body's changing demand for oxygen. Blood flow is also affected when someone suffers a severe injury or sudden illness—the heart beats faster and stronger to adjust to increased oxygen demand.

Regardless of the cause of shock, any significant decrease in body fluids affects the function of the heart. The heart will initially speed up to compensate for loss of body fluids and eventually will fail to beat rhythmically. The pulse may become irregular or be absent altogether.

The blood vessels act as pipelines, transporting oxygen and nutrients to all parts of the body and removing wastes. For the circulatory system to function properly, blood vessels must remain intact, preventing loss of blood volume. Normally, blood vessels decrease or increase the flow of blood to different areas of the body by constricting (decreasing their diameter) or dilating (increasing their diameter). This activity ensures that blood reaches the areas of the body that need it most, such as the vital organs. Injuries or illnesses, especially those that affect the brain and spinal cord, can cause blood vessels to lose this ability to change size. Blood vessels can also be affected if the nervous system is damaged by injury, infection, drugs or poisons.

If the heart is damaged, it cannot circulate blood properly. If blood vessels are damaged, the body cannot adjust blood flow. Regardless of the cause, when body cells receive inadequate oxygen, the result is shock. **Table 9-1** summarizes common types of shock and their causes.

When shock occurs, the body attempts to prioritize its needs for blood by ensuring adequate flow

Table 9-1   Common Types and Causes of Shock

TYPE	CAUSE
Anaphylactic	Life-threatening allergic reaction to a substance; may cause airway to swell, affecting ability to breathe; can occur from insect stings or from foods and drugs.
Cardiogenic	Failure of the heart to effectively circulate blood to all parts of the body; occurs with heart attack.
Hypovolemic	Severe bleeding or loss of blood plasma; occurs with internal or external wounds or burns or with severe fluid loss, as from vomiting and diarrhea.
Neurogenic	A disruption of the autonomic nervous system, which results in the blood vessels expanding and creating a drop in blood pressure; can be caused by fluid loss, trauma to the nervous system or emotional shock. Fainting is an example of neurogenic shock.
Septic	Toxins caused by a severe infection cause the blood vessels to dilate (expand).

to the vital organs. The body reduces the amount of blood circulating to the less important tissues of the arms, legs and skin. This reduction in blood circulation to the skin causes the skin of a person in shock to appear pale or ashen and feel cool. In later stages of shock, the skin, especially the lips and under the nails, may appear blue from a prolonged lack of oxygen. Increased sweating is also a natural reaction to stress caused by injury or illness, which makes the skin feel moist.

Signals

Although you may not always be able to determine the cause of shock, remember that shock is a life-threatening condition. You should learn to recognize the signals of shock.

The signals of shock include—

▶   Restlessness or irritability.
▶   Altered consciousness.

▶ Pale or ashen, bluish, cool or moist skin.
▶ Rapid breathing.
▶ Rapid and weak pulse.
▶ Excessive thirst.
▶ Nausea or vomiting.

Shock is a life-threatening condition. If any of these signals are present, assume the victim has a potentially life-threatening injury or illness. Give appropriate care.

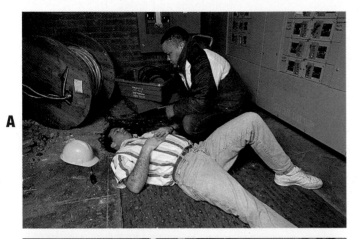

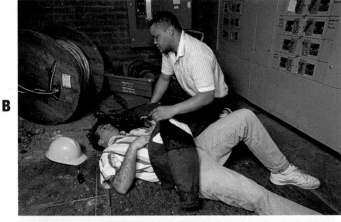

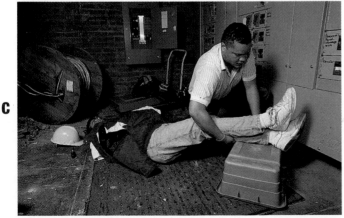

Figure 9-2 **A,** Monitor the victim's airway and breathing. **B,** Keep the victim from getting chilled or overheated. **C,** Elevate the victim's legs to keep blood circulating to the vital organs.

Care

Follow the emergency action steps: **CHECK—CALL—CARE. CHECK** the scene for safety and then the victim. **CALL** 9-1-1 or the local emergency number. **CARE** for the conditions you find (**Fig. 9-2, A**). Any specific care you give for life-threatening conditions will help to minimize the effects of shock. Make the victim as comfortable as possible. Helping the victim rest comfortably is important because pain can intensify the body's stress and accelerate the progression of shock. Keep the victim from getting chilled or overheated (**Fig. 9-2, B**). (In cooler environments this includes insulating the victim from the ground.) Watch for changes in the victim's level of consciousness, breathing rate and skin appearance.

You can further help the victim manage the effects of shock if you—

▶ Help the victim lie down on his or her back.
▶ Elevate the legs about 12 inches to help blood circulate to the vital organs (**Fig. 9-2, C**).
▶ Do not elevate the legs—
  • If the victim is nauseated or having trouble breathing.
  • If you suspect head, neck or back injuries or possible broken bones involving the hips or legs.
  • If moving causes more pain. If you are unsure of the victim's condition or if it is painful for him or her to move, leave the victim lying flat.
▶ Do not give the victim anything to eat or drink, even though he or she is likely to be thirsty. The victim's condition may be severe enough to require surgery, in which case it is better if the stomach is empty.

Special Considerations

Shock in Children

The signals of shock may be harder to detect in children. Suspect that shock may develop if a child is experiencing severe vomiting or diarrhea for an extended period of time (1 day). Replacing the fluids lost through vomiting or diarrhea is critical. Do not hesitate to call 9-1-1 or the local emergency number for a child who has developed severe vomiting or diarrhea.

Shock: The Domino Effect

- An injury causes severe bleeding.
- The heart attempts to compensate for the disruption of blood flow by beating faster.
- The victim first has a rapid pulse. More blood is lost. As blood volume drops, the pulse becomes weak or hard to find.
- The increased workload on the heart results in an increased oxygen demand. Therefore, breathing becomes faster.
- To maintain circulation of blood to the vital organs, blood vessels constrict in the arms, legs and skin. Therefore, the skin appears pale or ashen and feels cool.
- In response to the stress, the body perspires heavily and the skin feels moist.
- Because tissues of the arms and legs are now without oxygen, cells start to die.
- The brain now sends a signal to return blood to the arms and legs in an attempt to balance blood flow between these body parts and the vital organs.
- Vital organs now are not receiving adequate oxygen.
- The heart tries to compensate by beating even faster.
- More blood is lost and the victim's condition worsens.
- Without oxygen, the vital organs fail to function properly.
- As the brain is affected, the victim becomes restless, drowsy and eventually loses consciousness.
- As the heart is affected, it beats irregularly, resulting in an irregular pulse. The rhythm then becomes chaotic and the heart fails to circulate blood.
- There are no longer signs of life.
- When the heart stops, breathing stops.
- The body's continuous attempt to compensate for severe blood loss eventually results in death.

SUMMARY

Do not wait for shock to develop before giving care to a victim of injury or sudden illness. Always follow the general care steps for any emergency to minimize the progression of shock. Care for life-threatening conditions, such as breathing emergencies or severe external bleeding, before caring for non-life-threatening conditions. Remember that the key to managing shock effectively is calling 9-1-1 or the local emergency number and giving care as soon as possible.

APPLICATION QUESTIONS

1. Why did the woman go into shock?

2. What steps could the man have taken to minimize shock until EMS personnel arrived?

STUDY QUESTIONS

Circle T if the statement is true, F if it is false.

1. Shock is a condition resulting only from severe blood loss.   T   F

2. List four signals of shock.

3. List two conditions that frequently result in shock.

Use the following scenario to answer question 4.

Tara saw her brother Daren fall out of the tree he was climbing. When she reached him, he was lying on the ground, conscious but in pain. One leg was strangely twisted. Tara ran into the house, called 9-1-1 and told the call taker what had happened. Then she ran back to Daren, who was pale, sweating and appeared restless.

4. What can Tara do to care for Daren until EMS personnel arrive?

In questions 5 through 9, circle the letter of the correct answer.

5. Which of the following can cause shock?

    a. Bleeding
    b. Bee sting
    c. Heart attack
    d. All of the above

6. When shock occurs, the body prioritizes its need for blood. Where does it send blood first?

    a. The arms and legs
    b. The brain, heart and lungs
    c. The skin
    d. The spinal cord

7. Why does the skin appear pale during shock?

    a. Constriction of blood vessels near the skin's surface
    b. The majority of blood being sent to vital organs
    c. Profuse sweating
    d. a and b

8. Which of the following are included in the care for shock?

    a. Controlling bleeding when present
    b. Monitoring airway, breathing and circulation
    c. Helping the victim rest comfortably
    d. All of the above

9. Which body systems are affected by shock?

    a. Circulatory and respiratory
    b. All body systems
    c. Circulatory, respiratory and nervous
    d. Respiratory and nervous

10. Why is shock a life-threatening condition?

11. Why does elevating the victim's legs help to manage shock?

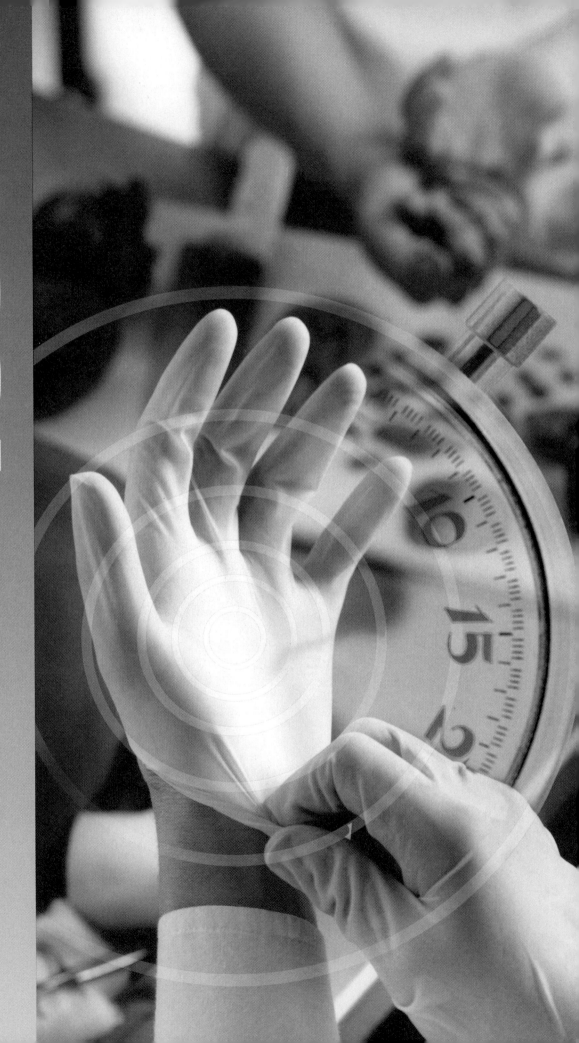

Part
FOUR

INJURIES

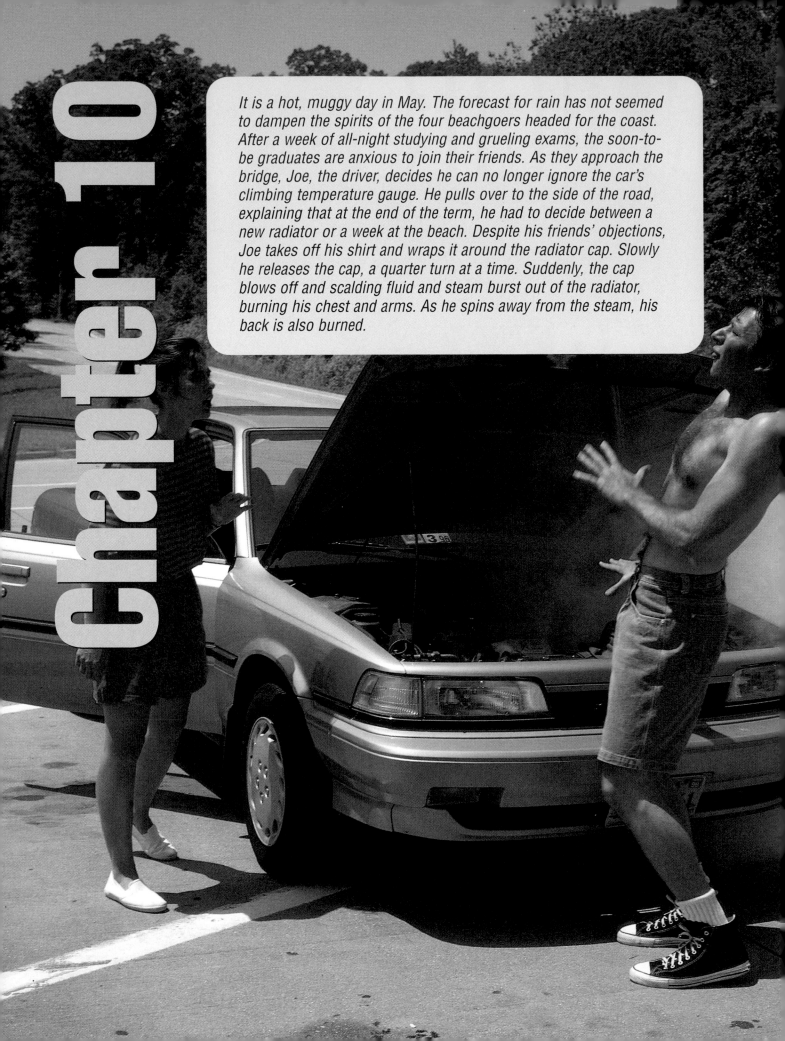

Chapter 10

It is a hot, muggy day in May. The forecast for rain has not seemed to dampen the spirits of the four beachgoers headed for the coast. After a week of all-night studying and grueling exams, the soon-to-be graduates are anxious to join their friends. As they approach the bridge, Joe, the driver, decides he can no longer ignore the car's climbing temperature gauge. He pulls over to the side of the road, explaining that at the end of the term, he had to decide between a new radiator or a week at the beach. Despite his friends' objections, Joe takes off his shirt and wraps it around the radiator cap. Slowly he releases the cap, a quarter turn at a time. Suddenly, the cap blows off and scalding fluid and steam burst out of the radiator, burning his chest and arms. As he spins away from the steam, his back is also burned.

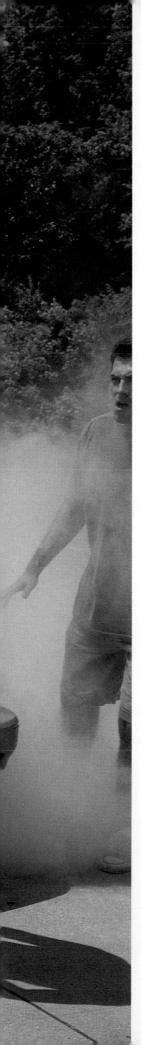

Soft Tissue Injuries

Objectives

After reading this chapter, you should be able to—

■ List two signals of closed wounds.

■ List four main types of open wounds.

■ Describe how to care for open and closed wounds.

■ Describe how to prevent infection in an open wound.

■ Describe how burns are classified.

■ Describe the signals of a critical burn.

■ List four signals of an infected wound.

■ Describe how to care for thermal, chemical, electrical and radiation burns.

After reading this chapter and completing the class activities, you should be able to—

■ Demonstrate how to control external bleeding.

Introduction

An infant falls and bruises his arm while learning to walk, a toddler scrapes her knee while learning to run, a child needs stitches in his chin after he falls off the "monkey bars" on the playground, another child gets a black eye in a fist fight, a teenager suffers a sunburn after a weekend at the beach and an adult cuts a hand while working in a woodshop. What do these injuries have in common? They are all soft tissue injuries.

*The **soft tissues** include the layers of skin, fat and muscle that protect the underlying body structures (**Fig. 10-1**). Most soft tissue injuries involve the outer layers of tissue. Organs, also composed of soft tissue, are vulnerable to damage from blunt trauma and penetrating forces. Fortunately, most soft tissue injuries are minor, requiring little attention. However, some soft tissue injuries can be severe and require immediate medical attention. In this chapter, you will learn how to recognize and care for various types of soft tissue injuries.*

WHAT ARE SOFT TISSUES?

The skin is composed of layers. The two primary layers of the skin are the outer layer, the **epidermis,** that provides a barrier to bacteria and other organisms that can cause infection, and a deeper layer, called the **dermis,** that contains the nerves, hair roots, sweat and oil glands and blood vessels. Because the skin is well supplied with blood vessels and nerves, most soft tissue injuries are likely to bleed and be painful. The **hypodermis,** located beneath the epidermis and dermis, contains fat, blood vessels and connective tissues. This layer insulates the body to help maintain body temperature. The fat layer also stores energy. The amount of fat varies among the different parts of the body and from person to person.

The muscles lie beneath the fat layer and comprise the largest segment of the body's soft tissues. Although the muscles are considered soft tissues, muscle injuries are discussed more thoroughly in Chapter 11.

TYPES OF SOFT TISSUE INJURIES

Wounds

A **wound** is defined as any physical injury involving a break in the layers of the skin. Wounds are typically classified as either closed or open. In a **closed wound,** the outer layer of skin is intact and the

KEY TERMS

Bandage: Material used to wrap or cover a part of the body; commonly used to hold a dressing or splint in place.

Burn: An injury to the skin or to other body tissues caused by heat, chemicals, electricity or radiation.

Closed wound: An injury that does not break the skin and in which soft tissue damage occurs beneath the skin.

Critical burn: Any burn that is potentially life threatening, disabling or disfiguring.

Deep burn: A burn that involves the two lower layers of skin, the dermis and the hypodermis,

and may destroy underlying structures; it can be life threatening.

Dressing: A pad placed directly over a wound to absorb blood and other body fluids and to prevent infection.

Open wound: An injury resulting in a break in the skin's surface.

Soft tissues: Body structures that include the layers of skin, fat and muscles.

Superficial burn: A burn involving only the top layer of skin, the epidermis, characterized by dry, red skin.

Wound: An injury to the soft tissues.

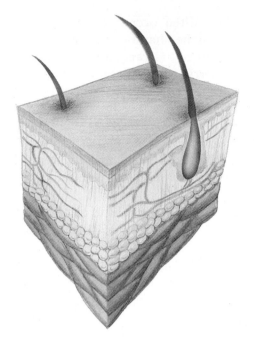

Figure 10-1 The soft tissues include the layers of skin, fat and muscle.

damage lies below the surface. A closed wound may bleed internally. With an *open wound,* the outer layer of skin is broken. External bleeding is often a factor when treating open wounds.

Closed Wounds

The simplest closed wound is a bruise, also called a **contusion** (**Fig. 10-2**). Bruises result when the body is subjected to a force, such as when you bump your leg on a table or chair. This bump or blow results in

damage to soft tissue layers and vessels beneath the skin, causing internal bleeding. When blood and other fluids seep into the surrounding tissues, the area discolors and swells. The amount of discoloration and swelling varies depending on the severity of the injury. At first, the area may only appear red. Over time, more blood and other fluids leak into the area, causing the area to turn dark red or purple. A significant violent force can cause injuries involving larger blood vessels and the deeper layers of muscle tissue. These injuries can result in profuse bleeding beneath the skin.

Care for Closed Wounds

Many closed wounds do not require special medical care. You can use direct pressure on the area to decrease bleeding that occurs beneath the skin. Elevating the injured part helps reduce swelling. Applying cold can be effective early on in helping control both pain and swelling. When applying ice or a chemical cold pack, place a gauze pad, a towel or other thin cloth between the source of the cold and the victim's skin (**Fig. 10-3**). Leave the ice or cold pack on the victim no more the 20 minutes. Then remove it for 20 minutes, and replace it.

However, do not assume that all closed wounds are minor injuries. Take the time to evaluate whether more serious injuries could be present. Seek immediate medical attention if—

▶ A victim complains of severe pain or cannot move a body part without pain.
▶ You think the force that caused the injury was great enough to cause serious damage.

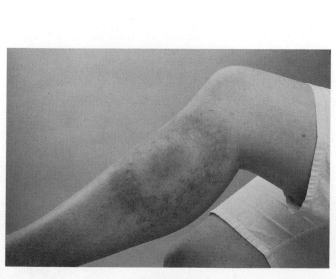

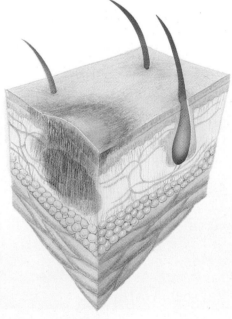

Figure 10-2 The simplest closed wound is a bruise.

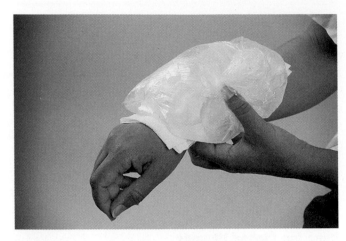

Figure 10-3 For a closed wound, apply ice to help control pain and swelling.

Open Wounds

In an open wound, the break in the skin can be as minor as a scrape of the surface layers or as severe as a deep penetration. The amount of bleeding depends on the location and severity of the injury.

The following are the four main types of open wounds:

▸ Abrasions
▸ Lacerations
▸ Avulsions
▸ Punctures

An **abrasion** is the most common type of open wound. It is characterized by skin that has been rubbed or scraped away (**Fig. 10-4**). This type of skin damage often occurs when a child falls and scrapes his or her hands or knees. An abrasion is sometimes called a scrape, a rug burn, a road rash or a strawberry. An abrasion is usually painful because scraping of the outer skin layers exposes sensitive nerve endings. Bleeding is not severe and is easily controlled, since only the small capillaries are damaged. Dirt and other matter can easily become embedded in the skin, making it especially important to clean the wound to prevent infection and aid healing.

A **laceration** is a cut. The cut may have either jagged or smooth edges (**Fig. 10-5**). Lacerations are commonly caused by sharp objects, such as knives, scissors or broken glass. A laceration can also result when a blunt force splits the skin. This splitting often occurs in areas where bone lies directly underneath the skin's surface, such as the chin bone or skull. Deep lacerations can also affect the layers of fat and muscle, damaging both nerves and blood vessels. Lacerations usually bleed freely and, depending on the structures involved, can bleed heavily. Lacerations are not always painful because damaged nerves cannot transmit pain signals to the brain. Lacerations can easily become infected if not cared for properly.

An **avulsion** is an injury in which a portion of the skin and sometimes other soft tissue is partially or completely torn away (**Fig. 10-6**). A partially avulsed piece of skin may remain attached but hangs like a flap. Bleeding is usually significant because avulsions often involve deeper soft tissue lay-

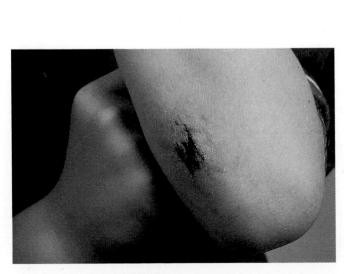

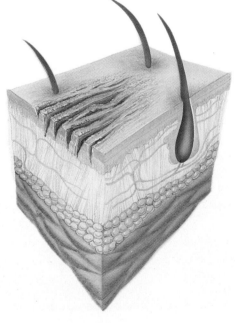

Figure 10-4 Abrasions can be painful, but bleeding is easily controlled.

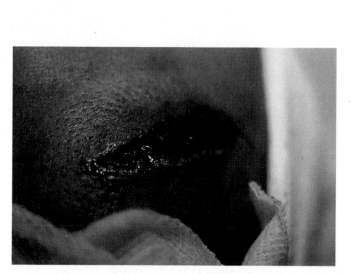

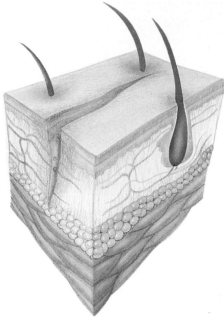

Figure 10-5   A laceration may have jagged or smooth edges.

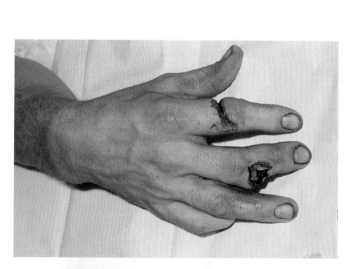

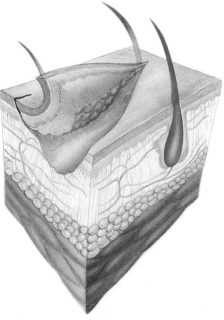

Figure 10-6   In an avulsion, part of the skin and other soft tissue is torn away.

ers. Sometimes a body part, such as a finger, may be severed (**Fig. 10-7**). Such an injury is called an **amputation**. Although damage to the tissue is severe when a body part is severed, bleeding is usually not as bad as you might expect. The blood vessels usually constrict and retract (pull in) at the point of injury, slowing bleeding and making it relatively easy to control with direct pressure. In the past, a completely severed body part could not be successfully reattached. With today's medical technology, reattachment is often successful.

A **puncture wound** results when the skin is pierced with a pointed object, such as a nail, a piece of glass, a splinter or a knife (**Fig. 10-8**). A gunshot wound is also a puncture wound. Because the skin usually closes around the penetrating object, external bleeding is generally not severe. However, internal bleeding can be severe if the penetrating object damages major blood vessels or internal organs. An object that remains embedded in the open wound is called an **embedded object** (**Fig. 10-9**). An object may also pass completely through a body part,

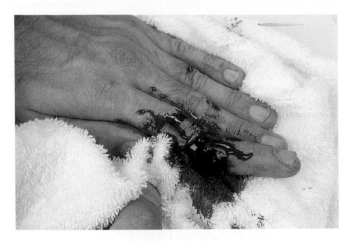

Figure 10-7 In a severe avulsion, a body part may be completely severed.

creating two open wounds—one at the entry point and one at the exit point.

Care for Open Wounds

Dressings and Bandages

All open wounds need some type of covering to help control bleeding and prevent infection. These coverings are commonly referred to as dressings and bandages, and there are many types.

Dressings are pads placed directly on the wound to absorb blood and other fluids and to prevent infection. To minimize the chance of infection, dressings should be sterile. Most dressings are porous, allowing air to circulate to the wound to promote healing. Standard dressings include vary-ing sizes of cotton gauze, commonly ranging from 2 to 4 inches square. Much larger dressings are used to cover very large wounds and multiple wounds in one body area. Some dressings have nonstick surfaces to prevent the dressing from sticking to the wound (**Fig. 10-10**).

An **occlusive dressing** is a bandage or dressing that closes a wound or damaged area of the body and prevents it from being exposed to the air (**Fig. 10-11**). By preventing exposure to the air, occlusive dressings help prevent infection. Occlusive dressings help keep in medications that are applied to the affected area. They also help keep in heat, body fluids and moisture. Occlusive dressing comes from the Latin word "occludere" meaning "to close up," and the Old French word "dresser" meaning "to arrange." Put the words together and you have "to arrange to close up." An example of an occlusive dressing is plastic wrap. This type of dressing is used for certain chest and abdominal injuries that will be discussed in Chapter 14.

A *bandage* is any material that is used to wrap or cover any part of the body. Bandages are used to hold dressings in place, to apply pressure to control bleeding, to protect a wound from dirt and infection and to provide support to an injured limb or body part. Any bandage applied snugly to create pressure on a wound or an injury is called a **pressure bandage**. Many different types of bandages are available commercially (**Fig. 10-12**).

A common type of bandage is a commercially made **adhesive compress** or adhesive bandage (**Fig. 10-13**). Available in assorted sizes, adhesive bandages consist of a small pad of nonstick gauze

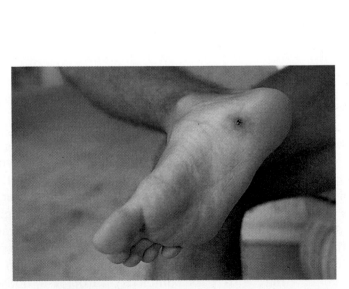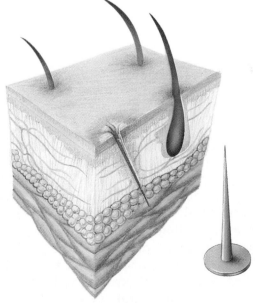

Figure 10-8 A puncture wound results when skin is pierced by a pointed object.

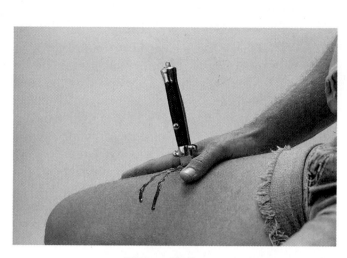

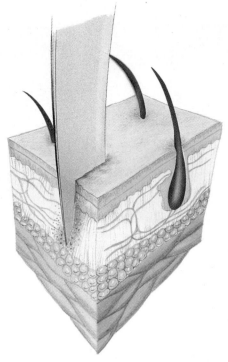

Figure 10-9   An object can become embedded in a wound.

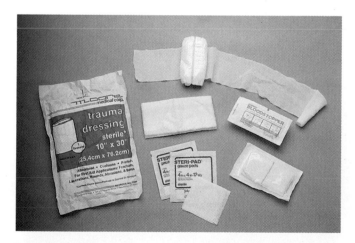

Figure 10-10   Dressings are pads placed directly on the wound. They come in various sizes. Some have surfaces that will not stick to a wound.

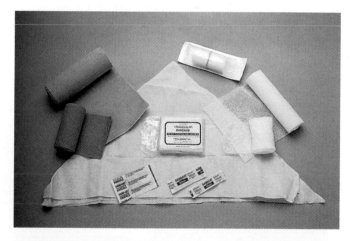

Figure 10-12   Different types of bandages are used to hold dressings in place, apply pressure to a wound, protect the wound from infection and provide support to an injured area.

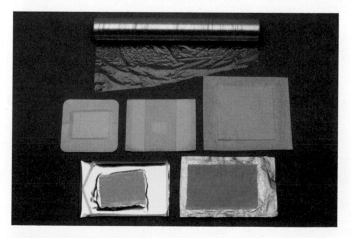

Figure 10-11   Occlusive dressings are designed to prevent air from passing through.

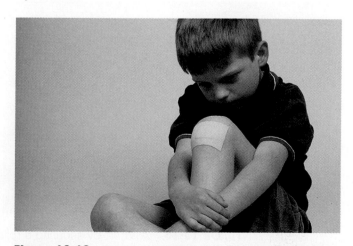

Figure 10-13   A common type of bandage is an adhesive compress.

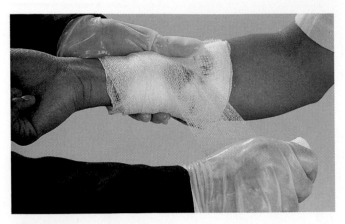

Figure 10-14   Roller bandages can be used to secure a dressing in place.

on a strip of adhesive tape that is applied directly to minor wounds.

The **bandage compress** is a thick gauze dressing attached to a bandage that is tied in place. Bandage compresses are specially designed to help control severe bleeding and usually come in sterile packages.

A **roller bandage** is usually made of gauze or gauze-like material. Roller bandages are available in assorted widths from ½ to 12 inches (1.3 to 30.5 centimeters) and lengths from 5 to 10 yards (4.6 to 9.1 meters). A roller bandage is generally wrapped around the body part. It can be tied or taped in place. A roller bandage may also be used to hold a dressing in place, secure a splint or control external bleeding (**Fig. 10-14**). Follow these general guidelines when applying a roller bandage:

▶ Check for feeling, warmth and color of the area below the injury site, especially fingers and toes, before and after applying the bandage.

▶ Secure the end of the bandage in place with a turn of the bandage. Wrap the bandage around the body part until the dressing is completely covered and the bandage extends several inches beyond the dressing. Tie or tape the bandage in place (**Fig. 10-15, _A-C_**).

▶ Do not cover fingers or toes. By keeping these parts uncovered, you will be able to see if the bandage is too tight (**Fig. 10-15, _D_**). If fingers or toes become cold or begin to turn pale, blue or ashen, the bandage is too tight and should be loosened slightly.

▶ If blood soaks through the bandage, apply additional dressings and another bandage. Do

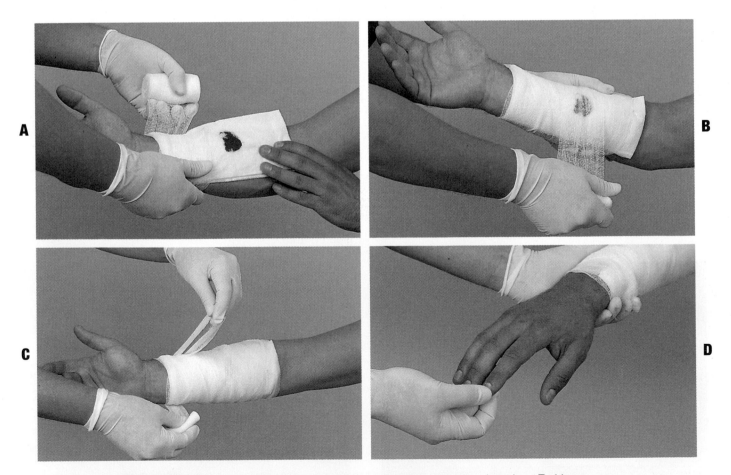

Figure 10-15   A, Start by securing a roller bandage over the dressing. **B,** Use overlapping turns to cover the dressing completely. **C,** Tie or tape the bandage in place. **D,** Check the fingers for feeling, warmth and color.

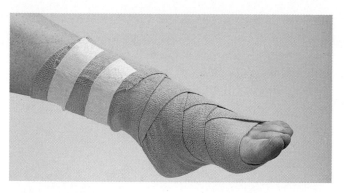

Figure 10-16 Elastic bandages can be applied to control swelling or support an injured limb.

not remove the blood-soaked bandages and dressings. Disturbing them may disrupt the formation of a clot and restart the bleeding.

Elastic bandages, sometimes called elastic wraps, are designed to keep continuous pressure on a body part. Elastic bandages are available in 2-, 3-, 4- and 6-inch (3.1, 7.6, 10.2 and 15.2 centimeter) widths. When properly applied, an elastic bandage can effectively control swelling or support an injured limb as in the care for an elapid (coral)

snakebite (**Fig. 10-16**). However, an improperly applied elastic bandage can restrict blood flow, which is not only painful but can also cause tissue damage if not corrected. Always check the area above and below the injury site for warmth and color, especially fingers and toes, after you have applied an elastic roller bandage. **Figure 10-17,** *A-D* shows some simple ways to ensure proper application of elastic roller bandages.

Care for Minor Open Wounds

In minor open wounds, such as abrasions, damage is only superficial and bleeding is minimal. To care for a minor open wound, follow these general guidelines:

▸ Use a barrier between your hand and the wound. If readily available, put on disposable gloves and place a sterile dressing on the wound.
▸ Apply direct pressure for a few minutes to control any bleeding.
▸ Wash the wound thoroughly with soap and water. If possible, irrigate an abrasion for 5 minutes with clean, running tap water.

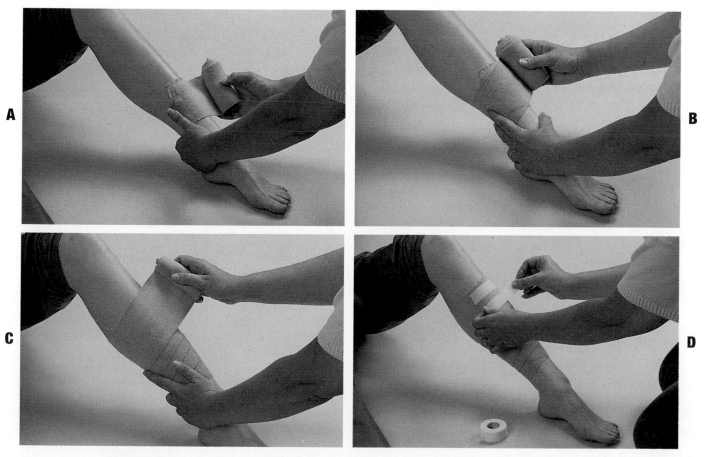

Figure 10-17   **A,** Start the elastic bandage at the point farthest from the heart. **B,** Anchor the bandage. **C,** Wrap the bandage using overlapping turns. **D,** Tape the end of the bandage in place.

▶ Apply triple antibiotic ointment or cream to a minor wound if the person has no known allergies or sensitivities to the medication.

▶ Cover the wound with a new sterile dressing and a bandage (or with an adhesive bandage) if it is still bleeding slightly or if the area of the wound is likely to come into contact with dirt or germs.

▶ Wash your hands immediately after giving care.

If it is only a splinter in the surface of the skin, it can be removed with tweezers.

▶ After removing the splinter from the skin, wash the area with soap and water, rinsing the area with cold tap water for about 5 minutes.

▶ After drying the area, apply a triple antibiotic ointment or cream to the area, if there are no known allergies or sensitivities to the medication.

▶ Cover it to keep it clean.

If the splinter is in the eye, do not attempt to remove it. Call 9-1-1 or the local emergency number.

Care for Major Open Wounds

A major open wound has severe bleeding, deep destruction of tissue or a deeply embedded object. To care for a major open wound, follow these general guidelines:

▶ Call 9-1-1 or the local emergency number.

▶ Put on disposable gloves. If blood has the potential to splatter, you may need to wear eye protection.

▶ Control external bleeding using the general steps below:
  • Cover the wound with a dressing and press firmly against the wound with a gloved hand.
  • Apply a pressure bandage over the dressing to maintain pressure on the wound and to hold the dressing in place.
  • If blood soaks through the bandage, do not remove the blood-soaked bandages; add more pads and bandages to help absorb the blood and continue to apply pressure.

▶ Monitor airway and breathing. Observe the victim closely for signals that may indicate that the victim's condition is worsening, such as faster or slower breathing, changes in skin color and restlessness.

▶ Take steps to minimize shock.

▶ Keep the victim from getting chilled or overheated.

▶ Have the victim rest comfortably and reassure him or her.

▶ Wash your hands immediately after giving care.

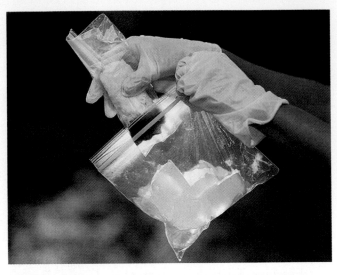

Figure 10-18   Wrap a severed body part in sterile gauze, put it in a plastic bag and put the bag on ice.

If the victim has an avulsion in which a body part has been completely severed—

▶ Call 9-1-1 or the local emergency number.

▶ Put on disposable gloves.

▶ Wrap the severed body part in sterile gauze or any clean material, such as a washcloth.

▶ Place the wrapped part in a plastic bag. Keep the body part cool by placing the bag on ice (**Fig. 10-18**). Do not place the bag on dry ice or in ice water.

▶ Make sure the part is transported to the medical facility with the victim.

If the victim has an embedded object in the wound—

▶ Put on disposable gloves.

▶ Do not remove the object.

▶ Use bulky dressings to stabilize the object. Any movement of the object can result in further tissue damage (**Fig. 10-19, A**).

▶ Control bleeding by bandaging the dressing in place around the object (**Fig. 10-19, B**).

▶ Call 9-1-1 or the local emergency number if not already done so.

▶ Wash your hands immediately after giving care.

Burns

Burns are a special kind of soft tissue injury. Burns account for about 25 percent of all soft tissue injuries. Thermal burns—burns caused by heat—are the most common.

Burns first destroy the epidermis, the top layer of skin. As the burn progresses, the dermis, or second layer, is injured or destroyed. Burns break the skin and thus can cause infection, fluid loss and loss

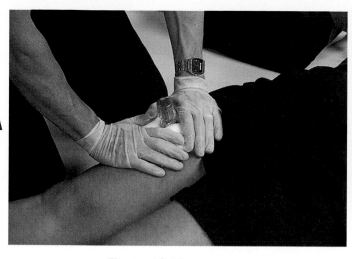 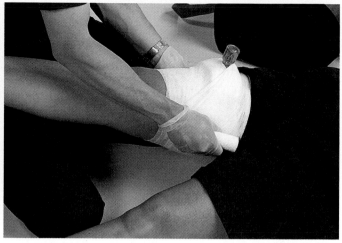

Figure 10-19   **A,** Use bulky dressings to support an embedded object. **B,** Use bandages over the dressing to control bleeding.

A STITCH IN TIME

It can be difficult to judge when a wound requires stitches. A general rule of thumb is that stitches are needed when the edges of skin do not fall together, the laceration involves the face or when any wound is over ½ inch long. Stitches speed the healing process, lessen the chances of infection and improve the look of scars. A health-care provider should apply stitches within the first few hours after the injury. The following major injuries always require medical attention and often need stitches:

- Bleeding from an artery or bleeding that is difficult to control
- Deep cuts or avulsions that show the muscle or bone, involve joints, such as the elbows, gape widely or involve the hands, feet or face
- Large punctures
- Large embedded objects
- Some human and animal bites
- Wounds that, if left unattended, could leave a conspicuous scar, such as those that involve the lip or eyebrow

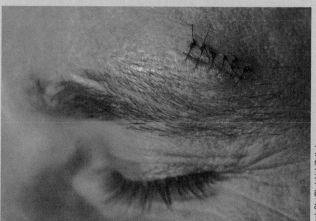

If you are caring for a wound and think it may need stitches, it probably does. If you are not sure, check with a health-care provider immediately. It can be dangerous to close a wound after a delay because of the probability of infection. To care for stitches, follow the instructions of your health-care provider. If the wound gets red or swollen or if pus begins to form, notify your health-care provider.

    Stitches are usually removed in 3 to 14 days, depending on where the wound is located. Some stitches dissolve naturally and do not require removal.

of body temperature control. Burns can also damage the respiratory system and the eyes. The severity of a burn depends on—

▶ The temperature of the source of the burn.
▶ The length of exposure to the source.
▶ The location of the burn.
▶ The extent of the burn.
▶ The victim's age and medical condition.

Because their skin is thinner and more delicate, older adults and young children are particularly susceptible to severe burns. People with chronic medical problems also tend to have more complications from severe burns, especially if they are not well nourished or have heart or kidney problems. People with nerve damage resulting from paralysis or other medical conditions may have no sensation; therefore, they become burned more easily because they do not feel heat.

Burns are classified by their source, such as heat, chemicals, electricity or radiation. They are also classified by depth. The deeper the burn, the more severe it is. Generally, burns are classified into two categories: *superficial* (first degree) *burns* and *deep burns.* Deep burns are further classified into **partial-thickness** (second degree) and **full-thickness** (third degree) **burns.**

Superficial Burns

A superficial burn (first degree) involves only the top layer of skin (**Fig. 10-20**). The skin is red and dry, and the burn is usually painful. The area may swell. Mild sunburn is an example of a superficial burn. Superficial burns generally heal in 5 to 6 days without permanent scarring.

Partial-Thickness Burns

A partial-thickness burn (second degree) involves both the epidermis and the dermis (**Fig. 10-21**). These injuries may look red and have blisters. The blisters may open and weep clear fluid, making the skin appear wet. The burned skin may look mottled (blotched). These burns are usually painful, and the area often swells. The burn usually heals in 3 or 4 weeks. Scarring may occur.

Full-Thickness Burns

A full-thickness burn (third degree) destroys all the layers of skin, as well as any or all of the underlying structures—fat, muscles, bones and nerves. These burns look brown or charred (black), with the tissues underneath sometimes appearing white (**Fig. 10-22**). They can be either extremely painful or relatively painless if the burn destroyed nerve endings in the skin. A third-degree burn is often life threatening and can take longer to heal or result in scarring.

Identifying Critical Burns

A *critical burn* requires the attention of medical professionals. Critical burns are potentially life threatening, disfiguring and disabling. Knowing whether you should call 9-1-1 or the local emer-

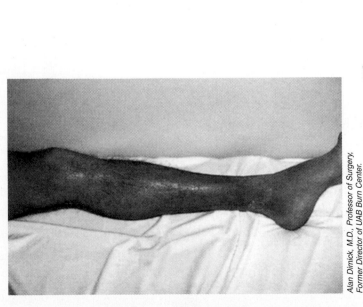

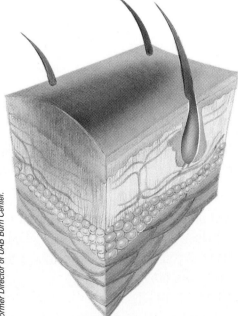

Alan Dimick, M.D., Professor of Surgery, Former Director of UAB Burn Center.

Figure 10-20 A superficial (first degree) burn.

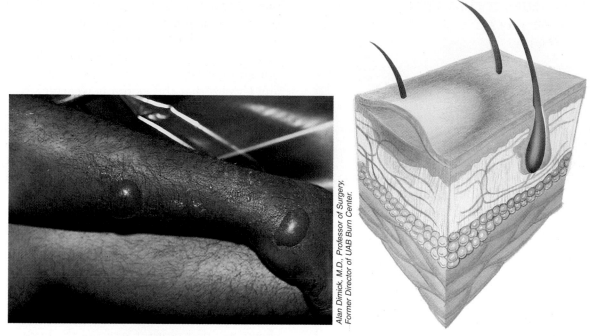

Figure 10-21 A partial-thickness (second degree) burn.

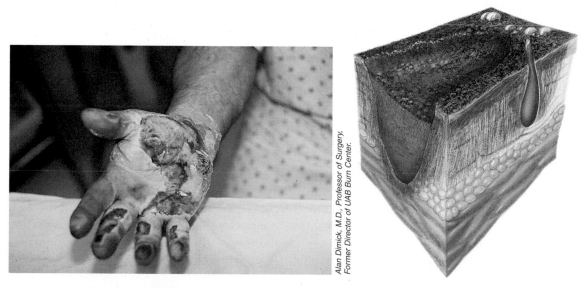

Figure 10-22 A full-thickness (third degree) burn.

gency number for a burn is often difficult. It is not always easy or possible to assess the severity of a burn immediately after injury. Even superficial burns to large areas of the body or to certain body parts can be critical. You cannot judge severity of a burn by the pain the victim feels because nerve endings may be destroyed. Call 9-1-1 or the local emergency number if the victim—

▶ Has trouble breathing.
▶ Has burns covering more than one body part or a large surface area.
▶ Has suspected burns to the airway. Note burns around the mouth and nose.

▶ Has burns to the head, neck, hands, feet or genitals (**Fig. 10-23**).
▶ Has a full-thickness burn and is younger than age 5 or older than age 60.
▶ Has a burn resulting from chemicals, explosions or electricity.

Care for Burns

Follow these basic steps when caring for a burn:

▶ Check the scene for safety.
▶ Stop the burning by removing the victim from the source of the burn.

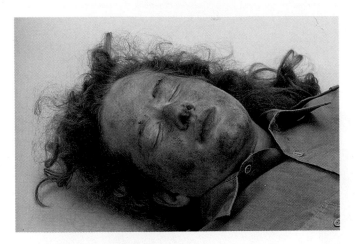

Figure 10-23 A critical burn to the face.

▸ Check for life-threatening conditions.
▸ Cool the burn with large amounts of cold running water.
▸ Cover the burn loosely with a sterile dressing.
▸ Prevent infection.
▸ Take steps to minimize shock.
▸ Keep the victim from getting chilled or overheated.
▸ Comfort and reassure the victim.

Even after the source of heat has been removed, soft tissue will continue to burn for minutes afterwards, causing more damage. Therefore, it is essential to cool any burned areas immediately with large amounts of cold water (**Fig. 10-24, A**). Do not use ice or ice water except on a small, superficial burn and then for no more than 10 minutes. Ice causes the body to lose heat and further damages delicate tissues. Use whatever resources are available—a tub, shower or garden hose. You can apply clean soaked towels, sheets or other wet cloths to a

burned face or other area that cannot be immersed. Be sure to keep these compresses cool and moist by adding more water. Otherwise, the compresses will quickly absorb the heat from the skin's surface, dry out and perhaps stick to the burned area. Remove any jewelry that the victim is wearing.

Allow several minutes for the burned area to cool. If pain continues when the area is removed from the water, continue cooling. When the burn is cool, remove all clothing from the area by carefully pulling or cutting material away. Do not try to remove any clothing that is sticking to skin.

Cover the burned area to keep out air and help reduce pain (**Fig. 10-24, B**). Use dry, sterile dressings if possible and loosely bandage them in place. Do not touch a burn with anything except a clean covering. The bandage should not put pressure on the burn surface. If the burn covers a large area of the body, cover the burned area with clean, dry sheets or other cloth. Covering the burn also helps to prevent infection. Do not try to clean a severe burn.

Do *not put ointments, butter, oil or other commercial or home remedies on blisters, deep burns or burns that may require medical attention*. Oils and ointments seal in heat, do not relieve pain well and will have to be removed by medical personnel. Other home remedies can contaminate open skin areas, causing infection. Do not break blisters. Intact skin helps prevent infection.

For minor superficial burns, care for the burned area as you would for an open wound. Cool the area. Wash the area with soap and water, and keep the area clean. Apply a triple antibiotic ointment if the person has no known allergies or sensitivities to the medication, and watch for signals of infection. A pharmacist or physician may be able to recom-

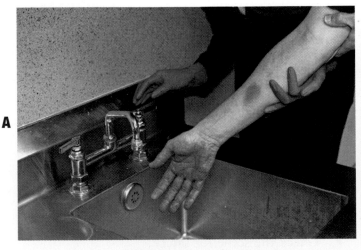

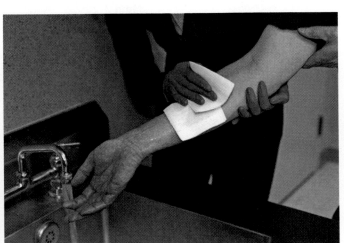

Figure 10-24 **A,** Large amounts of cool water are essential to cool burned areas.
B, Cover the burned area.

mend products that are effective in caring for superficial burns, such as sunburn.

Partial-thickness and full-thickness burns can cause shock as a result of pain and loss of body fluids. Have the victim lie down unless he or she is having trouble breathing. Elevate burned areas above the level of the heart, if possible. Burn victims have a tendency to become chilled. Help the victim maintain normal body temperature by protecting him or her from drafts.

Special Considerations

Burns can also be caused by chemicals, electricity and radiation. These burns have special requirements for care.

Chemical Burns

Chemical burns are common in industrial settings but also occur in the home. Typically, burns result from chemicals that are strong acids or alkalis. Cleaning solutions, such as household bleach, drain cleaners, toilet bowl cleaners, paint strippers, and lawn or garden chemicals are common sources of chemicals that can eat away or destroy tissues. These substances can quickly injure the skin.

As with heat burns, the stronger the chemical and the longer the contact, the more severe the burn. The chemical will continue to burn as long as it is on the skin. You must remove the chemical from the body as quickly as possible and call 9-1-1 or the local emergency number. Flush the burn with large amounts of cool, running water (**Fig. 10-25**). Continue flushing the burn for at least 20 minutes or until EMS personnel arrive. If the chemical is dry or in a powdered form, brush the chemical from the skin with a gloved hand or a piece of cloth. Then flush the residue from the skin with large amounts

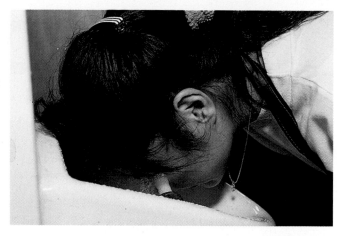

Figure 10-26   Flush the affected eye with cool water in the case of a chemical burn to the eye. Some facilities may have special eyewash stations.

of clean running tap water (under pressure) for at least <u>20 minutes.</u> Do not use a forceful flow of water from a hose; the force may further damage burned skin. If possible, have the victim remove contaminated clothes to prevent further contamination while you continue to flush the area.

If an eye is burned by a chemical, flush the affected eye with water until EMS personnel arrive. Tip the head so that the affected eye is lower than the unaffected eye as you flush (**Fig. 10-26**). This position helps prevent the chemical from getting into the unharmed eye. Flush from the nose outward. If both eyes are affected, direct the flow to the bridge of the nose and flush both eyes from the inner corner outward. Be aware that chemicals can be inhaled, potentially damaging the airway or lungs. Call 9-1-1 or the local emergency number if you believe chemicals have been inhaled. Let the call taker know if you believe chemicals have been inhaled.

Electrical Burns

The human body is a good conductor of electricity. When someone comes in contact with an electrical source, such as a power line, a malfunctioning household appliance or lightning, he or she conducts the electricity through the body. Electrical resistance of body parts produces heat, which can cause burn injuries (**Fig. 10-27, p. 196**). The severity of an electrical burn depends on the type and amount of contact, the current's path through the body and how long the contact lasted. Electrical burns are often deep. The victim may have an entrance wound and an exit wound where the current left the body. Although these wounds may look superficial, the tissues below may be severely damaged.

Electrical injuries cause problems in addition to burns. Electricity running through the body

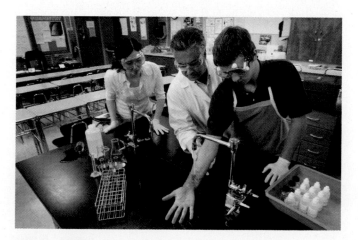

Figure 10-25   Flush a chemical burn with large amounts of cool running water.

STRIKING DISTANCE

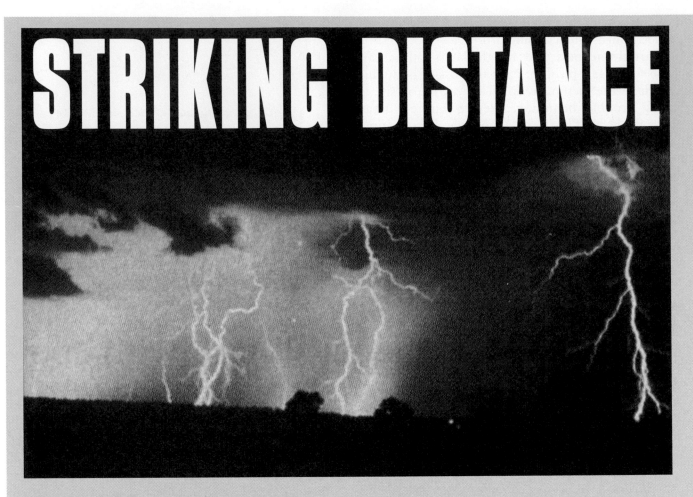

In medieval times, people believed that ringing church bells would dissipate lightning during thunderstorms. It was an unfortunate superstition for the bell ringers. Over one period of 33 years, lightning struck 386 church steeples and 103 bell ringers died (Kessler E).

Church bell ringers have dropped off the list of people most likely to be struck during a thunderstorm, but lightning strikes remain extremely dangerous. On average, lightning causes more deaths annually in the United States than any other weather hazard, including blizzards, hurricanes, floods, tornadoes, earthquakes and volcanic eruptions. The National Weather Service estimates that lightning kills nearly 100 people annually and injures about 300 others.

Lightning occurs when particles of water, ice and air moving inside storm clouds lose electrons. Eventually, the cloud becomes divided into layers of positive and negative particles. Most electrical currents run between the layers inside the cloud. However, occasionally, the negative charge flashes toward the ground, which has a positive charge. An electrical current snakes back and forth between the ground and the cloud many times in the seconds that we see a flash crackle down from the sky. Anything tall—a tower, a tree or a person—becomes a path for the electrical current.

Traveling at speeds up to 300 miles per second, a lightning strike can hurl a person through the air, burn his or her clothes off and sometimes cause the heart to stop beating. The most severe lightning strikes carry up to 50 million volts of electricity, enough to light 13,000 homes. Lightning can "flash" over a person's body, or, in its more dangerous path, it can travel through blood vessels and nerves to reach the ground.

Besides burns, lightning can also cause neurological damage, fractures and loss of hearing or eyesight. The victim sometimes acts confused and may describe the episode as getting hit on the head or hearing an explosion.

Use common sense around thunderstorms. If you see a storm approaching in the distance, do not wait until you are drenched to seek shelter. If a thunderstorm threatens, the National Weather Service advises you to—

- Postpone activities promptly. Do not wait for rain. Many people take shelter from the rain, but most people struck by lightning are not in the rain!
- Go quickly inside a completely enclosed building, not a carport, open garage or covered patio. If no enclosed building is convenient, a cave is a good option outside, but move as far as possible from the cave entrance.
- Watch cloud patterns and conditions for signals of an approaching storm.
- Designate safe locations and move or evacuate to a safe location at the first sound of thunder. Every 5 seconds between the flash of lightning and the sound (bang) of thunder equals 1 mile of distance.
- Use the 30-30 rule where visibility is good and there is nothing obstructing your view of the thunderstorm. When you see lightning, count the time until you hear thunder. If that time is 30 seconds or less, the thunderstorm is within 6 miles of you and is dangerous. Seek shelter immediately. The threat of lightning continues for a much longer period than most people realize. Wait at least 30 minutes after the last clap of thunder before leaving shelter. Do not be fooled by sunshine or blue sky! If inside during a storm, keep away from windows. Injuries may occur from flying debris or glass if a window breaks.

- Do not shower during a thunderstorm. Water and metal are both excellent conductors of electricity.
- Do not use a telephone, mobile phone or radio transmitter except for emergencies.

If you are caught in a storm outdoors and cannot find shelter, avoid—

- *Water.*
- *High ground.*
- *Open spaces.*
- All metal objects including electric wires, fences, machinery, motors, power tools, etc.
- Unsafe places, such as underneath canopies, small picnic or rain shelters or near trees.

Where possible, find shelter in a substantial building or in a fully enclosed metal vehicle, such as a hardtop car, truck or a van, with the windows completely shut.

If lightning is striking nearby when you are outside, you should—

- Crouch down. Put feet together. Place hands over ears to minimize hearing damage from thunder.

Avoid proximity to other people. Maintain a minimum distance of 15 feet between people. If there is a tornado alert, go to the location specified. This may be the basement or the lowest interior level of a building.

SOURCES

Kessler E: *The thunderstorm in human affairs,* Norman, Oklahoma, University of Oklahoma, 1983.

National Weather Service. *www.lightningsafety.noaa.gov/outdoors.htm.* Accessed 10/25/04.

Randall T: "50 million volts may crash through a lightning victim," *The Chicago Tribune,* Section 2D, August 13, 1989, p.1.

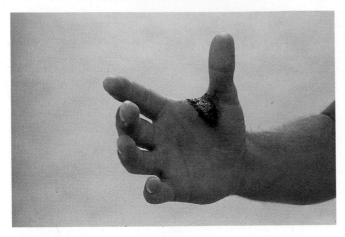

Figure 10-27 An electrical burn may severely damage underlying tissues.

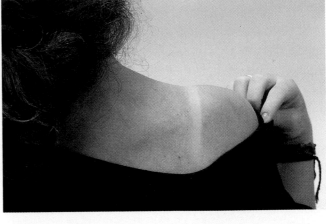

Figure 10-28 Solar radiation burns can be painful.

can make the heart beat erratically. As a result, the victim's heart or breathing may stop. The victim may also have fractured bones caused by strong muscle spasms. The signals of electrical injury include—

▶ Unconsciousness.
▶ Dazed, confused behavior.
▶ Obvious burns on the skin's surface.
▶ Trouble breathing or no breathing.
▶ Burns both where the current entered and where it exited the body, often on the hand or foot.

Suspect a possible electrical injury if you hear a sudden loud pop or bang or see an unexpected flash. Never go near a person with an electrical burn until you are sure the person is not still in contact with the power source. In case of high-voltage electrocution, such as that caused by down power lines, call 9-1-1 or the local emergency number. All people with electric shock require advanced medical care.

To care for a victim of an electrical injury, make sure the scene is safe. Turn off the power at its source and care for any life-threatening conditions. Electrocution can cause cardiac and breathing emergencies. Be prepared to give CPR or defibrillation, and care for shock and thermal burns.

In your check for non-life-threatening conditions, look for two burn sites, one where the current entered and one where it exited. Check for additional injuries, such as fractures.

Cover any burn injuries with a dry, sterile dressing and give care for shock.

Radiation Burns

The solar radiation of the sun and other types of radiation can cause burns. Solar burns are similar to heat burns. Usually solar burns are mild but can be painful (**Fig. 10-28**). They may blister, involving more than one layer of skin. Care for sunburns as you would any other burn. Cool the burn and protect the burned area from further damage by staying out of the sun. Do not break blisters. Intact skin helps prevent infection. People are rarely exposed to other types of radiation unless working in special settings, such as certain medical, industrial or research facilities. If you work in such settings, you should be informed of the risks and will be required to take precautions to prevent overexposure. Training is also provided to teach you how to prevent and respond to radiation emergencies.

INFECTION

Any break in the skin can provide an entry point for disease-producing microorganisms. Even a small, seemingly minor laceration or abrasion has the potential to become infected. An infection can range from being merely unpleasant to life threatening.

Preventing Infection

The best initial defense against infection is to cleanse the area thoroughly. For minor wounds, wash the area with plenty of soap and water. Most types of soaps are effective in removing harmful bacteria. Wounds that require medical attention be-

An Ounce of Prevention

A serious infection can cause severe medical problems. One such infection is tetanus, caused by the microorganism *Clostridium tetani*. This microorganism, commonly found in soil and feces of cows and horses, can infect many kinds of wounds. This probably explains why the cavalry in the American Civil War had higher rates of tetanus than the infantry. Worldwide, about 1 million people contract tetanus annually, with 20 to 50 percent of the cases resulting in death. In the United States, only 25 cases were reported in 2002.

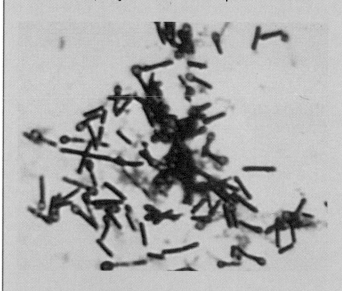

Tetanus is introduced into the body through a puncture wound, abrasion, laceration or burn. Because the organism multiplies in an environment that is low in oxygen, puncture wounds and other deep wounds are at particular risk for tetanus infection. The organism produces a powerful toxin, one of the most lethal poisons known, that affects the central nervous system and specific muscles. People injecting themselves with drugs, burn victims and people recovering from surgery have an increased risk of contracting the disease. Newborn babies can be infected through the stump of the umbilical cord.

Signals of tetanus include difficulty swallowing, irritability, headache, fever and muscle spasms near the infected area. As the infection progresses, it can affect other muscles, such as those in the jaw, causing the condition called "lockjaw." Once tetanus gets into the nervous system, its effects are irreversible.

The best way to prevent tetanus is to be immunized against it and then receive periodic booster shots. Immunizations assist the natural function of the immune system by building up antibodies, which are disease-fighting proteins that help protect the body against specific bacteria. Because the effects of immunization do not last a lifetime, booster shots help maintain the antibodies that protect against tetanus. Booster shots are recommended every 5 to 10 years or whenever a wound has been contaminated by dirt or an object, such as a rusty nail, that causes a puncture wound. Most infants or young children in this country receive an immunization known as DTaP, which includes the tetanus toxoid. About 70 percent of a sample of Americans 6 years of age or older were found to have antibodies in their systems that protect against tetanus. By age 60 to 69, however, the level of antibodies dropped to less than 50 percent and to about 30 percent by age 70. Fifty-nine percent of tetanus cases and 75 percent of deaths from tetanus occur in people 60 years of age or older.

The first line of defense against tetanus is to thoroughly clean an open wound. Clean a minor wound with soap and water, and apply an antibiotic ointment and a clean or sterile dressing. Major wounds should be cleaned and treated at a medical facility. If signals of wound infection develop, seek medical attention immediately. Infected wounds of the face, neck and head should receive immediate medical care, because the tetanus toxin can travel rapidly to the brain. A health-care provider will determine whether a tetanus shot is needed, depending on the victim's immunization status. Always contact your health-care provider if you do not remember the date of your last tetanus immunization or booster shot.

SOURCE
Sanford JP: "Tetanus—forgotten but not gone," *New England Journal of Medicine* 332(12):812-813.

cause of more extensive tissue damage or bleeding do not need be washed immediately. It is more important to control bleeding.

Puncture wounds do not bleed profusely and more readily become infected. Objects penetrating the soft tissues carry microorganisms that cause infections. Of particular danger is the microorganism that causes tetanus. Tetanus is a disease caused by bacteria that produces a powerful poison in the body. This poison enters the nervous system and can cause muscle paralysis (also known as "lockjaw"). Once tetanus reaches the nervous system, its effects are highly dangerous and can be fatal. However, in many cases, **tetanus** can now be successfully treated with **antitoxins.**

One of the ways to prevent tetanus is through immunization. Like all immunizations, the tetanus immunization helps the immune system defend against the invading pathogens that cause the disease. The immune system is the body system responsible for fighting off infection. Immunizations assist the natural function of the immune system by building up antibodies. Antibodies are disease-fighting proteins, which help protect the body against specific infections. The tetanus immunization is usually given in infancy. However, the effect of the immunization eventually wears off. Everyone should receive a booster shot at least every 10 years or whenever a wound is contaminated by dirt or an object, such as a rusty nail, that causes a puncture wound.

Signals

You can easily recognize the signals of an infection. The area around the wound becomes swollen and red. The area may feel warm or throb with pain. Some wounds have a pus discharge (**Fig. 10-29**). More serious infections may cause a person to develop a fever and feel ill. Red streaks may develop that progress from the wound in the direction of the heart.

Care

Care for an infected wound by keeping the area clean, elevating the area and applying warm, wet compresses and an antibiotic ointment. Change coverings over the wound daily. If a fever or red streaks develop, the infection is worsening. Contact your health-care provider to determine what additional care is necessary.

SUMMARY

Caring for wounds involves a few simple steps. You need to control bleeding and minimize the risk of infection. Remember that with minor wounds, your primary concern is to cleanse the wound to prevent infection. With major wounds, you should control

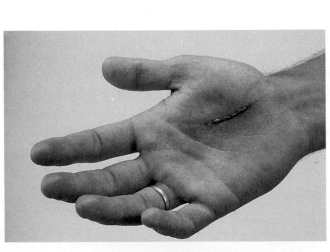
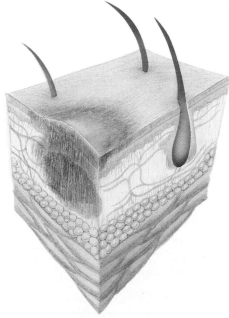

Figure 10-29   Close-up of palm of hand with infected cut.

the bleeding quickly and seek medical attention. Wear disposable gloves or use a barrier, such as plastic wrap, dressings or clean folded cloth, to avoid contact with blood. Dressings and bandages, when correctly applied, help control bleeding, reduce pain and minimize the danger of infection.

Burns damage the layers of the skin and sometimes the internal structures as well. Heat, chemicals, electricity and radiation all cause burns. When caring for a burn victim, always first ensure your personal safety. When the scene is safe, approach the victim, check for life-threatening conditions and for non-life-threatening conditions, if necessary. Follow the steps for burn care. In addition, always check for inhalation injury if the person has a heat or chemical burn. With electrical burns and victims of a lightning strike, check carefully for additional conditions, such as trouble breathing, cardiac arrest and fractures.

APPLICATION QUESTIONS

1. Which type of burn has Joe sustained? Why do you think so?

2. Will Joe's burns require medical attention? Why or why not?

3. What steps would you take to care for Joe's burns?

STUDY QUESTIONS

1. Match each term with the correct definition.

   a. Soft tissue
   b. Open wound
   c. Critical burn
   d. Bandages
   e. Closed wound
   f. Deep burn

   _____ Any burn that is potentially life threatening, disabling or disfiguring.

   _____ A burn that destroys skin and underlying tissues.

   _____ The layers of the skin, fat and muscles.

   _____ Wrappings that hold dressings in place.

   _____ Injury resulting in tissue damage beneath the skin's surface, while the skin remains intact.

   _____ Injury resulting in a break in the skin's surface.

2. Match each type of injury to its example.

   a. Abrasion
   b. Puncture
   c. Avulsion
   d. Contusion

   _____ Torn earlobe

   _____ Black eye

   _____ Scraped knee

   _____ Gunshot wound

3. Match each type of wound with the appropriate care.

   a. A major open wound
   b. A minor open wound
   c. A major open wound with an embedded object
   d. A severed body part

   _____ Cover with dressing and pressure bandage.

   _____ Wash the wound thoroughly with soap and water.

   _____ Wrap and place in plastic bag and then on ice.

   _____ Use bulky dressings to stabilize.

4. List four signals of infection.

5. List two purposes of bandaging.

6. List and describe four types of open wounds.

7. List four sources of burns.

8. Describe the following types of burns:

   a. Superficial burn
   b. Partial-thickness burn
   c. Full-thickness burn

In questions 9 through 24, circle the letter of the correct answer.

9. To prevent infection of a minor open wound you should—

   a. Wash the area with soap and water.
   b. Apply a pressure bandage.
   c. Remove all jewelry.
   d. Wrap the affected area with moist sterile dressings.

10. A signal of an infected open wound is—

    a. Red streaks from the wound in the direction of the heart.
    b. Swelling and redness around the wound.
    c. The affected area is cool to the touch
    d. Fever and chills.

11. Which should you do to care for an infected wound?

    a. Keep the area clean.
    b. Apply warm, wet compresses and a triple antibiotic ointment.
    c. Elevate the injured area.
    d. All of the above.

12. Which statement applies to all open wounds?

    a. They always bleed heavily.
    b. They are at risk for infection.
    c. They must always be cleaned immediately.
    d. They are life threatening.

13. Which distinguishes major open wounds from minor open wounds?

    a. The amount of dirt in the wound
    b. The depth of tissue damage
    c. The amount of pain that the victim is experiencing
    d. The amount of blood lost

14. Which should you do in caring for a major open wound?

    a. Apply direct pressure with a dressing to control bleeding.
    b. Wash the wound.
    c. Apply an occlusive dressing.
    d. Apply an antibiotic ointment.

15. Which should you do when caring for an injury in which the body part has been completely severed?

    a. Place the part directly on ice.
    b. Seek medical assistance and make sure the part is transported with the victim.
    c. Wash the body part thoroughly with soap and water.
    d. Secure it back in place using sterile roller bandages.

16. It is important to keep your immunizations up to date because—

    a. They provide lifetime protection against all threats of infection.
    b. They prepare your body to defend against certain infections.
    c. They stimulate the body to produce more blood.
    d. They eliminate the need to clean the wound.

17. A 6-year-old girl falls on a sharp object. The object is sticking out of her leg. What should you do?

    a. Allow the area to bleed freely.
    b. Remove the object and control bleeding.
    c. Wash the wound with soap and water.
    d. Stabilize the object in the position in which you find it.

18. Which is the step you should take to control external bleeding (minor)?

    a. Elevate the injured area.
    b. Apply direct pressure.
    c. Apply a pressure point.
    d. Apply a tourniquet.

19. Which could swelling and discoloration indicate?

    a. A closed wound
    b. Damage to underlying structures
    c. Internal bleeding
    d. All of the above

20. Which action would you take when caring for a minor closed wound?

    a. Use a warm compress over the wound.
    b. Apply cold and elevate the injured area.
    c. Keep the injured area below the level of the heart.
    d. Call 9-1-1 or the local emergency number.

21. What is the first step you should take when caring for an electrical burn?

    a. Check for life-threatening conditions.
    b. Make sure the scene is safe (the power source is turned off).
    c. Look for an entry and exit wound.
    d. Check for non-life-threatening conditions.

22. Which burns require professional medical attention?

    a. Burns that cover more than one body part.
    b. Burns whose victims are having trouble breathing.
    c. Burns resulting from electricity, explosions or chemicals.
    d. All of the above.

23. The chemist at the lab table near you spills a liquid corrosive chemical on his arm. Which would you do first?

    a. Remove the chemical with a clean cloth.
    b. Put a sterile dressing over the burn site.
    c. Flush the burn with water.
    d. Have the victim remove contaminated clothes.

24. Luke's grandmother was burned on one leg and foot when a pan of boiling water tipped off the stove. Which should Luke have done first to care for her?

    a. Put ice on the burned area.
    b. Put a dry, sterile dressing on the burned area.
    c. Help her put her foot and leg in the bathtub and flood it with cool water.
    d. Wash the area and then apply a burn ointment.

Answers are listed in Appendix A.

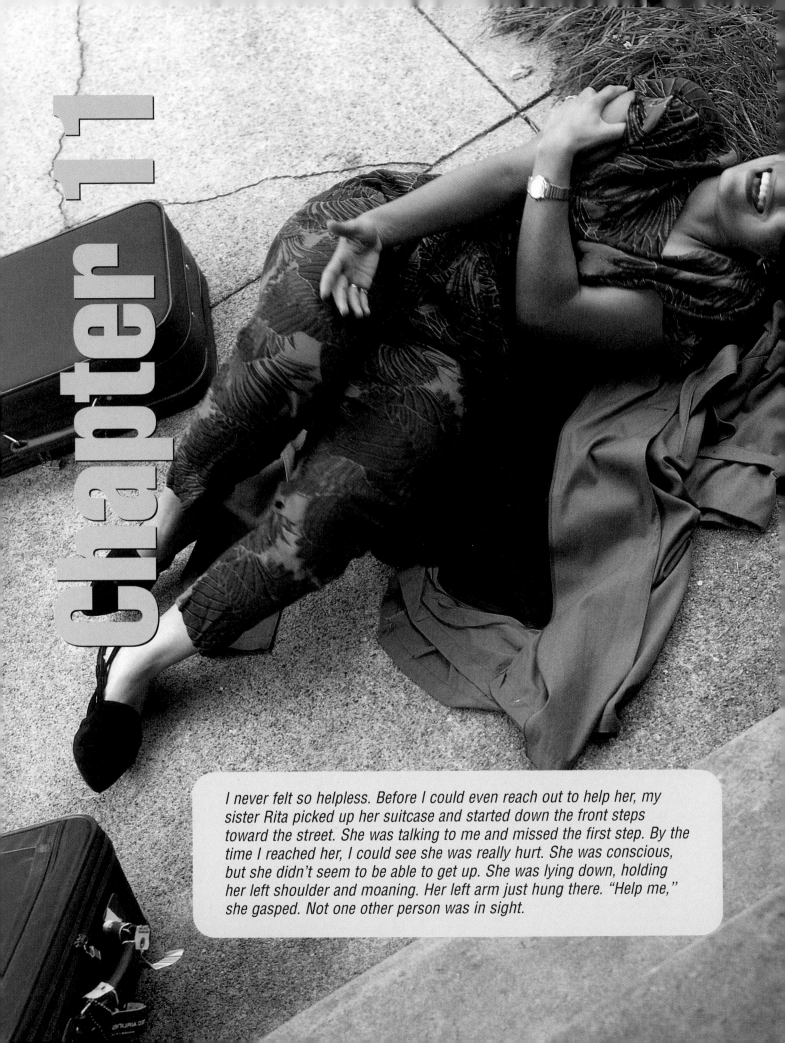

Chapter 11

I never felt so helpless. Before I could even reach out to help her, my sister Rita picked up her suitcase and started down the front steps toward the street. She was talking to me and missed the first step. By the time I reached her, I could see she was really hurt. She was conscious, but she didn't seem to be able to get up. She was lying down, holding her left shoulder and moaning. Her left arm just hung there. "Help me," she gasped. Not one other person was in sight.

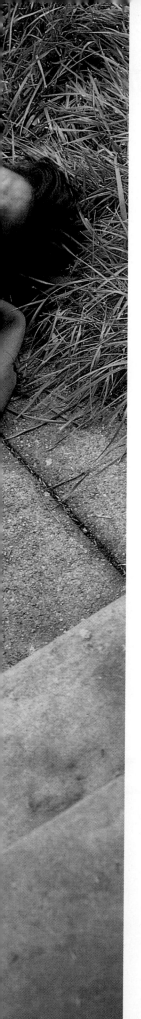

Musculoskeletal Injuries

Objectives

After reading this chapter, you should be able to—

■ *Identify four types of mechanical forces that can act upon the body and how these forces can lead to injury.*

■ *Identify four basic types of musculoskeletal injuries.*

■ *List eight signals of a serious musculoskeletal injury.*

■ *Describe the general care for musculoskeletal injuries.*

■ *List the five purposes for immobilizing a musculoskeletal injury.*

■ *List four principles of splinting.*

Introduction

Injuries to the musculoskeletal system are common. Millions of people at home, at work or at play injure their muscles, bones or joints. No age group is exempt. A person may fall and bruise his or her hip. A person who braces a hand against a dashboard in a car crash may injure the bones at the shoulder, disabling the arm. A person who falls while skiing may twist a leg, tearing the supportive tissues of a knee and making it impossible to stand or move.

Although musculoskeletal injuries are almost always painful, they are rarely life threatening when cared for properly. However, when not recognized and taken care of properly, musculoskeletal injuries can have serious consequences and even result in permanent disability or death. In this chapter, you will learn how to recognize and care for musculoskeletal injuries. Developing a better understanding of the structure and function of the body's framework will help you assess musculoskeletal injuries and give appropriate care.

THE MUSCULOSKELETAL SYSTEM

The musculoskeletal system is made up of muscles and bones that form the skeleton, as well as connective tissues, tendons and ligaments. Together, these structures give the body shape, form and stability. Bones and muscles connect to form various body segments. They work together to provide body movement.

Muscles

Muscles are soft tissues that are able to contract and relax. The body has over 600 muscles (**Fig. 11-1**). Most are *skeletal muscles,* which attach to the bones. Skeletal muscles account for most of your lean body weight (body weight without excess fat). All body movements result from skeletal muscles contracting and relaxing. Through a pathway of nerves, the brain directs muscles to contract, causing movement. Skeletal muscle actions are under our conscious control. Because you move them voluntarily, skeletal muscles are also called voluntary muscles. Skeletal muscles also protect the bones, nerves and blood vessels.

Most skeletal muscles are anchored to bone at each end by strong, cordlike, fibrous tissues called *tendons.* Muscles and their adjoining tendons extend across joints. When the brain sends a command to move, nerve impulses travel through the spinal cord and nerve pathways to the individual muscles and stimulate the muscle fibers to contract.

KEY TERMS

Bone: Dense, hard tissue that forms the skeleton.
Dislocation: The displacement of a bone from its normal position at a joint.
Fracture: A break or disruption in bone tissue.
Immobilize: Keep an injured body part from moving by using a splint or other method.
Joint: A structure where two or more bones are joined.
Ligament: A fibrous band that holds bones together at a joint.
Muscle: A soft tissue that contracts and relaxes to create movement.

Skeletal muscles: Muscles that attach to the bones.
Splint: A device used to immobilize body parts; to immobilize body parts with such a device.
Sprain: The stretching and tearing of ligaments and other soft tissue structures at a joint.
Strain: The stretching and tearing of muscles and tendons.
Tendon: A cordlike, fibrous band that attaches muscle to bone.

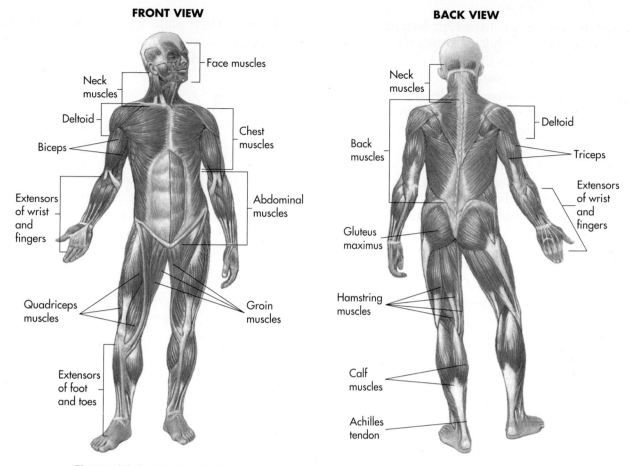

FRONT VIEW

Face muscles

Neck muscles

Deltoid

Biceps

Chest muscles

Extensors of wrist and fingers

Abdominal muscles

Quadriceps muscles

Groin muscles

Extensors of foot and toes

BACK VIEW

Neck muscles

Back muscles

Deltoid

Triceps

Extensors of wrist and fingers

Gluteus maximus

Hamstring muscles

Calf muscles

Achilles tendon

Figure 11-1   The body has over 600 muscles, most of them attached to bones by strong tissues called tendons. The shortening and lengthening of the muscles are what make the body move.

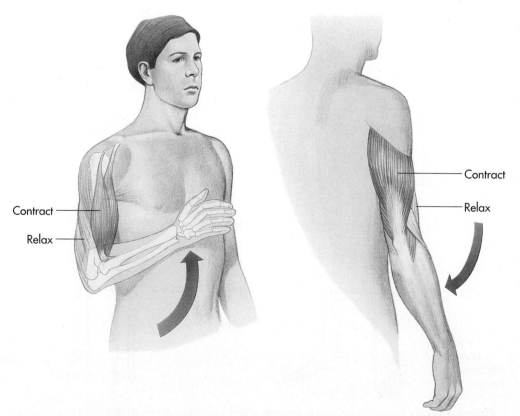

Contract

Relax

Contract

Relax

Figure 11-2   Movement occurs when one group of muscles contracts and an opposing group of muscles relaxes.

When the muscle fibers contract, pulling the ends of the muscle closer together, the muscles pull the bones, causing motion at the joint.

Muscles in a group often pull at the same time. For instance, the hamstring muscles are a group of muscles at the back of the thigh. When the hamstrings contract, the leg bends at the knee joint. The biceps are a group of muscles at the front of the upper arm. When the biceps contract, the arm bends at the elbow joint. Generally, when one group of muscles contracts, another group of muscles on the opposite side of the body part relaxes (**Fig. 11-2**). Even simple tasks, such as bending to pick up an object from the floor, involve a complex series of movements in which different muscle groups contract and relax.

Injuries to the brain, spinal cord or nerves can affect muscle control. A loss of muscle movement is called **paralysis.** Less serious or isolated muscle in-

juries may affect only strength because adjacent muscles can often do double duty and take over for the injured muscle.

The Skeleton

The skeleton is formed by over 200 bones of various sizes and shapes (**Fig. 11-3**). These bones shape the skeleton, giving each body part a characteristic form. The skeleton protects vital organs and other soft tissues. The skull protects the brain (**Fig. 11-4, _A_**). The ribs protect the heart and lungs (**Fig. 11-4, _B_**). The **spinal cord** is protected by the canal formed by the bones that form the spinal column (**Fig. 11-4, _C_**). Two or more bones come together to form joints. _Ligaments_, fibrous bands that hold bones together at joints, give the skeleton stability and, with the muscles, help maintain posture.

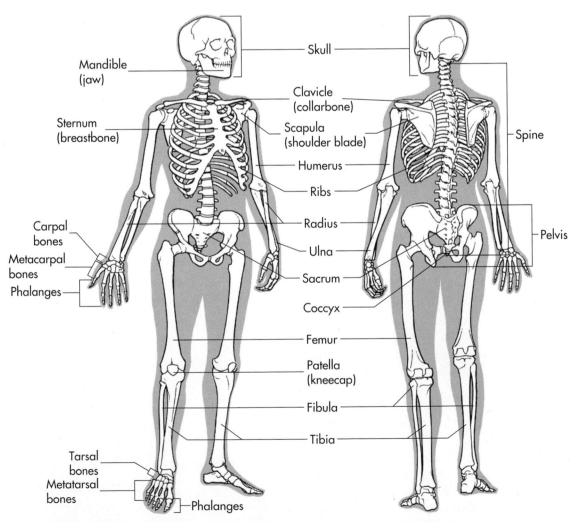

Figure 11-3 Over 200 bones in various sizes and shapes form the skeleton. The skeleton protects many of the organs inside the body.

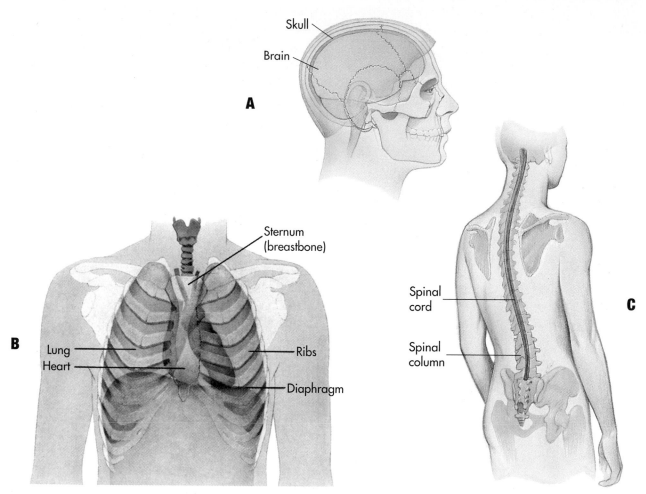

Figure 11–4   **A,** The immovable bones of the skull protect the brain. **B,** The rib cage protects the heart and lungs. **C,** The spinal cord is protected by the vertebrae.

Bones

Bones are hard, dense **tissues.** The strong, rigid structure of bones helps them to withstand stresses that cause injuries. The shape of bones depends on what the bones do and the stresses placed on them. For instance, although similar to the bones of the arms, the bones of the legs are much larger and stronger because they carry the body's weight (**Fig. 11-5**).

Bones have a rich supply of blood and nerves. Some bones store and manufacture red blood cells and supply them to the circulating blood. Bone injuries can bleed and are usually painful. The bleeding can become life threatening if not properly cared for. Bones heal by developing new bone cells within a fibrous network of tissue that forms between the broken bone ends. Bone is the only body tissue that can regenerate in this way.

Bones weaken with age. Young children's are softer and more porous than adults' bones, so they bend and break more easily. At puberty, a child's

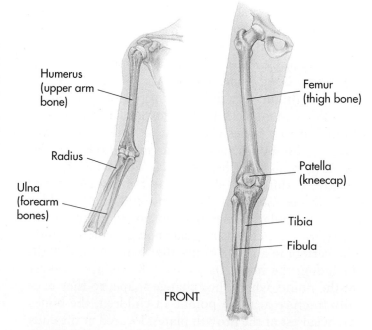

Figure 11-5   Leg bones are larger and stronger than arm bones because they carry the body's weight.

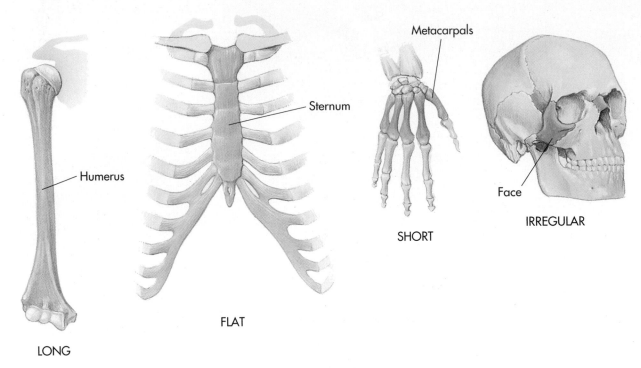

Figure 11-6   Bones vary in shape and size. Bones are weakest at the points where they change shape and usually fracture at these points.

bones become as hard as an adult's. As people age, their bones lose mass and density and bones are more likely to give way to even everyday stresses, which can cause significant injuries. For instance, an elderly person with significant bone loss can easily break the strongest bone in the body, the femur (thigh bone), just by pivoting his or her weight on one leg. The gradual, progressive weakening of bone is called **osteoporosis.**

Bones are classified as long, short, flat or irregular (**Fig. 11-6**). Long bones are longer than they are wide. Long bones include the bones of the upper arm (humerus), the forearm (radius and ulna), the thigh (femur) and the lower leg (tibia and fibula). Short bones are about as wide as they are long. Short bones include the small bones of the hand (carpals) and feet (tarsals). Flat bones have a relatively thin, flat shape. Flat bones include the breastbone (sternum), the ribs and the shoulder blade (scapula). Bones that do not fit in the other categories are called irregular bones, which include the vertebrae and the bones that make up the skull, including the bones of the face. Bones are weakest at the points where they change shape, so they usually fracture at these points. In children, the bones are weakest at the growth plates, located at the ends of long bones.

Joints

A *joint* is formed by the ends of two or more bones coming together at one place. Most joints allow motion. However, the ends of the bones at some joints are fused together, which restricts motion. Fused bones, such as the bones of the skull, form solid structures that protect their contents (**Fig. 11-7**).

Joints that allow movement are held together by tough, fibrous connective tissues called ligaments (**Fig. 11-8**). Ligaments resist joint movement. Joints surrounded by ligaments have restricted movement; joints that have few ligaments move more freely. For instance, the shoulder joint, with few ligaments, allows greater motion than the hip joint, although their structures are similar.

Joints that move more freely, such as the ankle and shoulder, have less natural support, which makes them more prone to injury. However, all joints have a normal range of movement. When a joint is forced beyond its normal range, ligaments stretch and tear, making the joint unstable. Unstable joints can be disabling, particularly when they are weight bearing, such as the knee or ankle. Unstable joints are also prone to re-injury and often develop arthritis in later years.

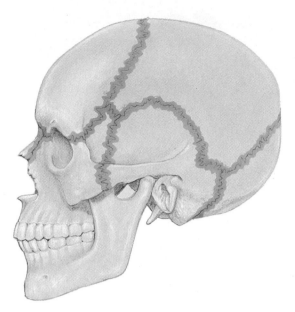

Figure 11-7   Fused bones, such as bones of the skull, form solid structures that protect their contents.

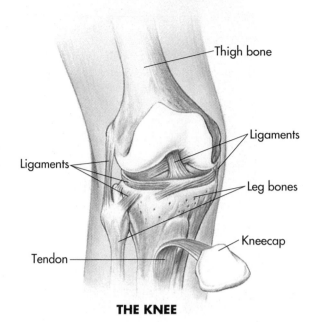

THE KNEE

Figure 11-8   A typical joint consists of two or more bones held together by ligaments.

INJURIES TO THE MUSCULOSKELETAL SYSTEM

Injuries to the musculoskeletal system are most commonly caused by mechanical forms of energy but can also occur from heat, chemical or electrical energy. Mechanical energy produces direct, indirect, twisting and contracting forces (**Fig. 11-9**). These forces can injure the structures of the musculoskeletal system. A direct force is the force of an object striking the body and causing injury at the point of impact. Direct forces can either be blunt or penetrating. For example, a fist striking the chin can break the jaw, or penetrating objects, such as bullets and knives, can injure structures beneath the skin at the point where they penetrate.

An indirect force travels through the body and causes injury to a body part away from the point of impact. For example, a fall on an outstretched hand may result in an injury to the shoulder or collarbone.

In twisting, one part of the body stays in one position while another part of the body turns. The twisting action can force body parts beyond their normal range of motion, causing injury. For example, if a ski and its binding keep the lower leg in one position while the body falls in another, the knee may be forced beyond its normal range of motion, causing injury. Twisting injuries are not always this complex. Twisting injuries more often occur from simply stepping off a curb (ankle) or turning to reach for an out-of-the-way object (back).

Sudden or powerful muscle contractions can result in musculoskeletal injuries. These injuries commonly occur in sports activities, such as throwing a ball a long distance without properly warming up or sprinting when out of shape. However, our daily routines also require sudden and powerful muscle contractions, such as when we suddenly turn to catch a heavy object like a falling child. Although infrequent, sudden and powerful muscle contractions can even pull a piece of bone away from the point at which it is normally attached.

Types of Musculoskeletal Injuries

The four basic types of musculoskeletal injuries are fracture, dislocation, sprain and strain. Injuries to the musculoskeletal system can be classified according to the body structures that are damaged. Some injuries may involve damage to more than one structure. For example, a direct blow to the knee may injure both ligaments and bones. Injuries are also classified by the nature and extent of the damage.

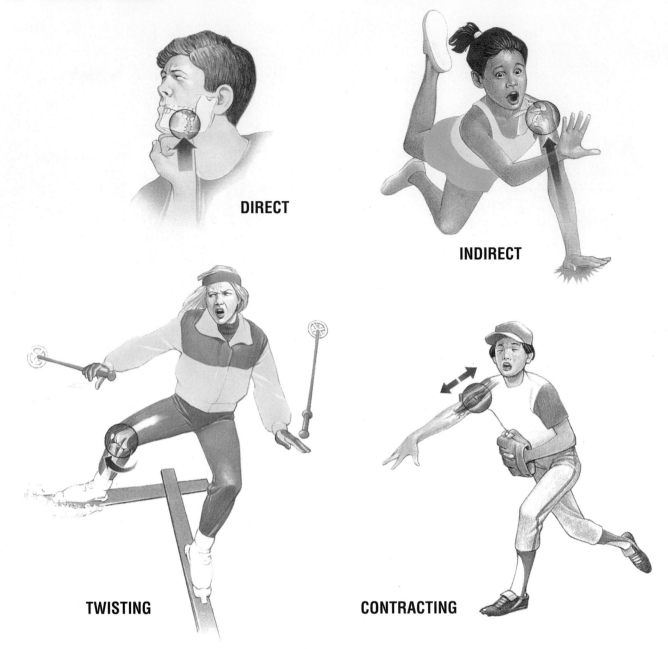

DIRECT

INDIRECT

TWISTING

CONTRACTING

Figure 11-9 Four forces—direct, indirect, twisting and contracting—cause 76 percent of all musculoskeletal injuries.

Fracture

A *fracture* is a break or disruption in bone tissue. Fractures include bones that are chipped or cracked, as well as bones that are broken all the way through (**Fig. 11-10**). Direct and indirect forces commonly cause fractures. However, if strong enough, twisting forces and strong muscle contractions can cause a fracture.

Fractures are classified as open or closed. **Open fractures** occur when the skin over the fracture site is broken. An example of an open fracture is when a limb is severely angulated or bent, causing bone ends to tear the skin and surrounding soft tissues.

Another example is when an object penetrates the skin and breaks the bone. Bone ends do not have to be visible in an open fracture. **Closed fractures** leave the skin unbroken and are more common than open fractures. Open fractures are more serious than closed fractures because of the risks of severe blood loss and infection. Although fractures are rarely an immediate threat to life, any fracture involving a large bone, such as the femur or pelvis, can cause severe shock because bones and soft tissue may bleed heavily.

Fractures are not always obvious unless a telltale sign, such as an open wound with protruding

The Breaking Point

Osteoporosis is a degenerative bone disorder. Research estimates indicate that among individuals over 50, osteoporosis can strike at any age. It is estimated that one out of every two women and one in four men will be affected by osteoporosis in their lifetime. Fair-skinned women with ancestors from northern Europe, the British Isles, Japan or China are genetically predisposed to osteoporosis. Inactive people are more susceptible to osteoporosis.

Osteoporosis occurs when the calcium content of bones decreases. Normally, bones are hard, dense tissues that endure tremendous stresses. Bone-building cells constantly repair damage that occurs as a result of everyday stresses, keeping bones strong. Calcium is vital to bone growth, development and repair. When the calcium content of bones decreases, bones become frail, less dense and less able to repair the normal damage they incur.

This loss of density and strength leaves bones more susceptible to fractures. Where once tremendous force was necessary to cause a fracture, fractures now may occur with little or no aggravation, especially to hips, vertebrae and wrists. Spontaneous fractures occur without trauma. The victim may be taking a walk or washing dishes when the fracture occurs. Some hip fractures thought to be caused by falls are actually spontaneous fractures that caused the victim's fall.

Osteoporosis can begin as early as age 30 to 35. The amount of calcium absorbed from the diet naturally declines with age, making calcium intake increasingly important. When calcium in the diet is inadequate, calcium in bones is withdrawn and used by the body to meet its other needs, leaving bones weakened.

Building strong bones before age 35 is the key to preventing osteoporosis. Calcium and exercise are necessary to bone building. The United States recommended daily allowance (U.S. RDA) ranges from 1000 to 2000 milligrams of calcium each day for adults over the age of 18. Three to four daily servings of low-fat dairy products should provide adequate calcium. Vitamin D is also necessary because it aids in absorption of calcium. Exposure to sunshine allows the body to make vitamin D. Fifteen minutes of sunshine on the hands and face of a young, light-skinned individual are enough to supply the RDA of vitamin D per day. Dark-skinned people and people over the age of 65 need more sun exposure. People who do not receive adequate sun exposure need to consume vitamin D. The best sources are vitamin-fortified milk and fatty fish such as tuna, salmon and eel.

Calcium supplements combined with vitamin D are available for those who do not take in adequate calcium. However, before taking a calcium supplement, consult your health-care provider. Many advertised calcium supplements are ineffective because they do not dissolve well in the body.

Exercise seems to increase bone density and the activity of bone-building cells. Regular exercise may reduce the rate of bone loss by promoting new bone formation and may stimulate the skeletal system to repair itself. An effective exercise program, such as aerobics, jogging or walking, involves the weight-bearing muscles of the legs. If you have any questions regarding your health and osteoporosis, consult a health-care provider.

bone ends or a severely deformed body part, is present. But the way in which the injury occurred is often enough to suggest a possible fracture.

Dislocation

A *dislocation* is a displacement or separation of a bone from its normal position at a joint (**Fig. 11-11**). As with a fracture, a dislocation can be caused by severe direct, indirect or twisting forces. A force violent enough to cause a dislocation can also cause a fracture, as well as cause damage to nearby nerves and blood vessels. Some joints, such as the shoulder or finger, dislocate easily because their bones and ligaments are small and fragile (**Fig. 11-12**). Other joints, such as joints of the elbow or spine, are well protected because of the shape of the bones and the way they fit together; therefore, they dislocate less easily.

Sprain

A *sprain* is the partial or complete tearing or stretching of ligaments and other tissues at a joint (**Fig.11-13, A**). A sprain usually results when the bones that form a joint are forced beyond their normal range of motion. The more ligaments that are torn, the more severe the injury. The sudden, violent forcing of a joint beyond its range of motion can completely rupture ligaments and even dislocate the bones. Severe sprains may also involve a fracture of the bones that form the joint. Ligaments may pull bone away from their point of attachment. Young children are more likely to have a

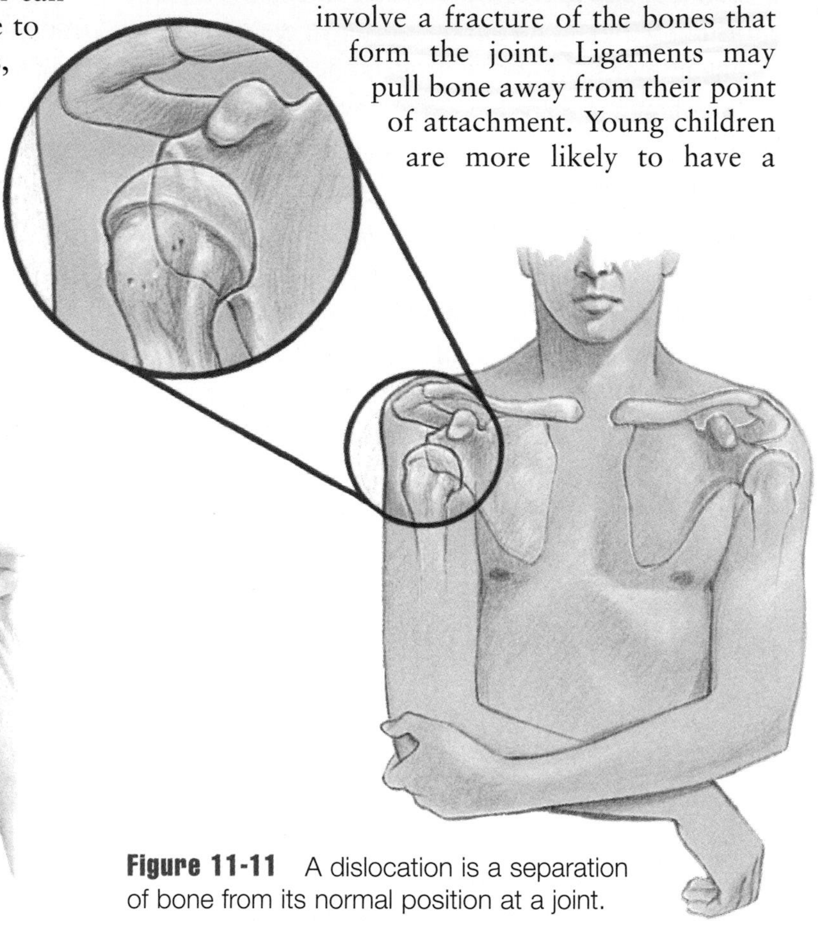

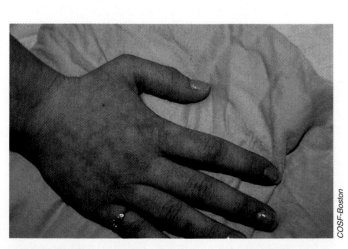

Figure 11-11   A dislocation is a separation of bone from its normal position at a joint.

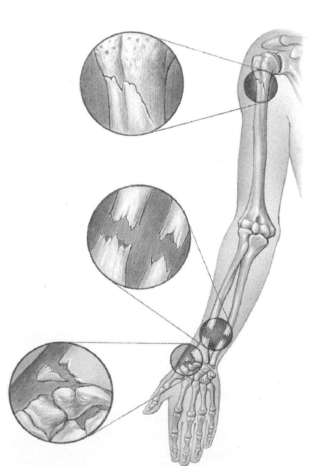

Figure 11-10   Fractures include chipped or cracked bones and bones broken all the way through.

Figure 11-12   Obvious deformity in thumb (dislocation).

fracture than a sprain because their ligaments are stronger than their bones.

Mild sprains, which stretch ligament fibers, generally heal quickly. The victim may have only a brief period of pain or discomfort and quickly return to activity with little or no soreness. For this reason, people often neglect sprains and the joint is often re-injured. Severe sprains or sprains that involve a fracture usually cause pain when the joint is moved or used. The weight-bearing joints of the ankle and knee and the joints of the fingers and wrist are those most commonly sprained.

Surprisingly, a sprain can be more disabling than a fracture. When fractures heal, they usually leave the bone as strong as it was before, or stronger, decreasing the likelihood that a second break will occur at the same spot. On the other hand, ligaments cannot regenerate. If the stretched or torn ligaments are not repaired, they render the joint less stable and may impede motion. The injured area may also be more susceptible to re-injury.

Figure 11-13 **A,** Injuries to joints are usually sprains. **B,** Injuries to the soft tissue between joints, the muscles and tendons, are strains.

Strain

A *strain* is a stretching and tearing of muscle fibers or tendons (**Fig. 11-13,** *B*). A strain is sometimes called a muscle pull or tear. Because tendons are tougher and stronger than muscles, tears usually occur in the muscle itself or where the muscle attaches to the tendon. Strains often result from overexertion, such as lifting something too heavy or working a muscle too hard. They can also result from sudden or uncoordinated movement. Strains commonly involve the muscles in the neck or back, the front or back of the thigh or the back of the lower

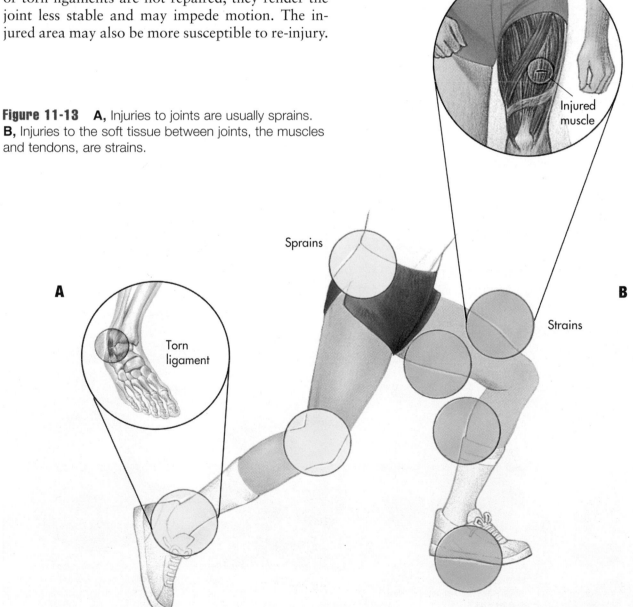

Heat or Cold?

Spring is the season of flowers, trees, strains and sprains. Almost as soon as armchair athletes come out of hibernation to become intramural heroes, emergency departments see an increase in sprained ankles, twisted knees and strained backs. So what do you do when you attempt the first slide of the softball season and wind up injured? Should you apply heat or apply cold?

The answer is both. First cold, then heat. And this treatment is the same whether the injury is a strain or a sprain.

How cold helps initially

When a person twists an ankle or strains his or her back, the tissues underneath the skin are injured. Blood and fluids seep out from the torn blood vessels and cause swelling to occur at the site of the injury. Your initial first aid objective is to keep the injured area cool to help control internal bleeding and reduce pain. Cold causes the broken blood vessels to constrict, limiting the blood and fluid that seep out. Cold also reduces muscle spasms and numbs the nerve endings.

How heat helps repair the tissue

A health-care provider will most likely advise applying ice periodically to the injury for about 48 hours or until the swelling goes away. After that, applying heat is often the more appropriate care. Heat speeds up chemical reactions needed to repair the tissue. White blood cells move in to rid the body of infections, and other cells begin the repair process, expediting proper healing of the injury. Applying heat too early, however, can cause swelling to increase, delaying healing. If you are unsure whether to use cold or heat on an injured area, always apply cold until you can consult a health-care provider.

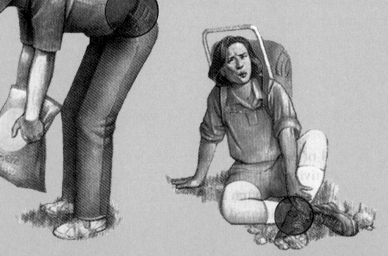

STRAIN **SPRAIN**

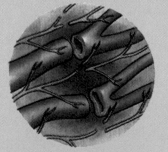

An injury causes damage to blood vessels, causing bleeding in the injured areas. Injury irritates nerve endings, causing pain.

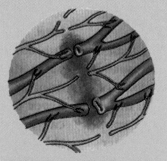

Applying ice or a cold pack constricts vessels, showing bleeding that causes the injury to swell. Cold deadens nerve endings relieving pain.

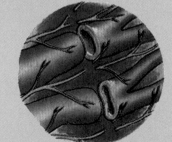

Applying heat dilates blood vessels, increasing blood flow to the injured area. Nerve endings become more sensitive.

leg. Strains of the neck and lower back can be particularly painful and therefore disabling.

Like sprains, strains are often neglected, which commonly leads to re-injury. Strains sometimes recur chronically, especially to the muscles of the neck, lower back and the back of the thigh. Neck and back problems are two of the leading causes of absenteeism from work, accounting annually for billions of dollars in workers' compensation claims and lost productivity.

Usually only a trained medical professional can tell the difference between a sprain, strain, fracture or dislocation. However, you do not need to know what kind of injury it is to give the appropriate care. The primary goal of care is to prevent further injury and get medical attention for the victim.

Checking for Musculoskeletal Injuries

You identify and care for injuries to the musculoskeletal system during the check for non-life-threatening conditions. Because musculoskeletal injuries look alike, you may have difficulty determining exactly what type of injury has occurred. Do not worry if you cannot identify the exact type of injury. It is more important to give proper care. As you check the victim, think about how the body normally looks and feels. Ask how the injury happened and if there are any areas that are painful. Visually inspect the entire body, beginning with the head. Compare the two sides of the body. Then, carefully check each body part. Do not ask the victim to move any areas in which he or she has pain or discomfort or if you suspect injury to the head, neck or back. Start with the neck, followed by the shoulders, the chest and so on. As you conduct the check, look for clues that may indicate a musculoskeletal injury.

Signals

Always suspect a serious injury when any of the following signals are present:

- Deformity
- Moderate or severe pain or discomfort, swelling and discoloration
- Inability to move or use the affected body part
- Bone fragments protruding from a wound
- Victim feels bones grating or felt or heard a snap or pop at the time of injury

- Loss of circulation or sensation in an **extremity** (the shoulders to the fingers; the hips to the toes)
- Tingling, cold or bluish color below the site of the injury
- Cause of the injury, such as a fall or vehicle crash, suggests the injury may be severe

Obvious deformity is often a signal of fracture or dislocation (**Fig. 11-14**). Abnormal lumps, ridges, depressions or unusual angles in body parts are types of deformities you may see. Dislocations are generally more obvious than other musculoskeletal injuries because the joint appears deformed. The displaced bone end often causes an abnormal lump, ridge or depression. Comparing the injured part to an uninjured part may help you detect a deformity.

Pain, swelling and discoloration of the skin commonly occur with any significant musculoskeletal injury. The injured area may be painful to touch and to move. Swelling and discoloration of the skin surrounding the injury are caused by bleeding from damaged blood vessels and tissues in the injured area. Swelling may appear rapidly at the site of injury, develop gradually or not appear at all. At first, the skin may only look red. As blood seeps to the skin's surface, the area begins to look bruised.

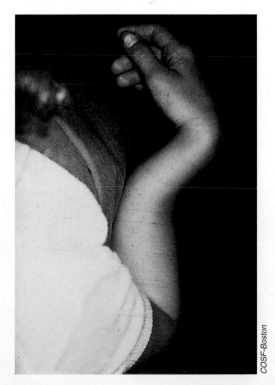

Figure 11-14   Serious bone or joint injuries may appear deformed.

COSF–Boston

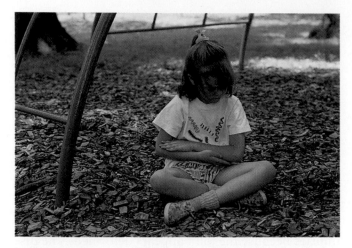

Figure 11-15 A victim with a broken bone will usually support the injured area in a comfortable position.

A victim's inability to move or use an injured part may also indicate a significant injury. The victim may tell you he or she is unable to move the part or that moving the injured part is simply too painful. Often, the muscles of an affected area contract in an attempt to hold the injured part in place. This muscle contraction helps to reduce pain and prevent further injury. Similarly, a victim often supports the injured part in the most comfortable position (**Fig. 11-15**). To manage musculoskeletal injuries, avoid any use of an injured body part that causes pain.

A lack of sensation in the affected part can also indicate serious injury or injury in another area. Fingers or toes, for example, can lose sensation if the arm or leg is injured. Also, check the victim's skin below the injured site for feeling, warmth and color (**Fig. 11-16**). Skin that is cold to the touch or bluish in color indicates a lack of or reduced circulation.

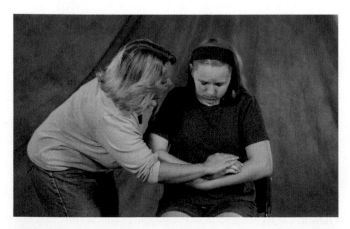

Figure 11-16 Check for feeling, warmth and color below the site of the injury.

Care

CHECK for any life-threatening conditions and give appropriate care. CALL 9-1-1 or the local emergency number if necessary. Then check for any non-life-threatening conditions and care for any other injuries.

CALL 9-1-1 or the local emergency number if—

▶ The injury involves the head, neck or back.
▶ The injury impairs walking or breathing.
▶ You see or suspect a fracture or dislocation.
▶ You see or suspect multiple musculoskeletal injuries.

The general care for musculoskeletal injuries includes following *RICE*: rest, immobilization, cold and elevation (**Fig. 11-17**).

Rest

Avoid any movements or activities that cause pain. Do not move or straighten the injured area. Help the victim find the most comfortable position. If you suspect injuries to the head, neck or back, it is best not to move the victim if the victim is unresponsive and has difficulty breathing. If you are alone and have to leave to get help, place the victim in a modified H.A.IN.E.S. (High Arm IN Endangered Spine) recovery position.

Immobilization

If you suspect a serious musculoskeletal injury, you must *immobilize* the injured part (keep it from moving) before giving additional care, such as applying ice or elevation. The purposes of immobilizing an injury are to—

▶ Lessen pain.
▶ Prevent further damage to soft tissues.
▶ Reduce the risk of serious bleeding.

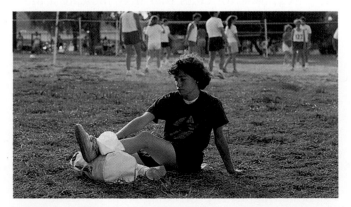

Figure 11-17 General care for all musculoskeletal injuries is similar. Remember rest, immobilization, cold and elevation.

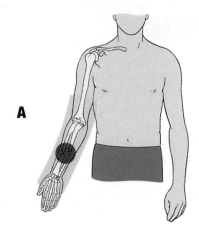 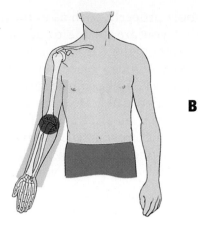

Figure 11-18 A, To immobilize a bone, the splint must include the joints above and below the fracture. **B,** To immobilize a joint, the splint must include the bones above and below the injured joint.

▶ Reduce the possibility of loss of circulation to the injured part.

▶ Prevent closed fractures from becoming open fractures.

You can immobilize an injured part by applying a splint, sling or bandages to keep the injured body part from moving. A *splint* is a device that maintains an injured part in place. An effective splint must extend above and below the injury site (**Fig. 11-18,** *A* and *B*). For instance, to immobilize a fractured bone, the splint must include the joints above and below the fracture. To immobilize a sprained or dislocated joint, the splint must include the bones above and below the injured joint.

When using a splint, follow these basic principles:

▶ Splint only if you have to move the injured person and you can do so without causing more pain and discomfort to the victim.

▶ Splint an injury in the position in which you find it. Do not move, straighten or bend the injured part.

▶ Splint the injured area and the joints or bones above and below the injury site.

▶ Check for proper circulation (feeling, warmth and color) before and after splinting.

Keep the victim as comfortable as possible, and avoid overheating or chilling. Monitor the victim's ABCs. Chapter 12 discusses splinting in detail.

Cold

Cold helps reduce swelling and eases pain and discomfort. You can make an ice pack by placing ice in a plastic bag and wrapping it with a towel or cloth or by using a large bag of frozen vegetables, such as peas. Place a layer of gauze or cloth between the source of cold and the skin to prevent damage to the skin. Leave an ice or a cold pack on the victim for no longer than 20 minutes. Remove the ice pack for 20 minutes. Reapply a new ice pack for an additional 20 minutes. Do not apply a cold pack to an open fracture. This could put pressure on the open fracture site, which could cause discomfort to the victim and possibly make the injury worse.

Elevation

Elevating the injured area helps slow the flow of blood, reducing swelling. If possible, elevate the injured area above the level of the heart. *Do not attempt to elevate a part you suspect is fractured or dislocated unless it has been immobilized or if it causes the victim more pain.*

CONSIDERATIONS FOR TRANSPORTING A VICTIM

Some musculoskeletal injuries are obviously minor and do not require professional medical care. Others may require you to call 9-1-1 or the local emergency number. If you discover a life-threatening emergency or think that one might develop, call 9-1-1 or the local emergency number and wait for help. Always call 9-1-1 or the local emergency number for any injury involving severe bleeding; suspected injuries to the head, neck or back; and possible serious injuries that may be difficult to transport properly, such as to the back, hip or legs, or that you are unable to adequately immobilize. Remember that fractures of large bones and severe sprains can bleed severely and are likely to cause shock. Some injuries are not serious enough for you to call EMS personnel but still require professional medical care. If you decide to transport the victim yourself, always splint the injury before moving the victim. If possible, have someone else drive you so that you can continue to give care.

SUMMARY

Sometimes it is difficult to tell whether an injury is a fracture, dislocation, sprain or strain. Because you cannot be sure which type of injury a victim might have, always care for the injury as if it were serious. If EMS personnel are on the way, do not move the victim. Control any bleeding. Take steps to minimize shock and monitor ABCs. If you need to transport the victim to a medical facility, be sure to immobilize the injury before moving the victim.

APPLICATION QUESTIONS

1. What types of musculoskeletal injuries could Rita have as a result of her fall?

3. What can Rita's sister do to make her more comfortable?

2. What would indicate that Rita's injury is severe?

4. Should her sister call EMS personnel? Why or why not?

STUDY QUESTIONS

1. Match each item with the correct definition.

a. Bone
b. Dislocation
c. Fracture
d. Joint
e. Ligaments
f. Muscle

g. Skeletal muscles
h. Splint
i. Sprain
j. Strain
k. Tendon

_____ Device used to keep body parts from moving.

_____ Displacement of a bone from its normal position at a joint.

_____ Tissue that contracts and relaxes to create movement.

_____ Broken bone.

_____ Dense, hard tissue that forms the skeleton.

_____ Injury that stretches and tears ligaments and other soft tissues at joints.

_____ Fibrous band attaching muscle to bone.

_____ Structure formed where two or more bones meet.

_____ Injury that stretches and tears muscles and tendons.

_____ Muscles that attach to bones.

_____ Fibrous bands holding bones together at joints.

2. List three common signals of musculoskeletal injuries.

3. List four principles of splinting.

In questions 4 through 8, circle the letter of the correct answer.

4. Which should you do when caring for an injured joint?

a. Have the victim immediately move the injured area.
b. Straighten the injured area before splinting.
c. Apply cold to the injured area.
d. Keep the injured area below the level of the heart.

5. Signals of a serious musculoskeletal injury include—

   a. Feeling, warmth and color below the site of the injury.
   b. Deformity or bone fragments protruding from a wound.
   c. The victim was hit in the thigh by a softball.
   d. Ability to move the injured area.

6. You find a person lying quietly on the ground. Her right leg is twisted at an unusual angle and you can see protruding bones and blood. Which do you do first?

   a. Straighten the leg.
   b. Check for life-threatening conditions.
   c. Use direct pressure to stop the bleeding.
   d. Look for material to use to immobilize the injured area.

7. Why should you immobilize a musculoskeletal injury?

   a. To prevent further injury to soft tissues
   b. To eliminate all discomfort or pain
   c. To control serious bleeding
   d. To help the victim to heal

8. Which step would you take before **and** after splinting an injury?

   a. Tell the victim to move the injured area.
   b. Check for feeling, warmth and color.
   c. Slide the splint down to extend below the injured area.
   d. Elevate the legs 8 inches.

Answers are listed in Appendix A.

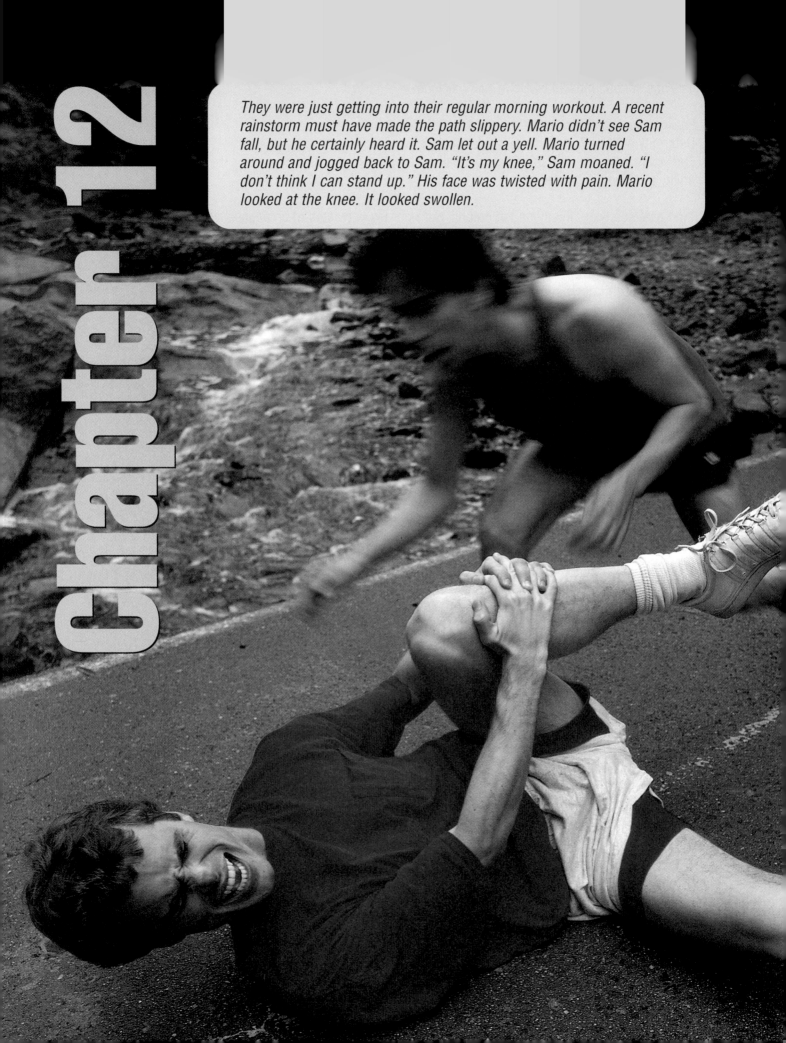

Chapter 12

They were just getting into their regular morning workout. A recent rainstorm must have made the path slippery. Mario didn't see Sam fall, but he certainly heard it. Sam let out a yell. Mario turned around and jogged back to Sam. "It's my knee," Sam moaned. "I don't think I can stand up." His face was twisted with pain. Mario looked at the knee. It looked swollen.

Injuries to the Extremities

Objectives

After reading this chapter, you should be able to—

■ *Describe how to care for injuries to the shoulder, upper arm and elbow.*

■ *Describe how to care for injuries to the forearm, wrist and hand.*

■ *List three specific signals of a fractured thigh bone.*

■ *Describe how to care for injuries to the thigh, lower leg and knee.*

■ *Describe how to care for injuries to the ankle and foot.*

After reading this chapter and completing the class activities, you should be able to demonstrate—

■ *How to effectively immobilize an injured extremity using an anatomic, soft or rigid splint.*

■ *How to effectively immobilize an upper extremity injury using a sling and a binder.*

Introduction

*Injuries to an **extremity**—an arm or leg—
are quite common. They can range from a
simple bruise to a dangerous or severely
painful injury, such as a fracture of the femur
(**thigh bone**). The prompt care you give can
help prevent further pain, damage and a lifelong disability.*

IMMOBILIZING EXTREMITY INJURIES

If you suspect a serious musculoskeletal injury, you
must immobilize the injured part before giving additional care, such as applying ice or elevating the
injured extremity. To immobilize an extremity injury, you can use a splint. There are three types of
splints—soft, rigid and anatomic. Soft splints include folded blankets, towels, pillows and a sling or
folded triangular bandages (cravat) (**Fig. 12-1**).
Rigid splints include boards, metal strips and folded
magazines or newspapers (**Fig. 12-2**). Anatomic
splints use the body as a splint. For example, an
arm can be splinted to the chest. An injured leg can
be splinted to the uninjured leg (**Fig. 12-3**). Remember, splint only if you must move the victim
and you can do so without causing more pain or
discomfort.

Splints are commercially made or can be improvised from materials at hand. Commercial splints
include padded board splints, air splints and spe-

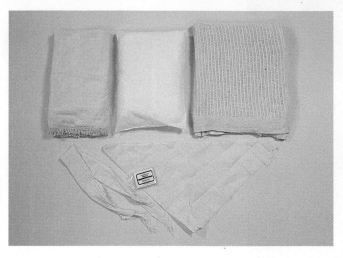

Figure 12-1 Soft splints include folded blankets, towels, pillows and a sling or cravat.

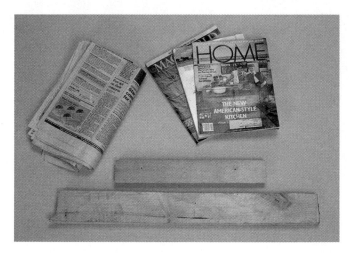

Figure 12-2 Rigid splints include boards, metal strips and folded magazines or newspapers.

KEY TERMS

Arm: The part of the upper extremity from the
shoulder to the hand.

Extremity: The shoulder to the fingers; the hip to
the toes.

Forearm: The part of the upper extremity from the
elbow to the wrist.

Leg: The part of the lower extremity from the
pelvis to the ankle.

Lower extremity: The parts of the body from the
hip to the toes.

Lower leg: The part of the lower extremity from
the knee to the ankle.

Thigh: The part of the lower extremity from the
pelvis to the knee.

Upper arm: The part of the upper extremity from
the shoulder to the elbow.

Upper extremity: The parts of the body from the
shoulder to the fingers.

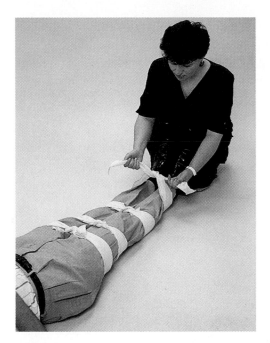

Figure 12-3   An injured leg can be splinted to the uninjured leg.

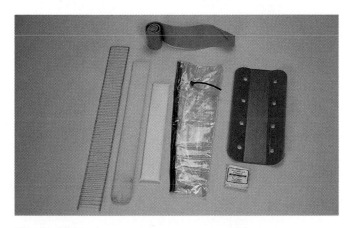

Figure 12-4   Commercial splints.

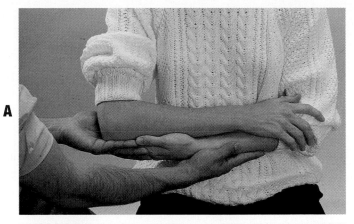

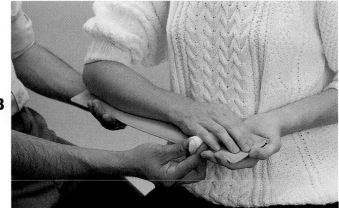

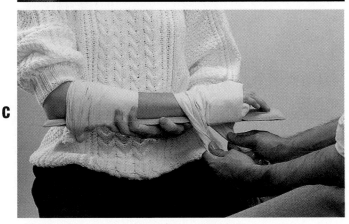

Figure 12-5   A, Support the arm above and below the injury site. The victim can help you. **B,** Pad a rigid splint to conform to the injured body part. **C,** Secure the splint in place.

cially designed flexible splints (**Fig. 12-4**). As a citizen responder, you are more likely to have access to triangular bandages to make **cravats** or other materials you can use to make a soft or anatomic splint.

To splint an injured body part—

1. Support the injured part in the position in which you find it. If possible, have the victim or a bystander help you (**Fig. 12-5, A**).
2. Cover any open wounds with a dressing and bandage to help control bleeding and prevent infection. Use direct pressure unless the bleeding is located directly over the suspected fracture. Wear disposable gloves or use a protective barrier.
3. Check the area below the injury site for feeling, warmth and color.

4. Apply the splint to immobilize the joints or bones above and below an injured area. If you are using a rigid splint, pad the splint so that it is contoured to the injured part (**Fig. 12-5, B**). This padding will help prevent further injury.
5. Secure the splint in place with cravats, roller bandages or other wide strips of cloth (**Fig. 12-5, C**). Avoid securing the splint directly over an open wound or the injury.

FRONT VIEW

BACK VIEW

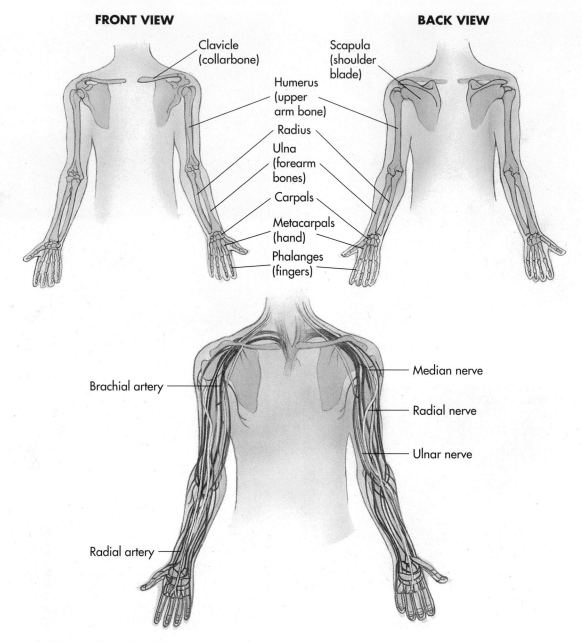

Figure 12-6 The upper extremities include the bones of the arms and hands, nerves and blood vessels.

6. Recheck below the injury site for feeling, warmth and color. Loosen the splint if the victim complains of numbness or if the area below the injury site is discolored or becomes cold.

7. Elevate the splinted part if doing so does not cause the victim discomfort.

After the injury has been immobilized, apply ice or a cold pack to the injured area. This will help minimize pain and swelling. Be sure to place gauze or cloth between the source of cold and the skin. Help the victim rest in the most comfortable position and reassure him or her. Prevent him or her from becoming chilled or overheated. Determine what additional care is needed. Continue to monitor the victim's level of consciousness, breathing, skin color and temperature. Be alert for any signals, such as changes in breathing rate, skin color or level of consciousness, that may indicate the victim's condition is worsening. Take steps to minimize shock.

SIGNALS OF SERIOUS EXTREMITY INJURIES

The extremities consist of bones, soft tissues, blood vessels and nerves. They are subject to various kinds of injury. Injury can affect the soft tissues, resulting in open or closed wounds. Injury can also affect the musculoskeletal system, resulting in sprains, strains, fractures or dislocations. Signals of a serious extremity injury include—

▶ Pain or tenderness.
▶ Swelling.
▶ Discoloration.
▶ Deformity of the limb.
▶ Inability to move or use the limb.
▶ Severe external bleeding.
▶ Loss of sensation, feeling or tingling.
▶ A limb that is cold to the touch.

UPPER EXTREMITY INJURIES

The term *upper extremity,* or *arm,* describes the parts of the body from the shoulders to the fingers. The bones of the upper extremities include the collarbone (clavicle), shoulder blade (scapula), bone from the shoulder to the elbow (humerus), *forearm* (**radius** and **ulna**), wrist (**carpals**), hand (**metacarpals**) and fingers (**phalanges**). **Figure 12-6** shows the major structures of the upper extremities.

The upper extremities are the most commonly injured areas of the body. The most frequent cause of injury is falling on the hand of an outstretched arm. Because a falling person instinctively tries to break his or her fall by extending the arms and hands, these areas receive the force of the body's weight, which can cause a serious injury.

Shoulder Injuries

The shoulder consists of three bones that meet to form the shoulder joint. These bones are the clavicle, scapula and humerus. The most common shoulder injuries are sprains. However, injuries to the shoulder may also involve a fracture or dislocation of one or more of these bones.

The most frequently injured bone of the shoulder is the **clavicle.** Clavicle injuries are more common in children than adults. Typically, the clavicle is fractured or separates from its normal position at

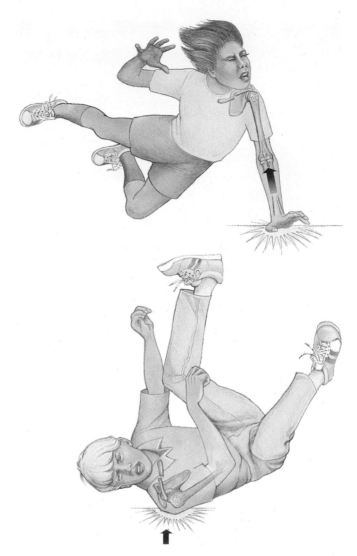

Figure 12-7   A clavicle fracture is commonly caused by a fall.

either end of the bone as a result of a fall (**Fig. 12-7**). An injury commonly occurs when the impact from a fall forces the outer end of the clavicle to separate from the joint where it touches the scapula. The victim usually feels pain in the shoulder area, which may radiate down the upper extremity. A person with a clavicle injury usually attempts to ease the pain by holding the arm against the chest (**Fig. 12-8**). The clavicle lies directly over major blood vessels and nerves to the upper extremity. It is especially important to immobilize a fractured clavicle promptly to prevent injury to these structures.

Scapula fractures are not common. A fracture of the scapula typically results from a violent force, such as a fall from a height or being hit by a car. Because it takes great force to fracture the scapula, you should look for additional injuries to the head,

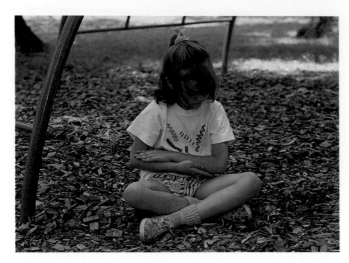

Figure 12-8 A victim with an injured clavicle will usually support the arm against the chest

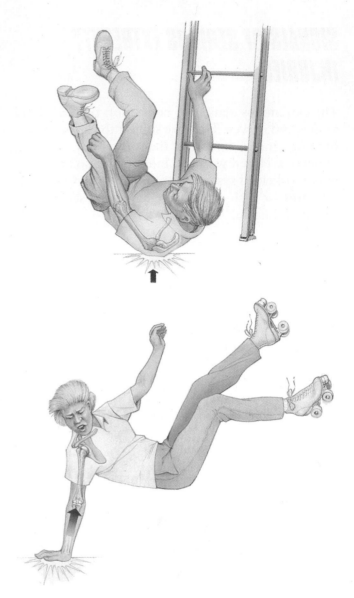

Figure 12-9 Dislocations are usually the result of a fall.

neck, back or chest cavity. The most significant signals of a fractured scapula are extreme pain and the inability to move the shoulder. If the chest cavity is injured, the victim may have trouble breathing.

A dislocation of the shoulder joint is another common type of shoulder injury. Like fractures, dislocations often result from falls or direct blows when the arm is in the throwing position. Such dislocations happen frequently in sports, such as football and rugby, when a player attempts to break a fall with an outstretched arm or gets tackled with the arm positioned away from the body (**Fig. 12-9**). This movement can result in ligaments tearing, which displaces bones. Shoulder dislocations are painful and can often be identified by deformity. As with other shoulder injuries, the victim often tries to minimize the pain by holding the upper extremity in the most comfortable position.

Care for Shoulder Injuries

To care for shoulder injuries, support the injured part. If an injured person is holding the forearm securely against the chest, do not change the position. Holding the arm against the chest is an effective method of immobilization. Allow the person to continue to support the upper extremity in the position in which he or she is holding it, usually the most comfortable position. Control any external bleeding with direct pressure. Use direct pressure unless the bleeding is located directly over the suspected fracture. Always wear disposable gloves or use another protective barrier. If the person is holding the upper extremity away from the body, use a pillow, rolled blanket or similar object to fill the gap between the upper extremity and chest to provide

support for the injured area. Splint the upper extremity in place (**Fig. 12-10**). Remember to check for feeling, warmth and color before and after applying the splint. Place the upper extremity in a sling and bind it to the chest with cravats to further stabilize the injury. Apply ice or cold pack. Take steps to minimize shock.

Upper Arm Injuries

The *upper arm* is the area that extends from the shoulder to the elbow. The bone of the upper arm is the **humerus.** The humerus is the largest bone in the arm.

The humerus can be fractured at any point, although it is usually fractured at the upper end near the shoulder or in the middle of the bone. The up-

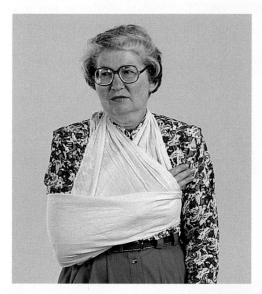

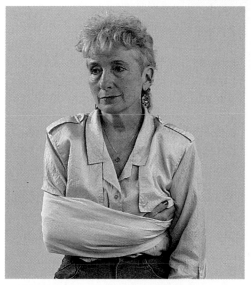 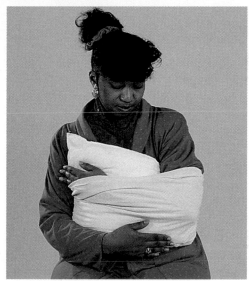

Figure 12-10 Splint the arm against the chest in the position the victim is holding it, using a sling, cravat, small pillow or a rolled blanket when necessary.

per end of the humerus often fractures in the elderly and in young children as a result of a fall. Breaks in the middle of the bone mostly occur in young adults. When the humerus is fractured, the blood vessels and nerves supplying the entire upper extremity may be damaged. Most humerus fractures are very painful and the victim will most likely not be able to use the injured arm. Do not permit the victim to use the arm. A humerus fracture can also cause considerable deformity.

Care for Upper Arm Injuries

Care for upper arm injuries in the same way as for shoulder injuries. Support the injured area. Allow the person to continue to support the upper ex-

tremity in the position in which he or she is holding it. Control any external bleeding. Place the upper extremity in a sling and bind it to the chest with cravats to further stabilize the injury. You can also use a rigid splint, if one is available, to provide support to the injured area (**Fig. 12-11**). Remember to check for feeling, warmth and color before and after applying the splint. Apply ice or a cold pack. Take steps to minimize shock.

Elbow Injuries

The elbow is a joint formed by the humerus and the two bones of the forearm, the **radius** and the **ulna**. Injuries to the elbow can cause permanent disabil-

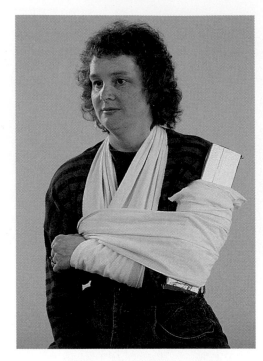

Figure 12-11 A short, padded splint can provide additional support for an injury to the upper arm.

ity, because all the nerves and blood vessels to the forearm and hand go through the elbow. Therefore, treat elbow injuries seriously.

Like other joints, the elbow can be sprained, fractured or dislocated. Injuries to a joint like the elbow can be made worse by movement because movement can easily damage the nerves and blood vessels located in the elbow. An injured elbow may be in a bent or straight position.

Care for Elbow Injuries

To give care for elbow injuries, support the injured area. Allow the person to continue to support the upper extremity in the position in which he or she is holding it. Control any external bleeding. Splint the arm from the shoulder to the wrist in the best way possible in the position you find it. The simplest way is to place the arm in a sling and secure it to the chest. If placing the arm in a sling is not possible, immobilize the elbow with a rigid splint and two cravats. If the elbow is bent, apply the splint diagonally across the underside of the arm (**Fig. 12-12, A**). The splint should extend several inches beyond the wrist and shoulder. If the elbow is straight, apply the splint along the arm. Secure the splint at the wrist and upper arm with cravats or roller bandages (**Fig. 12-12, B**). If a

splint is not available, secure the arm to the body using two cravats (**Fig. 12-12, C**). Always be sure the knots are tied against the splint and not directly on the arm. Remember to check for feeling, warmth and color before and after applying the splint. Apply ice or a cold pack. Take steps to minimize shock.

Forearm, Wrist and Hand Injuries

The forearm is the area between the elbow and the wrist. The wrist is a joint formed by the hand and forearm. Injuries to the wrist may involve one or both of the two forearm bones, the radius and ulna. The hand consists of many small bones—the carpals, metacarpals and phalanges. Serious injuries to the wrists and hands can significantly impact a person's daily activities.

If a person falls on an outstretched upper extremity, both forearm bones may break. When both forearm bones fracture, the arm may look s-shaped (**Fig. 12-13**). Because the radial artery and nerve are close to these bones, a fracture may cause severe bleeding or a loss of movement in the wrist and hand. The wrist is a common site of sprains and fractures. It is often difficult to tell the extent of the injury.

Because the hands are used in so many daily activities, they are susceptible to injury. Most injuries to the hands and fingers involve minor soft tissue damage. However, a serious injury may damage nerves, blood vessels and bones. Home, recreational and industrial mishaps often produce lacerations, avulsions, burns and fractures of the hands.

Care for Forearm, Wrist and Hand Injuries

To give care for forearm, wrist or hand injuries, support the injured area and control any external bleeding. You can support an injured forearm or wrist by placing a soft or rigid splint underneath the forearm, making sure that it extends beyond both the hand and elbow. If you are using a rigid splint, pad the splint and place a roll of gauze or a similar object in the palm to keep the palm and fingers in a normal position. Check the fingers for feeling, warmth and color before and after splinting. Secure the splint with cravats or a roller bandage (**Fig. 12-14, A**). Put the arm in a sling and secure it to the chest with cravats (**Fig. 12-14, B**). Apply ice or a cold pack and elevate. Take steps to minimize shock.

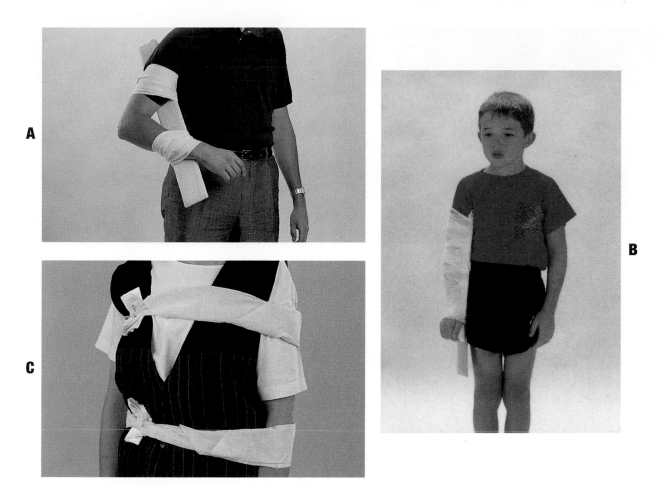

Figure 12-12   A, If the elbow is bent, apply the splint diagonally across the under-side of the arm. **B,** If the arm is straight, apply the splint along the underside of the arm. **C,** If a splint is not available, secure the arm to the body using two cravats.

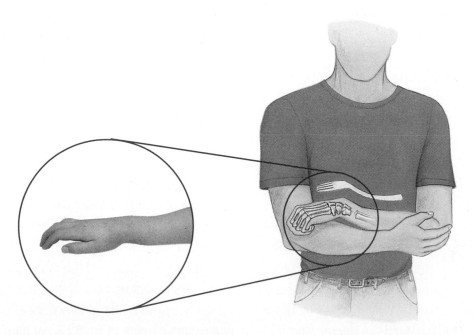

Figure 12-13   Fractures of both forearm bones often have a characteristic s-shaped deformity.

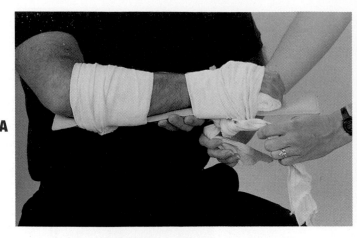
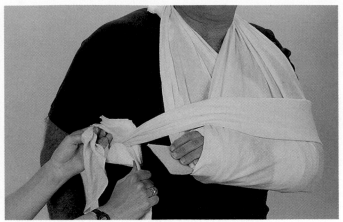

Figure 12-14   A, If the forearm is fractured, place a splint under the forearm and secure it with two cravats. **B,** Put the arm in a sling and secure it to the chest with cravats.

Carpal Tunnel Syndrome

Elaine W. was a 14-year-old violin student when she first noticed problems with her hands. After long practice sessions, she felt a strange tingling sensation in the fingers of her left hand. Soon, she was experiencing pain so severe that it woke her up at night. Then, she states, "I woke up one November morning and I couldn't move my left hand at all." Frightened, she consulted her physician, who diagnosed her with carpal tunnel syndrome. When rest and splinting did not alleviate her symptoms, Elaine had surgery to correct the problem. Although the surgery eliminated the pain and tingling, she still—some years later—has trouble holding things. "Wet dishes are the worst," she says. And at work, she uses a pencil to tap out words on her computer.

Elaine is just one of many Americans who suffer from carpal tunnel syndrome, a painful and debilitating irritation of the nerves and tendons in the wrist. The area for which the syndrome is named—the carpal tunnel—is the passageway formed by tendons and bones through which the nerves that supply the hand travel. When a person performs repetitive hand motion for long periods of time without rest, such as long typing sessions, assembly-line tasks or, in Elaine's case, practicing the violin, the nerves can become irritated, resulting in pain and numbness. Carpal tunnel syndrome is now the most commonly reported on-the-job injury. If untreated, it can cause permanent disability.

The first signals of carpal tunnel syndrome include hand and wrist pain and numbness. People with the syndrome describe the pain as an "electric" sensation that may radiate to the arm, shoulder and back. In time, the sufferer may lose grip strength in the hand, making even everyday tasks awkward or impossible.

Although carpal tunnel syndrome is not a new condition (it was first described in 1854), it has only recently become a serious occupational hazard. One U.S. legislator describes carpal tunnel syndrome as "the industrial disease of the Information Age." If employers do not do something about it, some experts foresee that half of every dollar earned by companies may go to treat carpal tunnel syndrome and its related disorders.

For a hand or finger injury, place a bulky dressing in the palm of the victim's hand and wrap the hand with a roller bandage (**Fig. 12-15**). For a possible fractured or dislocated finger, you can make a rigid splint by taping the injured area to a small object, such as an ice cream stick or tongue depressor (**Fig. 12-16**). You can also tape the injured finger to the finger next to it. Do not attempt to put the bones back into place if you suspect a finger or thumb dislocation. Apply ice or a cold pack and elevate injuries to the forearm, wrist and hand. Take steps to minimize shock.

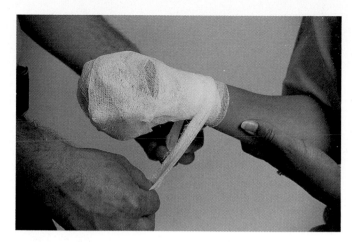

Figure 12-15   A bulky dressing is an effective splint for a hand or finger injury.

Many of today's occupations involve constant repetitive motions of the hand and wrist done at faster and faster speeds. Technical innovations—from grocery store scanners to computer keyboards—also contribute to the increase in carpal tunnel syndrome.

What can be done to treat carpal tunnel syndrome? Individuals with the syndrome are treated with physical therapy and elaborate wrist splints that immobilize the affected area. Sometimes surgery is needed to correct the nerve damage. These treatments are often not effective in alleviating all the signals, and sufferers must learn to live with their disability.

Because of the surge in carpal tunnel syndrome cases, the Occupational Safety and Health Administration (OSHA) has drafted guidelines for certain occupations, such as meatpacking, designed to prevent the onset of the syndrome. Specially designed desks, chairs and other office equipment for typists and data entry

clerks take some of the stress off wrists and hands. In some companies, typists are required to take rest breaks.

These guidelines make sense for those who find themselves working at a keyboard for long hours or who perform the same task over and over. Identify early signals and take steps to prevent wrist strain. Take frequent breaks, and for the marathon typist, make sure your chair is comfortable and that you can reach the keyboard without straining. Your wrists will thank you.

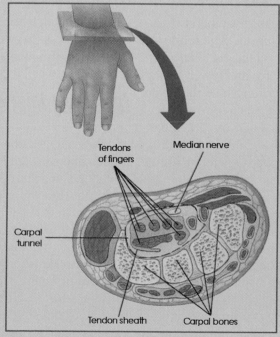

Tendons of fingers

Median nerve

Carpal tunnel

Tendon sheath

Carpal bones

SOURCES

CTS: Relief at hand, The University of California Berkeley Wellness Letter 11(4): 7, 1995.

Centers for Disease Control, "Carpal Tunnel Syndrome" www.cdc.gov/niosh/ctsfs.html. Accessed 10/15/04.

Gabor A: On-the-job-straining: repetitive motion is the Information Age's hottest hazard, US News and World Report 108(20): 51-53, 1990.

Katz RT: Carpal tunnel syndrome: a practical review, American Family Physician 49(6): 1371-1382, 1994.

Treating for carpal tunnel syndrome, Lancet 338 (8765): 479-481, 1991.

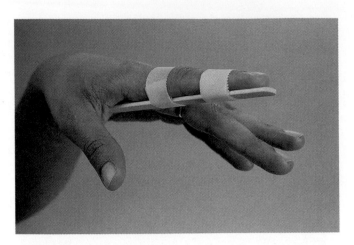

Figure 12-16 An ice cream stick can be used to splint a finger injury.

LOWER EXTREMITY INJURIES

Injuries to the *leg*, or *lower extremity*—the part of the body from the hip (pelvis) to the toes—can involve both soft tissue and musculoskeletal damage. The lower extremity includes the pelvic bones, thigh bone (femur), kneecap (**patella**), two bones in the *lower leg* (**tibia** and **fibula**), bones of the ankle (**tarsals**), foot (**metatarsals**) and toes (**phalanges**). **Figure 12-17** shows the major structures of the lower extremities.

Thigh Injuries

The *thigh* is the lower extremity from the pelvis to the knee. The thigh contains the **femur**. The femur is the largest bone in the body. The **femoral arteries** are the major supplier of blood to the lower extremities. Because of the size and strength of the femur, a significant amount of force is required to cause a fracture. When the femur is fractured, the blood vessels and nerves may be damaged. If a femoral artery is damaged, the blood loss can be life threatening.

Thigh injuries range from bruises and torn muscles to severe injuries, such as fractures or dislocations. Most femur fractures involve the upper end of the bone where the femur meets the pelvis at the hip joint (**Fig. 12-18**). Although the hip joint is not involved, such injuries are often called hip fractures.

A fracture of the femur usually produces a characteristic deformity. Because the thigh muscles are so strong, they pull the ends of the broken bone together, causing them to overlap. This pulling may cause the injured leg to be noticeably shorter than the other leg. The injured leg may also be turned outward (**Fig. 12-19**). Other signals of a fractured femur include severe pain and inability to move the lower extremity. Do not attempt to splint a suspected femur fracture (this requires special training and equipment). A fractured femur is a serious life-threatening injury that requires immediate medical attention.

Care for Thigh Injuries

Initial care for a victim with a serious injury to the thigh is to support the injured area and stop any external bleeding. Call 9-1-1 or the local emergency number immediately. EMS personnel are much better prepared to care for and transport a victim with a serious lower extremity injury. While waiting for EMS personnel to arrive, immobilize the injured area and help the victim rest in the most comfortable position. If the victim's lower extremity is supported by the ground, do not move it. Rather, use rolled towels or blankets to support the leg in the position in which you found it. A fractured femur can result in serious internal bleeding. The likelihood of shock is considerable. Therefore, take steps to minimize shock. Keep the person lying down and try to keep him or her calm. Keep the person from becoming chilled or overheated, and make sure to call 9-1-1 or the local emergency number. Monitor breathing. Notice how the victim's skin looks and feels, and watch for changes in the victim's level of consciousness. See Chapter 9 for more detailed information on shock.

Lower Leg Injuries

The lower leg is the area between the knee and the ankle. The tibia and fibula are the two bones in the lower leg. A fracture in the lower leg may involve the tibia, the fibula or both bones. Sometimes both are fractured simultaneously. However, a blow to the outside of the lower leg can cause an isolated fracture of the smaller bone (fibula). Because these two bones lie just beneath the skin, open fractures are common (**Fig. 12-20**). Lower leg fractures may cause a severe deformity in which the lower leg is bent at an unusual angle (angulated), as well as pain and inability to move the leg.

FRONT VIEW

BACK VIEW

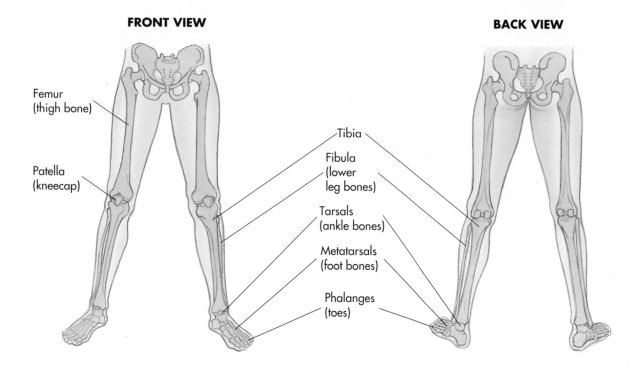

Femur
(thigh bone)

Patella
(kneecap)

Tibia

Fibula
(lower
leg bones)

Tarsals
(ankle bones)

Metatarsals
(foot bones)

Phalanges
(toes)

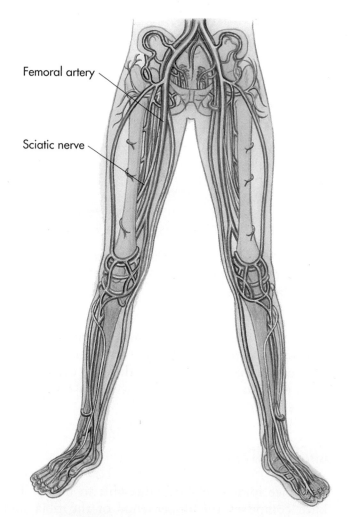

Femoral artery

Sciatic nerve

Figure 12-17   The lower extremities.

Care for Lower Leg Injuries

Support the injured area and control any external bleeding. Call 9-1-1 or the local emergency number immediately. While waiting for EMS personnel to arrive, immobilize the injured area and help the victim rest in the most comfortable position. Do not forget that the ground acts as an adequate splint. If the victim's lower extremity is supported by the

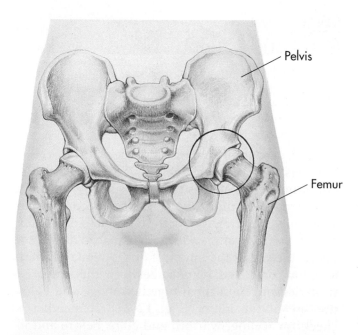

Pelvis

Femur

Figure 12-18   The upper end of the femur meets the pelvis at the hip joint.

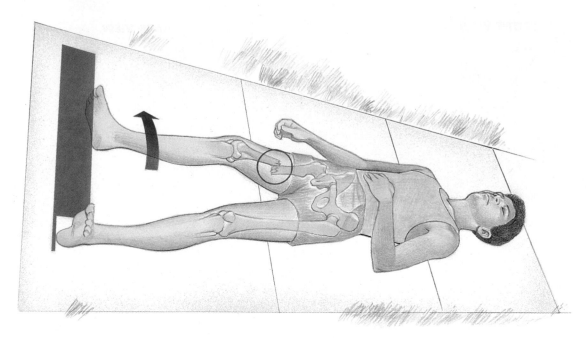

Figure 12-19 A fractured femur often produces a characteristic deformity. The injured leg is shorter than the uninjured leg and may be turned outward.

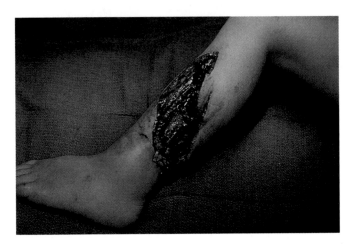

Figure 12-20 A fracture of the lower leg can be an open fracture.

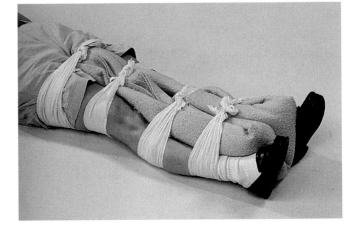

Figure 12-21 To splint an injured leg, secure the injured leg to the uninjured leg with cravats. A pillow or rolled blanket can be placed between the legs.

ground, do not move it. Rather, use rolled towels or blankets to support the leg in the position in which you found it. In other situations, such as when you must transport the person, you can secure the injured lower extremity to the uninjured lower extremity with several wide cravats placed above and below the site of the injury. If one is available, place a pillow or rolled blanket between the lower extremities and bind them together above and below the site of the injury (**Fig. 12-21**). Remember to check for feeling, warmth and color before and after applying the splint. Do not be surprised if EMS personnel later remove the splint and apply a more rigid splint or a mechanical device called a traction splint. This device reduces the deformity of the lower extremity by applying traction to overcome the pull of the thigh muscles that are causing the bone ends to overlap. Apply ice or a cold pack. Take steps to minimize shock.

Knee Injuries

The knee joint is highly vulnerable to injury. The knee comprises the upper ends of the tibia and fibula, the lower end of the femur and the patella. The patella is a free-floating bone that moves on the lower front surface of the thigh bone.

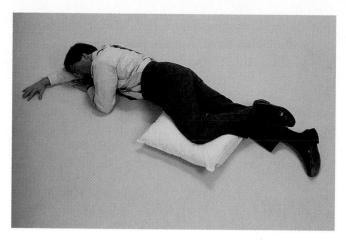

Figure 12-22   Support a knee injury in the bent position if the victim cannot straighten the knee.

Sprains, fractures and dislocations of the knee are common in athletic activities that involve quick movements or exert unusual force on the knee. Deep lacerations in the area of the knee can cause severe joint infections. The patella is very vulnerable to bruises and lacerations, as well as dislocations. Violent forces to the front of the knee, such as those caused by hitting the dashboard of a motor vehicle or falling and landing on bent knees, can fracture the kneecap.

Care for Knee Injuries

To care for an injured knee, support the injured area and control any external bleeding. If the knee is bent and cannot be straightened without pain, you can support it on a pillow or folded blanket in the bent position (**Fig. 12-22**). If the knee is on the ground, the ground will provide adequate support. Call 9-1-1 or the local emergency number to have the victim transported to a medical facility for examination. Help the victim to rest in the most comfortable position until EMS personnel arrive. If you decide to splint the injured area and the knee is straight, you can secure it to the uninjured leg as you might do for an injury of the thigh or lower leg. Check feeling, warmth and color before and after splinting. Apply ice or a cold pack. Take steps to minimize shock.

Ankle and Foot Injuries

The foot consists of many small bones—the tarsals, metatarsals and phalanges. The ankle is a joint formed by the foot and the lower leg. Ankle and foot injuries are commonly caused by twisting

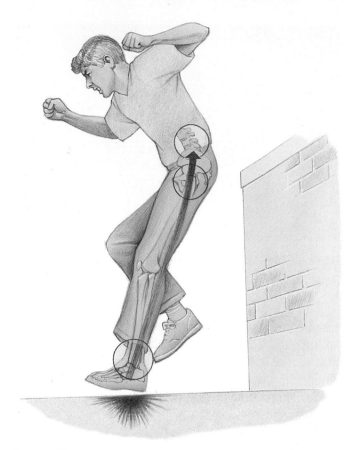

Figure 12-23   In a jump or fall from a height, the impact can be transmitted up the legs, causing injuries to the thigh, pelvis, head, neck or back.

forces. Injuries range from minor sprains with little swelling and pain to fractures and dislocations.

Many common ankle and foot injuries are caused by severe twisting forces that occur when the foot turns in or out at the ankle as a person steps down from a height, such as a curb or step. Fractures of the feet and ankles can occur from forcefully landing on the heel. The force of the impact may also be transmitted up the lower extremities. This transmitted force can result in an injury elsewhere in the body (**Fig. 12-23**). Always suspect that a victim who has fallen or jumped from a height may also have additional injuries to the thigh, pelvis, head, neck or back. Foot injuries may also involve the toes. Although toe injuries are painful, they are rarely serious.

Care for Foot Injuries

Care for ankle and foot injuries by supporting the injured area and controlling any external bleeding. Immobilize the ankle and foot by using a soft splint, such as a pillow or rolled blanket. Check the toes

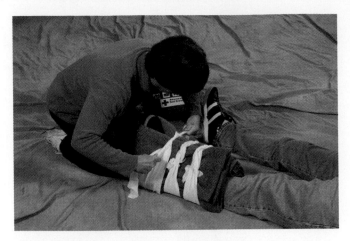

Figure 12-24 An injured ankle can be immobilized with a pillow or rolled blanket secured with two or three cravats.

for feeling, warmth and color before and after splinting. Wrap the injured area with the soft splint, and secure it with two or three cravats (**Fig. 12-24**). Then elevate the injured ankle or foot to help reduce the swelling. Apply ice or a cold pack. Suspect that any victim who has fallen or jumped from a height may also have injuries elsewhere.

As with other musculoskeletal injuries, you cannot always distinguish between minor and severe injuries. You should initially care for all lower leg injuries as if they are serious. If the victim cannot bear weight on the injured area or the joint looks swollen and too painful to move, call 9-1-1 or the local emergency number.

SUMMARY

You can care for musculoskeletal and soft tissue injuries to the extremities by giving care that focuses on minimizing pain, shock and further damage to the injured area. Immobilize the injured area, apply ice or a cold pack and take steps to minimize shock. Control any external bleeding. Reassure the victim. Care for any life-threatening conditions and call 9-1-1 or the local emergency number if necessary.

APPLICATION QUESTIONS

1. Could Sam have sustained a serious injury? Why or why not?

2. What steps should Mario take to help Sam?

STUDY QUESTIONS

1. Match each term with the correct definition.

   a. Upper arm   c. Thigh
   b. Forearm   d. Lower leg

   _____ The part of the lower extremity from the pelvis to the knee.

   _____ The part of the upper extremity from the elbow to the wrist.

   _____ The part of the lower extremity from the knee to the ankle.

   _____ The part of the upper extremity from the shoulder to the elbow.

2. Identify the most frequent cause of upper extremity injuries.

Base your answers for questions 3 through 5 on the scenario below.

A person attempting to leap a 4-foot gate catches one foot on the gate and falls hard on the other side. He appears to be unable to get up. He says his left leg and arm both hurt. When you check him, you find that he is unable to move the leg, which is beginning to swell. The left arm looks deformed at the shoulder, and he has no sensation in the fingers of that arm. The arm is beginning to look bruised and is painful. He says he feels a little nauseated and dizzy, and he has a scrape on his hand.

3. What type of injury does the victim have?

4. Identify the signals that support your answer.

5. Describe the steps you would take to help the victim.

6. List two specific signals of a fractured femur.

7. List three types of splints used to immobilize an extremity.

In questions 8 and 9, circle the letter of the correct answer.

8. A man who has fallen down a steep flight of stairs is clutching his right arm to his chest. He says his shoulder hurts, and he cannot move his arm. How should you care for him?

   a. Give him some ice and tell him to go home.
   b. Immobilize the arm in the position you found it.
   c. Tell him to move the arm back to its normal position.
   d. Check the stairs to see what caused him to trip.

9. A child has fallen from a bicycle onto the pavement and landed on her elbow. The elbow is bent and the girl says she cannot move it. What do you do after calling 9-1-1 or the local emergency number?

   a. Straighten the elbow and splint it.
   b. Drive her to the hospital.
   c. Immobilize the elbow in the bent position.
   d. Ask her to continue to try to move the elbow.

10. An elderly woman has tripped and fallen over some gardening tools. She is lying on the ground, conscious and breathing. Her lower leg is bleeding profusely from a gash and seems to be bent at an odd angle. List the steps of care you should give.

Answers are listed in Appendix A.

SKILL SHEET   Applying An Anatomic Splint

Check the scene and the victim. Call 9-1-1 or the local emergency number, if necessary. *Remember: Always obtain consent and follow standard precautions to prevent disease transmission. Use protective equipment (disposable gloves and breathing barriers). Wash your hands immediately after giving care.*

If you decide to use an anatomic splint to immobilize the injury...

Step 1

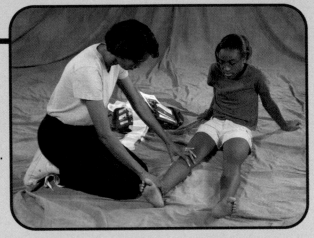

Support the injured area.

- Support the injured area above and below the injury site.
- Let the ground support the injured area whenever possible, or have the victim or bystander help you.

Step 2

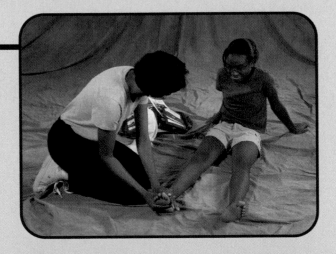

Check for feeling, warmth and color.

- Check for feeling, warmth and color below the injury.
- If you are not able to check warmth and color because a sock or shoe is in place, check for feeling (sensation).

Step 3

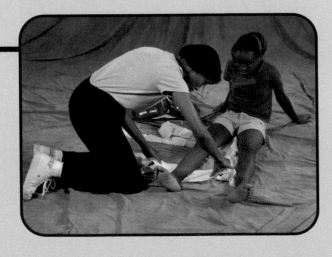

Place several folded triangular bandages above and below the injured area.

- Thread several triangular bandages underneath the legs at the knee or ankle.
- Position triangular bandages by sliding them underneath the legs.
- Do not position a bandage at the injury site.

Step 4

Place the uninjured area next to the injured area.

- Carefully move the uninjured leg next to the injured leg.

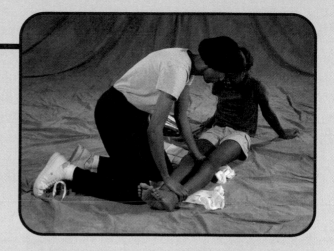

Step 5

Tie triangular bandages securely.

- Tie ends of each triangular bandage together with knots. Check to see that triangular bandages are snug but not too tight.
- If more than one finger fits under the bandages, tighten bandages.
- The splint should be snug but not so tight that blood flow is impaired.

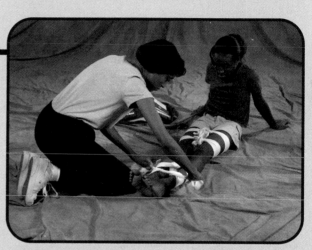

Step 6

Recheck for feeling, warmth and color.

- If the area below the injury is bluish or cool, loosen the splint.
- If you are not able to check warmth and color because a sock or shoe is in place, check for feeling (sensation).
- Reassure the victim and, if necessary, take steps to minimize shock.

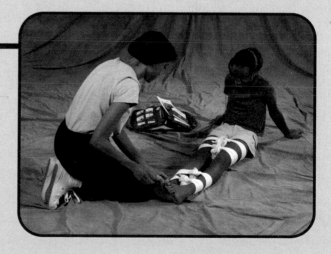

SKILL SHEET   Applying a Soft Splint

Check the scene and the victim. Call 9-1-1 or the local emergency number, if necessary. *Remember: Always obtain consent and follow standard precautions to prevent disease transmission. Use protective equipment (disposable gloves and breathing barriers). Wash your hands immediately after giving care.*

If you decide to use a soft splint to immobilize the injury...

Step 1

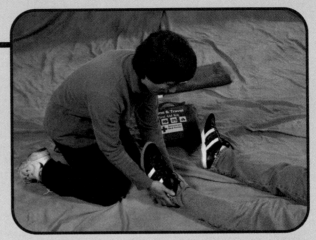

Support the injured area.

- Support the injured area above and below the injury site.
- Let the ground support the injured area whenever possible, or have the victim or a bystander help you.

Step 2

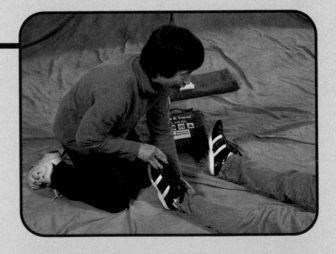

Check for feeling, warmth and color.

- Check for feeling, warmth, and color below the injury.
- If you are not able to check warmth and color because a sock or shoe is in place, check for feeling (sensation).

Step 3

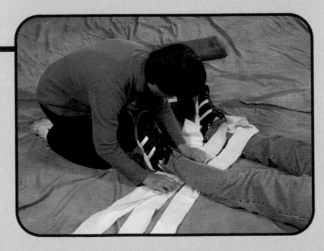

Place several folded triangular bandages above and below the injured area.

- Slide two folded triangular bandages underneath the injured area at the ankle and lower calf and position them above and below the injured area.
- Do not position a bandage at the injury site.

Step 4

Gently wrap a soft object (a folded blanket or pillow) around the injured area.

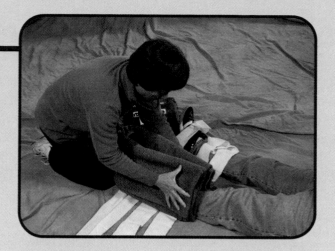

Step 5

Tie triangular bandages securely with knots.

- Tie bandages around the foot, from the heel to the front of the ankle.
- Check to see that triangular bandages are snug but not too tight.
- If more than one finger fits under the bandages, tighten bandages.
- The splint should fit snugly but not so tightly that blood flow is impaired.

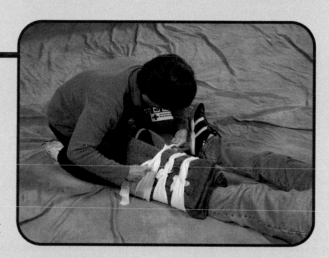

Step 6

Recheck for feeling, warmth and color.

- If area below the injury is bluish or cool, loosen the splint.
- If you are not able to check warmth and color because a sock or shoe is in place, check for feeling (sensation).
- Reassure the victim and, if necessary, take steps to minimize shock.

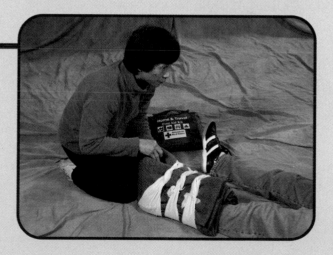

SKILL SHEET   Applying a Rigid Splint

Check the scene and the victim. Call 9-1-1 or the local emergency number, if necessary. *Remember: Always obtain consent and follow standard precautions to prevent disease transmission. Use protective equipment (disposable gloves and breathing barriers). Wash your hands immediately after giving care.*

If you decide to use a rigid splint to immobilize an injury...

Step 1

Support the injured area.

- Support the injured area above and below the injury site.
- Let the victim support the injured area or have a bystander help you.

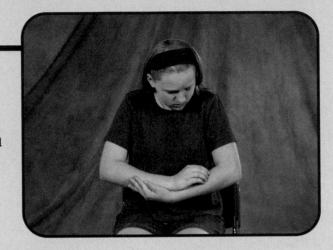

Step 2

Check for feeling, warmth and color.

- Check for feeling, warmth, and color below the site of the injury.

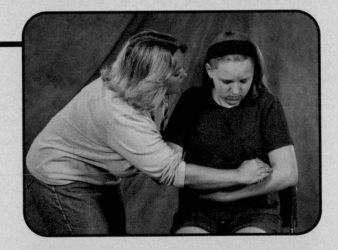

Step 3

Place the rigid splint under the injured area and the joints above and below the injured area.

- Have the victim or a bystander hold the splint in place.
- Pad the splint to keep the injured area in a natural position.

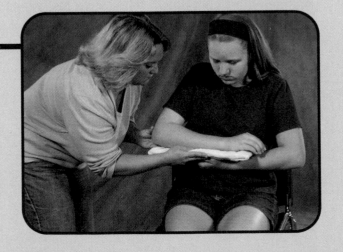

Step 4

Tie several folded triangular bandages above and below the injured area.

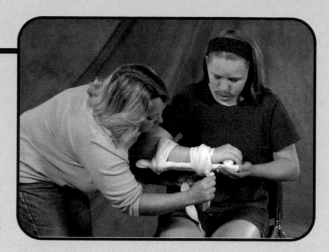

- Do not position a bandage at the injury site.
- Check to see that triangular bandages are snug but not too tight.
- If more than one finger fits under the bandages, tighten the bandages.
- The splint should fit snugly but not so tightly that blood flow is impaired.

Step 5

Recheck for feeling, warmth and color.

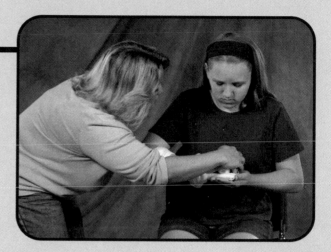

- If the area below the injury is bluish or cool, loosen the splint.
- Reassure the victim and, if necessary, take steps to minimize shock.

If a rigid splint is used on a forearm, you must also immobilize the elbow. Bind the arm to the chest using folded triangular bandages, or apply a sling.

SKILL SHEET   Applying a Sling and Binder

Check the scene and the victim. Call 9-1-1 or the local emergency number, if necessary. *Remember: Always obtain consent and follow standard precautions to prevent disease transmission. Use protective equipment (disposable gloves and breathing barriers). Wash your hands immediately after giving care.*

If you decide to use a sling and binder to immobilize the injury…

Step 1

Support the injured area.

- Support the injured area above and below the injury site.
- Let the victim support the injured area or have a bystander help you.

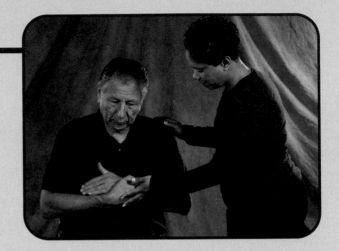

Step 2

Check for feeling, warmth and color.

- Check for feeling, warmth, and color below the site of the injury.

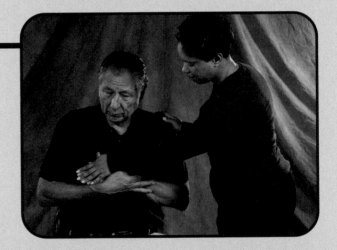

Step 3

Place a triangular bandage under the injured arm, across the chest and over the uninjured shoulder to form a sling.

- Position the point of the triangular bandage at the elbow.
- Bring the other end across the chest and over the opposite shoulder.

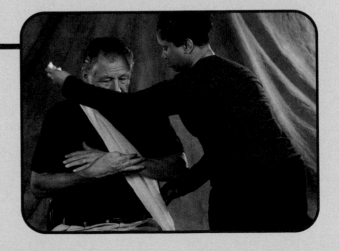

Step 4

Tie the ends of the sling.

- Tie the ends of the triangular bandage at the side of the neck opposite the injury.
- Place a gauze pad under the knot to make the knot more comfortable.

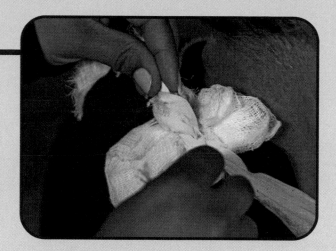

Step 5

Bind the injured area to the chest with a folded triangular bandage.

- Bind the injured arm to the chest using a folded triangular bandage.
- Tie the ends of the binder on the side opposite the injured area.
- Place a gauze pad under the knot to make the knot more comfortable.
- The splint should fit snugly but not so tightly that blood flow is impaired.

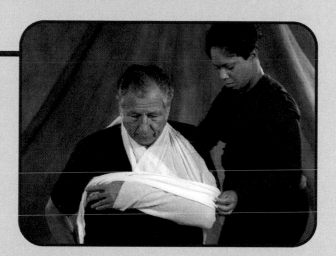

Step 6

Recheck for feeling, warmth and color.

- If the area below the injury is bluish or cool, loosen the splint.
- Reassure the victim and, if necessary, take steps to minimize shock.

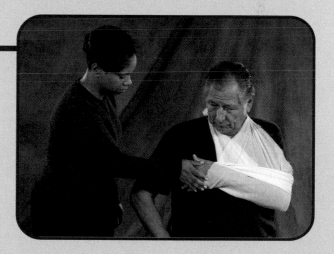

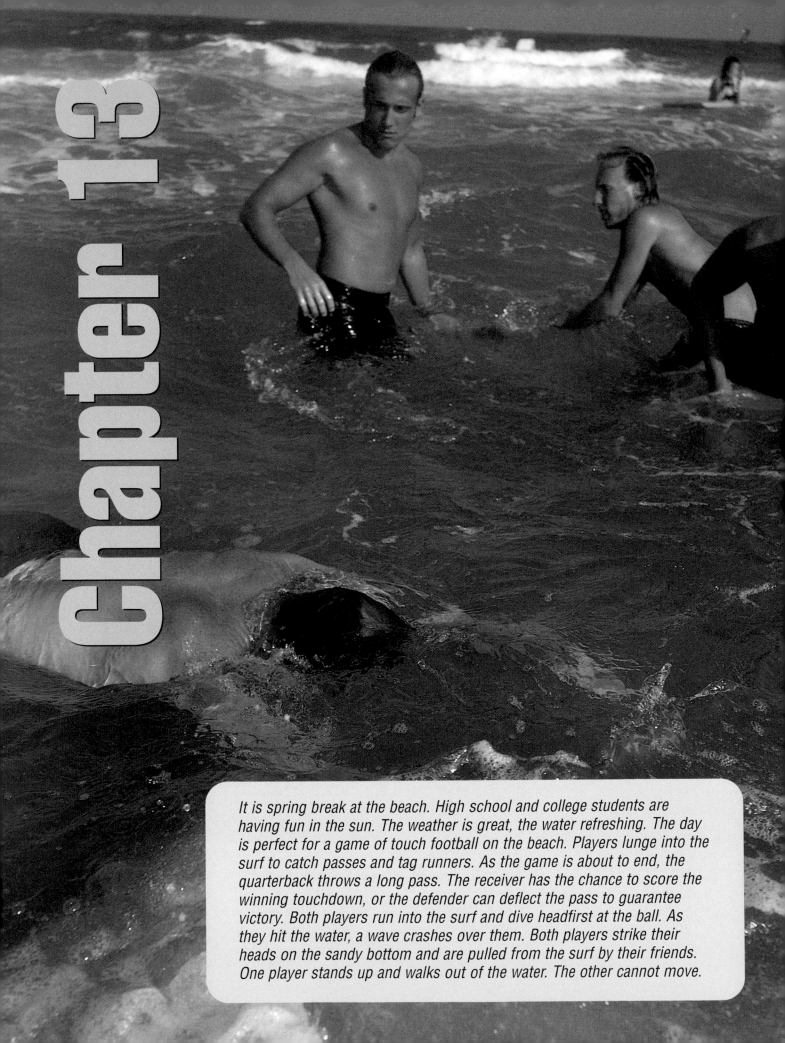

Chapter 13

It is spring break at the beach. High school and college students are having fun in the sun. The weather is great, the water refreshing. The day is perfect for a game of touch football on the beach. Players lunge into the surf to catch passes and tag runners. As the game is about to end, the quarterback throws a long pass. The receiver has the chance to score the winning touchdown, or the defender can deflect the pass to guarantee victory. Both players run into the surf and dive headfirst at the ball. As they hit the water, a wave crashes over them. Both players strike their heads on the sandy bottom and are pulled from the surf by their friends. One player stands up and walks out of the water. The other cannot move.

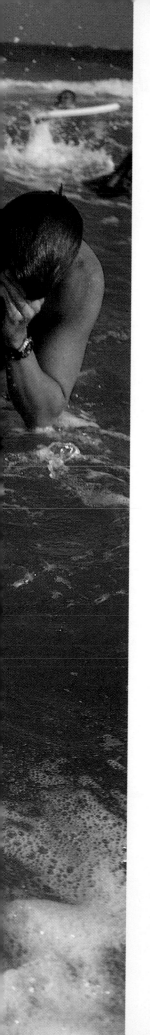

Injuries to the Head, Neck and Back

Objectives

After reading this chapter, you should be able to—

■ *Identify the most common causes of head, neck and back injuries.*

■ *List nine situations that might indicate serious head, neck and back injuries.*

■ *List the signals of head, neck and back injuries.*

■ *Describe how to effectively minimize movement of the victim's head, neck and back.*

■ *Know the situations in which you would hold the victim's head in the position found.*

■ *Describe how to care for specific injuries to the head, face, neck and lower back.*

Introduction

Each year, nearly 11,000 people in the United States are hospitalized with an injury to the head or to the most vulnerable part of the neck and back region—the spine. Most of these victims are males between the ages of 15 and 30.

Motor vehicle collisions account for nearly half of all head, neck and back injuries. Other causes include falls, injuries from sports and recreational activities and violent acts, such as assault. **Figure 13-1** *shows the most common causes of spinal injuries.*

Today, hundreds of thousands of permanently disabled victims of head, neck or back injury live in the United States. These survivors have a wide range of physical and mental impairments, including paralysis, speech and memory problems and behavioral disorders. Fortunately, prompt care can often prevent head, neck and back injuries from resulting in death or disability. In this chapter, you will learn how to recognize when a head, neck or back injury may be serious. You will also learn how to give appropriate care to minimize the effects of these injuries.

RECOGNIZING SERIOUS HEAD, NECK AND BACK INJURIES

Injuries to the head, neck or back often damage both bone and soft tissue, including brain tissue and the spinal cord. It is usually difficult to determine the extent of damage in head, neck and back injuries, so treat all such injuries as serious.

The Head

The head contains the brain, special sense organs, the mouth and nose and related structures. It is formed by the skull and the face. The broad, flat bones of the skull are fused together to form a hollow shell. This hollow shell, the cranial cavity, contains the brain. The face is on the front of the skull. The bones of the face include the bones of the cheek, forehead, nose and jaw.

The Brain

Injuries to the head can affect the brain. The brain can be bruised or lacerated when extreme force causes it to move in the skull, stretching and tearing tissue or bumping against the skull. Extreme force, or trauma, can fracture the thick bones of the skull. The major concern with skull fractures is damage to the brain. Blood from a ruptured vessel in the brain can accumulate within the skull (**Fig. 13-2**). Because the skull contains very little free space, bleeding can build up pressure that can further damage brain tissue.

K E Y   T E R M S

Concussion: An injury to the brain caused by a violent blow to the head, followed by a temporary impairment of brain function, usually without permanent damage to the brain.

Manual stabilization: A technique used to minimize movement of the victim's head and neck and keep them in line with the body to protect the spine while giving care.

Spinal cord: A bundle of nerves extending from the base of the skull to the lower back, protected by the spine.

Spine: A strong, flexible column of vertebrae, extending from the base of the skull to the tip of the tailbone (coccyx), that supports the head and the trunk and encases and protects the spinal cord; also called the spinal column or the vertebral column.

Vertebrae: The 33 bones of the spine.

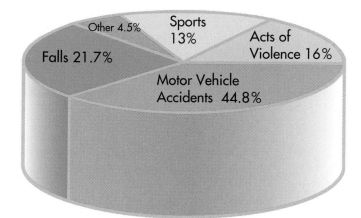

SPINAL CORD INJURIES

Figure 13-1 Motor vehicle accidents account for nearly half of all spinal injuries.

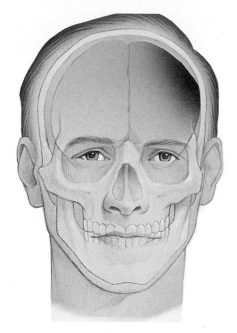

Figure 13-2 Injuries to the head can rupture blood vessels in the brain. Pressure builds within the skull as blood accumulates, causing brain injury.

Bleeding within the skull can occur rapidly or slowly over a period of days. This bleeding will affect the brain, resulting in changes in consciousness. Unconsciousness, semiconsciousness or drifting in and out of consciousness is often the first and most important signal of a serious head injury.

The Face

The face contains both bones and soft tissues. Although some injuries to the face are minor, many can be life threatening. With a facial injury, consider that the force that caused it may have been sufficiently strong to fracture facial bones and damage the brain or the spine. Facial injuries can also affect the airway and the victim's ability to breathe.

The Neck

The neck, which contains the larynx and part of the trachea, also contains major blood vessels, muscles and tendons and cervical bones of the spine. Any injury to the neck must be considered serious. The neck can be injured by crushing or penetrating forces, by sharp-edged objects that can lacerate tissues and blood vessels or by forces that cause the neck to stretch or bend too far. Injuries to muscles, bones and nerves can result in severe pain and headaches.

The Back

The back is made up of soft tissue, bones, cartilage, nerves, muscles, tendons and ligaments. It supports the skull, shoulder bones, ribs and pelvis and protects the spinal cord and other vital organs. The part of the back that is most susceptible to severe injury is the spine.

The Spine

The *spine* is a strong, flexible column of vertebrae, extending from the base of the skull to the tip of the tailbone. The spine supports the head and the trunk and protects the spinal cord. The spine is also called the **spinal column** or **vertebral column**. The spine consists of small bones, *vertebrae,* with circular openings. The vertebrae are separated from each other by cushions of cartilage called disks **(Fig. 13-3, A)**. This cartilage acts as a shock absorber when a person walks, runs or jumps. The *spinal cord,* a bundle of nerves, runs through the hollow part of the vertebrae. Nerve branches extend to various parts of the body through openings on the sides of the vertebrae.

The spine is divided into five regions: the cervical (neck) region, the thoracic (upper and middle back) region, the lumbar (lower back) region, the sacrum (the lower part of the spine) and the coccyx

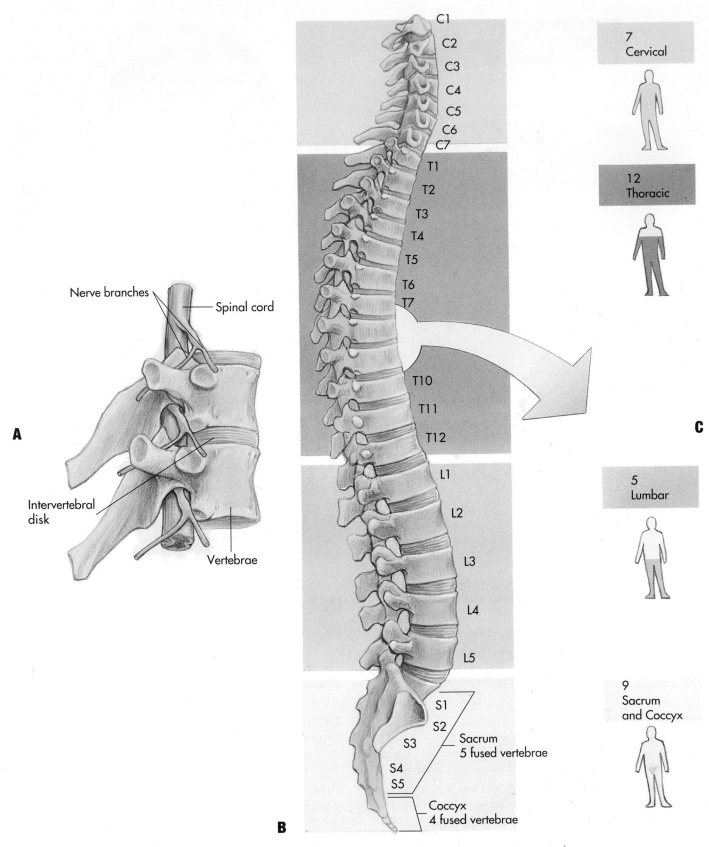

Figure 13-3 **A,** Vertebrae are separated by cushions of cartilage called disks. **B** and **C,** The spine is divided into five regions. Traumatic injury to a region of the spine can paralyze specific body areas.

(tailbone), which is the small triangular bone at the lower end of the spinal column (**Fig. 13-3, B**).

Injuries to the spine often fracture the vertebrae and sprain the ligaments. These injuries usually heal without problems. With severe injuries, however, the vertebrae may shift and compress or sever the spinal cord. Both can cause temporary or permanent paralysis, even death. The parts of the body that are paralyzed depend on which area of the spinal cord is damaged (**Fig. 13-3, C**).

Checking The Scene

Evaluate the scene for clues as to whether a head, neck or back injury may have occurred.

Check the scene and think about the forces involved in the injury. Strong forces are likely to cause severe injury to the head, neck and back. For example, a driver whose head hits and breaks a car windshield in a crash may receive a potentially serious head, neck or back injury. Similarly, a swimmer who dives into shallow water and hits his or her head on the bottom may sustain a serious injury (**Fig. 13-4**).

You should consider the possibility of a serious head, neck or back injury in the following situations:

▶ Any motor vehicle crash
▶ A fall from a height greater than the victim's standing height
▶ Victim complains of neck or back pain.
▶ Victim has tingling or weakness in extremities.
▶ Victim is not fully alert.
▶ Victim appears to be intoxicated.
▶ Victim appears to be frail or over 65 years of age

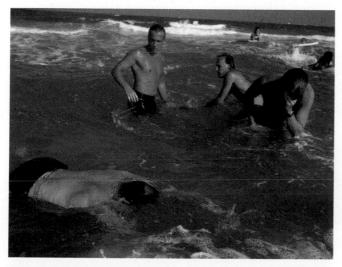

Figure 13-4   Check the scene for clues as to whether a head, neck or back injury has occurred.

Signals

When you are checking a victim with a suspected head, neck or back injury, look for any swollen or bruised areas, but do not put direct pressure on any area that is swollen, depressed or soft. You may also find certain signals that indicate a serious injury. These signals include—

▶ Changes in the level of consciousness.
▶ Severe pain or pressure in the head, neck or back.
▶ Tingling or loss of sensation in the extremities.
▶ Partial or complete loss of movement of any body part.
▶ Unusual bumps or depressions on the head or neck.
▶ Sudden loss of memory.
▶ Blood or other fluids in the ears or nose.
▶ Profuse external bleeding of the head, neck or back.
▶ Seizures in a person who does not have a seizure disorder.
▶ Impaired breathing or impaired vision as a result of injury.
▶ Nausea or vomiting.
▶ Persistent headache.
▶ Loss of balance.
▶ Bruising of the head, especially around the eyes or behind the ears.

These signals may be obvious or develop later. Alone, these signals do not always suggest a serious head, neck or back injury, but they may when combined with the cause of the injury. Regardless of the situation, always call 9-1-1 or the local emergency number when you suspect a serious head, neck or back injury.

Care

Head, neck and back injuries can become life-threatening emergencies. A serious injury to the head or neck can cause a victim to stop breathing. Call 9-1-1 or the local emergency number. Always give the following care while waiting for EMS personnel to arrive:

▶ Minimize movement of the head, neck and back. Because excessive movement of the head, neck or back can damage the spinal cord irreversibly, keep the victim as still as possible until EMS personnel arrive. Use a technique called manual stabilization to minimize movement of the head and neck.

▶ Check for life-threatening conditions. Be sure to maintain an open airway.

▶ Monitor consciousness and breathing.

▶ Control any external bleeding with direct pressure unless the bleeding is located directly over a suspected fracture. Wear disposable gloves or use another barrier.

▶ Maintain normal body temperature.

Manual Stabilization

To perform *manual stabilization,* place your hands on both sides of the victim's head. Gently hold the person's head, in the position in which you found it and support it in that position until EMS personnel arrive. Try to keep the person from moving his or her lower body, since this movement will change the position of the head and neck. Keeping the head in the position you find it helps prevent further damage to the spinal column. The way in

which you perform this technique depends upon the position in which you find the victim (**Fig. 13-5,** *A-C*). Manual stabilization can be performed on victims who are lying down, sitting or standing.

Do not attempt to align the head and lower body. If the head is sharply turned to one side, DO NOT move it. Support it in the position found. Place the person in a modified H.A.IN.E.S. recovery position if a head, neck or back injury is suspected and you are unable to maintain an open airway or if you have to leave to get help or an AED.

Check for Life-Threatening Conditions

As you learned in Chapter 5, you do not always have to roll the victim onto his or her back to check breathing. A cry of pain, chest movement as a result of inhaling and exhaling or the sound of breathing tells you the victim is breathing, so you may not need to move him or her to check. If the victim

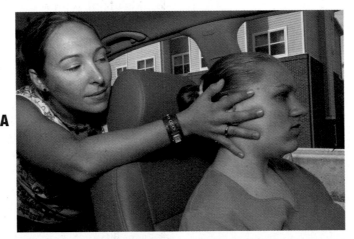

A

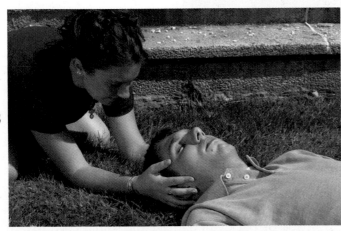

B

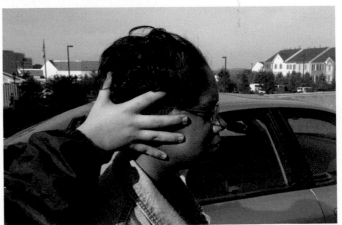

C

Figure 13-5 **A-C,** Support the victim's head in the position in which you find the victim, using manual stabilization.

is breathing normally, support him or her in the position in which you found him or her. If the victim is not breathing or you cannot tell, roll the victim gently onto his or her back, but avoid twisting the spine. To open the airway and give rescue breaths, gently lift the chin to open the airway as described in Chapter 6 to avoid moving the head or neck.

If the victim begins to vomit, carefully roll him or her onto one side to keep the airway clear. This is more easily done by two people in order to maintain manual stabilization and minimize movement of the victim's head, neck and back. Ask another responder to help move the victim's body while you maintain manual stabilization (**Fig. 13-6**).

Monitor Consciousness and Breathing

While stabilizing the head and neck, observe the victim's level of consciousness and breathing. A serious injury can result in changes in consciousness. The victim may give inappropriate responses to name, time, place or when describing what happened. He or she may speak incoherently (in a way that cannot be understood). The victim may be drowsy, appear to lapse into sleep and then suddenly awaken or completely lose consciousness. Breathing may become rapid or irregular. Because injury to the head or neck can paralyze chest nerves and muscles, breathing can stop.

Control External Bleeding

Some head and neck injuries involve soft tissue damage. Because many blood vessels are located in the head and two major arteries (the carotid arter-

ies) and the jugular veins are located in the neck, the victim can lose a significant amount of blood quickly. If the victim is bleeding externally, control it promptly with dressings, direct pressure and bandages. Do not apply pressure to both carotid arteries simultaneously, and do not put a bandage around the neck. Doing so could cut off or seriously diminish the oxygen supply to the brain.

Maintain Normal Body Temperature

A serious injury to the head or spine can disrupt the body's normal heating or cooling mechanism. When this disruption occurs, the victim is more susceptible to shock. For example, a victim suffering a serious head, neck or back injury while outside on a cold day will be more likely to develop hypothermia because the normal shivering response to rewarm the body may not work. For this reason, it is important to take steps to minimize shock by keeping the victim from becoming chilled or overheated.

SPECIFIC INJURIES

The head is easily injured because it lacks the padding of muscle and fat found in other areas of the body. You can feel bone just beneath the surface of the skin over most of the head, including the chin, cheekbones and scalp (**Fig. 13-7**). When you are checking a victim with a suspected head injury,

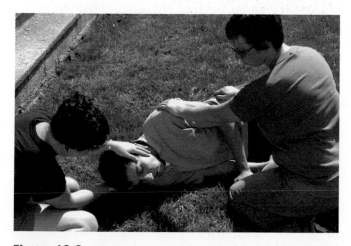

Figure 13-6 Maintain manual stabilization while rolling the victim's body.

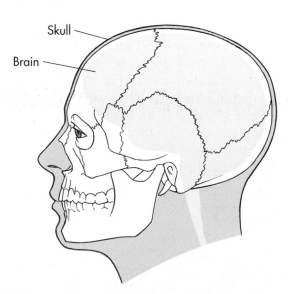

Figure 13-7 The head is easily injured because it lacks the padding of muscle and fat found in other areas of the body.

look for any swollen or bruised areas, but do not put direct pressure on any area that is swollen, depressed or soft.

Concussion

A *concussion* is a temporary impairment of brain function. Any significant force to the head can cause a concussion. It usually does not result in permanent physical damage to brain tissue. In most cases, the victim loses consciousness for only an instant and may say that he or she "blacked out" or "saw stars." A concussion sometimes results in a loss of consciousness for longer periods of time. Other times, a victim may be confused or have **amnesia** (loss of memory). Anyone suspected of having a concussion should be examined by a health-care provider. If the condition occurred during a sporting event, the victim should not return to participation until after seeing a health-care provider.

Scalp Injury

Scalp bleeding can be minor or severe. However, minor lacerations can bleed heavily because the scalp contains many blood vessels. If the victim has an open wound, control the bleeding with direct pressure. Apply several dressings and hold them in place with your gloved hand. If gloves are not available, use a protective barrier. Be sure to press gently at first because the skull may be fractured. If you feel a depression, spongy area or bone fragments, do not put direct pressure on the wound. Attempt to control bleeding with pressure on the area around the wound (**Fig. 13-8**). Secure the dressings with a roller bandage or triangular bandage (**Fig. 13-9, *A* and *B***). Call 9-1-1 or the local emergency number if you are unsure about the extent of the injury. EMS personnel will be better able to evaluate the injury.

Cheek Injury

Injury to the cheek usually involves only soft tissue. You may have to control bleeding on either the outside, inside or both sides of the cheek. The victim can swallow blood with bleeding inside the cheek. If the victim swallows enough blood, nausea or vomiting can result, which would complicate the situation.

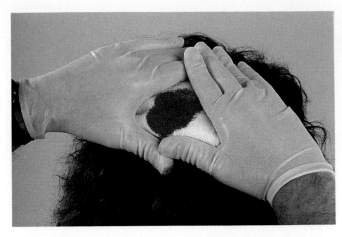

Figure 13-8 To avoid putting pressure on a deep scalp wound, apply pressure around the wound.

Begin by examining both the outside and inside of the cheek. To control bleeding, place several dressings, folded or rolled, inside the mouth, against the cheek. The victim may be able to hold these dressings in place, or you may have to hold them with your gloved hand. If there is external bleeding, place dressings on the outside of the cheek and apply direct pressure (**Fig. 13-10, *A* and *B***).

If an object passes completely through the cheek and becomes embedded and you cannot control bleeding with the object in place, the object should be removed so that you can control bleeding and keep the airway clear. *This circumstance is the only exception to the general rule not to remove embedded objects from the body.* An embedded object in the cheek cannot be easily stabilized, makes control of bleeding more difficult and may become dislodged and obstruct the airway. You can remove the object by pulling it out in the same direction it entered. Once the object is removed, fold or roll several dressings and place them inside the mouth. Also, apply dressings to the outside of the cheek. Be sure not to obstruct the airway. Place the victim in a seated position leaning slightly forward so that blood will not drain into the throat. As with any serious bleeding or embedded object, call 9-1-1 or the local emergency number.

Nose Injury

Nose injuries are usually caused by a blow from a blunt object. A nosebleed often results. High blood pressure, changes in altitude or dry air can also cause nosebleeds. In most cases, you can con-

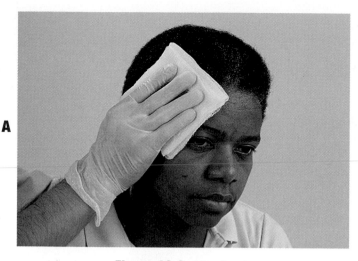

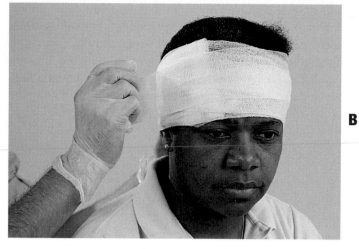

Figure 13-9   A, Apply pressure to control bleeding from a scalp wound. **B,** Then secure dressings with a bandage.

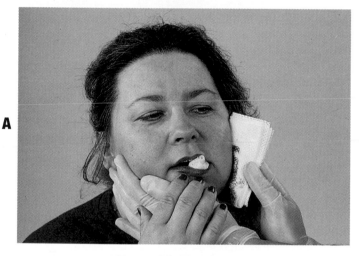

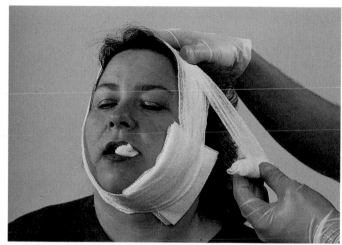

Figure 13-10   A, To control bleeding inside the cheek, place folded dressings inside the mouth against the wound. **B,** To control bleeding outside the cheek, use dressings to apply pressure directly to the wound. Bandage so as not to restrict breathing.

trol bleeding by having the victim sit with the head slightly forward while pinching the nostrils together (**Fig. 13-11**). Have the victim apply this pressure for about 10 minutes. Other methods of controlling bleeding include applying an ice pack to the bridge of the nose or putting pressure on the upper lip just beneath the nose. Keep the victim leaning slightly forward so that blood does not drain into the throat and cause the victim to vomit.

Once you have controlled the bleeding, tell the victim to avoid rubbing, blowing or picking the nose, which could restart the bleeding. You may suggest applying a little petroleum jelly inside the nostril later to help keep the mucous membranes in

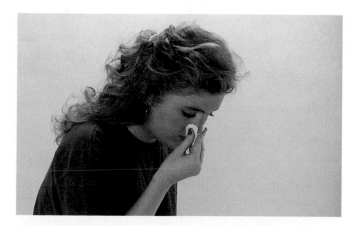

Figure 13-11 To control a nosebleed, have the victim lean forward and pinch the nostrils together until bleeding stops.

the nostril moist. You should seek additional medical care if the nosebleed continues after you use the techniques described, if bleeding recurs or if the victim says the bleeding is the result of high blood pressure. If the victim loses consciousness, place the victim on his or her side to allow blood to drain from the nose and mouth. Call 9-1-1 or the local emergency number immediately.

If you think an object is in the nostril, look into the nostril. If you see the object and can easily grasp it, while wearing disposable gloves, then do so. However, do not probe the nostril with your finger or another object. This may push the object farther into the nose and cause bleeding, block the airway or make it more difficult to remove later. If the object cannot be removed easily, the victim should receive advanced medical care.

Eye Injury

Injuries to the eye can involve the bone and soft tissue surrounding the eye or the eyeball. Blunt objects, like a fist or a baseball, may injure the eye area, or a smaller object may penetrate the eyeball. Injuries that penetrate the eyeball are very serious and can cause blindness.

Care for open or closed wounds around the eyeball as you would for any other soft tissue injury. Never put direct pressure on the eyeball. Follow these guidelines when giving care for an eye with an embedded object:

1. Place the victim on his or her back.
2. Do not attempt to remove any object embedded in the eye.
3. Wearing disposable gloves, place a sterile dressing around the object.
4. Stabilize any embedded object as best you can. You can stabilize the object by placing a paper cup around the object to support it (**Fig. 13-12, A**).
5. Bandage loosely and do not put pressure on the injured eye/eyeball (**Fig. 13-12, B**).
6. Seek immediate medical attention.

Foreign bodies, such as dirt, sand or slivers of wood or metal, that get in the eye are irritating and can cause significant damage. The eye immediately produces tears in an attempt to flush out such objects. Pain from the irritation is often severe. The victim may have difficulty opening the eye because light further irritates it.

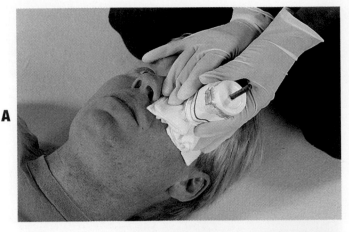

A

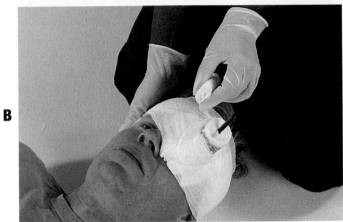

B

Figure 13-12 A, Support the object with a paper cup. **B,** Carefully bandage the cup in place.

First, try to remove the foreign body by telling the victim to blink several times. Then try gently flushing the eye with water. If the object remains, the victim should receive more advanced medical care. The eye should be continuously flushed until EMS personnel arrive. Flushing the eye with water is also appropriate if the victim has any chemical in the eye (**Fig. 13-13**).

Ear Injury

External injuries to the ear are common. Open wounds, such as lacerations or abrasions, can result from recreational injuries, for example, being struck by a racquetball or falling off a bike. An avulsion of the ear may occur when a pierced earring catches on something and tears away from the ear. You can control bleeding from the soft tissues of the ear by applying direct pressure to the affected area with a gloved hand or other barrier.

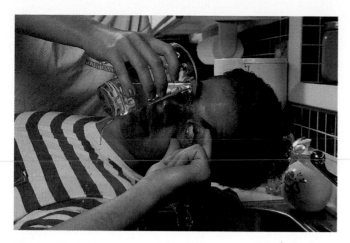

Figure 13-13   If chemicals enter the eye, flush the eye continuously with water.

The ear can also be injured internally. A direct blow to the head may rupture the eardrum. Sudden pressure changes, such as those caused by an explosion or a deep-water dive, can also injure the ear internally. The victim may lose hearing or balance or experience inner ear pain. These injuries require more advanced medical care.

A foreign object, such as dirt, an insect or cotton, can easily become lodged in the ear canal. If you can easily see and grasp the object, remove it. Do not try to remove any object by using a pin, toothpick or a similar sharp item. You could force the object farther back or puncture the eardrum. Sometimes you can remove the object if you pull down on the earlobe, tilt the head to the side and shake or gently strike the head on the affected side. If you cannot easily remove the object, the victim should seek more advanced medical care.

If the victim has a serious head injury, blood or other fluid may be in the ear canal or may be draining from the ear. Do not attempt to stop this drainage with direct pressure. Instead, just cover the ear lightly with a sterile dressing. Call 9-1-1 or the local emergency number.

Mouth, Jaw and Neck Injuries

Your primary concern for any injury to the mouth, jaw or neck is to ensure that the airway is open. Such injuries may cause trouble breathing if blood or loose teeth obstruct the airway. A swollen or crushed trachea may also obstruct breathing.

If you do not suspect a serious head, neck or back injury, place the victim in a seated position with the head tilted slightly forward to allow any blood to drain. If this position is not possible, place the victim on his or her side to allow blood to drain from the mouth.

For injuries that penetrate the lip, place a rolled dressing between the lip and the gum. You can place another dressing on the outer surface of the lip. If the tongue is bleeding, apply a dressing and direct pressure with a gloved hand. Applying ice or a cold pack to the lips or tongue can help reduce swelling and ease pain. Place gauze between the source of cold and the tongue. If the bleeding cannot be controlled easily, the victim should seek medical attention.

If the injury knocked out one or more of the victim's teeth, control the bleeding and save the tooth or teeth for replantation. If the person is conscious and able to cooperate, rinse out the mouth with cold tap water, if available. To control the bleeding, roll a sterile dressing and insert it into the space left by the missing tooth or teeth. Have the victim bite down on the dressing to maintain pressure (**Fig. 13-14**). Carefully pick up the tooth by the crown (*not at the root end*). If dirty, gently rinse off the root of the tooth in water. Do not scrub the tooth or remove any attached tissue fragments.

Opinions vary as to how the tooth should be saved. One option is to place the dislodged tooth or teeth in the injured person's mouth. This method, however, is not always the best approach because a crying child could **aspirate** the tooth or the tooth

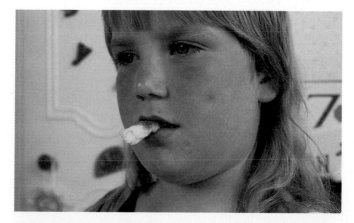

Figure 13-14   If a tooth is knocked out, place a sterile dressing directly in the space left by the tooth. Tell the victim to bite down.

could otherwise become an airway obstruction. The tooth could also be swallowed with blood or saliva. In addition, you may need to control serious bleeding in the mouth. Because of these concerns, simply place the tooth in a closed container of cool, fresh milk until it reaches the dentist. If milk is not available, use water. If the injury is severe enough to call 9-1-1 or the local emergency number, give the tooth to EMS personnel when they arrive. If the injury is not severe enough to call 9-1-1 or the local emergency number, the victim should immediately see a dentist who can replant the tooth within 30 minutes to an hour after the injury. For the tooth to be successfully replanted, time is critical.

Injuries serious enough to fracture or dislocate the jaw can also cause other head or neck injuries. Call 9-1-1 or the local emergency number. Be sure to maintain an open airway. Check inside the

Now Smile

Knocked-out teeth no longer spell doom for pearly whites. Most dentists can successfully replant a knocked-out tooth if they can do so quickly and if the tooth is properly handled. Replanting a tooth is similar to replanting a tree. On each tooth, tiny root fibers called periodontal fibers attach to the jawbone to hold the tooth in place. Inside the tooth, a canal filled with bundles of blood vessels and nerves runs from the tooth into the jawbone and surrounding tissues.

"When these fibers and tissues are torn from the socket, it is important that they be replaced within an hour," says American Academy of Pediatric Dentists expert, Dr. J. Bogart. Generally, the sooner the tooth is replanted, the greater the chance it will survive. The knocked-out tooth must be handled carefully to protect the fragile tissues. Be careful to pick up the tooth by the chewing edge (crown), not the root. Do not rub or handle the root part of the tooth. It is best to preserve the tooth by placing it in a closed container of cool, fresh milk until it reaches the dentist. Because milk is not always available at an injury scene, water may be substituted.

A dentist or emergency room will clean the tooth, taking care not to damage the root fibers. The tooth is then placed back into the socket and secured with

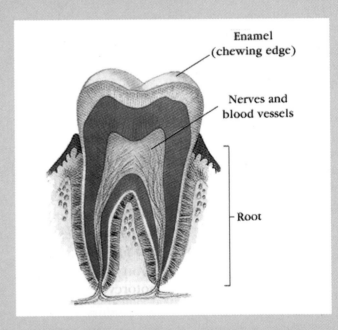

Enamel (chewing edge)

Nerves and blood vessels

Root

special splinting devices. The devices keep the tooth stable for 2 to 3 weeks while the fibers reattach to the jawbone. The bundles of blood vessels and nerves grow back within 6 weeks.

SOURCES
American College of Emergency Physicians, *Dental Emergencies.* www.acep.org. Accessed 10/25/04.
American Dental Association, *Dental Emergencies and Injuries.* www.ada.org/public/manage/emergencies.asp. Accessed 10/25/04.
Bogart J, DDS: Executive Director, American Academy of Pediatric Dentists. Interview April 1990.
Medford H, DDS: Acute care of an avulsed tooth, *Annals of Emergency Medicine* 11:559-61, 1982.

mouth for bleeding. Control bleeding as you would for other head injuries. Minimize movement of the head, neck or back.

A soft tissue injury to the neck can produce severe bleeding and swelling that may result in airway obstruction. Because the spine may also be involved, care for a serious neck injury as you would a possible spinal injury. If the victim has struck his or her neck on a steering wheel or run into a clothesline, the injury can be devastating. The trachea may be crushed or collapsed, causing an airway obstruction that requires immediate medical attention. While waiting for EMS personnel to arrive, try to keep the victim from moving, and encourage him or her to breathe slowly. Control any external bleeding with direct pressure, wearing a glove or using another barrier. Be careful not to apply pressure that constricts both carotid arteries. For a large laceration to the neck, apply an occlusive dressing to avoid the possibility of air getting into a vein.

Lower Back Injury

Certain injuries to the neck and back are not life-threatening but can be extremely painful and temporarily disabling and may occur without warning. These injuries usually occur from forcing the back beyond its limits in strength or flexibility. Using improper lifting techniques when lifting or moving heavy objects is one way to injure the back. Working in a cramped space in a bent-over or awkward position may cause back pain, as can sitting or standing in one position for a long period of time. Often acute back pain that develops suddenly is a result of one of the following causes:

- Ligament pulls and muscle strains—violent movement or unaccustomed effort stretches or tears muscles in the back or neck, or the ligaments that bind together or surround each section of the spine.
- Vertebrae displacement—twisting movement causes two vertebrae to slip out of place, and facets (bony projections) lock in a position that puts pressure on a nerve or irritates the joint, often causing muscles to go into spasm.
- Slipped (prolapsed) disk—pressure and wear and tear on one of the cartilage disks that separate the vertebrae cause the soft center of the disk to protrude through the disk's outer layer.

This center part presses on a nerve, often causing muscles to spasm.

Signals of lower back injury include—

- Shooting pain in the lower back.
- Sharp pain in one leg.
- Sharp pain and tightness across the lower back.
- A sudden, sharp pain in the back and a feeling that something snapped.
- Inability to bend over without pain.

Regardless of the possible cause of back pain, call 9-1-1 or the local emergency number immediately if the victim has any of the following accompanying signals:

- Numbness or tingling in any extremity
- Difficulty moving
- Loss of bladder or bowel control

These signals indicate possible damage to the spinal cord. Wait for EMS personnel to arrive and keep the victim warm and quiet.

A person with pain in one side of the small of the back who also has a fever or feels ill should call a physician. The victim may have a kidney infection. Older adults with back pain may have a life-threatening emergency—an aortic **aneurysm.** For older adults with severe back pain, call 9-1-1 or the local emergency number.

Because the care for lower back injury varies depending on the nature of the injury, the victim should consult a physician. Cold treatment is usually recommended for musculoskeletal injuries initially, followed by heat treatment. Bed rest and pain-relieving medications, such as acetaminophen or ibuprofen, generally provide relief for strains and muscle spasms. Exercises are frequently recommended to strengthen the back and abdominal muscles after the pain has gone and should only be done at the direction of a physician or physical therapist.

PREVENTING HEAD, NECK OR BACK INJURIES

Injuries to the head, neck or back are a major cause of death, disability and disfigurement. However, many such injuries can be prevented. By using safety practices in all areas of your life, you can help reduce risks to yourself and to others around you.

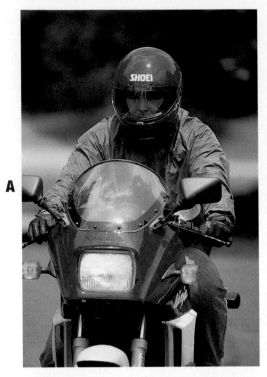

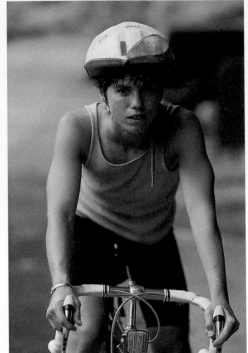

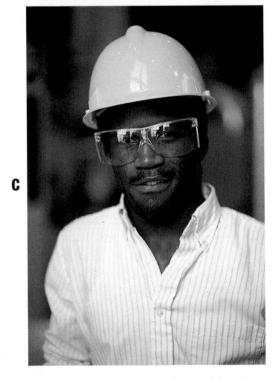

Figure 13-15 **A-C,** Wearing a helmet helps protect against head, neck or back injuries.

Safety practices that can help prevent injuries to the head, neck and back include—

▶ Wearing safety belts (lap and shoulder restraints) and placing children in car safety seats.
▶ When appropriate, wearing approved helmets, eyewear, faceguards and mouthguards (**Fig. 13-15,** *A-C*).

▶ Taking steps to prevent falls.
▶ Obeying rules in sports and recreational activities.
▶ Avoiding inappropriate use of alcohol and other drugs.
▶ Inspecting work and recreational equipment periodically.
▶ Thinking and talking about safety.

SUMMARY

In this chapter, you have learned how to recognize and care for serious head, neck and back injuries; specific injuries to the head and neck; and lower back problems. Like injuries elsewhere on the body, injuries to the head, neck and back often involve both soft tissue and bone. Often the cause of the injury is the best indicator of whether or not it is serious. If you have any doubts about the seriousness of an injury, call 9-1-1 or your local emergency number.

APPLICATION QUESTION

1. Is it safe to assume that the football player who walks out of the water does not have a head, neck or back injury? Why or why not?

STUDY QUESTIONS

1. Match each term with the correct definition.

    a. Concussion
    b. Manual stabilization
    c. Spinal column
    d. Spinal cord
    e. Vertebrae

    _____ Technique used to minimize movement of the victim's head and neck while giving care.

    _____ Head injury that usually does not permanently damage the brain.

    _____ Column of vertebrae extending from the base of the skull to the tip of the tailbone.

    _____ The 33 bones of the spinal column.

    _____ A bundle of nerves extending from the base of the skull to the lower back, protected by the spinal column

2. List five situations that might result in serious head, neck or back injuries.

3. List six signals of head, neck or back injuries.

4. List five ways to prevent head, neck or back injuries.

5. List the steps of care for an eye injury in which the eyeball has been penetrated.

In questions 6 through 13, circle the letter of the correct answer.

6. Which are the most common causes of serious head, neck and back injury?

    a. Motor vehicle accidents
    b. Sports-related injuries
    c. Falls
    d. Violence

7. Serious injuries to the head, neck or back can damage—

    a. Soft tissues.
    b. Nerve tissues.
    c. Bones.
    d. All of the above.

8. Which of the following situations would cause you to suspect a serious head, neck or back injury?

   a. A man complains of lower back pain after working out in the gym.
   b. Two people bump their heads together while reaching for a piece of paper on the floor.
   c. A high school football player is holding his neck after making a tackle.
   d. A child trips and falls onto her hands and knees.

9. Which should you do when caring for a victim of suspected head, neck or back injury?

   a. Help support the injured area by walking the victim to the nearest wall.
   b. Call the victim's physician for additional care.
   c. Check for life-threatening conditions and maintain an open airway.
   d. Have the victim lie flat and elevate the legs 8-12 inches.

10. At the scene of a car crash, a victim has blood seeping from his ears. Which should you do?

   a. Loosely cover the ears with a sterile dressing.
   b. Do nothing; this is a normal finding in a head injury.
   c. Collect the fluid in a sterile container for analysis.
   d. Pack the ears with sterile dressings to prevent further fluid loss.

11. Which is your primary concern when caring for an injury to the mouth or neck?

   a. Infection
   b. Airway obstruction
   c. Swelling
   d. Scarring

12. Caring for a penetrating injury to the eyeball includes—

   a. Placing direct pressure on the eyeball.
   b. Removing the object.
   c. Washing the affected eye.
   d. Stabilizing the object.

13. Which is a signal of an injured ear?

   a. Hearing loss
   b. Loss of balance
   c. Inner ear pain
   d. All of the above

14. As you begin to apply direct pressure to control bleeding for a scalp injury, you notice a depression of the skull in the area of the bleeding. What should you do next?

15. What should you do for a victim of suspected head, neck or back injury whom you find lying on his side, moaning in pain?

Answers are listed in Appendix A

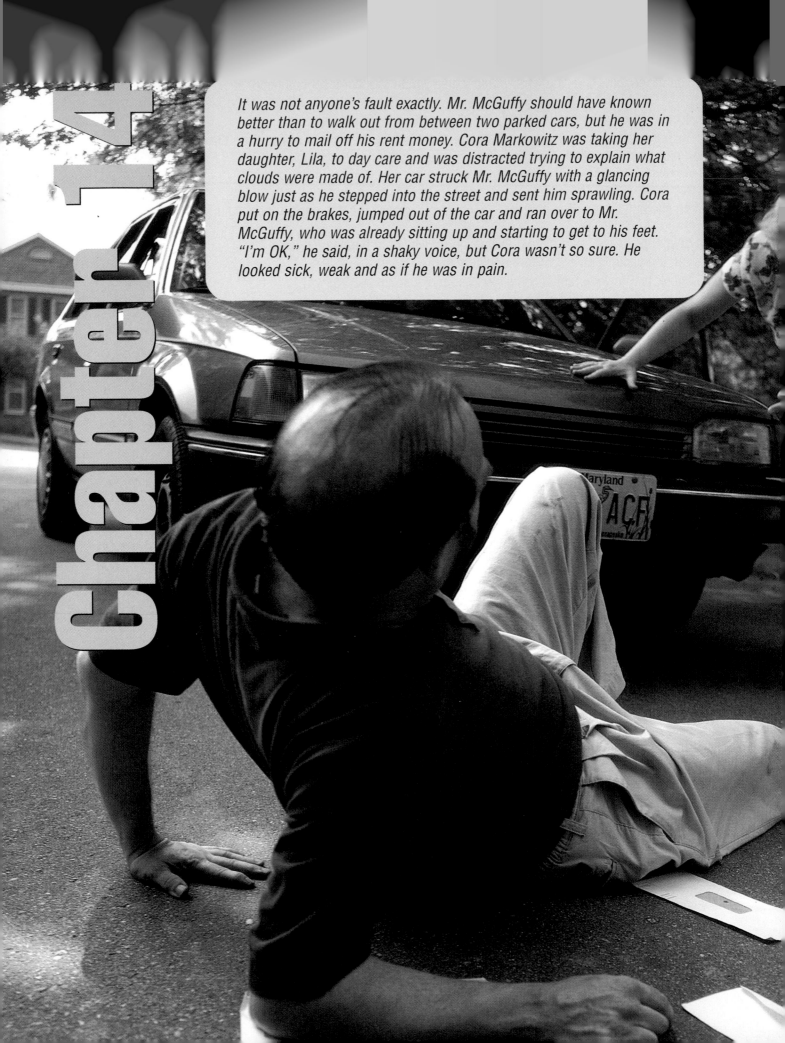

chapter 14

It was not anyone's fault exactly. Mr. McGuffy should have known better than to walk out from between two parked cars, but he was in a hurry to mail off his rent money. Cora Markowitz was taking her daughter, Lila, to day care and was distracted trying to explain what clouds were made of. Her car struck Mr. McGuffy with a glancing blow just as he stepped into the street and sent him sprawling. Cora put on the brakes, jumped out of the car and ran over to Mr. McGuffy, who was already sitting up and starting to get to his feet. "I'm OK," he said, in a shaky voice, but Cora wasn't so sure. He looked sick, weak and as if he was in pain.

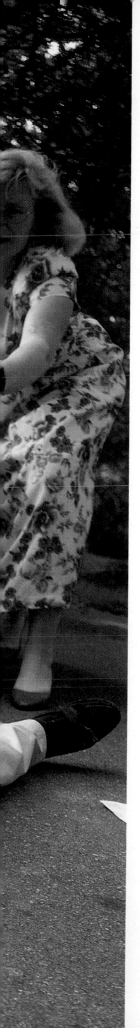

Injuries to the Chest, Abdomen and Pelvis

Objectives

After reading this chapter, you should be able to—

- *Explain why injuries to the chest, abdomen and pelvis can be fatal.*

- *List the seven signals of chest injury.*

- *Describe how to care for rib fractures.*

- *Describe how to care for a sucking chest wound.*

- *List the signals of serious abdominal and pelvic injuries.*

- *Describe the care for open and closed abdominal and pelvic injuries.*

- *Describe how to care for injuries to the genitals.*

Introduction

Many injuries to the chest and abdomen involve only soft tissues. Often these injuries, like those that occur elsewhere on the body, are only minor cuts, scrapes, burns and bruises. Occasionally, severe injuries occur, such as fractures or injuries to organs that cause severe bleeding or impair breathing. Fractures and lacerations often occur in motor vehicle collisions to occupants not wearing seat belts. Falls, sports mishaps and other forms of trauma, the violent force or mechanism that can cause injury, may also cause such injuries.

Injuries to the pelvis may be minor soft tissue injuries or serious injuries to bone and internal structures. The pelvis is the lower part of the trunk, containing part of the intestines, bladder and reproductive organs. It includes a group of large bones that forms a protective girdle around the organs inside. A great force is required to cause serious injury to the pelvic bones.

Because the chest, abdomen and pelvis contain many organs important to life, injury to these areas can be fatal. You may recall from the previous chapter that a force capable of causing severe injury in these areas may also cause injury to the spine.

General care for these injuries includes—
▸ Calling 9-1-1 or the local emergency number.
▸ Limiting movement.
▸ Monitoring breathing and signs of life.
▸ Controlling bleeding.
▸ Minimizing shock.

This chapter describes the signals of different injuries to the chest, abdomen and pelvis and the care you would give for them. In all cases, follow the Emergency Action Steps. Check the scene and the victim. Call 9-1-1 or the local emergency number. Care for the victim. Care for all life-threatening injuries first. All the injuries described in this chapter are serious and require advanced medical care. Always call 9-1-1 or the local emergency number immediately.

INJURIES TO THE CHEST

The *chest* is the upper part of the trunk. The chest is shaped by 12 pairs of ribs. Ten of the pairs attach to the *sternum* (breastbone) in front and to the spine in back. Two pairs, the floating ribs, attach only to the spine. The *rib cage,* formed by the ribs, the sternum and the spine, protects vital organs, such as the heart, major blood vessels and the lungs (**Fig. 14-1**). Also in the chest are the esophagus, the trachea and the muscles of respiration.

Chest injuries are a leading cause of trauma deaths each year. Injuries to the chest may result from a wide variety of causes, such as motor vehicle accidents, falls, sports mishaps and crushing or penetrating forces (**Fig. 14-2**). Chest injuries may involve the bones that form the chest cavity or they may involve the organs or other structures in the cavity itself.

KEY TERMS

Abdomen: The middle part of the trunk, containing the stomach, liver, intestines and spleen.
Chest: The upper part of the trunk, containing the heart, major blood vessels and lungs.
Genitals: The external reproductive organs.
Pelvis: The lower part of the trunk, containing the intestines, bladder and internal reproductive organs.

Rib cage: The cage of bones formed by the 12 pairs of ribs, the sternum and the spine.
Sternum: The long, flat bone in the middle of the front of the rib cage; also called the breastbone.

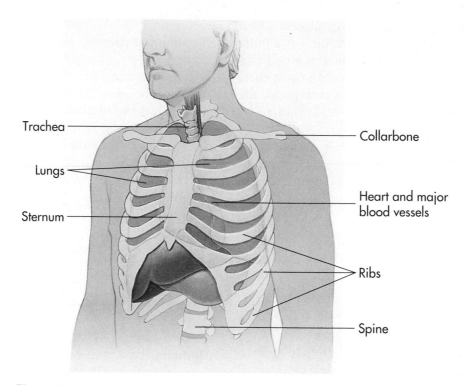

Figure 14-1   The rib cage surrounds and protects several vital organs.

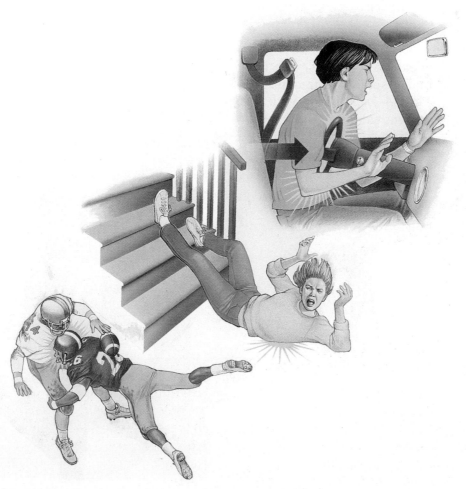

Figure 14-2   About one-third of the deaths from motor vehicle collisions involve chest injuries. Crushing forces, falls and sports mishaps can also lead to chest injuries.

Chest wounds are either open or closed. Open chest wounds occur when an object, such as a knife or bullet, penetrates the chest wall. Fractured ribs may break through the skin to cause an open chest injury. A closed chest wound does not break the skin. Closed chest wounds are generally caused by blunt objects, such as steering wheels.

You may recognize some of the signals of a serious chest injury from previous discussions of respiratory distress, soft tissue injuries and musculoskeletal injuries. They include—

▶ Trouble breathing.
▶ Severe pain at the site of the injury.
▶ Flushed, pale, ashen or bluish skin.
▶ Obvious deformity, such as that caused by a fracture.
▶ Coughing up blood (may be bright red or dark like coffee grounds).
▶ Bruising at the site of a blunt injury, such as that caused by a seat belt.
▶ A "sucking" noise or distinct sound when the victim breathes.

Rib Fractures

Rib fractures are usually caused by direct force to the chest. Although painful, a simple rib fracture is rarely life threatening (**Fig. 14-3**). A victim with a fractured rib generally remains calm, but his or her breathing is shallow because normal or deep breathing is painful. The victim will usually attempt to ease the pain by supporting the injured area with a hand or arm. Rib fractures are less common in children because children's ribs are so flexible that they bend rather than break. However, the forces that can cause a rib fracture in adults can severely bruise the lung tissue of children, which can be a life-threatening injury. Look for signals, such as what caused the injury, bruising on the chest and trouble breathing, to determine if a child has potential chest injury.

Care for Rib Fractures

If you suspect a fractured rib, have the victim rest in a position that will make breathing easier. Do not move the victim if you suspect a head, neck or back injury. Call 9-1-1 or the local emergency number. Binding the victim's upper arm to the chest on the injured side will help support the injured area and make breathing more comfortable. You can use an object such as a pillow or rolled blanket to support and immobilize the area (**Fig. 14-4**). Monitor breathing and skin condition, and take steps to minimize shock.

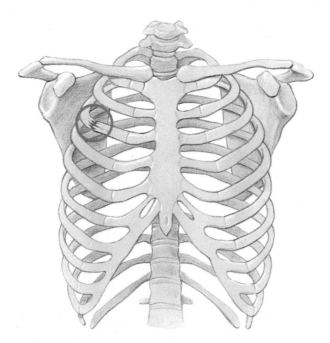

Figure 14-3 A simple rib fracture is painful but rarely life threatening.

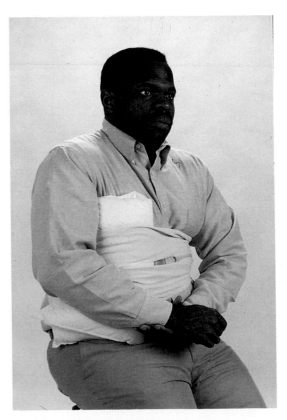

Figure 14-4 When a rib fracture occurs, use a pillow or folded blanket to support and immobilize the injured area.

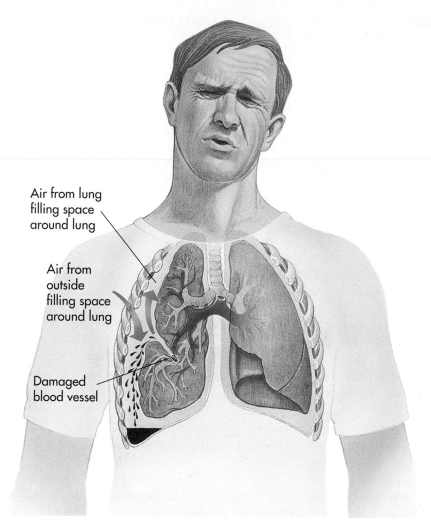

Air from lung filling space around lung

Air from outside filling space around lung

Damaged blood vessel

Figure 14-5 A puncture wound that penetrates the lung or the chest cavity surrounding the lung allows air to go in and out of the cavity.

Puncture Wounds

Puncture wounds to the chest range from minor to life threatening. Stab and gunshot wounds are examples of puncture injuries. The penetrating object can injure any structure or organ within the chest, including the lungs. A puncture injury can allow air to enter the chest through the wound. Air in the chest cavity does not allow the lungs to function normally.

Puncture wounds cause varying degrees of internal or external bleeding. A puncture wound to the chest is a life-threatening injury. If the injury penetrates the rib cage, air can pass freely in and out of the chest cavity, and the victim cannot breathe normally. With each breath the victim takes, you hear a sucking sound coming from the wound. This sound is the primary signal of a penetrating chest injury called a sucking chest wound (**Fig. 14-5**). Without proper care, the victim's condi-

tion will worsen. The affected lung or lungs will fail to function, and breathing will become more difficult. Call 9-1-1 or the local emergency number.

Care for Puncture Wounds

To care for a sucking chest wound, cover the wound with a large **occlusive dressing,** a dressing that does not allow air to pass through it. A piece of plastic wrap or a plastic bag folded several times and placed over the wound makes an effective occlusive dressing. Tape the dressing in place, except for one side or corner that remains loose. A taped-down dressing keeps air from entering the wound when the victim inhales, and having an open corner allows air to escape when the victim exhales (**Fig. 14-6**). If these materials are not available to use as dressings, use a folded cloth. Call 9-1-1 or the local emergency number. Take steps to minimize shock.

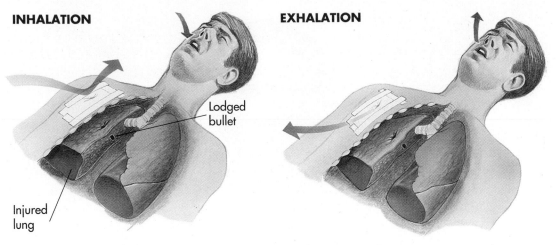

INHALATION

EXHALATION

Lodged bullet

Injured lung

Figure 14-6   An occlusive dressing with one loose corner keeps air from entering the wound when the victim inhales and allows air to escape when the victim exhales. This helps keep the injured lung from collapsing.

INJURIES TO THE ABDOMEN

The *abdomen* is the area immediately under the chest and above the pelvis. The upper abdomen is partially protected by the lower ribs and spine. It is protected in back by the spine. The muscles of the back and abdomen also help protect vital internal organs such as the liver, spleen and stomach (**Fig. 14-7**). These vital organs are easily injured and tend to bleed profusely when injured. The liver and spleen are less protected in children because the major part of the organ is positioned below the rib cage and the abdominal muscles are not as strong as those of adults.

Located in the upper right part of the abdomen, the liver is protected somewhat by the lower ribs. However, it is delicate and can be torn by blows from blunt objects or penetrated by a fractured rib. The resulting bleeding can be severe and can quickly be fatal. When the liver is injured, bile can leak into the abdomen, which can cause severe irritation and infection.

The spleen is located behind the stomach and is protected somewhat by the lower left ribs. Like the liver, this organ is easily damaged. The spleen may rupture when the abdomen is struck forcefully by a blunt object. Because the spleen stores blood, an injury to the spleen can cause a

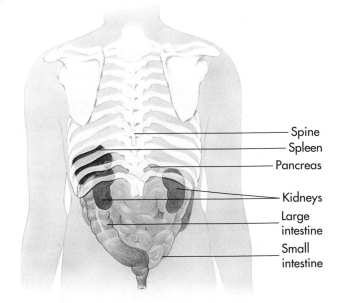

FRONT VIEW

BACK VIEW

Liver
Stomach
Gallbladder
Large intestine
Small intestine

Spine
Spleen
Pancreas
Kidneys
Large intestine
Small intestine

Figure 14-7   Unlike the organs of the chest or pelvis, organs in the abdominal cavity are relatively unprotected by bones.

severe loss of blood in a short time and can be life threatening.

The stomach is one of the main digestive organs. The upper part of the stomach changes shape depending on its contents, the stage of digestion and the size and strength of the stomach muscles. The stomach can bleed severely when injured, and food contents may leak into the abdominal cavity and possibly cause infection.

Like a chest injury, an injury to the abdomen may be either open or closed. Injuries to the abdomen can be very painful. Even with a closed wound, the rupture of an organ can cause serious internal bleeding that results in shock. It is especially difficult to determine if a person has an internal abdominal injury if he or she is unconscious. Always suspect an abdominal injury in a victim who has multiple injuries. Signals of serious abdominal injury include—

▶ Severe pain.
▶ Bruising.
▶ External bleeding.
▶ Nausea.
▶ Vomiting (sometimes containing blood).
▶ Weakness.

▶ Thirst.
▶ Pain, tenderness or a tight feeling in the abdomen.
▶ Organs protruding from the abdomen.
▶ Rigid abdominal muscles.
▶ Other signals of shock.

Care for Injuries to the Abdomen

With a severe open injury, abdominal organs sometimes protrude through the wound (**Fig. 14-8, *A***). To care for an open wound to the abdomen, follow these steps:

▶ Call 9-1-1 or the local emergency number.
▶ Put on disposable gloves or use another barrier.
▶ Carefully position the victim on the back.
▶ Do not apply direct pressure.
▶ Do not push any protruding organs back in.
▶ Remove clothing from around the wound (**Fig. 14-8, *B***).
▶ Apply moist, sterile dressings loosely over the wound (**Fig. 14-8, *C***). (Warm tap water can be used.)
▶ Cover dressings loosely with plastic wrap, if available.

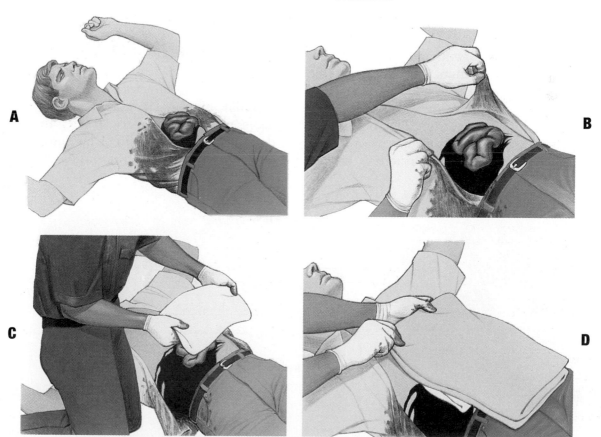

Figure 14-8   A, Severe injuries to the abdominal cavity can result in protruding organs. **B,** Carefully remove clothing from around the wound. **C,** Apply a large, moist, sterile dressing over the wound and cover it with plastic wrap. **D,** Place a folded towel over the dressing to maintain warmth.

▶ Cover dressings lightly with a folded towel to maintain warmth (**Fig. 14-8, D**).

Shock is likely to occur with a serious abdominal injury. Call 9-1-1 or the local emergency number immediately, and take steps to minimize shock. Keep the victim from becoming chilled or overheated, and monitor breathing and how the skin looks and feels until EMS personnel arrive.

To care for a closed abdominal injury—

▶ Call 9-1-1 or the local emergency number.
▶ Carefully position the victim on the back unless you suspect injury to the head, neck or back.
▶ Bend the victim's knees slightly. This position allows the muscles of the abdomen to relax. If moving the victim's legs causes pain, leave them straight.
▶ Place rolled-up blankets or pillows under the victim's knees.
▶ Take steps to minimize shock. Keep the victim from becoming chilled or overheated, and monitor breathing and how the skin looks and feels until EMS personnel arrive.

INJURIES TO THE PELVIS

The *pelvis* is the lower part of the trunk. It contains the bladder, reproductive organs and part of the large intestine, including the rectum. Major arteries (the femoral arteries) and nerves pass through the pelvis. The organs within the pelvis are well protected on the sides and back but not in front (**Fig. 14-9**).

Injuries to the pelvis may include fractures to the pelvic bone and damage to structures within.

Fractured bones may puncture or lacerate these structures, or they can be injured when struck a forceful blow by blunt or penetrating objects. An injury to the pelvis sometimes involves the **genitals,** the external reproductive organs. Genital injuries are either closed wounds, such as a bruise, or open wounds, such as an avulsion or laceration. Any injury to the genitals is extremely painful.

Signals of pelvic injury are the same as those for an abdominal injury. These signals include—

▶ Severe pain.
▶ Bruising.
▶ External bleeding.
▶ Nausea.
▶ Vomiting (sometimes containing blood).
▶ Weakness.
▶ Thirst.
▶ Pain, tenderness or a tight feeling in the area.
▶ Protruding organs.
▶ Rigid abdominal muscles.
▶ Other signals of shock.

Certain pelvic injuries may also cause loss of sensation in the legs or inability to move them. This loss of sensation or movement may indicate an injury to the lower spine.

Care for Injuries to the Pelvis

Care for pelvic injuries is similar to that for abdominal injuries. Do not move the victim unless necessary. If possible, try to keep the victim lying flat. Otherwise, help him or her into a comfortable position. Control any external bleeding, and cover

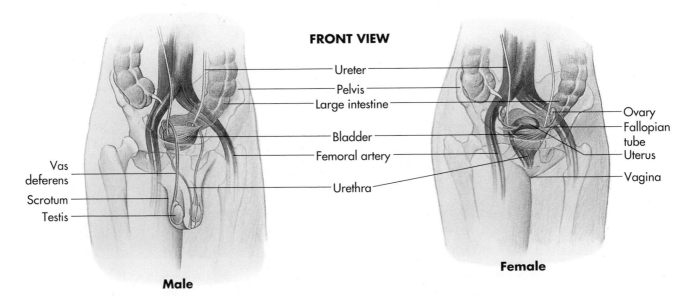

FRONT VIEW

Ureter
Pelvis
Large intestine
Bladder
Femoral artery
Urethra

Vas deferens
Scrotum
Testis

Ovary
Fallopian tube
Uterus
Vagina

Male

Female

Figure 14-9 The internal structures of the pelvis are well protected on the sides and back, but not in front.

any protruding organs. Always call 9-1-1 or the local emergency number and take steps to minimize shock. Major bleeding can occur with pelvic injuries.

Any injury to the genitals is extremely painful. Care for a closed wound to the genitals as you would for any closed wound. If the injury is an open wound, apply a sterile dressing and direct pressure with your gloved hand or the victim's hand or use a barrier. If any parts are completely avulsed, wrap them as described in Chapter 10, and make sure they are transported with the victim. Injuries to the genital area can be embarrassing for both the victim and the responder. Explain briefly what you are going to do, then do it. Do not act in a timid or hesitant manner. Hesitation or shyness will only make the situation more difficult for you and the victim.

SUMMARY

Injuries to the chest, abdomen or pelvis can be serious. They can damage soft tissues, bones and internal organs. Although many injuries are immediately obvious, some may be detected only as the victim's condition worsens over time. Watch for the signals of serious injuries that require medical attention.

Care for any life-threatening conditions, and then give any additional care needed for specific injuries. Always call 9-1-1 or the local emergency number as soon as possible. Have the victim remain as still as possible. For open wounds to the chest, abdomen or pelvis, control bleeding. If you suspect a fracture, immobilize the injured part. Use occlusive dressings for sucking chest wounds and open abdominal wounds when these materials are available. Your actions can make the difference in the victim's chance of survival.

APPLICATION QUESTION

1. What steps should Cora take to care for Mr. McGuffy?

STUDY QUESTIONS

1. Match each term with the correct definition.

   a. Abdomen
   b. Chest
   c. Genitals
   d. Pelvis
   e. Sternum

   _____ External reproductive organs.

   _____ The middle part of the trunk, containing the stomach, liver and spleen.

   _____ The upper part of the trunk, containing the heart, major blood vessels and lungs.

   _____ Long, flat bone in the middle of the front of the rib cage, also called the breastbone.

   _____ The lower part of the trunk, containing the intestines, bladder and reproductive organs.

2. List five general steps of care for injuries to the chest, abdomen and pelvis.

3. List four signals of chest injury.

4. A horse being loaded into a trailer kicks a man in the chest. He is clutching the left side of his chest and says it hurts to breathe. What type of injury would you suspect he has, and what care should you give?

5. Name the primary signal of a sucking chest wound.

6. List four signals of abdominal and pelvic injury.

In question 7, circle the letter of the correct answer.

7. Care for injuries to the chest, abdomen and pelvis includes—

   a. Watching for changes in a victim's breathing.
   b. Controlling internal bleeding.
   c. Giving the victim fluids.
   d. Minimizing bystander activity.

Base your answers for questions 8 through 10 on the scenario below.

You arrive at the local convenience store late Saturday night to satisfy your frozen yogurt craving. As you enter, you notice drops of blood on the floor. A robbery has just occurred—the store clerk appears to have been beaten and stabbed. He is conscious but in considerable pain and is having trouble breathing. You hear a sucking sound when he breathes.

8. What type of injury does the victim have?

9. Identify the signals that support your answer in question 8.

10. Describe the steps you would take to help the victim.

Answers are listed in Appendix A.

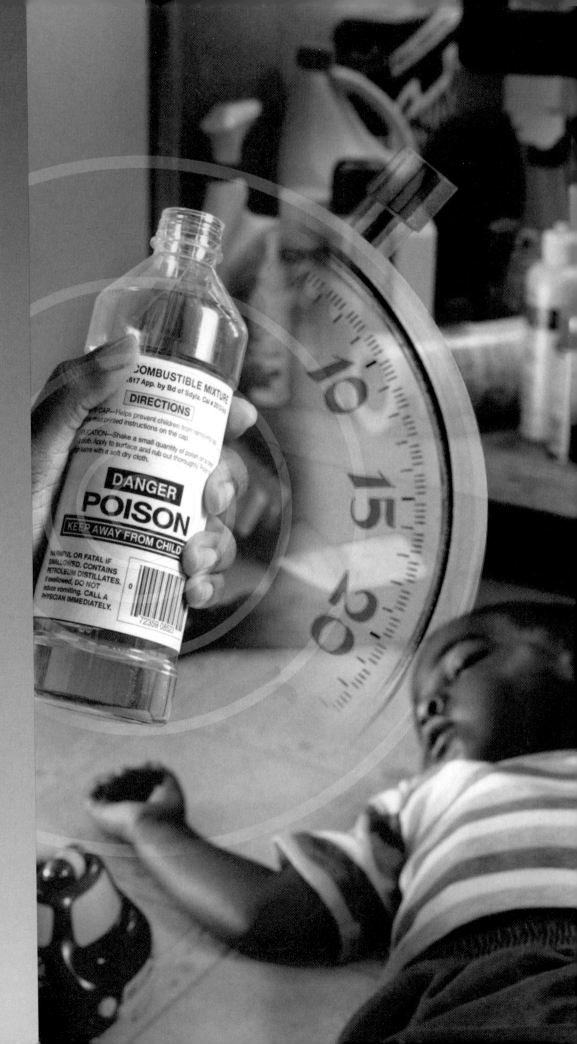

MEDICAL EMERGENCIES

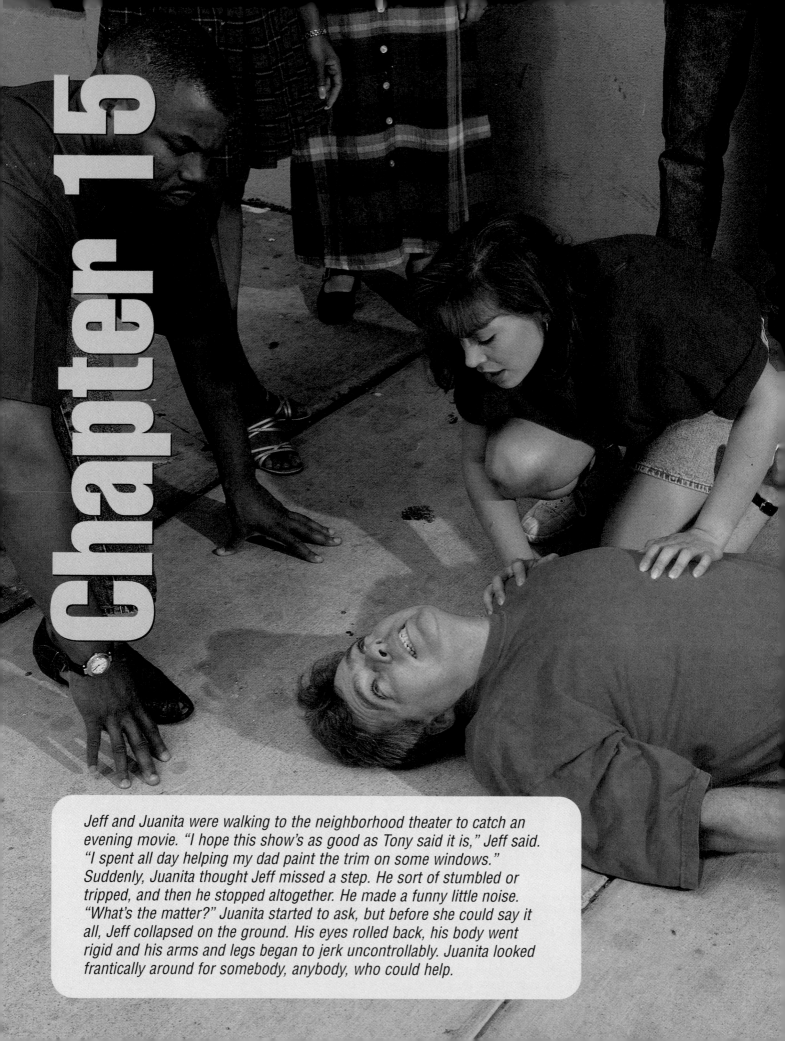

Chapter 15

Jeff and Juanita were walking to the neighborhood theater to catch an evening movie. "I hope this show's as good as Tony said it is," Jeff said. "I spent all day helping my dad paint the trim on some windows." Suddenly, Juanita thought Jeff missed a step. He sort of stumbled or tripped, and then he stopped altogether. He made a funny little noise. "What's the matter?" Juanita started to ask, but before she could say it all, Jeff collapsed on the ground. His eyes rolled back, his body went rigid and his arms and legs began to jerk uncontrollably. Juanita looked frantically around for somebody, anybody, who could help.

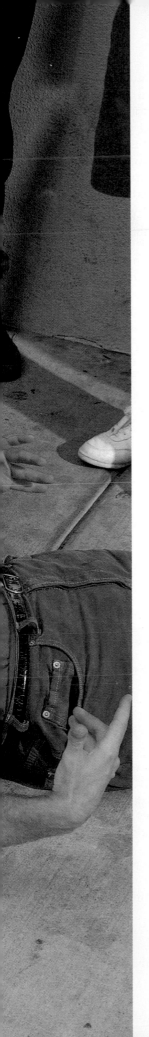

Sudden Illness

Objectives

After reading this chapter, you should be able to—

- List the general guidelines for giving care to a victim of a sudden illness.

- Recognize the signals of a sudden illness.

- Describe how to care for a victim who faints.

- Describe how to care for a victim of a diabetic emergency.

- Describe how to care for a victim having a seizure.

- Describe how to care for a victim of a stroke.

- Identify five ways to reduce the risk of a stroke or transient ischemic attack (TIA).

Introduction

While some illnesses develop over time, others can strike without a moment's notice. However, if you look closely, you may see the signals of a developing sudden illness. You may hear the person describe his or her signals or you may notice a change in the person's appearance. By knowing the signals of sudden illness and paying careful attention to details at the emergency scene, you can determine how best to help a victim of sudden illness.

SPECIFIC SUDDEN ILLNESSES

Sudden illnesses become evident in a variety of ways. Many different conditions, such as a diabetic emergency, stroke, seizures, poisoning, heart attack and shock, can all cause a change in a person's level of consciousness. A victim of sudden illness may faint or complain of feeling light-headed, dizzy or weak. He or she may feel nauseated or may vomit. Breathing, pulse, body temperature and skin color may change. A person who looks or feels ill generally is ill.

Sudden illness may result from a condition that has a rapid and intense onset and then subsides quickly (**acute**), or it may result from a persistent condition that continues over a long period of time (**chronic**). In an emergency, you may not know what caused the illness. However, you do not need to know the exact cause to give appropriate care to the victim.

In this chapter, you will learn that following the emergency action steps: CHECK—CALL—CARE is all you need to do to give first aid to a victim of sudden illness.

Faced with a person who has an unknown illness, you may not be sure whether to call 9-1-1 or the local emergency number. In some cases, such as fainting, the condition is momentary and the person immediately recovers. In this situation, activating the EMS system may not be necessary. However, if the problem is not resolved quickly or if you have any doubts about its severity, always call 9-1-1 or the local emergency number for help. It is better to err on the side of caution. Refer to Chapter 5 for conditions and situations in which you should call 9-1-1 or the local emergency number.

Some of the sudden illnesses you may encounter include—

▶ Fainting.
▶ Diabetic emergencies.
▶ Seizures.
▶ Stroke.
▶ Poisoning.
▶ Heart attack.
▶ Shock.

K E Y   T E R M S

Diabetes mellitus: A condition in which the body does not produce enough insulin, or does not use insulin effectively enough, to regulate the amount of sugar (glucose) in the bloodstream; often referred to simply as diabetes.

Diabetic emergency: A situation in which a person becomes ill because of an imbalance of sugar (glucose) and insulin in the bloodstream.

Epilepsy: A chronic condition characterized by seizures that may vary in type and duration; can usually be controlled by medication.

Fainting: A partial or complete loss of consciousness resulting from a temporary reduction of blood flow to the brain.

Glucose: A simple sugar found in certain foods, especially fruits, and a major source of energy for all living organisms.

Hyperglycemia: A condition in which too much sugar (glucose) is in the bloodstream and the insulin level in the body is too low.

Hypoglycemia: A condition in which too little sugar (glucose) is in the bloodstream and the insulin level in the body is too high.

Insulin: A hormone produced in the pancreas that enables the body to use sugar (glucose) for energy; frequently used to treat diabetes.

Seizure: An irregularity in the brain's electrical activity often marked by loss of consciousness and uncontrollable muscle movement; also called a convulsion.

Stroke: A disruption of blood flow to a part of the brain, which may cause permanent damage to brain tissue; also called a cerebrovascular accident (CVA).

Transient ischemic attack (TIA): A temporary episode that, like a stroke, is caused by a disruption of blood flow to the brain; sometimes called a mini-stroke.

Follow these general guidelines for care:

▶ Do no further harm.
▶ Monitor breathing and consciousness.
▶ Help the victim rest in the most comfortable position.
▶ Keep the victim from getting chilled or overheated.
▶ Reassure the victim.
▶ Give any specific care needed.

Depending on the condition in which you find the victim, you may be able to do little more than help him or her rest comfortably until EMS personnel arrive. However, knowing enough about sudden illness to recognize when to call 9-1-1 or the local emergency number is your top priority as a citizen responder.

Fainting

One of the most common sudden illnesses is fainting. *Fainting* (also known as **syncope**) is a partial or complete loss of consciousness. Fainting is caused by a temporary reduction of blood flow to the brain, such as when blood pools in the legs and lower body. When the brain is suddenly deprived of its normal blood flow, it momentarily shuts down and the person faints.

Fainting can be triggered by an emotionally stressful event, such as the sight of blood. It may be caused by pain, specific medical conditions such as heart disease, standing for long periods of time or overexertion. Some people, such as pregnant women or the elderly, are more likely than others to faint when suddenly changing positions, such as moving from sitting or lying down to standing (**Fig. 15-1**).

Any time changes inside the body momentarily reduce the blood flow to the brain, fainting may occur.

Fainting may occur with or without warning. Often, the change in level of consciousness may initially make the victim feel light-headed or dizzy. Because fainting is a form of shock, the victim may show signals of shock, such as pale, cool or moist skin (see Chapter 9). The victim may feel nauseated and complain of numbness or tingling in the fingers and toes. Other signals that precede fainting include—

▶ Sweating.
▶ Vomiting.
▶ Distortion or dimming of vision.
▶ Head or abdominal pain.

Some victims feel as though everything is going dark just before they lose consciousness.

Care for Fainting

Usually, fainting is a self-correcting condition. When the victim collapses, normal circulation to the brain resumes. The victim typically regains consciousness within a minute. Fainting itself does not usually harm the victim, but related injuries, such as from falling, may occur. If you can reach the person as he or she is starting to collapse, lower him or her to the ground or other flat surface. Position the victim on his or her back, and elevate the legs about 12 inches to keep blood circulating to the vital organs. If you are unsure of the victim's condition or if moving is painful for the victim, keep him or her lying flat. Loosen any restrictive clothing, such as a tie or collar (**Fig. 15-2**). Check for any other life-threatening and non-life-threatening conditions. Do

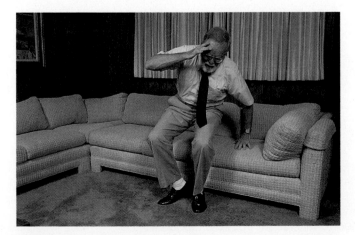

Figure 15-1 A sudden change in positions can sometimes trigger fainting.

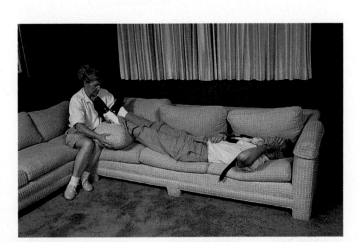

Figure 15-2 To care for fainting, place the victim on his back, elevate the feet and loosen any restrictive clothing, such as a tie or collar.

not give the victim anything to eat or drink. Also, do not slap the victim or splash water on his or her face. Splashing water could cause the victim to **aspirate** the water.

As long as the fainting victim recovers quickly and has no lasting signals, you may not need to call 9-1-1 or the local emergency number. However, it may be appropriate to have a bystander or family member take the victim to a physician or emergency department to determine if the fainting episode is linked to a more serious condition.

Diabetic Emergencies

The condition in which the body does not produce enough insulin or does not use insulin effectively is called *diabetes mellitus,* commonly known as diabetes. Diabetes mellitus is one of the leading causes of death and disability in the United States today. Consider the following facts and figures on diabetes:

▶ An estimated 18.2 million Americans currently have diabetes.
▶ Diabetes contributes to other conditions, such as blindness; kidney, heart, and periodontal (tooth) disease; and stroke.
▶ Direct costs associated with diabetes were $91.8 billion in 2002. For the same year, an additional $39.8 billion in indirect costs was attributed to disability, loss of work and premature mortality. For more information you can visit the American Diabetes Association's Web site at *www.diabetes.org.*

To function normally, body cells need sugar as a source of energy. Through the digestive process, the body breaks down food into simple sugars such as *glucose,* which are absorbed into the bloodstream. However, sugar cannot pass freely from the blood into the body cells. *Insulin,* a hormone produced in the pancreas, is needed for sugar to pass into the cells (**Fig. 15-3**). Without a proper balance of sugar and insulin, the cells will starve and the body will not function properly.

When diabetes is not properly controlled, one of two problems can occur—the victim can have too much or too little sugar in the bloodstream. This imbalance of sugar and insulin in the blood causes illness. A situation in which a victim becomes ill because of an imbalance of insulin and sugar in the bloodstream is called a *diabetic emergency.*

There are two major types of diabetes. In Type I diabetes (also known as insulin-dependent diabetes), the body produces little or no insulin. Since Type I diabetes tends to develop in childhood, it is commonly called juvenile diabetes. Most people who have Type I diabetes have to inject insulin into their bodies daily. In Type II diabetes, (also called non-insulin-dependent diabetes), the body produces insulin, but either the cells do not use the insulin effectively or not enough insulin is produced. Type II diabetes, which is much more common than Type I diabetes, is also known as adult onset diabetes because it usually occurs in adults. Most people who have Type II diabetes can regulate their blood glucose levels sufficiently through diet and do not require insulin injections.

Anyone who has diabetes must carefully monitor his or her diet and amount of exercise. People

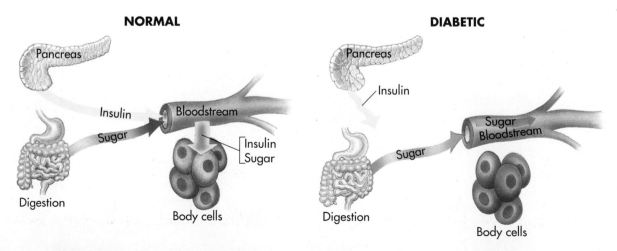

Figure 15-3 The hormone insulin is needed to take sugar from the blood into the body cells.

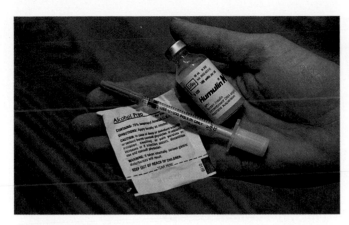

Figure 15-4   People who have insulin-dependent diabetes inject insulin to increase the amount of insulin in the body.

who have insulin-dependent diabetes (and occasionally those who have non-insulin-dependent diabetes) must also regulate their use of insulin (**Fig. 15-4**). When diet and exercise are not controlled, either of two problems can occur—too much or too little sugar in the body. This imbalance of sugar and insulin in the blood causes illness.

When the insulin level in the body is too low, the sugar level in the blood is high. This condition is called *hyperglycemia* (**Fig. 15-5, *A***). Sugar is present in the blood, but it cannot be transported from the blood into the cells without insulin. In this condition, body cells become starved for sugar. The body attempts to meet its need for energy by using other stored food and energy sources, such as fats.

However, converting fat to energy is less efficient, produces waste products and increases the acidity level in the blood, causing a condition called **diabetic ketoacidosis**. A victim with diabetic ketoacidosis becomes ill. He or she may have flushed, hot, dry skin and a sweet, fruity breath odor that can be mistaken for the smell of alcohol. The victim also may appear restless or agitated. If the condition is not treated promptly, **diabetic coma**, a life-threatening emergency, can occur.

On the other hand, when the insulin level in the body is too high, the person has a low blood sugar level. This condition is known as *hypoglycemia* (**Fig. 15-5, *B***). The blood sugar level can become too low if the diabetic—

▶ Takes too much insulin.
▶ Fails to eat adequately or due to sudden illness cannot keep food or liquids down.
▶ Overexercises and burns off sugar faster than normal.
▶ Experiences great emotional stress.

In this situation, sugar is used up rapidly, so not enough sugar is available for the brain to function properly. If left untreated, hypoglycemia may result in a life-threatening condition called **insulin shock**.

Many people who have diabetes have blood glucose monitors that can be used to check their blood sugar level if they are conscious. Many hypoglycemic and hyperglycemic episodes are now managed at home because of the rapid information these monitors provide.

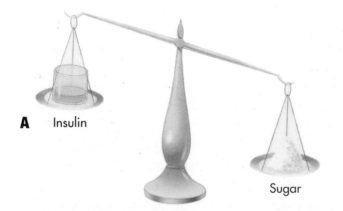

A   Insulin

Sugar

DIABETIC COMA (HYPERGLYCEMIA)

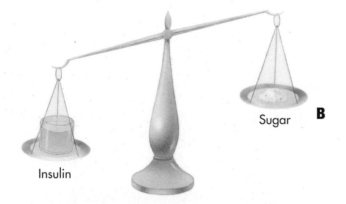

Insulin

Sugar   B

INSULIN REACTION (HYPOGLYCEMIA)

Figure 15-5   A, Hyperglycemia occurs when there is insufficient insulin in the body, causing a high level of sugar in the blood. **B,** Hypoglycemia occurs when the insulin level in the body is high, causing a low level of sugar in the blood.

Innovations in the Treatment of Diabetes

Diabetes has no cure and is one of the leading causes of death and disability in the United States. In an effort to save lives and reduce medical costs, companies, researchers and physicians have devoted their resources to developing innovative ways to treat diabetes. The following information provides insight on medicines and technologies used to treat diabetes.

Oral Medications

Oral medications to control diabetes work in one of three ways. They either stimulate the pancreas to release more insulin, increase the body's sensitivity to the insulin that is already present or slow the breakdown of foods (especially starches) into glucose. Only people with Type II diabetes can use pills to manage their diabetes. These medications work most effectively when used in combination with meal planning and exercise.

Minimally Invasive and Noninvasive Glucose Monitors

Many patients who have diabetes find it inconvenient or difficult to puncture their fingers several times a day to monitor their blood glucose levels. Several companies have developed noninvasive devices that would eliminate the need to puncture the skin.

Potential ways to determine blood glucose levels include—

- Shining a beam of light onto the skin or through body tissues.
- Measuring the energy waves (infrared radiation) emitted by the body.
- Applying radio waves to the fingertips.
- Using ultrasound.
- Checking the thickness (viscosity) of fluids in tissue underneath the skin.

Hopefully, like the process of sterilizing syringes before an injection, sticking a finger to test a blood glucose level will soon fade into history.

Insulin Replacement Therapy

Most people who need insulin take insulin shots. Other ways to take insulin include insulin pens, insulin jet injectors and insulin pumps. Someday people with diabetes may no longer need needles or shots to take insulin. Researchers are testing new ways to deliver insulin into the bloodstream.

There are more than 20 types of insulin products available. The decision as to which insulin to choose is based on an individual's lifestyle, a physician's preference and experience and the person's blood sugar levels. Among the criteria considered in choosing insulin are—

- How soon it starts working (onset).
- When it works the hardest (peak time).
- How long it lasts in the body (duration).

External Insulin Pumps

Some people who have diabetes wear an external insulin pump, about the size of a deck of cards, that weighs about 3 ounces and can be worn on a belt or carried in a pocket. The pump is programmed to give insulin throughout the day and can give additional amounts in a short time if needed, such as after a meal. Frequent blood glucose monitoring is essential to determine approximate insulin dosages and to ensure that insulin is delivered.

Pancreatic Islet Cell Transplantation

The pancreas makes insulin and enzymes that help the body digest food. Spread over the pancreas are cells called the islets of Langerhans. Islets consist of two types of cells: alpha cells, which make glucagon,

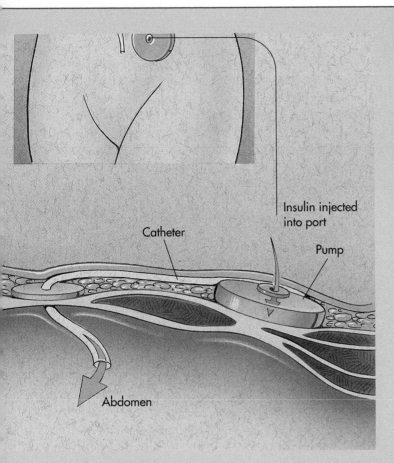

Catheter

Insulin injected
into port

Pump

Abdomen

currently under way and results will be announced in several years.

Rejection is the biggest problem of the transplant. A variety of immunosuppressive drugs are needed to keep the transplanted islets functioning.

Researchers do not fully know what long-term effects this procedure may have. Although very encouraging, more research is needed to answer questions about how long the islets will survive and how often the transplantation procedure will be successful.

a hormone that raises the level of glucose (sugar) in the blood, and beta cells, which make insulin. Insulin is a hormone that helps the body use glucose for energy. If beta cells do not produce enough insulin, diabetes will develop.

Researchers at the University of Alberta in Edmonton, Canada, are using a procedure called the Edmonton protocol to transplant pancreatic islets into people with Type I diabetes. Islets are taken from a donor pancreas and transferred into another person. Once transplanted, the beta cells begin to make and release insulin. Researchers hope that islet transplantation will help people with Type I diabetes live without daily injections of insulin.

According to the Immune Tolerance Network, as of June 2003, about 50 percent of the patients have remained insulin-free up to 1 year after receiving a transplant. A clinical trial of the Edmonton protocol is

REFERENCES AND SOURCES:

American Diabetes Association. *www.diabetes.org*

FDA Consumer Drug Information. *www.fda.gov/cder/consumerinfo/default.htm*

Juvenile Diabetes Foundation International. *www.jdrf.org*

National Center for Chronic Disease Prevention and Health Promotion Centers for Disease Control and Prevention.
  www.cdc.gov/nccdphp/bb_diabetes/index.htm

National Diabetes Education Program. *www.ndep.nih.gov*

National Diabetes Information Clearinghouse (NDIC).
  www.diabetes.niddk.nih.gov/dm/pubs/medicines_ez/specific.htm. Accessed 08/12/04.

National Diabetes Information Clearinghouse (NDIC).
  www.diabetes.niddk.nih.gov/dm/pubs/insulin/index.htm Accessed 08/12/04.

National Diabetes Information Clearinghouse (NDIC).
  www.diabetes.niddk.nih.gov/dm/pubs/pancreaticislet.htm. Accessed 08/12/04.

National Institute of Diabetes and Digestive and Kidney Diseases of the National Institutes of Health. *www.niddk.nih.gov/*

U.S. Food and Drug Administration FDA. *www.fda.gov/diabetes/glucose.html.* Accessed 08/15/04.

U.S. Food and Drug Administration FDA. *www.fda.gov/diabetes/insulin.html.* Accessed 08/12/04.

U.S. Food and Drug Administration FDA. *www.fda.gov/diabetes/insulin.html.* Accessed 08/12/04.

Signals of Diabetic Emergencies

Although hyperglycemia and hypoglycemia are different conditions, their major signals are similar. These include—

▸ Changes in level of consciousness, including dizziness, drowsiness and confusion.
▸ Irregular breathing.
▸ Abnormal pulse (rapid or weak).
▸ Feeling or looking ill.

It is not important for you to differentiate between hyperglycemia and hypoglycemia because the basic care for both of these diabetic emergencies is the same.

Care for Diabetic Emergencies

First, check and care for any life-threatening conditions. If the victim is conscious, check for non-life-threatening conditions by looking for anything visibly wrong. Ask if he or she has diabetes, or look for a medical ID tag or bracelet. If the victim tells you that he or she has diabetes and exhibits the signals above, then suspect a diabetic emergency. If the conscious victim can take food or fluids, give him or her sugar (**Fig. 15-6**). Most candy, fruit juices and nondiet soft drinks contain enough sugar to begin to reverse hypoglycemia. Common table sugar, either dry or dissolved in a glass of water, also works well to return the victim's blood sugar to an acceptable level. If the victim's problem is low blood sugar (hypoglycemia), the sugar you give will help quickly. If the victim's blood sugar level is already too high (hyperglycemia), the additional sugar will do no further harm. Often, a person who

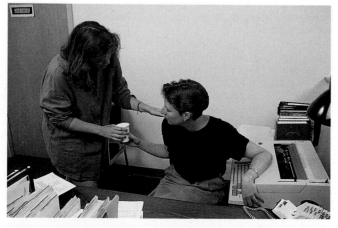

Figure 15-6 If a victim of a diabetic emergency is conscious, give him or her food or fluids containing sugar.

has diabetes will know what is wrong and will ask for something with sugar in it. He or she may carry a readily available source of sugar for such situations. If the victim is conscious but does not feel better approximately 5 minutes after taking sugar, call 9-1-1 or the local emergency number immediately. If the victim is unconscious, call 9-1-1 or the local emergency number immediately. Do not give the victim anything by mouth. Instead, monitor signs of life and breathing and keep him or her from getting chilled or overheated.

Seizures

When the normal functions of the brain are disrupted by injury, disease, fever, poisoning or infection, the electrical activity of the brain becomes irregular. This irregularity can cause a loss of body control known as a *seizure.*

Seizures may be caused by an acute or chronic condition. The chronic condition is known as *epilepsy.* Today about 2.3 million Americans are affected by epilepsy. Epilepsy is usually controlled with medication. Most people who are seizure-free for 2 to 5 years can be taken off medication. The most clearly established risk factors for epilepsy are severe head trauma, central nervous system infections, a stroke or having a family member who has epilepsy. A large proportion of new cases of epilepsy among the elderly is due to stroke. Stroke is discussed later in this chapter.

Before a seizure occurs, the victim may experience an aura. An aura is an unusual sensation or feeling, such as a visual hallucination; a strange sound, taste or smell; or an urgent need to get to safety. If the victim recognizes the aura, he or she may have time to tell bystanders and sit down before the seizure occurs.

Seizures generally last 1 to 3 minutes and can produce a wide range of signals. When a victim has a seizure, breathing may become irregular and even stop temporarily. The victim may drool, the eyes may roll upward and the body may become rigid. The victim may also urinate or defecate. Seizures that cause the victim to experience mild blackouts that others may mistake for daydreaming are commonly known as nonconvulsive seizures because the body remains relatively still during the episode. More severe seizures, known as convulsive seizures, may cause the victim to experience sudden, uncontrolled muscular contractions (convulsions), lasting several minutes.

Care for Seizures

Although a seizure may be frightening to watch, you can easily help care for the person. Remember that he or she cannot control the seizure and the violent muscular contractions that may occur, so do not try to stop the seizure. Do not hold or restrain the person, because doing so can cause musculoskeletal injuries. As always, stay calm so that you can give the most appropriate care.

Your objectives for care are to protect the victim from injury and maintain an open airway. First, move nearby objects, such as furniture, that might cause injury. Protect the person's head by placing a thin cushion, such as folded clothing, beneath it. If possible, loosen any clothing that may restrict breathing.

Do not try to place anything in the person's mouth or between his or her teeth. Contrary to the myth, people having seizures do not swallow their tongues. Seizure victims rarely bite their tongues or cheeks with enough force to cause any significant bleeding. However, some blood may be present. Position the victim on his or her side as soon as the seizure ends, which will help blood or other fluids drain out of the mouth. Avoid direct contact with any blood by using an appropriate barrier, such as disposable gloves.

When the seizure is over, the victim will probably be drowsy and disoriented and will need to rest. If breathing becomes abnormal during the seizure, it usually returns to normal soon afterward. Be sure to check for life-threatening conditions. Look for non-life-threatening conditions, checking to see if the victim was injured during the seizure. Be reassuring and comforting. If the seizure occurred in public, the victim may be embarrassed and self-conscious. Try to provide a measure of privacy for the person. Ask bystanders not to crowd around the person. If possible, take the victim to a nearby place, away from bystanders, to rest. If moving the victim to a more secluded location is not possible, use your body or an object, such as a blanket, to shield the victim from onlookers. Stay with the victim until he or she is fully conscious and aware of his or her surroundings.

Although most victims of seizure recover within a few minutes after the seizure ends, actual recovery time depends on the type and severity of the seizure. If the victim is known to have periodic seizures, you probably will not need to call 9-1-1 or the local emergency number immediately. However, call 9-1-1 or the local emergency number for any of the following situations—

- The seizure lasts more than 5 minutes.
- The victim has repeated seizures, one after another, without regaining consciousness in between.
- The victim appears to be injured.
- The victim is not known to have a predisposing condition, such as epilepsy, that could have brought on the seizure.
- The victim is pregnant.
- The victim is an infant or child who is experiencing an initial febrile seizure (*see below*).
- The victim is known to have diabetes.
- The seizure takes place in water.
- The victim fails to regain consciousness after the seizure.

Febrile Seizure

Infants and young children may be at risk for epilepsy, as well as for seizures brought on by a rapid increase in body temperature, known as **febrile seizures**. Febrile seizures usually affect young people younger than the age of 18 and are most common in children younger than age 5. Febrile seizures are typically triggered by infections of the ear, throat or digestive system and are most likely to occur when the infant or child runs a rectal fever of over 102° F (38.9° C). A victim experiencing a febrile seizure may experience some or all of the following signals:

- A sudden rise in body temperature
- A change in level of consciousness
- Rhythmic jerking of the head and limbs
- Urinating or defecating
- Confusion
- Drowsiness
- Crying out
- Becoming rigid
- Holding the breath
- Rolling the eyes upward

Care for an infant or child who experiences a febrile seizure is similar to the care for any other seizure victim. Immediately after a febrile seizure, cool the body. Cool the body by removing excess clothing and giving the victim a sponge bath in lukewarm water. Be careful not to cool the infant or child too much, because this could bring on another seizure. Contact your physician before using a medication, such as acetaminophen, to control fever. Giving aspirin to a feverish infant or child under age 19 has been linked to **Reye's syndrome,** an illness that affects the brain and other internal organs.

Parents should stay calm and carefully observe the child. To prevent accidental injury, the child should be placed on a protected surface such as the floor or ground. The child should not be held or restrained during a convulsion. To prevent choking, the child should be placed on his or her side or stomach. When possible, the parent should gently remove all objects in the child's mouth. The parent should never place anything in the child's mouth during a convulsion. Objects placed in the mouth can be broken and obstruct the child's airway. If the seizure lasts longer than 10 minutes, the child should be taken immediately to the nearest medical facility for further treatment. Once the seizure has ended, the child should be taken to his or her doctor to check for the source of the fever. This is especially urgent if the child shows signals of stiff neck, extreme lethargy or abundant vomiting. If the child has a febrile seizure at a later date that ends quickly and is associated with another illness, the child should be checked by a physician or taken to an emergency department as soon as possible.

Stroke

A *stroke,* also called a cerebrovascular accident (CVA) or "brain attack", is a disruption of blood flow to a part of the brain, causing permanent damage to brain tissue. Most commonly, a stroke is caused by a blood clot, called a **thrombus** or **embolus,** that forms or lodges in the arteries that supply blood to the brain. Another common cause of stroke is bleeding from a ruptured artery in the brain caused by a head injury, high blood pressure or an **aneurysm**—a weak area in the wall of an artery that balloons out and can rupture (**Fig. 15-7**).

Fat deposits lining an artery (**atherosclerosis**) may also cause stroke. Less commonly, a tumor or swelling from a head injury may compress an artery and cause a stroke.

A *transient ischemic attack (TIA),* often referred to as a "mini-stroke," is a temporary episode that, like a stroke, is caused by a disruption in blood flow to a part of the brain. However, unlike a stroke, the signals of TIA disappear within a few minutes or hours of its onset. Although the indicators of TIA disappear quickly, the victim is not out of danger at that point. In fact, someone who experiences TIA has a greater chance of having a stroke in the future than someone who has not had a TIA. Because you cannot distinguish a stroke from a TIA, remember to call 9-1-1 or the local emergency number immediately when any signals of stroke appear.

Risk Factors

The risk factors for stroke and TIA are similar to those for heart disease (see Chapter 7). Some risk factors are beyond your control, such as age, gender, or family history of stroke, TIA, diabetes or heart disease.

Hypertension (**high blood pressure**) increases your risk of stroke by approximately seven times over that of someone who does not have hypertension. High blood pressure puts pressure on arteries and makes them more likely to burst. Even mild hypertension can increase your risk of stroke. Have your blood pressure checked regularly and, if it is high, follow your physician's advice on how to lower it. You can often control high blood pressure by losing weight, changing your diet, exercising routinely and managing stress. If those measures are not sufficient, your physician may prescribe medication.

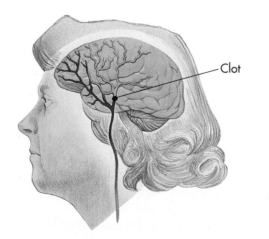
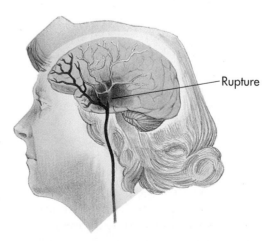

Figure 15-7 A stroke can be caused by a blood clot or bleeding from a ruptured artery in the brain.

Cigarette smoking is another major risk factor of stroke. Smoking is linked to heart disease and cancer, as well as to stroke. Smoking increases blood pressure and makes blood more likely to clot. If you smoke and would like to quit, many techniques and support systems are available to help you. Your physician or local health department can assist you. The benefits of not smoking begin as soon as you stop, and some of smoking's damage may actually be reversible. Approximately 10 years after a person has stopped smoking, his or her risk of stroke is the same as the risk for a person who has never smoked. Even if you do not smoke, be aware that inhaling secondhand smoke (from other smokers) is detrimental to your health. Avoid long-term exposure to cigarette smoke and protect children from this danger as well.

Diets that are high in saturated fats and cholesterol can increase your risk of stroke by causing fatty materials to build up on the walls of your blood vessels. Foods high in cholesterol include egg yolks and organ meats, such as liver and kidneys. Saturated fats are found in beef, lamb, veal, pork, ham, whole milk and whole-milk products. Moderating your intake of these foods can help prevent stroke.

Diabetes is another major risk factor for stroke. If you have been diagnosed with diabetes, follow your physician's advice about how to control it. If untreated, diabetes can cause damage to the blood vessels throughout the body.

By paying attention to the signals of stroke and reporting them to your physician, you can prevent damage before it occurs. Experiencing a TIA is the clearest warning that a stroke may occur. Do not ignore its stroke-like signals, even if they disappear completely within minutes or hours.

Prevention

You can help prevent stroke if you—

▸ Control your blood pressure.
▸ Do not smoke.
▸ Eat a healthy diet.
▸ Exercise regularly.
▸ Control diabetes.

Regular exercise reduces your chances of stroke by strengthening the heart and improving blood circulation. Exercise also helps in weight control. Being overweight increases the chance of developing high blood pressure, heart disease and atherosclerosis.

FAST Recognition of Stroke

For a brain attack, think FAST!

F Face—Weakness on one side of the face.
  ▪ Ask the person to smile. This will show if there is drooping or weakness in the muscles on one side of the face.

A Arm—Weakness or numbness in one arm.
  ▪ Ask the person to raise both arms to find out if there is weakness in the limbs.

S Speech—Slurred speech or trouble speaking.
  ▪ Ask the person to speak a simple sentence to listen for slurred or distorted speech. Example: "I have the lunch orders ready."

T Time—Time to call 9-1-1 or the local emergency number if you see any of these signals.
  ▪ Note the time that the signals began and call 9-1-1 or the local emergency number right away.

The FAST mnemonic is based on the Cincinnati Pre-Hospital Stroke Scale, which was originally developed for emergency medical services (EMS) workers in 1997. The scale was designed to help paramedics identify strokes in the field, so that they can prepare the emergency room before they arrive. The FAST method for public awareness has been in use in the community in Cincinnati, Ohio since 1999, and has since been used in several other variations of the message. It was validated by researchers at the University of North Carolina in 2003.

Sudden Signals of a Stroke

As with other sudden illnesses, the primary signals of a stroke or TIA are looking or feeling ill or displaying abnormal behavior. Other signals of stroke come on suddenly, including sudden weakness and numbness of the face, arm or leg. Usually, weakness or numbness occurs only on one side of the body. The victim may have difficulty talking or being understood when speaking. Vision may be blurred or dimmed; the pupils of the eyes may be of unequal size. The victim may also experience a sudden, severe headache; dizziness, confusion or change in mood; or ringing in the ears. The victim may drool, become unconscious or lose bowel or bladder control.

The Brain Makes a Comeback

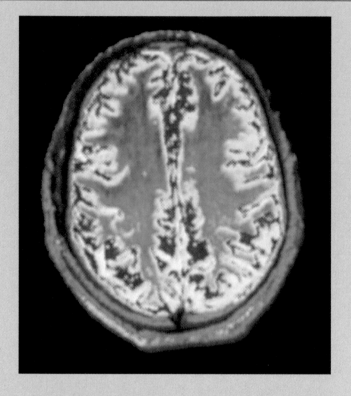

About 700,000 Americans will have a stroke this year. Neuroscientists are puzzled by the random effects of stroke. Each stroke survivor has a unique, perplexing set of problems, and physicians find recovery equally unpredictable.

A stroke occurs when blood flow to the brain is cut off. The most common, accounting for about 88 percent, is an ischemic stroke, caused by a blood clot that blocks a blood vessel or artery in the brain. The other major, but less common type, is a hemorrhagic stroke, caused when a blood vessel in the brain ruptures and spills blood into the surrounding tissue. Brain cells in the area begin to die because they stop getting the oxygen and nutrients needed to function or they are killed by the vessel's rupture and sudden blood spill.

Ongoing research has provided physicians with acute and preventive treatments. The most common treatment for stroke is medication or drug therapy. The most popular classes of drugs used to prevent or treat stroke are *antithrombotics (antiplatelet agents and anticoagulants), thrombolytics* and *neuroprotective agents.*

Ischemic Stroke: Treated by removing obstruction and restoring blood flow to the brain.

Acute Treatment

- **Clot-busters (such as t-PA)**
  A promising treatment for ischemic stroke is the FDA-approved clot-busting drug t-PA, which must be administered within a 3-hour window from the onset of signals to be most effective.

Preventive Treatment

- **Anticoagulants/Antiplatelets**
  Antiplatelet agents such as aspirin, and anticoagulants such as warfarin or heparin interfere with the blood's ability to clot and can play an important role in preventing stroke.

- **Thrombolytic**
  Used to treat an ongoing, acute ischemic stroke, these drugs halt the stroke by dissolving the blood clot that is blocking blood flow to the brain. *Recombinant tissue plasminogen activator (rt-PA)* can be effective if given intravenously within 3 hours of the first signal of a stroke, but it should be used only after a physician has confirmed that the victim has suffered an ischemic stroke.

Care for a Stroke

Call 9-1-1 or the local emergency number immediately. If the victim is unconscious, make sure that he or she has an open airway and care for any life-threatening conditions. If fluid or vomit is in the victim's mouth, position him or her on one side to allow any fluids to drain out of the mouth (**Fig. 15-8**).

When possible, position the victim's affected (paralyzed) side down. Doing so will prevent further injury and aid breathing. You may have to remove some fluids or vomit from the mouth by using one of your fingers. Stay with the victim and monitor his or her breathing and signs of life.

If the victim is conscious, check for non-life-threatening conditions. If you see signals of a

- **Neuroprotectants**
  Medications that protect the brain from secondary injury caused by stroke. Although only a few neuroprotectants are FDA-approved for use at this time, many are in clinical trials.
- **Carotid Endarterectomy**
  A procedure in which blood vessel blockage is surgically removed from the carotid artery.
- **Angioplasty and Stents**
  Physicians sometimes use balloon angioplasty and implantable steel screens called stents to treat cardiovascular disease in which mechanical devices are used to remedy fatty buildup clogging the vessel.

Hemorrhagic Stroke: Physicians introduce an obstruction to prevent rupture and bleeding of aneurysms and arteriovenous malformations.

- **Surgical Intervention**
  For hemorrhagic stroke, surgical treatment is often recommended to either place a metal clip at the base, called the neck, of the aneurysm or to remove the abnormal vessels comprising an arteriovenous malformation (AVM).
- **Endovascular Procedures (such as coils).**
  Endovascular procedures are less invasive and involve the use of a catheter introduced through a major artery in the leg or arm, guided to the aneurysm or AVM where it deposits a mechanical agent, such as a coil, to prevent rupture.

Strokes still present many mysteries, but scientists are learning more about stroke every day. With about 4.8 million stroke survivors alive today, physicians and patients are hopeful that new drugs and treatments may eventually eliminate the long-term effects. Knowing the warning signals and acting

quickly greatly increase the chances of receiving the most effective treatment for any type of stroke.

For more information on neurological disorders or advances in research visit the following organizations:

American Health Assistance Foundation
www.ahaf.org

American Stroke Association:
A Division of American Heart Association
www.strokeassociation.org

Brain Aneurysm Foundation
www.bafound.org

Children's Hemiplegia and Stroke Association (CHASA)
www.hemikids.org

Hazel K. Goddess Fund for Stroke Research in Women
www.thegoddessfund.org

National Aphasia Association
www.aphasia.org

National Institute of Neurological Disorders and Stroke
www.ninds.nih.gov

National Stroke Association
www.stroke.org

SOURCES
American Stroke Association. *www.strokeassociation.org*
American Heart Association. *Heart Disease and Stroke Statistics—*
    2004 Update. Dallas, Tex., 2003. *www.americanheart.org*
National Institute of Neurological Disorders and Stroke. *www.ninds.nih.gov*
"Stroke: Hope Through Research", NINDS. Publication date July 2004.

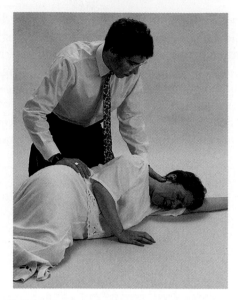

Figure 15-8   Position a victim on the side to help fluids or vomit drain from the victim's mouth.

stroke, call 9-1-1 or the local emergency number immediately. A stroke can make the victim fearful and anxious. Often, he or she does not understand what has happened. Offer comfort and reassurance. Have the victim rest in a comfortable position. Do not give him or her anything to eat or drink. Although a stroke may cause the victim to experience difficulty speaking, he or she can usually understand what you say. If the victim is unable to speak, you may have to use nonverbal forms of communication, such as hand squeezing or eye blinking, and communicate in forms that require a yes-or-no response (squeeze or blink once for "yes," twice for "no.")

In the past, a stroke almost always caused irreversible brain damage. Today, new medications and medical procedures can limit or reduce the damage caused by stroke. Many of these new treatments are time-sensitive; therefore, you should immediately call 9-1-1 or the local emergency number to get the best care for the victim.

SUMMARY

Sudden illness can strike anyone at any time. Even if you do not know the cause of the illness, you can still give proper care. Recognizing the signals of sudden illness, such as changes in consciousness, profuse sweating, confusion and weakness, will help you determine the necessary care to give the victim until EMS personnel arrive.

APPLICATION QUESTIONS

1. What were the signals of Jeff's illness?

2. What could Juanita do to help Jeff during and after the seizure?

3. What should Juanita consider in her decision whether to call 9-1-1 or the local emergency number?

STUDY QUESTIONS

1. Match each term with the correct definition.

   a. Diabetic emergency   f. Insulin
   b. Epilepsy   g. Seizure
   c. Fainting   h. Stroke
   d. Hyperglycemia   i. Transient ischemic attack (TIA)
   e. Hypoglycemia

   _____ A hormone that enables the cells to use sugar.

   _____ A temporary reduction of blood flow to the brain, resulting in loss of consciousness.

   _____ A disruption of blood flow to the brain that causes brain tissue damage.

   _____ A disruption of the brain's electrical activity, which may cause loss of consciousness and body control.

   _____ A condition in which too little sugar is in the bloodstream.

   _____ A condition in which too much sugar is in the bloodstream.

   _____ A chronic condition characterized by seizures and usually controlled by medication.

   _____ A temporary disruption of blood flow to the brain; sometimes called a mini-stroke.

   _____ A situation in which a person becomes ill because of an imbalance of sugar (glucose) and insulin in the bloodstream.

2. List four general signals of a sudden illness.

3. List four general guidelines of care that should be applied in any sudden illness.

4. List six instances in which you should call 9-1-1 or the local emergency number for a seizure victim.

5. List six ways to decrease the risk of stroke or TIA.

6. Describe how to care for a seizure victim once the seizure is over.

7. What signals of sudden illness do you find in the scenario that follows? Circle the signals in the scenario below.

I was at the grocery store with my grandmother. As the butcher reached over the counter to hand her a package of steaks, my grandmother stumbled toward a nearby chair. She sat in the chair, looking confused. I noticed that she was sweating profusely and her pupils were different sizes. I stood beside her and asked if I could help. At first, she didn't seem to recognize me. Then she mumbled something to me. I could not understand her very well, but I think she was telling me that she felt weak and wanted me to let her rest for a few minutes.

8. What care would you give for the grandmother in the scenario?

In questions 9 through 16, circle the letter of the correct answer.

9. If you were caring for someone who looked pale, was unconscious and was breathing irregularly, what should you do?

   a. Call 9-1-1 or the local emergency number.
   b. Inject the victim with insulin.
   c. Give sugar to the victim.
   d. Let the victim rest for a while.

10. A friend who has diabetes is drowsy and seems confused. He is not sure if he took his insulin today. What should you do?

   a. Suggest he rest for an hour or so.
   b. Tell him to take his insulin.
   c. Tell him to eat or drink something with sugar in it.
   d. Check his breathing and signs of life.

11. Your father has diabetes. He also suffered a stroke a year ago. You find him lying on the floor, unconscious. What should you do after calling 9-1-1 or the local emergency number?

   a. Call his physician.
   b. Lift his head up and try to give him a sugary drink.
   c. Check for breathing, signs of life and severe bleeding.
   d. Inject him with insulin yourself, while waiting for EMS personnel to arrive.

12. In caring for the victim of a seizure, you should—

   a. Move any objects that might cause injury.
   b. Try to hold the victim still.
   c. Place a spoon between the person's teeth.
   d. Splash the person's face with water.

13. To reduce the risk of aspiration of blood or other fluids in a seizure victim—

   a. Place an object between the victim's teeth.
   b. Position the victim on his or her side after the seizure ends.
   c. Place a thick object, such as a rolled blanket, under the victim's head.
   d. Move the victim into a sitting position.

14. Controlling high blood pressure reduces your risk of—

    a. Heart disease, stroke and TIA.
    b. Seizure.
    c. Diabetes.
    d. Epilepsy.

15. At the office, your boss complains that she has had a severe headache for several hours. Her speech suddenly becomes slurred. She loses her balance and falls to the floor. What should you do?

    a. Give her two aspirin.
    b. Help her find and take her high blood pressure medication.
    c. Call 9-1-1 or the local emergency number.
    d. Tell her to rest for a while.

16. Which of the following is (are) included in the care you give for fainting?

    a. If possible, help to lower the victim to the floor or other flat surface.
    b. If possible, elevate the legs.
    c. Give the victim something to eat or drink.
    d. a and b.

Answers are listed in Appendix A.

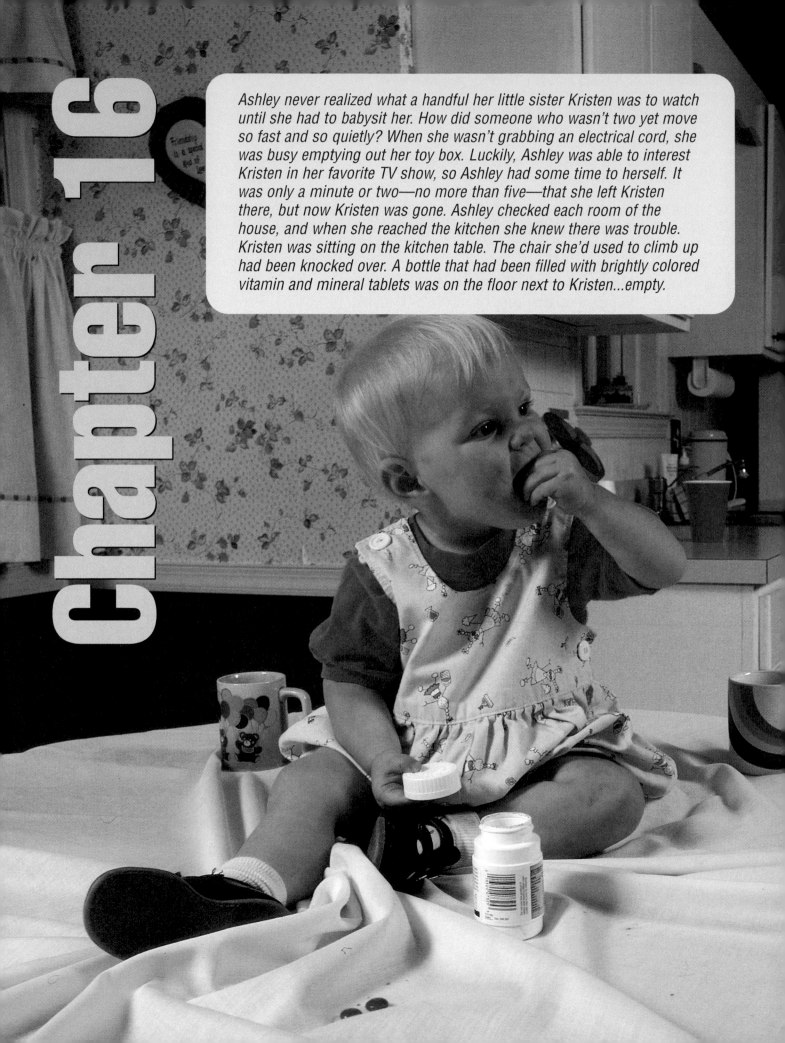

Ashley never realized what a handful her little sister Kristen was to watch until she had to babysit her. How did someone who wasn't two yet move so fast and so quietly? When she wasn't grabbing an electrical cord, she was busy emptying out her toy box. Luckily, Ashley was able to interest Kristen in her favorite TV show, so Ashley had some time to herself. It was only a minute or two—no more than five—that she left Kristen there, but now Kristen was gone. Ashley checked each room of the house, and when she reached the kitchen she knew there was trouble. Kristen was sitting on the kitchen table. The chair she'd used to climb up had been knocked over. A bottle that had been filled with brightly colored vitamin and mineral tablets was on the floor next to Kristen...empty.

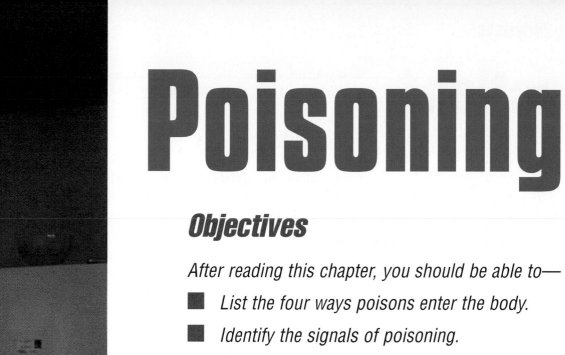

Poisoning

Objectives

After reading this chapter, you should be able to—

- ■ List the four ways poisons enter the body.
- ■ Identify the signals of poisoning.
- ■ Identify the general guidelines for care for any poisoning emergency.
- ■ Describe how to care for a victim of a poisoning.
- ■ Identify the signals of anaphylaxis.
- ■ List eight ways to prevent poisoning.

Introduction

Chapter 15 described sudden illnesses caused by conditions inside the body. Poisoning is also considered a sudden illness. However, unlike those conditions that have an internal cause, such as fainting and stroke, poisoning results when external substances enter the body. The substance could be a food that is swallowed, a pesticide that is absorbed through the skin, or venom that enters the body through a bite or sting. Even certain plants and foods can be poisonous. In this chapter and in Chapters 17 and 18, you will learn how to recognize and care for various kinds of poisoning emergencies.

Between 1 and 2 million poisonings occur each year in the United States. More than 90 percent of all poisonings take place in the home. Unintentional poisonings far outnumber intentional ones, and most unintentional poisonings occur in children younger than age 5.

HOW POISONS ENTER THE BODY

A *poison* is any substance that can cause injury, illness or death when introduced into the body. Poisons include solids, liquids, sprays and fumes (gases and vapors). A poison can enter the body in four ways: inhalation, ingestion, absorption and injection (**Fig. 16-1, *A* to *D***).

Inhalation

Poisoning by inhalation occurs when a person breathes in toxic fumes. Examples of *inhaled poisons* include—

- ▶ Gases, such as—
  - Carbon monoxide from an engine, kerosene heater or other sources of combustion.
  - Carbon dioxide, that can occur naturally from decomposition.
  - Nitrous oxide, used for medical purposes.
  - Chlorine, found in some commercial swimming facilities.
- ▶ Fumes from—
  - Household products, such as glues and paints.
  - Drugs, such as crack cocaine.

Ingestion

Ingestion means swallowing. *Ingested poisons* include foods, such as certain mushrooms and shellfish; drugs, such as alcohol; medications, such as aspirin; and household items such as cleaning products, pesticides and plants (**Fig. 16-2**).

Absorption

An *absorbed poison* enters the body after it comes in contact with the skin. Absorbed poisons come from plants, such as poison ivy, poison oak and poi-

KEY TERMS

Absorbed poison: A poison that enters the body after it comes in contact with the skin.

Anaphylaxis: A severe allergic reaction; a form of shock.

Ingested poison: A poison that is swallowed.

Inhaled poison: A poison that is breathed into the lungs.

Injected poison: A poison that enters the body through the skin through a bite, sting or as drugs or misused medications injected with a hypodermic needle.

Poison: Any substance that can cause injury, illness or death when introduced into the body in relatively small amounts.

Poison Control Center: A specialized health-care center that provides information in cases of poisoning or suspected poisoning emergencies.

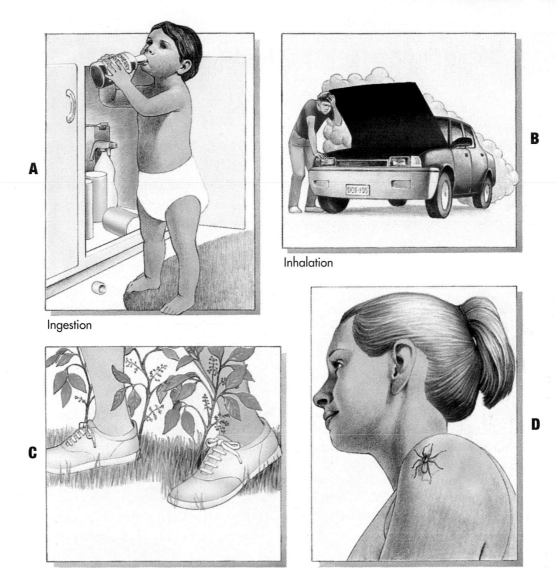

A

Ingestion

B

Inhalation

C

Absorption

D

Injection

Figure 16-1 A poison can enter the body in four ways: **A,** ingestion, **B,** inhalation, **C,** absorption and **D,** injection.

son sumac, as well as from fertilizers and pesticides used in lawn and plant care.

Injection

Injected poisons enter the body through the bites or stings of certain insects, spiders, ticks, marine life, animals and snakes, or as drugs or misused medications injected with a hypodermic needle. Poisoning from bites and stings is covered in Chapter 17.

Many substances that are not poisonous in small amounts are poisonous in larger amounts. Medications (prescription or over-the-counter) can be poisonous if they are not taken as prescribed or directed. You will learn more about abuse and misuse of medications in Chapter 18.

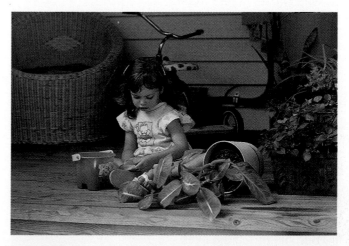

Figure 16-2 Many common household plants are poisonous.

Common Causes of Poisoning (by age group)

Younger than age 6	Ages 6 to 19	Older than age 19
Analgesic medications	Analgesic medications	Analgesic medications
Cleaning substances	Bites and stings	Antidepressant drugs
Cosmetics and personal care products	Cleaning substances	Bites and stings
Cough and cold remedies	Cosmetics	Chemicals
Gastrointestinal medications	Cough and cold remedies	Cleaning substances
Plants	Food products and food poisoning	Food products and food poisoning
Topical medications	Plants	Fumes and vapors
Vitamins	Stimulants and street drugs	Insecticides
		Sedatives and hallucinogenic drugs

SIGNALS OF POISONING

As you approach the victim, be aware of any unusual odors, flames, smoke, open or spilled containers, an open medicine cabinet, an overturned or damaged plant or other signals of poisoning. A victim of poisoning generally looks ill and displays signals common to other sudden illnesses. You may also suspect a poisoning based on any information you have from or about the victim. Also look for

any drug paraphernalia or empty containers at the scene. Never jeopardize your safety to enter a scene that you know or suspect may be unsafe. Instead, immediately call 9-1-1 or the local emergency number to assist any victims. If you have even a slight suspicion that the victim has been poisoned, seek medical assistance immediately. Signals of poisoning include—

▸ Nausea.
▸ Vomiting.
▸ Diarrhea.
▸ Chest or abdominal pain.
▸ Trouble breathing.
▸ Sweating.
▸ Changes in consciousness.
▸ Seizures.
▸ Headache.
▸ Dizziness.
▸ Weakness.
▸ Irregular pupil size.
▸ Burning or tearing eyes.
▸ Abnormal skin color.
▸ Burn injuries around the lips or tongue or on the skin.

Common Signals of Poisoning

Nausea
Vomiting
Diarrhea
Chest or abdominal pain
Trouble breathing
Sweating
Changes in consciousness
Seizures
Headache
Dizziness
Weakness
Irregular pupil size
Burning or tearing eyes
Abnormal skin color
Burns around the lips or tongue or on the skin

CARE FOR POISONING

The severity of a poisoning depends on the type and amount of the substance; how and where it entered the body; the time that elapsed since the poison entered the body; and the victim's size, weight, medical condition and age. Some poisons act quickly and produce characteristic signals while others act slowly and cannot be easily identified.

If you think someone has been poisoned, call the Poison Control Center (PCC) and follow their directions.

After you have checked the scene and determined that there has been a poisoning, follow these general care guidelines—

▸ Remove the person from the source of poison.
▸ Check the person's level of consciousness and signs of life.
▸ If there is a life-threatening condition found (e.g., a person who is unconscious, not breathing or a there is a change in consciousness), call 9-1-1 or the local emergency number first.
▸ Care for any life-threatening conditions.
▸ If the person is conscious, ask questions to get more information.
▸ Look for any containers and take them with you to the telephone (Fig. 16-3).
▸ Follow the directions of the Poison Control Center or the EMS.

Do not give the person anything to eat or drink unless medical professionals tell you to. If you do not know what the poison was and the person vomits, save some of the vomit. The hospital may analyze it to identify the poison.

Poison Control Centers

Poison control centers are specialized health-care centers that provide information in cases of poisoning or suspected poisoning emergencies. A network of poison control centers exists throughout the United States, as well as abroad. Some poison control centers are located in the emergency departments of large hospitals. Medical professionals in these centers have access to information about virtually all poisonous substances and can tell you how to care for someone who has been poisoned. You can obtain the phone number from your telephone directory, your physician, a local hospital or your local EMS system.

Poison control centers answer over 2 million poisoning calls each year. Since many poisonings can be cared for without the help of EMS personnel, poison control centers help prevent overburdening of the EMS system. If you think someone has been poisoned, call the national Poison Control Center at 800-222-1222.

For more information visit the American Association of Poison Control Centers Web site at *www.aapcc.org*.

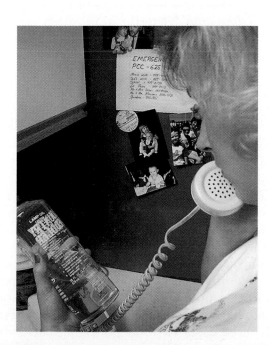

Figure 16-3 When you call EMS personnel, a call taker can link you with the Poison Control Center and send an ambulance if needed.

Inhaled Poisons

When giving care to a victim of poisoning, you need to follow precautions to ensure that you do not become poisoned as well. This is particularly true with inhaled poisons. Toxic fumes come from a variety of sources and may or may not have an odor. If you notice clues at the scene of an emergency that might lead you to suspect that toxic fumes are present, such as a strong smell of fuel or a hissing sound like gas escaping from a pipe or valve, you may not be able to reach the victim without risking your safety. In cases like this, be prepared to call 9-1-1 or the local emergency number instead of entering the scene. Let the EMS professional know what you have discovered, and only enter the scene if he or she tells you it is safe to do so.

A commonly inhaled poison is **carbon monoxide,** which is present in substances such as car exhaust and tobacco smoke. Carbon monoxide can also be produced by fires, defective cooking equipment, defective furnaces and kerosene heaters. Carbon monoxide is also found in indoor skating rinks and when charcoal is used indoors. It is a colorless, odorless gas. Carbon monoxide detectors, which work much like smoke detectors, are now available for use in homes.

A pale or bluish skin color, which indicates a lack of oxygen, may signal carbon monoxide poisoning. For years, people were taught that carbon monoxide poisoning was indicated by a cherry-red color of the skin and lips. However, new evidence shows that such redness occurs after most victims have died. It is highly lethal and can cause death after only a few minutes of exposure.

All victims of inhaled poison need oxygen as soon as possible. If you can remove the person from the source of the poison without endangering yourself, then do so. You can help a conscious victim by getting him or her to fresh air and then calling 9-1-1 or the local emergency number. If you find an unconscious victim, remove him or her from the scene if it is safe to do so and call 9-1-1 or the local emergency number. Then give care for any other life-threatening conditions.

Ingested Poisons

In some cases of ingested poisoning, the Poison Control Center may instruct you to induce vomiting. Vomiting may prevent the poison from moving to the small intestine, where most absorption takes place. *However, vomiting should be induced only if advised by a medical professional.*

The Poison Control Center or medical professional will advise you exactly how to induce vomiting. In some instances, vomiting should not be induced. These include when the victim—

▸ Is unconscious.
▸ Is having a seizure.
▸ Is pregnant (in the last trimester).
▸ Has ingested a corrosive substance, such as drain or oven cleaner or a petroleum product, such as kerosene or gasoline.
▸ Is known to have heart disease.

You can dilute some ingested poisons by giving the victim water to drink. Examples of such poisons are caustic or corrosive chemicals, such as acids, that can eat away or destroy tissues. Vomiting these corrosives could burn the esophagus, throat and mouth. Diluting the corrosive substance decreases the potential for burning and damaging tissues. **Do not** give the victim anything to eat or drink unless medical professionals tell you to do so.

Foods can be another type of ingested poison. The U.S. Centers for Disease Control and Prevention (CDC) estimates that 76 million people suffer food-borne illnesses each year in the United States. Approximately 325,000 people are hospitalized and more than 5000 die from food-borne illness. Two of the most common categories of food poisoning are bacterial food poisoning and chemical food poisoning (also known as environmental food poisoning). Bacterial food poisoning typically occurs when bacteria grow on food that is allowed to stand at room temperature after it is cooked. The bacteria release **toxins** into the food. Even when the food is reheated, the toxins may not be destroyed. Foods most likely to cause bacterial food poisoning are ham, tongue, sausage, dried meat, fish products, and dairy and dairy-based products. Chemical food poisoning typically occurs when foods with high acid content, such as fruit juices or sauerkraut, are stored in containers lined with zinc, cadmium or copper or in enameled metal pans. Another primary source of chemical food poisoning is lead, which may be found in pipes that supply drinking and cooking water.

Food Poisoning

One of the most common causes of food poisoning is the *Salmonella* bacteria, most often found in poultry and raw eggs. Proper handling and cooking of food can help prevent *Salmonella* poisoning. The most deadly type of food poisoning is botulism, which is caused by a bacterial toxin associated with home canning. Before opening a canned or bottled food, inspect the can or lid to see if it is swollen or if the "safety button" in the center of the lid has popped up (**Fig. 16-4**). If either has occurred, throw the food away.

The signals of food poisoning, which can begin between 1 and 48 hours after eating contaminated food, include nausea, vomiting, abdominal pain, diarrhea, fever and dehydration. Severe cases of food poisoning can result in shock or death, particularly in children, the elderly and those with an impaired immune system. Some victims of food poisoning may require antibiotic or antitoxin therapy. Fortunately, most cases of food poisoning can be prevented by proper cooking, refrigeration and sanitation procedures.

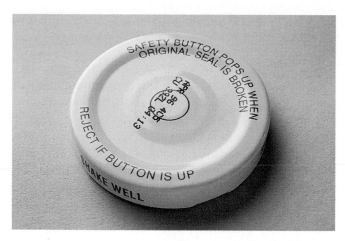

Figure 16-4 Inspect the safety button of the lid before opening a canned or bottled food.

Absorbed Poisons

People often come into contact with poisonous substances that can be absorbed into the body. Millions of people each year suffer irritating effects after touching or brushing against poisonous plants such as poison ivy, poison oak and poison sumac. Other poisons absorbed through the skin include dry and wet chemicals, such as those used in yard and garden maintenance, which may also burn the surface of the skin. To care for a victim who has come into contact with a poisonous plant, immediately rinse the affected area thoroughly with water (Fig. 16-5, *A*). Using soap cannot hurt, but soap may not do much to remove the poisonous plant oil that causes the allergic reaction. Before washing the affected area, you may need to have the victim remove any jewelry. This is only necessary if the jewelry is contaminated or if it constricts circulation due to swelling. If a rash or weeping lesion (an oozing sore) develops, seek advice from a pharmacist or physician about possible treatment. Medicated lotions may help soothe the area. **Antihistamines** may also help dry up the lesions and help stop or reduce itching. These over-the-counter products are available at a pharmacy or grocery store. If the condition worsens and large areas of the body or the face are affected, the victim should see a physician, who may administer **anti-inflammatory drugs,** such as **corticosteroids,** or other medications to relieve discomfort.

If the injury involves dry chemicals, brush off the chemicals using a gloved hand before flushing with tap water (under pressure). Be careful not to get the chemical on yourself or the person.

Safe Food Handling Tips

- Wash hands thoroughly with soap and water before preparing or handling food; between handling raw and cooked foods; and whenever handling food preparation surfaces, dishes and utensils.
- Thaw all frozen meats, poultry or fish in the refrigerator, not at room temperature.
- Never put cooked meats back onto a surface used to hold or store the meat before cooking unless the surface has been washed thoroughly.
- Rinse all raw fruits and vegetables thoroughly before use.
- Wash and dry tops of canned goods before opening.
- Keep cold foods in the refrigerator at or below 40° F (4° C).
- Be sure hot foods are heated to and kept at or above 140° F (60° C).
- Throw out all perishable foods not kept at safe hot or cold temperatures. Dispose of all perishable food left out at room temperature for 2 or more hours.
- Store dry foods such as flour, sugar and cereal in glass, plastic or metal containers with tight lids.
- Store all foods in containers that are clean, have tight-fitting covers and are insect- and rodent-resistant.
- Store food items away from nonfood items.

Use an inventory system to rotate and use up all food items.

Source: Centers for Disease Control Web site,
www.cdc.gov/ncidod.op/food.htm

If wet chemicals contact the skin, flush the area continuously with large amounts of cool running water. Continue flushing at least 20 minutes or until EMS personnel arrive.

If running water is not available, brush off dry chemicals, such as lime, with a gloved hand. Take care not to inhale any of the chemical or get any of the dry chemical in your eyes or the eyes of the victim or any bystanders. Many dry chemicals are activated by contact with water, but if continuous running water is available, it will flush the chemical from the skin before the activated chemical can do harm. Running water reduces the threat to you and quickly and easily removes the substance from the victim.

Injected Poisons

Insect and animal bites and stings are among the most common sources of injected poisons. Chapter 17 describes the general signals of stings and bites of insects, spiders, ticks, marine life, snakes, scorpions, animals and humans, as well as the appropriate care. Chapter 18 provides information about another common source of injected poisons—the use of injected drugs.

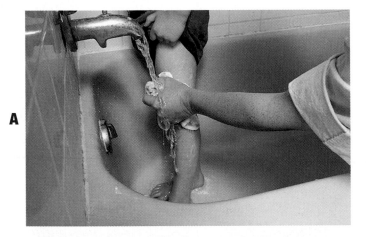

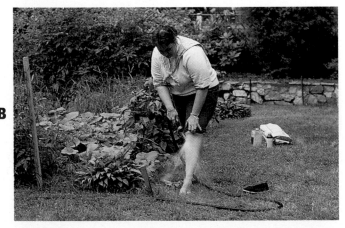

Figure 16-5 A, To care for skin contact with a poisonous plant, immediately rinse the affected area thoroughly with water. **B,** Whenever chemical poisons come in contact with the skin or eyes, flush the affected area continuously with large amounts of water.

ANAPHYLAXIS

Severe allergic reactions to poisons are rare. But when one occurs, it is truly a life-threatening medical emergency. This reaction is called *anaphylaxis* and was discussed in Chapter 6. Anaphylaxis is a form of shock. It can be caused by an insect bite or sting or contact with certain drugs, medications, foods and chemicals. Anaphylaxis can result from any of the four modes of poisoning described in this chapter.

Signals of Anaphylaxis

Anaphylaxis usually occurs suddenly, within seconds or minutes after the victim comes into contact with the poisonous substance. The skin or area of the body that came in contact with the substance usually swells and turns red (**Fig. 16-6**). Other signals include hives (reddish bumps on the skin), rash, itching and burning skin and eyes, weakness, nausea, vomiting, restlessness, dizziness, dilated pupils, slurred speech, chest discomfort or pain, weak or rapid pulse, and rapid or trouble breathing that includes coughing and wheezing. This trouble breathing can progress to an obstructed airway as the tongue, throat and bronchial passageways swell. Death from anaphylaxis usually occurs because the victim's breathing is severely impaired.

Care for Anaphylaxis

Call 9-1-1 or the local emergency number immediately. Anaphylaxis is a life-threatening condition. Monitor the victim's airway and breathing. Have the

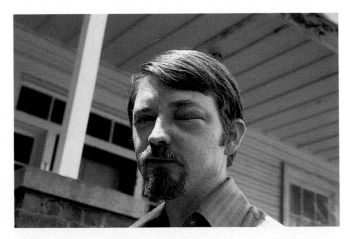

Figure 16-6 In anaphylaxis, the skin or area of the body usually swells and turns red.

Epinephrine Administration

Approximately two million people in the United States are at risk for anaphylaxis, and each year 400 to 800 people in the United States die from anaphylactic reactions. Insect stings; penicillin; aspirin; food additives, such as sulfites; and certain foods, such as shellfish, fish and nuts can trigger anaphylaxis in susceptible individuals. These reactions may be life threatening and require immediate care. A medical ID bracelet or necklace should be worn by the individual at risk. Some possible signs and symptoms in anaphylactic victims include:

- Swelling to the face, neck, hands, throat, tongue or any body part.
- Itching of tongue, armpits, groin or any body part.
- Dizziness.
- Redness or welts on the skin.
- Red watery eyes.
- Nausea, abdominal pain or vomiting.
- Rapid heart rate.
- **Difficulty breathing** or swallowing.
- Feeling of constriction in the throat or chest.

Epinephrine is a prescribed medication of choice to treat the signs and symptoms of these reactions. Call 9-1-1 or the local emergency number or summon more advanced medical personnel immediately.

If you know that a person has a prescribed epinephrine auto-injector and is unable to administer it him or herself, then you may help the person use it if you are trained and state and local regulations allow.

Note: Rescuers should follow local protocols or medical directives when applicable.

Use an epinephrine auto-injector when a victim:

- Relates a history of allergies or allergic reactions.
- Is having an allergic reaction.
- Requests assistance to administer epinephrine.
- Provides the epinephrine auto-injector.
- Has a family member who relates a victim history of allergies or allergic reactions and provides the victim's epinephrine auto-injector.

If the person is unconscious, has trouble breathing, complains of the throat tightening or explains that he or she is subject to severe allergic reactions, have someone call 9-1-1 or the local emergency number.

- Determine whether the person has already taken epinephrine or antihistamine. If so, **do not** administer another dose.
- Check the expiration date of the auto-injector. If it has expired, do not use it.
- If the medication is visible, confirm that the liquid is clear and not cloudy. If it is cloudy, do not use it.

Step 1: Locate the middle of one thigh or the upper arm to use as the injection site. Grasp the auto-injector firmly in your fist and pull off the safety cap with your other hand.

Step 2: Hold the (black) tip near the person's outer thigh so that the auto-injector is at a 90-degree angle to the thigh.

Step 3: Swing out then firmly jab the tip straight into the outer thigh. You will hear a click.

Step 4: Hold the auto-injector firmly in place for 10 seconds, then remove it from the thigh and massage the injection site for several seconds.

Re-evaluate the ABCs and observe response to epinephrine.

Step 5: Give the used auto-injector to the emergency medical services personnel when they arrive.

In all cases of epinephrine administration, follow-up care and transport to a medical facility is needed. The beneficial effect of epinephrine is relatively short in duration. Victims having a severe allergic reaction may require additional medications that can be administered only in a hospital.

SOURCE
American Red Cross Advisory Council on First Aid and Safety (ACFAS), Statement on Epinephrine Administration, 2001.

Poisonous Plants

By the time we are adults, most of us are aware that eating an unidentified mushroom can be a one-way ticket to the local hospital. We are rarely aware of the many poisonous plants in our homes and gardens. Of the approximately 30,000 known plant species, only about 700 are poisonous. But a number of these poisonous plants are not located in the rain forest or on some tropical island; they are quietly sitting in pots or vases in our living rooms.

Many poisonous household products now have some sort of warning label, but we are rarely warned about the dangers of a seemingly innocuous houseplant or shrub. Take, for example, lily-of-the-valley, with its delicate, sweet-scented, little white bells, which is a mainstay of bridal bouquets. If you were to nibble the stem, flowers, leaves or red berries of the plant, you would regret it. The effects of the poison in this plant include burning of the mouth and throat, vomiting, irregular heartbeat, coma and circulatory failure. In Africa, lily-of-the-valley plants have been used to poison the tips of arrows.

Be aware of certain plants associated with the holiday season. Holly berries, if eaten, are sufficiently toxic to cause illness, especially in a child. Eating mistletoe berries can result in vomiting, diarrhea, delirium, cardiovascular collapse and death. Skin contact with the sap of a poinsettia causes blistering. In fact, the sap of snow-on-the-mountain, a relative of the poinsettia, is so potent it has been used in place of a hot iron to brand cattle.

Several common houseplants are highly toxic. The philodendron is a popular plant for home and office because it flourishes without direct sunlight and needs little care. The philodendron and other plants in the same family have leaves of various sizes, shapes and colors. But the plants in this family all have one aspect in common: some parts contain needlelike crystals of a chemical—calcium oxalate—that become embedded in the mouth and tongue when plant parts are chewed, causing intense burning and severe swelling. The dieffenbachia, a large, handsome houseplant related to the philodendron, has large bright green leaves striped with white. It is also known as "dumb cane" because chewing the leaves can make the mouth and tongue so swollen that speaking is impossible. Another houseplant to be aware of is the Jerusalem cherry, whose red or orange fruit look like cherry tomatoes and are somewhat poisonous.

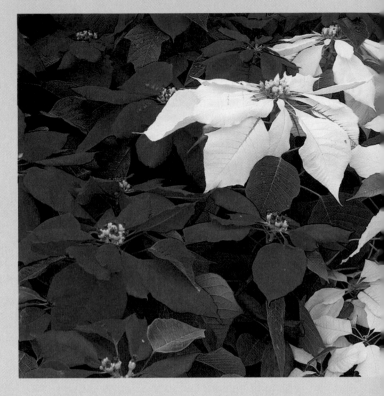

The most dangerous plant grown in the home or garden is oleander. In the United States, oleanders are grown as houseplants in the north and as outdoor shrubs in California, Florida and tropical areas. The leaves are stiff, narrow, dark green and shiny, and the flowers are pink, white or red. Drinking the water from a vase that has held oleander flowers can make a person violently ill, as will eating the leaves, stems or flowers. People have been poisoned from eating hot dogs roasted on sticks from an oleander bush as well as from inhaling smoke from the burning foliage.

A number of the plants we commonly grow in gardens are poisonous if eaten, for example, the bulbs and other parts of the narcissus, hyacinth and snowdrop. The berries of English ivy and yew can cause vomiting, stomach pain, headache, diarrhea and convulsions. Foxglove plants can cause heart failure. Eating the flowers of the lavender plant or the bulb of the autumn crocus can result in kidney damage, dehydration, abdominal pains and shock. The castor plant is grown mainly for the oil produced from its pleasant-tasting, shiny, black-and-brown seeds. It only takes one or two of those seeds, chewed and swallowed, to die.

Treat certain products of the orchard and vegetable garden with caution. The seeds inside the pits of peaches, apricots, cherries and other fruit contain potentially lethal cyanide. So do apple seeds. The leaves of rhubarb can damage the kidneys. Eating the raw shoots and berries of asparagus can result in unpleasant skin rashes and blisters. Even the potato plant is not entirely safe; all the green parts of the plant are poisonous, and so are green areas on potatoes themselves. Always cut away the green spots and sprouts on a potato before cooking, and do not expose uncooked potatoes to sunlight. The leaves and stems of the tomato plant, which is related to the potato, are also poisonous.

Other poisonous relatives of the potato include tobacco, jasmine and jimsonweed. Eating them can result in respiratory failure, headache, abdominal pain, delirium and weakness. Skin contact can cause severe skin irritation. Jimsonweed was named after the Jamestown, Virginia, settlement where, in 1676, some soldiers sent to put down an uprising were poisoned by cooked jimsonweed greens and fruit. A tall plant with thick stems, toothed leaves, trumpet-shaped white or lavender flowers, and a fruit encased in a green, spiny husk, jimsonweed grows wild in fields, along roadsides and sometimes in backyards and gardens. If eaten, it can cause

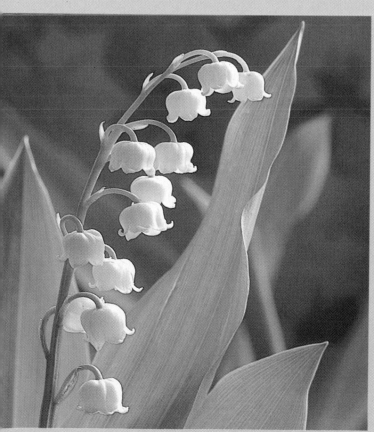

convulsions, hallucinations, coma and death. Other poisonous plants common in woods, fields, vacant lots or gardens include mountain laurel, deadly nightshade and Japanese honeysuckle.

The most violently toxic plant that grows wild in the Northern Hemisphere is the water hemlock. Hemlock acts on the central nervous system in about $\frac{1}{2}$ hour. The ancient Greeks used an extract from another hemlock plant, the poison hemlock, for executions, the most famous victim being the philosopher Socrates.

What precautions can you take to ensure against plant poisoning? First of all, learn about the plants you have in your home, office and garden. Nurseries and other places that sell house and garden plants rarely provide warnings about the possibilities of poisoning. Many poison control centers state that their most frequent calls concern children who have eaten plants. Keep plants you know are toxic out of reach of infants and small children (or better yet, keep toxic plants out of homes with children altogether); remove berries and leaves from the floor; and if you don't know whether a plant can be poisonous, consult a poison control center.

Do not store bulbs where they can be mistaken for onions. Clean up any clippings and leaves from garden work, but do not burn them, because poisonous plants, when burned, can produce poisonous smoke that is dangerous if inhaled. Do not bite into an unfamiliar seed, no matter where you find it. The rosary pea, a member of the pea family that grows in the tropics, produces a black and red seed that has been used in costume jewelry. People have died from chewing or swallowing only one rosary pea.

Learn about the weeds and wild plants that grow in your neighborhood, and never eat any part of a plant you cannot positively identify. Poison hemlock is also known as fool's parsley. If you have a yen to forage for wild plant foods, take a field identification course taught by someone credentialed in the subject. Do not rely on field guidebooks. Even the clearest photograph is no proof against mistaking a "safe" plant for an unsafe one, and that first bite of a water hemlock root that you mistook for a wild carrot could be your last.

SOURCES
Coil SM: *Poisonous plants*, New York, 1991, Franklin Watts.
Lerner C: *Dumb cane and daffodils: poisonous plants in the house and garden*, New York, 1990, William Morrow.
Westbrooks RG, Preacher JW: *Poisonous plants of eastern North America*, Columbia, South Carolina, 1986, University of South Carolina Press.
Woodward L: *Poisonous plants: a colorful field guide*, New York, 1985, Hippocrene Books.

victim rest in a comfortable position. This position is usually sitting upright or leaning forward. Comfort and reassure the victim until EMS personnel arrive, and continue to monitor the victim's condition.

People who know they are extremely allergic to certain substances may carry an anaphylaxis kit in case they have a severe allergic reaction. Such kits are available by prescription only. The kit contains a dose of the drug epinephrine (adrenaline) that can be injected into the body to counteract the anaphylactic reaction. If you are allergic to a substance, contact a doctor to discuss whether you need such a kit.

An **auto-injector** (Fig. 16-7) is another way to administer epinephrine. An auto-injector is a spring-loaded needle and syringe system with a single dose of epinephrine. Epinephrine is injected into the victim by firmly pushing the device against the victim's outer thigh. Like the anaphylaxis kit, an auto-injector is available only through a prescription.

In some cases you may need to assist the victim in using his or her kit. Assisting a victim with medication can include getting the pen or kit from a purse, car, home or out of a specially designed carrier or belt; taking it out of the plastic tube; or assisting the victim with the injection.

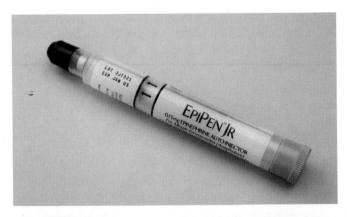

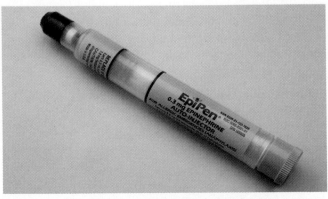

Figure 16-7 Epinephrine auto-injectors.

PREVENTING POISONING

The best approach to poisoning emergencies is to prevent them from occurring in the first place. Prevention is a simple principle, but often people do not take enough precautions. Of all the child poisoning cases reported, the vast majority occurred when the child was under the direct supervision of a parent or guardian. It takes only a brief lapse of supervision for a child to get into trouble. Children are naturally curious and can get into things in ways adults might not consider possible. Many substances commonly found in or around the house are poisonous. Children are especially vulnerable to these substances because of their tendency to put everything in their mouths. Extra care may be needed in monitoring the actions of children in homes that are not childproof. For example, in such homes, medications may not be stored in childproof containers.

When giving medication to a child, do so carefully. Medicine is not candy and should never be called candy to entice a child to take it. Cough syrup may look like a soft drink to children, and many coated medicine tablets look like candy. Some children's medicine has a pleasant candy flavor so that children will take it more easily. When giving any of these substances, make it clear to the child that it is medicine. Take care also to keep the medication out of reach of children.

By following these general guidelines, you will be able to prevent most poisoning emergencies:

▶ Keep all medications and household products well out of the reach of children. Special latches and clamps are available to keep children from opening cabinets. Use these or other methods to keep children from reaching any substances that may be poisonous. Consider all household or drugstore products to be potentially harmful.

▶ Use childproof safety caps on containers of medication and other potentially dangerous products.

▶ Keep products in their original containers, with the labels in place.

▶ Use poison symbols to identify dangerous substances, and teach children what the symbols mean.

▶ Dispose of outdated medications and household products properly and in a timely manner.

▶ Use potentially dangerous chemicals only in well-ventilated areas.

▶ Wear proper clothing when work or recreation may put you in contact with a poisonous substance (**Fig. 16-8**). Your employer must follow strict guidelines to protect you from coming into contact with poisonous substances in the workplace.

▶ Immediately wash those areas of the body that you suspect may have come into contact with a poison.

One of the best ways to prevent poisonings is to be aware of which common household items can be poisonous. These include, but are not limited to, acetaminophen, acids, ammonia, aspirin, bleach, cosmetics, detergents, drain cleaner, heating fuel, iodine, lye, lighter fluid, oven cleaner, paint, pesticides, toilet bowl cleaner, turpentine and weed killer. Some common household plants and garden shrubs are also poisonous.

SUMMARY

Poisoning can occur in any one of four ways: inhalation, ingestion, absorption and injection. The severity of a poisoning depends on the type and amount of the substance; how and where it entered the body; the time elapsed since the poison entered the body; and the victim's size, weight and age. For suspected poisonings, call the National Poison Control Center at (800) 222-1222. Poison control center personnel are specially trained to handle these types of emergencies. Call 9-1-1 or the local emergency number if the victim has any life-threatening conditions. Follow the directions of poison control center personnel or the EMS call taker.

Increasing your awareness and taking steps to reduce the risks is one of the best ways to prevent a poisoning emergency. Identify items in your environment, such as household cleaners, plants and medications, that may pose a danger to you, your family or co-workers. Learn to handle and store these items properly by following the manufacturer's directions.

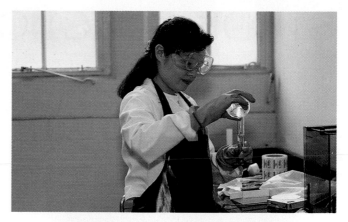

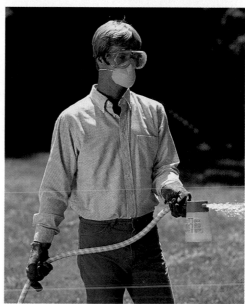

Figure 16-8   Wear proper clothing for any activities that may put you in contact with a poisonous substance.

APPLICATION QUESTIONS

1. What clues did Ashley find at the scene to alert her that Kristen may have been poisoned?

2. What should Ashley do to care for Kristen?

STUDY QUESTIONS

1. Match each term with the correct definition.

    a. Absorbed poison   d. Inhaled poison
    b. Anaphylaxis   e. Injected poison
    c. Ingested poison   f. Poison control center

    _____ A poison introduced into the body through bites, stings or a hypodermic needle.

    _____ A life-threatening allergic reaction.

    _____ A center staffed by professionals who can tell you how to give care in a poisoning emergency.

    _____ A poison that is swallowed.

    _____ A poison that enters the body through contact with the skin.

    _____ A poison that enters the body through breathing.

2. List at least six common signals of poisoning.

3. List four factors that determine the severity of poisoning.

4. Describe how to care for a person who has spilled a poisonous substance on his or her skin or has touched a poisonous plant, such as poison ivy.

5. Describe seven steps you can take to prevent poisoning emergencies in your home.

Base your answers for questions 6 through 8 on the scenario below.

Beth was putting fertilizer on her favorite rose bush. She looked down and saw a strange plant that appeared to be a weed. She leaned over and plucked the plant out of the ground with her bare hand. A little while later, her hands started itching and burning. Her fingers became swollen, and red bumps began to appear all over her forearm.

6. Identify the signals that indicate that a poisoning emergency has occurred.

7. What kind of care would you give Beth?

8. What could Beth have done to prevent this situation from happening?

In questions 9 and 10, circle the letter of the correct answer.

9. Your neighbor has accidentally swallowed some pesticide. He is conscious and alert. What should you do?

    a. Give him something to drink.
    b. Induce vomiting.
    c. Call the Poison Control Center.
    d. Have him lie down.

10. You walk into a room and find an unconscious child on the floor. There is an empty medicine bottle next to her. What should you do first?

    a. Call 9-1-1 or the local emergency number or the Poison Control Center.
    b. Give rescue breathing.
    c. Give her something to drink.
    d. Check the airway.

Answers are listed in Appendix A.

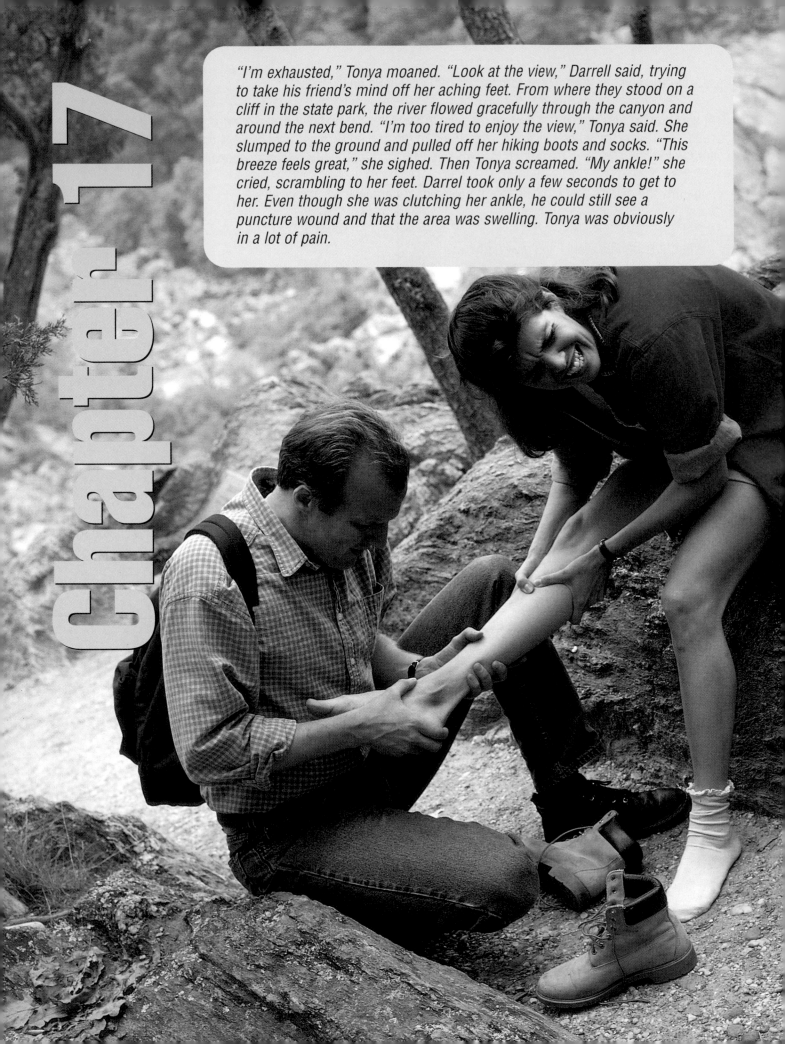

"I'm exhausted," Tonya moaned. "Look at the view," Darrell said, trying to take his friend's mind off her aching feet. From where they stood on a cliff in the state park, the river flowed gracefully through the canyon and around the next bend. "I'm too tired to enjoy the view," Tonya said. She slumped to the ground and pulled off her hiking boots and socks. "This breeze feels great," she sighed. Then Tonya screamed. "My ankle!" she cried, scrambling to her feet. Darrel took only a few seconds to get to her. Even though she was clutching her ankle, he could still see a puncture wound and that the area was swelling. Tonya was obviously in a lot of pain.

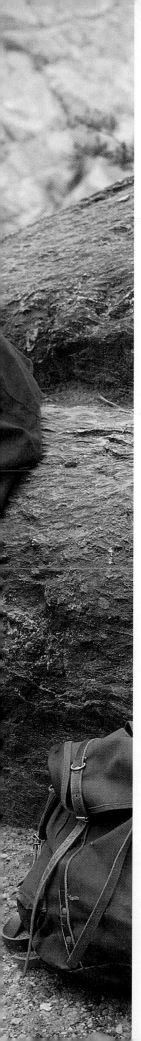

Bites and Stings

Objectives

After reading this chapter, you should be able to—

■ *Identify five signals of the most common types of bites and stings.*

■ *Describe how to care for insect, spider or scorpion stings.*

■ *Describe how to care for tick bites.*

■ *Describe how to care for snakebites.*

■ *Describe how to care for marine life bites or stings.*

■ *Describe how to care for domestic or wild animal bites.*

■ *Describe how to care for human bites.*

■ *Identify five ways to protect yourself from insect and tick bites.*

Introduction

Bites and stings are among the most common forms of injected poisonings. In this chapter, you will learn how to recognize, care for and prevent some of the most common types of bites and stings—those of insects, ticks, spiders and scorpions, marine life, snakes, domestic and wild animals and humans. Chapter 18 provides information on another common form of injected poisoning—injected drug misuse and abuse.

SIGNALS

As with other kinds of poisoning, poisons that are injected through bites and stings may produce various signals. Specific signals depend on factors such as the type and location of the bite or sting; the amount of poison injected; the time elapsed since the poisoning; and the victim's size, weight and age. Less severe reactions to bites and stings may trigger signals including—

▶ A bite or sting mark at the point of injection (entry site).
▶ A stinger, tentacle or venom sac remaining in or near the entry site.
▶ Redness at or around the entry site.
▶ Swelling at or around the entry site.
▶ Pain or tenderness at or around the entry site.

Severe allergic reactions to bites and stings may bring on a life-threatening condition, a form of shock known as anaphylaxis. The signals of and care for anaphylaxis are described in Chapters 6 and 16.

CARE FOR SPECIFIC BITES AND STINGS

The following sections provide detailed instructions on how to care for specific kinds of bites and stings. **Table 17-1** highlights this information.

Insects

Between .5 to 5 percent of the American population is severely allergic to substances in the venom of bees, wasps, hornets and yellow jackets. For highly allergic people, even one sting can result in anaphylaxis. Such highly allergic reactions account for the nearly 50 reported deaths that occur from insect stings each year. When highly allergic people are stung, call 9-1-1 or the local emergency number immediately for medical care. However, for most people, insect stings may be painful or uncomfortable but are not life threatening.

To give care for an insect sting, first examine the sting site to see if the stinger is in the skin. If the stinger is still present, remove it to prevent any further poisoning. Scrape the stinger away from the skin with your fingernail or the edge of a plastic card, such as a credit card (**Fig. 17-1**). Often the venom sac will still be attached to the stinger. Do not remove the stinger with tweezers, because this may put pressure on the venom sac, causing it to burst and release more venom into the skin.

Next, wash the site with soap and water. Cover the site to keep it clean. Apply an ice or cold pack to the area to reduce the pain and swelling. Place a layer of gauze or cloth between the source of cold and the skin to prevent skin damage. Observe the victim periodically for signals of an allergic reaction. Be sure to ask the victim if he or she has had any prior allergic reactions to insect bites or stings.

KEY TERMS

Antivenin: A substance used to counteract the poisonous effects of snake, spider or insect venom.
Lyme disease: An illness transmitted by a certain kind of infected tick; victims may or may not develop a rash.

Rabies: A disease caused by a virus transmitted through the saliva of infected mammals.
Rocky Mountain spotted fever: A disease transmitted by a certain kind of infected tick; victims develop a spotted rash.

Table 17-1 Caring for Bites and Stings

INSECT BITES AND STINGS	TICK BITES	SPIDER BITES	SCORPION STINGS	SNAKE BITES	MARINE LIFE STINGS	DOMESTIC AND WILD ANIMAL BITES	HUMAN BITES
SIGNALS:	**SIGNALS:**	**SIGNALS:**	**SIGNALS:**	**SIGNALS:**	**SIGNALS:**	**SIGNALS:**	**SIGNALS:**
Stinger may be present

Pain

Local swelling

Hives or rash

Nausea and vomiting

Trouble breathing | Bull's eye, spotted or black and blue rash around bite or on other body part

Fever and chills

Flu-like aches | Bite mark or blister

Local swelling

Pain or cramping

Nausea and vomiting

Trouble breathing and swallowing

Profuse sweating or salivation

Irregular heartbeat | Bite mark

Local swelling

Pain or cramping

Nausea and vomiting

Trouble breathing or swallowing

Profuse sweating or salivation

Irregular heartbeat | Bite mark

Severe pain and burning

Local swelling and discoloration | Possible marks

Pain

Local swelling | Bite mark

Bleeding

Pain | Bite mark

Bleeding

Pain |
| **CARE:** | **CARE:** | **CARE:** | **CARE:** | **CARE:** | **CARE:** | **CARE:** | **CARE:** |
| Remove stinger; scrape it away with a plastic card or finger nail.

Wash wound.

Cover wound.

Apply a cold pack.

Watch for signals of allergic reactions; take steps to minimize shock if they occur. | Remove tick with tweezers.

Wash the area with soap and warm water.

Apply antiseptic or triple antibiotic ointment to wound.

Watch for signals of infection.

Get medical attention if necessary. | If black widow or brown recluse—call 9-1-1 or local emergency number immediately to have antivenin administered and have wound cleaned. | Call 9-1-1 or local emergency number.

Wash wound.

Apply a cold pack.

Get medical care to have antivenin administered. | Call 9-1-1 or local emergency number.

Wash wound.

Immobilize bitten part and keep it lower than the heart.

Minimize victim's movement. | If jellyfish—soak area in either vinegar, alcohol or baking soda paste.

If stingray—immobilize and soak area in nonscalding hot water until pain goes away.

Clean and bandage wound.

Call 9-1-1 or local emergency number, if necessary. | If wound is minor—wash wound, control bleeding, apply triple antibiotic ointment and a dressing and get medical attention as soon as possible.

If wound is severe—call 9-1-1 or local emergency number, control bleeding and do not wash wound. | If wound is minor—wash wound, control bleeding, apply triple antibiotic ointment and a dressing and get medical attention as soon as possible.

If wound is severe—call 9-1-1 or local emergency number, control bleeding and do not wash wound. |

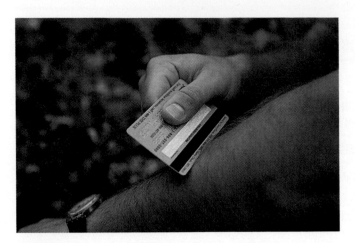

Figure 17-1 If someone is stung and a stinger is present, scrape it away from the skin with your fingernail or a plastic card, such as a credit card.

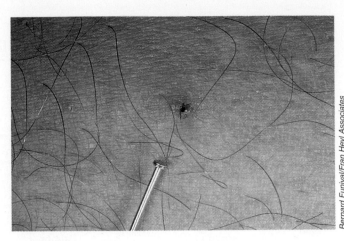

Figure 17-2 A deer tick can be as small as the head of a pin.

Ticks

Ticks can contract, carry and transmit disease to humans. *Rocky Mountain spotted fever* is caused by the transmission of microscopic bacteria from the wood tick or dog tick host to other warm-blooded animals, including humans. The disease gets part of its name from the spotted rash that appears after a victim becomes infected. The rash may first appear on wrists or ankles, then spreads rapidly to other parts of the body. Other signals of Rocky Mountain spotted fever include fever and chills, severe headache and joint and muscle aches.

Early treatment by medical professionals is important because untreated victims die from shock or kidney failure. Although the disease was first diagnosed in the western United States, Rocky Mountain spotted fever cases continue to be reported throughout North and South America today. Rocky Mountain spotted fever is sometimes known by various regional names, such as black fever, mountain fever, tick fever, spotted fever or pinta fever.

Lyme disease, or *Lyme borreliosis,* is another illness that people can get from the bite of an infected tick. Lyme disease is an illness that affects a growing number of people in the United States. It is spread primarily by a type of tick that commonly attaches itself to field mice and deer. It is sometimes called a deer tick. Like all ticks, it attaches itself to any warm-blooded animal that brushes by it, including humans. This tick is found around beaches and in wooded and grassy areas.

Deer ticks are very tiny and difficult to see, especially in the late spring and summer. They are much smaller than the common dog tick or wood tick. They can be as small as a poppy seed, the period at the end of this sentence or the head of a pin (**Fig. 17-2**). Even in the adult stage, they are only as large as a grape seed. A deer tick can attach itself and bite you without your knowledge. Many people who develop Lyme disease cannot recall having been bitten.

You can get Lyme disease from the bite of an infected tick at any time of the year. However, the risk is greatest between May and July, when ticks are most active and outdoor activities are at their peak. To protect yourself from tick bites, wear repellent and proper clothing, check and clean your clothes thoroughly after having been in wooded areas and use precautions when removing a tick.

The first signal of infection may appear a few days or a few weeks after a tick bite. Typically, a rash starts as a small red area at the site of the bite. It may spread up to 6 to 8 inches across (**Fig. 17-3**). In fair-skinned people, the center of the rash is lighter in color and the outer edges are raised and red, sometimes giving the rash a bull's-eye appearance. In dark-skinned people, the rash area may look black and blue, like a bruise. A rash can appear anywhere on the body, and more than one rash may appear on various body parts. However, you can even have Lyme disease without developing a rash.

Other signals of Lyme disease include fever and chills, headache, weakness or fatigue and flu-like joint and muscle aches. These signals may develop slowly and may not occur at the same time as a rash. The more severe signals of Lyme disease may appear weeks, months or even years after a tick bite.

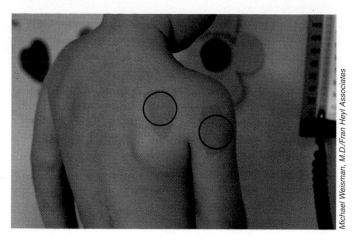

Figure 17-3 A person with Lyme disease may develop a rash.

Michael Weisman, M.D./Fran Heyl Associates

Lyme disease can get worse if it is not treated. In its advanced stages, Lyme disease may cause arthritis, numbness, memory loss, problems with vision or hearing, high fever and stiffness in the neck. Some of these signals could indicate brain or nervous system problems. An irregular or rapid heartbeat could occur, which can indicate heart problems.

If you find an embedded tick, with a gloved hand, grasp the tick with fine-tipped pointed, non-etched, non-rasped tweezers as close to the skin as possible and pull slowly and upward (**Fig. 17-4**). Do not try to burn the tick off. Do not apply petroleum jelly or nail polish to the tick. These remedies are not always effective in removing the tick and can cause further harm to the victim. If you cannot remove the tick, or if its mouth parts remain embedded, get medical care. Place the tick in a sealable

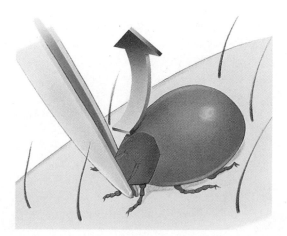

Figure 17-4 Remove a tick by pulling slowly, steadily and firmly with fine-tipped tweezers.

container for analysis. Wash the bite area with soap and warm water. Apply antiseptic or triple antibiotic ointment to help prevent infection. If rash, flulike signals or joint pain appears, seek medical attention. Wash your hands thoroughly. If you do not have tweezers, use a glove, plastic wrap, a piece of paper or a leaf to protect your fingers.

If you cannot remove the tick, obtain medical care. Even if you can remove the tick, you may want to let your physician know that you have been bitten by a tick in case you become ill within the following month or two. Mouth parts of adult ticks may sometimes remain in your skin, but these will not cause disease. Check the site periodically thereafter. If a rash or flulike signals develop, seek medical care. Redness at the site of a tick bite does not necessarily mean you are infected with a disease.

A physician will usually use antibiotics to treat Lyme disease and Rocky Mountain spotted fever. Antibiotics work best and most quickly when taken soon after the victim has been bitten. If you suspect you may have been infected with Lyme disease or Rocky Mountain spotted fever, do not delay seeking treatment. Treatment is slower and less effective in advanced stages.

Additional information on Lyme disease and Rocky Mountain spotted fever may be available from your state or local health department. You can also contact the American Lyme Disease Foundation, Inc., Web site *www.aldf.com.*

Spiders and Scorpions

Few spiders in the United States have venom that causes death. However, the bites of the black widow and brown recluse spiders can make you seriously ill and are occasionally fatal. These spiders live in most parts of the United States. You can identify them by the unique designs on their bodies. The black widow spider is black with a reddish hourglass shape on its underbody (**Fig. 17-5, A**). The brown recluse spider is light brown with a darker brown, violin-shaped marking on the top of its body (**Fig. 17-5, B**).

Both spiders prefer dark, out-of-the-way places where they are seldom disturbed. Bites usually occur on the hands and arms of people reaching into places, such as wood, rock and brush piles or rummaging in dark garages and attics. Often, the victim will not know that he or she has been bitten until signals develop.

The bite of the black widow spider is the more painful and often the more deadly of the two, especially in very young and elderly victims. The venom of a black widow spider is even deadlier than that of a rattlesnake, although the smaller amount of venom injected by the spider usually produces a less severe reaction than that of a snakebite.

The bite of a black widow spider usually causes a sharp pinprick pain, followed by a dull pain in the area of the bite. Other signals of this bite include muscular rigidity in the shoulders, back and abdomen; restlessness; anxiety; profuse sweating; weakness; and drooping eyelids.

A brown recluse spider bite may produce little or no pain initially, but localized pain develops an hour or more later. A blood-filled blister forms under the surface of the skin, sometimes in a target or bull's-eye pattern. Over time, the blister increases in size and eventually ruptures, leaving a black scar.

If the victim recognizes the spider as either a black widow or brown recluse, he or she should seek medical care as soon as possible. Health-care professionals will clean the wound and give medication to reduce the pain and inflammation. An *antivenin,* a substance used to counteract the poisonous effects of the venom, is available for black widow bites. Antivenin is used mostly for children and the elderly and is rarely necessary when bites occur in healthy adults.

Scorpions live in dry regions of the southwestern United States and Mexico. They are usually about 3 inches long and have 8 legs and a pair of crab-like pincers. At the end of the tail is a stinger, used to inject venom. Scorpions live in cool, damp places, such as basements, junk piles, woodpiles and under the bark of living or fallen trees. They are most active in the evening and at night, which is when most stings occur. Like spiders, only a few species of scorpions have a potentially fatal sting (**Fig. 17-6**). *However, because it is difficult to distinguish highly poisonous scorpions from the nonpoisonous scorpions, all scorpion stings should be treated as medical emergencies.*

Signals of spider bites and scorpion stings may include—

▶ A mark indicating a possible bite or sting.
▶ Severe pain in the sting or bite area.
▶ A blister, lesion or swelling at the entry site.

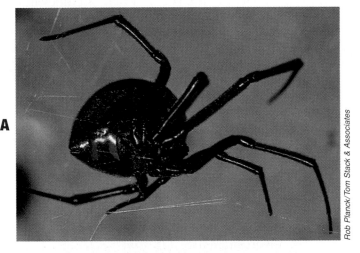

A

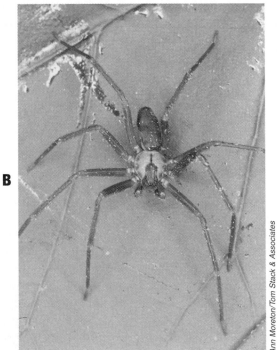

B

Ann Moreton/Tom Stack & Associates

Rob Planck/Tom Stack & Associates

Figure 17-5 **A,** The black widow spider and, **B,** brown recluse spider have characteristic markings.

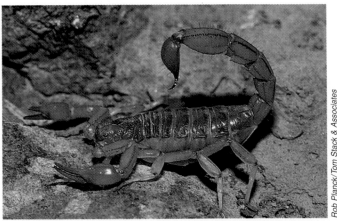

Rob Planck/Tom Stack & Associates

Figure 17-6 The stings of only a few species of scorpions found in the United States can be fatal.

▶ Nausea and vomiting.
▶ Trouble breathing or swallowing.
▶ Sweating or salivating profusely.
▶ Irregular heart rhythms.
▶ Muscle cramping or abdominal pain.

If a person is bitten by a spider (i.e., brown recluse or black widow) or stung by a scorpion, call 9-1-1 or the local emergency number. Wash the wound and apply an ice or a cold pack to the site to reduce swelling. Remember to place a layer of gauze or cloth between the source of cold and the skin to prevent skin damage.

Snakes

Few areas of medicine have provoked more controversy about care for an injury than snakebites. Snakebite care issues, such as whether to use a tourniquet, cut the wound, apply ice, when to apply suction, use electric shocks or capture the snake, have been discussed at length over the years. Of the estimated 7000 to 8000 people reported bitten by poisonous snakes annually in the United States, fewer than five die. **Figure 17-7** shows the four kinds of poisonous snakes found in the United States. Rattlesnakes account for most snakebites and nearly all deaths from snakebites. Most deaths occur because the victim has an allergic reaction, is in poor health or because too much time passes before the victim receives medical care. Although advice to citizen responders has varied greatly over the years, elaborate initial care is usually unnecessary because, in most cases, the victim can reach professional medical care within 30 minutes.

Signals that indicate a poisonous snakebite include—

▶ One or two distinct puncture wounds, which may or may not bleed. The exception is the coral snake, whose teeth leave a semicircular mark.

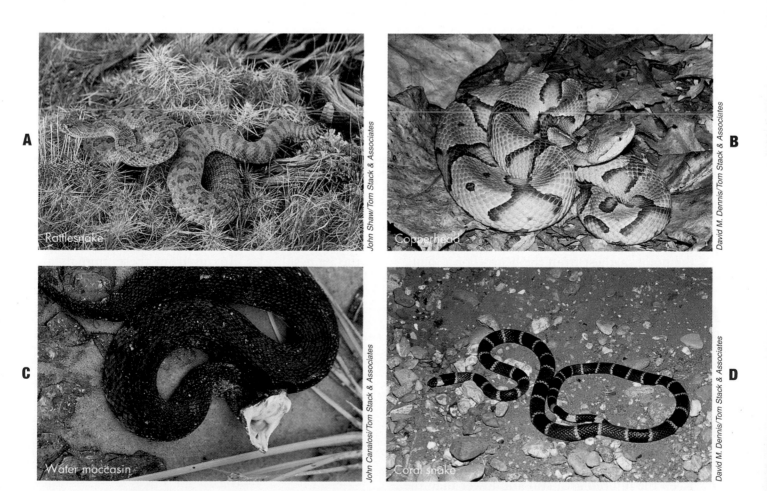

Figure 17-7 There are four kinds of poisonous snakes found in the United States: **A,** Rattlesnake. **B,** Copperhead. **C,** Water moccasin. **D,** Coral snake.

▸ Severe pain and burning at the wound site immediately after or within 4 hours of the incident.

▸ Swelling and discoloration at the wound site immediately after or within 4 hours of the incident.

To care for a bite from a pit viper, such as a rattlesnake, copperhead or cottonmouth, follow these steps—

▸ Call 9-1-1 or the local emergency number.

▸ Wash the wound.

▸ Keep the injured area still and lower than the heart. If possible, carry a person who must be taken to a medical facility or have him or her walk slowly.

▸ Do not apply ice.

▸ Do not cut the wound.

▸ Do not apply suction.

▸ Do not apply a tourniquet.

▸ Do not use electric shock, such as from a car battery.

Care for a bite from an elapid snake, such as a coral snake, is the same as for a pit viper, except that after washing the wound you should apply an elastic roller bandage by following these steps (see Chapter 10 for more information on using an elastic bandage)—

▸ Check for feeling, warmth and color of the limb beyond where you will be placing the bandage by noting changes in skin color and temperature.

▸ Place the end of the bandage against the skin and use overlapping turns.

▸ Gently stretch the bandage as you continue wrapping. The wrap should cover a long body section, such as an arm or a calf, beginning at the point farthest from the heart. For a joint like a knee or ankle, use figure-eight turns to support the joint.

▸ Always check the area above and below the injury site for feeling, warmth and color, especially fingers and toes, after you have applied an elastic roller bandage. By checking before and after bandaging, you will be able to tell if any tingling or numbness is from the bandaging or the injury.

▸ Check the snugness of the bandaging—a finger should easily, but not loosely, pass under the bandage.

▸ Keep the injured area still and lower than the heart. If possible, carry a person who must be taken to a medical facility or have him or her walk slowly.

▸ Do not apply ice.

▸ Do not cut the wound.

▸ Do not apply suction.

▸ Do not apply a tourniquet.

▸ Do not use electric shock, such as from a car battery.

Marine Life

The stings of some forms of marine life are not only painful but can also make you sick (**Fig. 17-8**). The side effects include allergic reactions that can cause breathing and heart problems and paralysis. If the sting occurs in water, move the person from the water to dry land as soon as possible. Call 9-1-1 or the local emergency number if the victim does not know what stung him or her, has a history of allergic reactions to marine life stings, is stung on the face or neck or starts to have trouble breathing.

If you know the sting is from a jellyfish, sea anemone or Portuguese man-of-war, soak the injured part in vinegar as soon as possible. Vinegar often works best to offset the toxin and reduce pain. Rubbing alcohol or a baking soda paste may also be used. Do not rub the wound or apply fresh water or ammonia, because these substances will increase pain. Meat tenderizer is no longer recommended because the active ingredient once used to reduce pain is no longer contained in most meat tenderizers.

If you know the sting is from a stingray, sea urchin or spiny fish, flush the wound with tap water. Ocean water may also be used. Immobilize the injured part, usually the foot, and soak the affected area in nonscalding hot water (as hot as the person can stand) for about 30 minutes or until the pain subsides. Toxins from these animals are heat-sensitive, and dramatic relief of local pain often occurs from one application of hot fluid. If hot water is not available, packing the area in hot sand may have a similar effect if the sand is hot enough. Then carefully clean the wound and apply a bandage. Watch for signals of infection, and check with a health-care provider to determine if a tetanus shot is needed. (Tetanus is discussed later in this chapter.)

Domestic and Wild Animals

The bite of a domestic or wild animal carries the risk of infection, as well as soft tissue injury. Dog bites are the most common of all bites from domes-

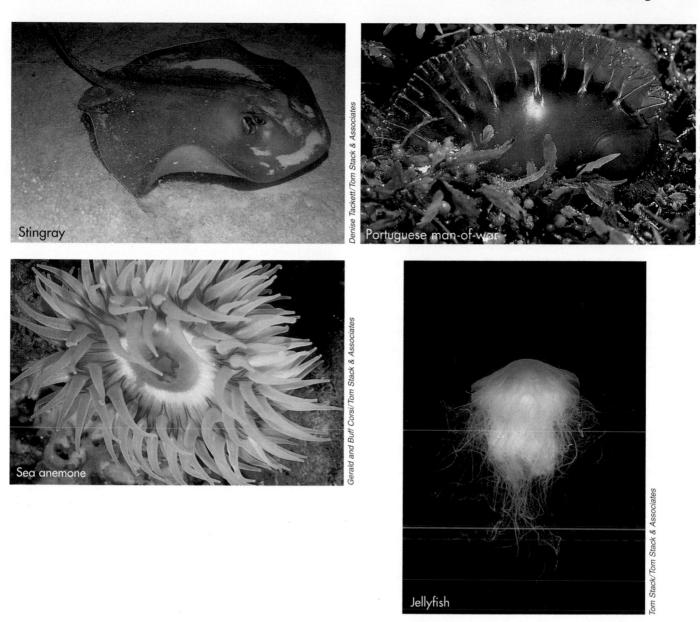

Figure 17-8 The painful sting of some marine animals can cause serious injury and illness.

tic or wild animals. One of the most serious possible infections is rabies. **Rabies** is a disease caused by a virus transmitted commonly through the saliva of diseased mammals, such as skunks, bats, raccoons, cats, dogs, cattle and foxes.

Animals with rabies may act in unusual ways. For example, nocturnal animals, such as raccoons, may be active in the daytime. A wild animal that usually tries to avoid humans may not run away when you approach. Rabid animals may salivate; appear partially paralyzed; or act irritable, aggressive or strangely quiet. To reduce your risk of becoming infected with rabies, do not pet or feed wild animals and do not touch the body of a dead wild animal.

If not treated, rabies is fatal. *Anyone bitten by a wild or domestic animal must get professional medical attention as soon as possible.* To prevent rabies from developing, the victim receives a series of vaccine injections to build up immunity. In the past, caring for rabies meant a lengthy series of painful injections that had many unpleasant side effects. The vaccines used now require fewer and less painful injections and have fewer side effects.

Tetanus is another potentially fatal infection. Tetanus is caused by the transmission of bacteria that produce a toxin, which can occur in wounds created by animal and human bites. The toxin associated with tetanus, which attacks the central nervous system, is one of the most deadly poisons known. Wounds to the face, head and neck are the most likely to be fatal because of the proximity of these areas to the brain.

Signals of tetanus are irritability, headache, fever and painful muscular spasms. One of the most common signals of tetanus is muscular stiffness in the jaw, which is why tetanus is sometimes known as "lockjaw." It can take anywhere from 3 days to 5 weeks before these signals occur. Eventually, if the condition is not treated, every muscle in the body goes into spasms. Care for tetanus includes prompt and thorough cleansing of the wound by a medical professional, followed by a series of immunization injections. Care for tetanus is discussed further in Chapter 10.

If someone is bitten by a wild or domestic animal, try to get him or her away from the animal without endangering yourself. Do not try to restrain or capture the animal. If the wound is minor, wash it with soap and water, control any bleeding, apply triple antibiotic ointment and a dressing and take the victim to a physician or medical facility. If the wound is bleeding heavily, control the bleeding but do not clean the wound. Seek medical care immediately. The wound will be properly cleaned at a medical facility.

Contact animal control authorities, if possible and if necessary, and provide a description of the animal and the area in which the animal was last seen. In some jurisdictions, if you need to contact EMS personnel about an animal wound, they will also contact animal control authorities.

Human Bites

Human bites are quite common. Human bites differ from other bites in that they may be more contaminated, tend to occur in higher-risk areas of the body (especially on the hands) and often receive delayed care. At least 42 different species of bacteria have been reported in human saliva, so it is not surprising that serious infection often follows a human bite. According to the Centers for Disease Control and Prevention (CDC), human bites are not considered to carry a risk of transmitting human immunodeficiency virus (HIV), the virus that causes the acquired immunodeficiency syndrome (AIDS). Children are often the inflictors and the recipients of human bite wounds.

As with animal bites, it is important to get the victim of a human bite to professional medical care as soon as possible so that antibiotic therapy can be prescribed, if necessary. If the wound is not severe, wash it with soap and water, control any bleeding, apply triple antibiotic ointment and a dressing and

take the victim to a physician or medical facility. If the bite is severe, control bleeding and call 9-1-1 or the local emergency number. The wound will be properly cleaned at a medical facility.

PREVENTING BITES AND STINGS

Preventing bites and stings from insects, spiders, ticks, snakes and scorpions is the best protection against the transmission of injected poisons. When in wooded or grassy areas, follow these general guidelines to prevent bites and stings:

▶ Apply insect or tick repellent according to label instructions.
▶ Wear sturdy hiking boots.
▶ Wear long-sleeved shirts and long pants.
▶ Tuck your pant legs into your socks or boots. Tuck your shirt into your pants.
▶ Wear light-colored clothing to make it easier to see tiny insects or ticks.
▶ Use a rubber band or tape the area where pants and socks meet to prevent ticks or other insects from getting under clothing.
▶ Inspect yourself carefully for insects or ticks after being outdoors or have someone else do it. If you are outdoors for a long period of time, check yourself several times during the day. Check especially in moist, hairy areas of the body (including the back of the neck and the scalp line).
▶ Shower immediately after coming indoors, using a washcloth to scrub off any insects or ticks. Carefully inspect yourself for embedded ticks and remove them appropriately.
▶ Keep an eye out for and avoid the nests of wasps, bees and hornets.
▶ If you have pets that go outdoors, spray them with repellent made for your type of pet. Apply the repellent according to the label, and check your pet for ticks often.
▶ When hiking in woods and fields, stay in the middle of trails. Avoid underbrush, fallen trees and tall grass.
▶ Avoid walking in areas known to be populated with snakes.
▶ Make noise as you walk through areas that may be populated with snakes, because many snakes will retreat if they detect your movement.
▶ If you encounter a snake, look around, because other snakes may be nearby. Turn around and walk away, back on the same path you were just on.

If you will be in a grassy or wooded area for a length of time or if you know the area is highly infested with insects or ticks, you may want to use a repellent. Diethyltolumide (DEET) is an active ingredient in many skin-applied repellents that are effective against ticks and other insects. Repellents containing DEET can be applied on exposed areas of skin and clothing. However, repellents containing permethrin, another common repellent, should be used only on clothing.

If you use a repellent, follow these general rules:

▶ Keep all repellents out of the reach of children.
▶ To apply repellent to the face, first spray it on your hands and then apply it from your hands to your face. Avoid sensitive areas, such as the lips, eyes and near the mouth.
▶ Never spray repellents containing permethrin on your skin or a child's skin.
▶ Never use repellents on a wound or on irritated skin.
▶ Never put repellents on children's hands. Children may put their hands in their eyes or mouth.
▶ Use repellents sparingly and according to label instructions. Heavier or more frequent applications will not increase effectiveness and may be toxic.
▶ Wash treated skin with soap and water and remove clothes that have been treated after you come indoors.
▶ If you suspect you are having an allergic reaction to a repellent, wash the treated skin immediately and call a physician.

To prevent stings from marine animals, you might consider wearing a wet suit or dry suit or protective footwear in the water—especially at times when or in areas where there is a high risk of such occurrences.

To prevent dog bites, the Humane Society of the United States offers the following guidelines:

▶ Do not run past a dog. The dog's natural instinct is to chase and catch prey.
▶ If a dog threatens you, do not scream. Avoid eye contact, try to remain motionless until the dog leaves, then back away slowly until the dog is out of sight.
▶ Do not approach a strange dog, especially one that is tied or confined.
▶ Always let a dog see and sniff you before you pet the animal.

Many of the dog bites that are reported in the United States each year could have been prevented by taking these precautions.

SUMMARY

Bites and stings are one of the most common types of injected poisonings. For suspected injected poisonings, call the local or national poison control center or local emergency number. Remember, the best way to avoid any kind of poisoning is to take steps to prevent it.

APPLICATION QUESTIONS

1. Given the details of the scenario, what do you think caused Tonya's injury?

2. How should Darrell care for Tonya's injury?

3. What should Darrell consider when deciding how to get professional medical help for Tonya?

4. What could Tonya have done to help prevent her injury?

STUDY QUESTIONS

1. Match each term with the correct definition.

   a. Injected poison
   b. Lyme disease
   c. Antivenin
   d. Rabies
   e. Rocky Mountain spotted fever

   _____ An illness people get from the bite of a specific type of infected tick; victims may or may not develop a rash.

   _____ A poison introduced into the body through bites, stings or a hypodermic needle.

   _____ A substance used to counteract the poisonous effects of snake, spider or insect venom.

   _____ A disease transmitted by a certain kind of tick; victims develop a spotted rash.

   _____ A disease caused by a virus transmitted through the saliva of infected mammals.

2. List the steps of care for a tick bite.

3. Describe at least four ways to prevent bites and stings.

4. List three signals of common types of bites and stings.

5. List the steps of care for a snakebite.

6. *You are playing with your 5-year-old sister at a neighborhood park. Suddenly, a dog runs out of the bushes, jumps on your sister and bites her on the cheek. The wound is deep and bleeding heavily.*

   What should you do? Write your answer on the lines below the scenario.

   _____

   _____

   _____

In questions 7 through 12, circle the letter of the correct answer.

7. In caring for a bee sting, what should you do?

    a. Remove the remaining stinger by scraping it from the skin.
    b. Remove the remaining stinger using tweezers.
    c. Pull the stinger out with your bare hands.
    d. Rub over the stinger with an alcohol swab.

8. When spending time outdoors in woods or tall grass, what should you do to prevent bites and stings?

    a. Wear light-colored clothing.
    b. Use insect or tick repellent.
    c. Tuck pant legs into boots or socks.
    d. All of the above.

9. Which of the following are signals of Lyme disease?

    a. Trouble breathing
    b. Headache, fever, weakness, joint and muscle pain
    c. Paralysis
    d. Sneezing

10. Which of the following should you do to care for a scorpion sting?

    a. Apply suction to the wound.
    b. Wash the wound and apply a cold pack.
    c. Call 9-1-1 or the local emergency number.
    d. b and c.

11. Which of the following should you apply to a jellyfish, sea anemone or Portuguese man-of-war sting?

    a. Vinegar
    b. Meat tenderizer
    c. Baking soda paste
    d. a or c

12. Which of the following should you do to care for a severe human bite?

    a. Wash the wound with an antiseptic.
    b. Control bleeding and follow standard precautions to prevent disease transmission.
    c. Call 9-1-1 or the local emergency number immediately.
    d. b and c.

Answers are listed in Appendix A.

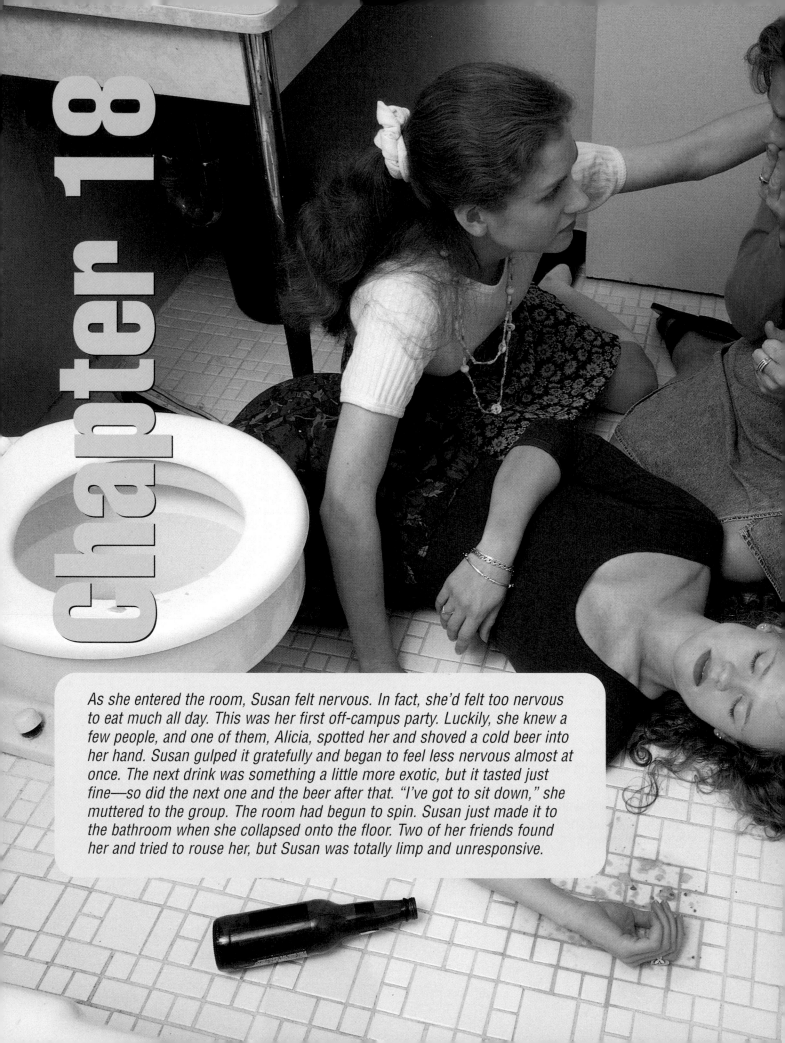

chapter 18

As she entered the room, Susan felt nervous. In fact, she'd felt too nervous to eat much all day. This was her first off-campus party. Luckily, she knew a few people, and one of them, Alicia, spotted her and shoved a cold beer into her hand. Susan gulped it gratefully and began to feel less nervous almost at once. The next drink was something a little more exotic, but it tasted just fine—so did the next one and the beer after that. "I've got to sit down," she muttered to the group. The room had begun to spin. Susan just made it to the bathroom when she collapsed onto the floor. Two of her friends found her and tried to rouse her, but Susan was totally limp and unresponsive.

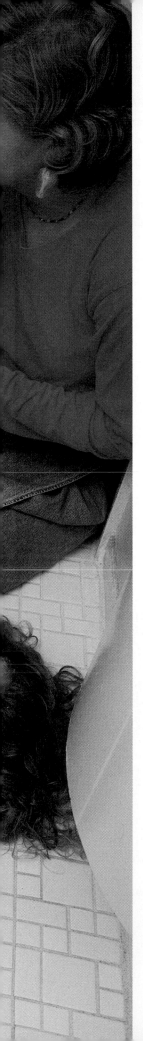

Substance Misuse and Abuse

Objectives

After reading this chapter, you should be able to—

■ *Identify the six main categories of commonly misused or abused substances.*

■ *Identify the signals that may indicate substance misuse or abuse.*

■ *Describe how to care for someone who you suspect or know is misusing or abusing a substance.*

■ *Explain how you can help prevent substance abuse or misuse.*

Introduction

Substance misuse *is the use of a substance for unintended purposes or for appropriate purposes but in improper amounts or doses.* Substance abuse *is the deliberate, persistent and excessive use of a substance without regard to health concerns or accepted medical practices. Substance abuse and misuse cost the United States billions of dollars each year in medical care, insurance and lost productivity. Even more important, however, are the lives lost or permanently impaired each year from injuries or medical emergencies related to substance abuse or misuse.*

Because of the publicity they receive, we tend to think of illegal drugs when we hear of substance abuse or misuse. However, legal substances are among those most often misused or abused. Such legal substances include nicotine (found in tobacco products), alcohol (found in beer, wine and liquor) and over-the-counter medications, such as aspirin, sleeping pills and diet pills.

This chapter will address how to recognize common forms of substance abuse and misuse, how to care for their victims and how to prevent substance misuse and abuse.

KEY TERMS

Addiction: The compulsive need to use a substance. Stopping use would cause the user to suffer mental, physical and emotional distress.

Cannabis products: Substances, such as marijuana and hashish, that are derived from the *Cannabis sativa* plant and can produce feelings of elation, distorted perceptions of time and space, and impaired motor coordination and judgment.

Dependency: When one using a drug becomes physically and psychologically addicted to the drug.

Depressants: Substances, such as tranquilizers and sleeping pills, that cause the central nervous system to slow down physical and mental activity.

Drug: Any substance, other than food or water, intended to affect the functions of the body.

Hallucinogens: Substances that affect mood, sensation, thought, emotion and self-awareness; alter perceptions of time and space; and produce hallucinations and delusions. Also known as psychedelics.

Inhalants: Substances, such as glue and paint thinners, inhaled to produce a mood-altering effect.

Medication: A drug given therapeutically to prevent or treat the effects of a disease or condition, or otherwise enhance mental or physical well-being.

Narcotics: Drugs that dull the senses and are prescribed to relieve pain.

Overdose: An excess use of a drug, resulting in adverse reactions ranging from mania and hysteria to coma and death. Specific reactions to an overdose include changes in blood pressure and heartbeat, sweating, vomiting and liver failure.

Stimulants: Substances that affect the central nervous system and increase physical and mental activity.

Substance abuse: The deliberate, persistent, excessive use of a substance without regard to health concerns or accepted medical practices.

Substance misuse: The use of a substance for unintended purposes, or for intended purposes but in improper amounts or doses.

Synergistic effect: The interaction of two or more drugs to produce a certain effect.

Tolerance: The body becomes resistant to a drug or other substance because of continued use.

Withdrawal: The condition produced when a person stops using or abusing a substance to which he or she is addicted.

EFFECTS OF SUBSTANCE MISUSE AND ABUSE

Substance abuse and misuse pose a very serious threat to the health of millions of Americans. According to the Drug Abuse Warning Network (DAWN), drug-related emergency department admissions are at an all-time high. The number of emergency department patients who say that they have used illegal substances has risen dramatically. The greatest increase is in the number of people who admit to using cocaine and crack—more than a 47 percent increase since 1995.

According to the *National Vital Statistics Reports*, over 40,000 Americans died as a result of drug- or alcohol-induced deaths in 2001. This figure does not include unintentional injuries, homicides and other causes indirectly related to drug use. Experts estimate that as many as two-thirds of all homicides and serious assaults occurring annually involve alcohol alone. Other problems directly or indirectly related to substance abuse include dropping out of school; adolescent pregnancy; suicide; involvement in crime; and transmission of the human immunodeficiency virus (HIV), the virus that causes acquired immunodeficiency syndrome (AIDS).

FORMS OF SUBSTANCE MISUSE AND ABUSE

Many substances that are abused or misused are not illegal. Other substances are legal only when prescribed by a physician. Some are illegal only for underage users (for example, alcohol). **Figure 18-1** shows some commonly misused and abused substances that are legal.

A *drug* is any substance, other than food or water, taken to affect body functions. A drug given therapeutically to prevent or treat the effects of a disease or condition or otherwise enhance mental or physical well-being is a *medication*. Any drug can cause *dependency*, when one using a drug becomes physically and psychologically addicted to the drug.

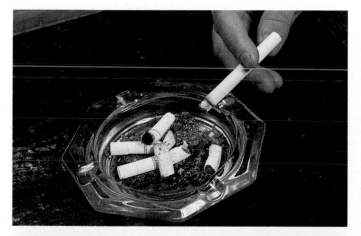
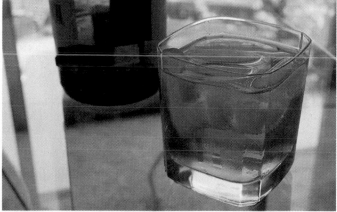
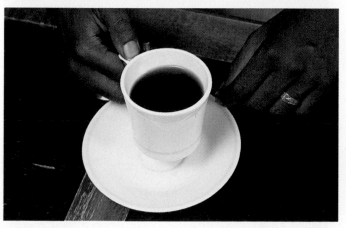
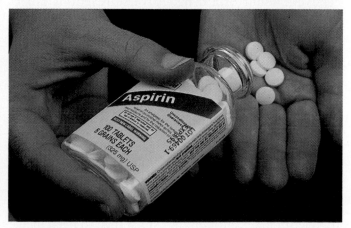

Figure 18-1   Misused and abused substances.

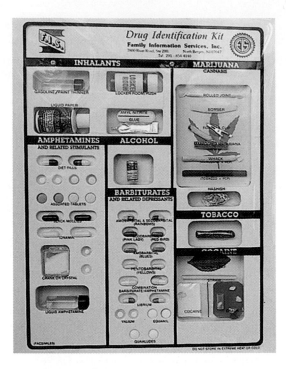
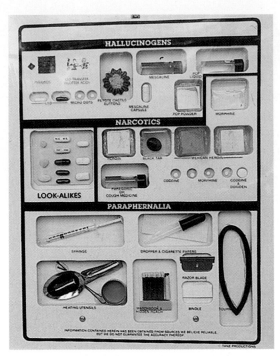

Figure 18-2 Substance abuse and misuse involve a broad range of improperly used legal and illegal substances.

The victim feels that he or she needs the drug to function normally. Those with a compulsive need for a substance and who would suffer mental, physical and emotional distress if they stopped taking it are said to have an *addiction* to that substance. **Figure 18-2** shows a variety of legal and illegal substances that are commonly misused.

When one continually uses a substance, its effects on the body decrease—the condition is called *tolerance.* The person then has to increase the dose and frequency of the substance to obtain the intended effect.

An *overdose* occurs when someone uses an excessive amount of a drug. Adverse reactions range from mania and hysteria to coma and death. Specific reactions include changes in blood pressure and heartbeat, sweating, vomiting and liver failure. An overdose may occur unintentionally if a person takes too much medication at one time, for example, when someone forgets that he or she took one dose of a medication and takes an additional dose too soon (**Fig. 18-3**).

An overdose may also be intentional, such as in suicide attempts. Sometimes the victim takes a sufficiently high dose of a substance to be certain to cause death. Other times, to gain attention or help, the victim takes enough of a substance to need medical attention but not enough to cause death.

The term *withdrawal* describes the condition produced when a person suddenly stops using or abusing a drug to which he or she is addicted. Stopping the use of a substance may occur as a deliberate decision or because the person is unable to obtain the specific drug. Withdrawal from certain substances, such as alcohol, can cause severe mental and physical discomfort. Because withdrawal may become a serious medical condition, medical professionals often oversee the process.

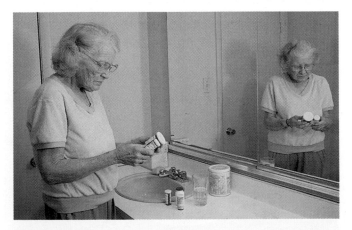

Figure 18-3 Overdose can occur when a person unintentionally takes an extra dose.

A heightened or exaggerated effect may be produced when two or more substances are used at the same time. This is called a *synergistic effect.* The drug most commonly used in combination with other drugs is alcohol.

MISUSED AND ABUSED SUBSTANCES

Substances are categorized according to their effects on the body. The six major categories are stimulants, hallucinogens, depressants, narcotics, inhalants and cannabis products. The category to which a substance belongs depends mostly on the way the substance is taken or the effects it has on the central nervous system. Some substances depress the nervous system, whereas others speed up its activity. Some are not easily categorized because they have various effects or may be taken in a variety of ways. **Table 18-1** lists commonly abused and misused substances.

Stimulants

Stimulants are drugs that affect the central nervous system by increasing physical and mental activity. They produce temporary feelings of alertness and prevention of fatigue. They are sometimes used for weight reduction because they also suppress appetite.

Many stimulants are ingested as pills, but some can be absorbed or inhaled. Amphetamines, dextroamphetamines and methamphetamines are stimulants. Their slang names include uppers, bennies, black beauties, speed, crystal, meth and crank. One dangerous stimulant is called ice. Ice is an extremely addictive, smokeable form of methamphetamine.

Cocaine is one of the most publicized and powerful stimulants. Cocaine can be taken into the body in different ways. The most common way is sniffing it in powder form, a practice known as snorting. In this method, the drug is absorbed into the blood through capillaries in the nose. A purer and more potent form of cocaine is crack. Crack is smoked. The vapors that are inhaled into the lungs reach the brain and cause almost immediate effects. Crack is highly addictive.

Interestingly, the most common stimulants in America are legal. Leading the list is caffeine, which is present in coffee, tea, many kinds of sodas, chocolate, diet pills and pills used to combat fatigue. The next most common stimulant is nicotine,

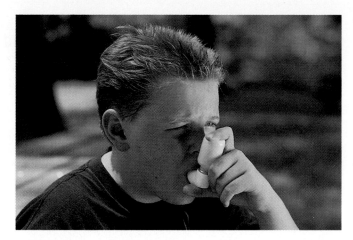

Figure 18-4   Medication used to treat asthma is a common legal stimulant.

found in tobacco products. Other stimulants used for medical purposes are asthma medications or decongestants that can be taken by mouth or inhaled (**Fig. 18-4**).

Hallucinogens

Hallucinogens, also known as psychedelics, are substances that cause changes in mood, sensation, thought, emotion and self-awareness. They alter one's perception of time and space and may produce visual, auditory and tactile delusions.

Hallucinogens often have physical effects similar to stimulants but are classified differently because of the other effects they produce. Hallucinogens sometimes cause what is called a "bad trip." A bad trip can involve intense fear, panic, paranoid delusions, vivid hallucinations, profound depression, tension and anxiety. The victim may be irrational and feel threatened by any attempt others make to help.

Among the most widely abused hallucinogens are lysergic acid diethylamide (LSD), called acid; psilocybin, called mushrooms; phencyclidine (PCP), called angel dust; and mescaline, called peyote, buttons or mesc. These substances are usually ingested, but PCP also can be inhaled.

Depressants

Depressants are substances that affect the central nervous system by decreasing physical and mental activity. Depressants are commonly used for med-

Table 18-1 Commonly Misused and Abused Substances

CATEGORY	SUBSTANCES	POSSIBLE EFFECTS
Stimulants	Caffeine Cocaine, crack cocaine Methamphetamines Amphetamines Dextroamphetamines Nicotine Over-the-counter diet aids Asthma treatments	Increase mental and physical activity, produce temporary feelings of alertness, prevent fatigue, suppress appetite.
Hallucinogens	LSD (lysergic acid diethylamide) PCP (phencyclidine) Mescaline Peyote Psilocybin	Cause changes in mood, sensation, thought, emotion and self-awareness; alter perceptions of time and space; may produce profound depression, tension and anxiety, as well as visual, auditory or tactile hallucinations.
Depressants	Barbiturates Narcotics Alcohol Antihistamines Sedatives Tranquilizers Over-the-counter sleep aids	Decrease mental and physical activity, alter consciousness, relieve anxiety and pain, promote sleep, depress respiration, relax muscles and impair coordination and judgment.
Narcotics	Morphine Codeine Heroin Methadone Opium	Relieve pain, may produce stupor or euphoria, may cause coma or death and are highly addictive.
Inhalants	Medical anesthetics Gasoline and kerosene Glues in organic cements Lighter fluid Paint and varnish thinners Aerosol propellants	Alter moods; may produce a partial or complete loss of feeling; may produce effects similar to drunkenness, such as slurred speech, lack of inhibitions and impaired motor coordination. Can also cause damage to the heart, lungs, brain and liver.

ical purposes. They relieve anxiety, promote sleep, depress respiration, relieve pain, relax muscles and impair coordination and judgment. Like other substances, the larger the dose or the stronger the substance, the greater its effects. Common depressants are barbiturates, benzodiazepines, narcotics and alcohol. Most depressants are ingested or injected.

Alcohol is the most widely used and abused substance in the United States (**Fig. 18-5**). In small

amounts, its effects may be fairly mild. In higher amounts, its effects can be toxic.

Alcohol is like other depressants in its effects and risks for overdose. Frequent drinkers may become dependent on the effects of alcohol and increasingly tolerant of those effects. Drinking alcohol frequently or in large amounts causes many unhealthy consequences. Alcohol poisoning can occur when a large amount of alcohol is consumed in

Table 18-1 Commonly Misused and Abused Substances (Continued)

CATEGORY	SUBSTANCES	POSSIBLE EFFECTS
Cannabis products	Hashish Marijuana THC (tetrahydrocannabinol)	Produce feelings of elation, increase appetite, distort perceptions of time and space and impair motor coordination and judgment. May irritate throat, redden eyes, increase pulse and cause dizziness.
Other	MDMA (methylenedioxymethamphetamine or ecstasy)	Elevate blood pressure and produce euphoria or erratic mood swings, rapid heartbeat, profuse sweating, agitation and sensory distortions.
	Anabolic steroids	Enhance physical performance, increase muscle mass and stimulate appetite and weight gain. Chronic use can cause sterility, disruption of normal growth, liver cancer, personality changes and aggressive behavior.
	Aspirin	Relieve minor pain and reduces fever. Can impair normal blood clotting and cause inflammation of the stomach and small intestine.
	Laxatives	Relieve constipation. Can cause uncontrolled diarrhea and dehydration.
	Decongestant nasal sprays	Relieve congestion and swelling of nasal passages. Chronic use can cause nosebleeds and changes in the lining of the nose, making breathing difficult without sprays.

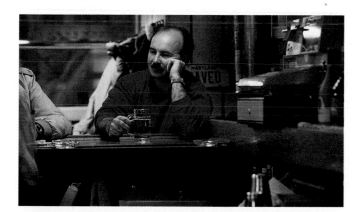

Figure 18-5   Alcohol is the most widely used and abused substance in the United States.

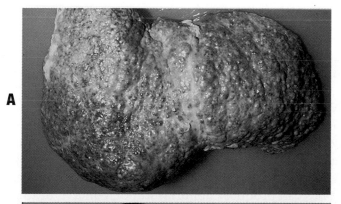

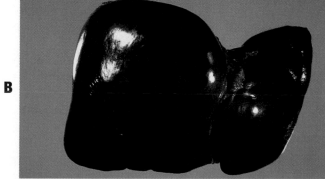

a short period of time. Alcohol poisoning can result in unconsciousness and, if untreated, death.

Chronic drinking can also affect the brain and cause a lack of coordination, memory loss and apathy. Other problems include liver disease, such as cirrhosis (**Fig. 18-6,** *A* and *B*). In addition, many psychological, family, social and work problems are related to chronic drinking.

Figure 18-6   **A,** Chronic drinking can result in cirrhosis, a disease of the liver. **B,** A healthy liver.

The Incalculable Cost of Alcohol Abuse

The hospital morgue is full: a teenager who drowned while boating, an elderly man who died of a chronic liver disease, and a woman who was shot by her boyfriend. The victims seem to share no connection other than that each body lies in the same morgue.

But there is a connection: alcohol.

Public health officials are seeing a growing number of injuries, illnesses and other social problems in which alcohol plays a role. More than 100,000 people die each year from alcohol-related causes. From the child abused by her alcoholic parent to the driver who drinks and causes a six-car pileup, our country feels the impact of alcohol abuse.

Each year, alcohol-related motor vehicle crashes result in approximately 17,500 deaths in the United States. According to the Centers for Disease Control and Prevention (CDC), alcohol impaired driving is the highest among drivers ages 21 to 24 years, and is a leading cause of death among persons ages 16 to 25 years. Nearly one-third of all drownings involve alcohol. In 2002, alcohol was involved in at least 39 percent of all boating fatalities, making alcohol the ninth leading cause of boating accidents.

Studies have shown that reckless and violent behavior have been linked to alcohol abuse. Nearly one-half of all homicides, one-third of all suicides and two-thirds of all assaults involve alcohol. One of the best predictors of violence is alcohol abuse. Crime and other social problems are also linked to alcohol. Social workers find alcohol abuse a factor in nearly 50 percent of child abuse cases. Alcohol abuse ranges from 20 percent to 45 percent among the homeless.

These personal and social consequences to alcohol abuse create a tremendous economic burden. According to the National Institute on Drug Abuse, the cost of alcohol addiction runs an estimated $118 billion annually. This cost is associated with

Narcotics

Narcotics, derived from opium, are drugs that work on the central nervous system to relieve pain. Narcotics are so powerful and highly addictive that all are illegal without a prescription, and some are not prescribed at all. When taken in large doses, narcotics can produce euphoria, stupor, coma or death. The most common natural narcotics are morphine and codeine. Most other narcotics, including heroin, are synthetic or semisynthetic.

Heroin abuse is associated with serious health conditions such as fatal overdoses, spontaneous abortion, collapsed veins and infectious diseases such as HIV and hepatitis B. Other possible effects of long-term abuse include infection of the heart lining and valves, abscesses and liver disease. In addition, street heroin may have additives that do not readily dissolve in the bloodstream, which could create a blockage in blood vessels leading to vital organs, such as the lungs, heart or brain.

One of the most detrimental effects of long-term heroin use is addiction. A person who uses heroin on a regular basis develops a tolerance for the drug and must use increasingly larger doses to achieve the same intensity of his or her first "rush." Over time, the person becomes physically dependent on the drug. In some cases, the dependency can be so strong that a person begins to experience signals of withdrawal within hours after his or her last dose.

Inhalants

Substances inhaled to produce mood-altering effects are called *inhalants*. Inhalants also depress the central nervous system. Inhalants include medical anesthetics, such as amyl nitrite and nitrous oxide (also known as laughing gas), as well as hydrocarbons, known as solvents. Solvents' effects are similar to those of alcohol. People who use solvents may aptime missed from work, reduced job productivity, medical bills, support for families and property damage.

In terms of economic cost, lives and productivity, alcohol abuse outdistances cocaine, heroin and all other drugs.

Health-care costs account for $15 billion to $20 billion of alcohol costs, and research documenting the detrimental health effects of alcohol is growing. Physicians now say that even moderate drinking increases risks of high blood pressure, cirrhosis of the liver and decreased motor development for children whose mothers drink while pregnant. Prolonged or heavy drinking can cause serious long-term effects, including risk of heart attack; many cancers; stroke; gastrointestinal bleeding; kidney failure; and problems of the nervous system, such as tremors and dementia.

SOURCES

Centers for Disease Control and Prevention. Behavioral Risk Factor Surveillance System survey data. U.S. Department of Health and Human Services, 1999, *www.cdc.gov/brfss*. Accessed 08/31/04.

Centers for Disease Control and Prevention, "Measures of Alcohol Consumption and Alcohol-Related Health Effects from Excessive Consumption," U.S. Department of Health and Human Services. *www.cdc.gov/alcohol/factsheets/general_information.htm*. Accessed 08/31/04.

National Center for Injury Prevention and Control, Water Related Injuries Fact Sheet, U.S. Department of Health and Human Services, *www.cdc.gov/ncipc/factsheets/drown.htm*. Accessed 08/31/04.

United States Coast Guard, Boating Statistics—2003, U.S. Department of Homeland Security. Accessed 10/08/04.

www.uscgboating.org/statistics/Boating_Statistics_2003.pdf. Accessed 12/14/04.

pear to be drunk. Solvents include toluene, found in glues; butane, found in lighter fluids; acetone, found in nail polish removers; fuels, such as gasoline and kerosene; and propellants, found in aerosol sprays.

The use of inhalants can damage the heart, lungs, brain and liver. Abusing specific solvents can also lead to irreversible hearing loss and uncontrollable spasms in the arms and legs.

Cannabis Products

Cannabis products, including marijuana, tetrahydrocannabinol, or THC, and hashish are all derived from the plant *Cannabis sativa.* Marijuana is the most widely used illicit drug in the United States. It is typically smoked in cigarette form or in a pipe. The effects include feelings of elation, distorted perceptions of time and space and impaired judgment and motor coordination. Marijuana irritates the throat; reddens the eyes; and causes a rapid pulse, dizziness and often an increased appetite. Depending on the dose, the user and many other factors, cannabis products can produce effects similar to those of other substances.

Marijuana, although illicit, has been used for some medicinal purposes. Marijuana or its legal synthetic versions are used as an antinausea medication for people who are undergoing chemotherapy for cancer, for treating glaucoma, for treating muscular weakness caused by multiple sclerosis, and to combat the weight loss caused by cancer and AIDS.

Other Substances

Some other substances do not fit neatly into these categories. These substances include designer drugs, steroids and over-the-counter substances that can be purchased without a prescription.

Designer Drugs

Designer drugs are variations of other substances, such as narcotics and amphetamines. Through simple and inexpensive methods, the molecular structure of substances produced for medicinal purposes can be modified by chemists to produce extremely potent and dangerous street drugs; hence the term designer drug. When the chemical makeup of a drug is altered, the user can experience a variety of unpredictable and dangerous effects. The chemist may have no knowledge of the effects a new designer drug might produce. One designer drug, a form of the commonly used surgical anesthetic fentanyl, can be made 2000 to 6000 times stronger than its original form.

One of the more commonly used designer drugs is methylenedioxymethamphetamine (MDMA), often called ecstasy. Although ecstasy is structurally related to stimulants and hallucinogens, its effects differ somewhat from either category. Ecstasy can evoke a euphoric high that makes it popular. Other signals of ecstasy use range from the stimulant-like effects of increased blood pressure, rapid heartbeat, profuse sweating and agitation to the hallucinogenic-like effects of paranoia, sensory distortion and erratic mood swings.

Anabolic Steroids

Anabolic steroids are drugs sometimes used by athletes to enhance performance and increase muscle mass (**Fig. 18-7**). Their medical uses include stimu-

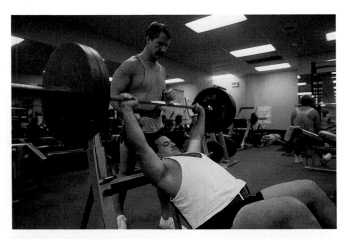

Figure 18-7 Anabolic steroids are drugs sometimes used by athletes to enhance performance and increase muscle mass.

lating weight gain for persons unable to gain weight naturally. They should not be confused with corticosteroids, which are used to counteract the toxic effects of and allergic reactions to absorbed poisons, such as poison ivy. Chronic use of anabolic steroids can lead to sterility, liver cancer and personality changes, such as aggressive behavior. Steroid use by younger people may also disrupt normal growth.

Over-the-Counter Substances

Aspirin, laxatives and nasal sprays are among the most commonly misused or abused over-the-counter substances. Aspirin is an effective minor pain reliever and fever reducer that is found in a variety of medicines. People use aspirin for many reasons and conditions. In recent years, cardiologists have praised the benefits of aspirin for the treatment of heart disease. As useful as aspirin is, misuse can have toxic effects on the body. Typically, aspirin can cause inflammation of the stomach and small intestine that results in bleeding ulcers. Aspirin can also impair normal blood clotting.

Laxatives are used to relieve constipation. They come in a variety of forms and strengths. If used improperly, laxatives can cause uncontrolled diarrhea that may result in dehydration. The very young and the elderly are particularly susceptible to dehydration.

The abuse of laxatives is frequently associated with attempted weight loss and eating disorders, such as anorexia nervosa or bulimia. **Anorexia nervosa** is a disorder that typically affects young women and is characterized by a long-term refusal to eat food with sufficient nutrients and calories. Anorexics typically use laxatives to keep from gaining weight. **Bulimia** is a condition in which victims gorge themselves with food, then purge by vomiting or using laxatives. For this reason, the behavior associated with bulimia is often referred to as "binging and purging." Anorexia nervosa and bulimia both have underlying psychological factors that contribute to their onset. The effect of both of these eating disorders is severe malnutrition, which can result in death.

Antihistamines, such as decongestant nasal sprays, can help relieve the congestion of colds or hay fever (**Fig. 18-8**). If misused, they can cause physical dependency. Using the spray over a long period can cause nosebleeds and changes in the lin-

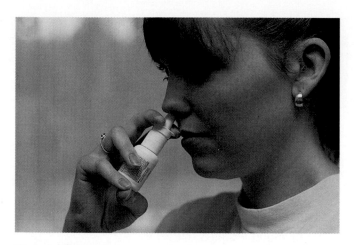

Figure 18-8 Antihistamines, such as nasal sprays, are used to relieve the congestion of colds and allergies but, if misused, can cause dependency.

ing of the nose that make breathing difficult without the spray.

SIGNALS OF SUBSTANCE MISUSE AND ABUSE

Many of the signals of substance misuse and abuse are similar to those of other medical emergencies. You should not necessarily assume that someone who is stumbling, is disoriented or has a fruity, alcohol-like odor on the breath is intoxicated by alcohol or other drugs. Instead, he or she may be a victim of a diabetic emergency (see Chapter 15).

The misuse or abuse of stimulants can have many unhealthy effects on the body, which mimic other conditions. For example, a stimulant overdose can cause moist or flushed skin, sweating, chills, nausea, vomiting, fever, headache, dizziness, rapid pulse, rapid breathing, high blood pressure and chest pain. In some instances, a stimulant overdose can cause respiratory distress, disrupt normal heart rhythms or cause death. The victim may appear very excited, restless, talkative or irritable or the victim may suddenly lose consciousness. Stimulant abuse can lead to addiction and can cause a heart attack or stroke.

Specific signals of hallucinogen abuse may include sudden mood changes and a flushed face. The victim may claim to see or hear something not present. He or she may be anxious and frightened.

Specific signals of depressant abuse may include drowsiness, confusion, slurred speech, slowed heart

and breathing rates and poor coordination. A person who abuses alcohol may smell of alcohol. A person who has consumed a great deal of alcohol in a short time may be unconscious or hard to arouse. The person may vomit violently.

Specific signals of alcohol withdrawal, a potentially dangerous condition, include confusion and restlessness, trembling, hallucinations and seizures.

CARE FOR SUBSTANCE MISUSE AND ABUSE

As in other medical emergencies, you do not have to diagnose substance misuse or abuse to give care. Follow these general principles as you would for any poisoning:

▶ Check the scene to be sure it is safe to help the person. Do not approach the victim if he or she is behaving in a threatening manner.
▶ Call 9-1-1, the local emergency number or the poison control center.
▶ Check for any life-threatening conditions.
▶ Care for any conditions you find.

Because many of the physical signals of substance abuse mimic other conditions, you should not assume that a victim has overdosed on a substance. Always check for life-threatening conditions and give care as you would for any victim of a sudden illness or injury.

People who misuse or abuse substances may become aggressive or uncooperative. If the person becomes agitated or makes the scene unsafe in any way, go to a safe place and wait for EMS personnel and the police. *Give care only if you feel the person is not a danger to you and others.*

If possible, interview the victim or bystanders to try to find out what substance was taken, how much was taken and when it was taken. You may be able to find clues that suggest the nature of the problem. Such clues may help you provide more complete information to EMS personnel. Look for containers, pill bottles, drug paraphernalia and signals of other medical problems. If you suspect that someone has used a designer drug, tell EMS personnel. Telling EMS personnel your suspicions is important because a person who has overdosed on a designer drug frequently may not respond to usual medical treatment.

Steroids: Body Meltdown

If you think using steroids is the way to get those sculpted, muscular bodies that are typical of body-builders and many professional athletes, think again. These drugs may build up bodies on the outside, but they can cause a body meltdown on the inside. Physicians and other public health officials warn of the dangers of steroid abuse and are particularly concerned about the long-term effects of high doses. Anabolic steroids are synthetic chemicals that mimic the hormone testosterone. Testosterone gives a male his masculine characteristics—deeper voice, beard and mustache and other sex characteristics. Anabolic steroids have several legitimate, legal uses. They are prescribed by physicians to treat skeletal and growth disorders, certain types of anemia, some kinds of breast cancer and to offset the negative effects of irradiation and chemotherapy.

Steroids are also used illegally to create proteins and other substances that build muscle tissue, which is why they are popular with some athletes and body-builders. In recent years, several professional athletes have made the headlines because of their abuse of steroids. Physicians are now getting a better idea of the devastating effects that illegal steroids can have on the body. The problem is that some young athletes and bodybuilders are listening to their gym buddies rather than their physicians. Steroids are being used in larger doses than ever before and at younger ages. Although both young males and females abuse steroids, the abuse of steroids among young males is becoming as prevalent as eating disorders have become in young females.

Before you listen to another person's justification of steroids, consider these effects:

- **Stunted growth.** In children, steroids cause the growth plates in the bones to close prematurely. As a teenager, you may have been destined to be 6-foot-4, but taking steroids can permanently stunt your growth.

- **Heart disease and stroke.** Steroids cause dangerous changes in cholesterol levels. One study found dramatic drops in the amount of good cholesterol or high-density lipoprotein (HDL), which helps remove the fatty deposits on the artery walls, in steroid users. The research also shows dramatic increases in bad cholesterol or low-density lipoprotein (LDL), which clogs the arteries and causes heart problems. Your steroid-doped body may look fine on the outside, but inside it may look like the body of a man in his 50s whose arteries are so clogged that he needs heart surgery.

- **Aggressive personality and psychological disorders.** Some people who take anabolic steroids become unnaturally aggressive. A few have devel-

PREVENTING SUBSTANCE ABUSE

Experts in the field of substance abuse generally agree that prevention efforts are far more cost effective than treatment. Yet, preventing substance abuse is a complex process that involves many underlying factors. Various approaches, including educating people about substances and their effects on health and attempting to instill fear of penalties, have not by themselves proved particularly effective. To be effective, prevention efforts must address the various underlying factors of and approaches to substance abuse.

The following factors may contribute to substance abuse:

▸ A lack of parental supervision.
▸ The breakdown of traditional family structures.

oped documentable mental disorders. In a *Sports Illustrated* article, a South Carolina football player described his nightmare with steroids. He described pulling a gun on a pizza delivery boy in his dorm and how his family intervened when he began threatening suicide. Many physicians feel the psychiatric effects of steroids may be their most threatening side effect.

- **Lowered white blood cell count.** Taking steroids also reduces the number of white blood cells in your body. With fewer white blood cells, your body has fewer antibodies to fight off infections, including cancers and other diseases.

- **Sexual dysfunction and disorders.** Synthetic steroids cause your body to cut off its own natural production of steroids, resulting in shrinking testicles in men. Women may grow facial hair, breast size may decrease and voice may become permanently deeper. In both sexes, steroids may cause sterility and reduced sexual interest.

- **Impaired liver function and liver disease.** Steroids seriously affect the liver's ability to function. They irritate the liver, causing tissue damage and an inability to clear bile. Physicians also have found blood-filled benign tumors in the livers of steroid users.

Steroids pose dangers beyond these physiological side effects. Because steroids are often sold on the black market, they are increasingly sold by drug traffickers who obtain their wares from unsanitary laboratories. Yet another danger comes from the fact that sharing needles to inject steroids increases the transmission of viruses such as HIV and hepatitis.

SOURCES

Altman L: New breakfast of champions: a recipe for victory or disaster?, *The New York Times*, November 20, 1988.

Chaikin T, Telander R: The nightmare of steroids, *Sports Illustrated*, 69:18, 1988.

National Institute on Drug Abuse. "Anabolic steroids: a threat to body and mind." National Institutes of Health, No. 94-3721,1991. *www.drugabuse.gov/ResearchReports/Steroids/AnabolicSteroids.html*. Accessed 09/01/04.

USA Today, Vol. 121, No. 2573, February 1993.

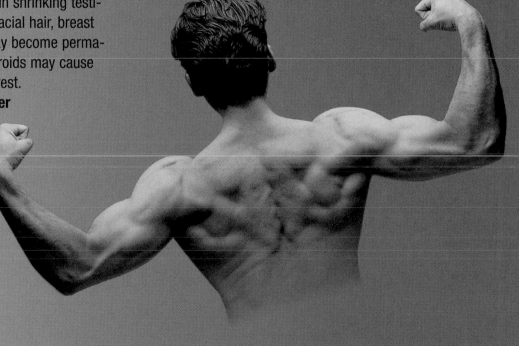

- A wish to escape unpleasant surroundings and stressful situations.
- The widespread availability of substances.
- Peer pressure and the basic need to belong.
- Low self-esteem, including feelings of guilt or shame.
- Media glamorization, especially of alcohol and tobacco, promoting the idea that using substances enhances fun and popularity.

- A history of substance abuse in the home or community environments.

Recognizing and understanding these factors may help prevent substance abuse.

SOURCES OF HELP FOR VICTIMS OF SUBSTANCE ABUSE

Al-Anon Family Group Headquarters, Inc.
www.al-anon.org

Alcoholics Anonymous
www.alcoholics-anonymous.org

Cocaine Anonymous
www.ca.org/phones.html

Mothers Against Drunk Driving (MADD)
www.madd.org.home

Narcotics Anonymous
www.na.org

National Council on Alcoholism and Drug Dependence Helpline
(800) 622-2255

Remove Intoxicated Drivers (RID)
www.crisny.org/not-for-profit/ridusa

Students Against Driving Drunk (SADD)
www.saddonline.com

U.S. Department of Health and Human Services Substance Abuse and Mental Health Services Administration
www.samhsa.gov/index.aspx

After a substance abuse emergency, the victim may need additional support to overcome addiction. If you know the victim, you may be able to help him or her contact one of the many agencies and organizations that offer ongoing assistance to victims of substance abuse. Community-based programs through schools and religious institutions provide access to hot lines and local support groups. Some of the resources listed above may have facilities or contacts in your area. Look on the internet or in the advertising pages of the telephone book under Counseling; Drug Abuse and Addiction Information; Social Service Organizations; or Clinics and Health Services for additional resources.

PREVENTING SUBSTANCE MISUSE

Some poisonings from medicines occur when the victims knowingly increase the dosage beyond what is directed. The best way to prevent such misuse is to take medications only as directed. On the other hand, many poisonings from medicinal substances are not intentional. The following guidelines can help prevent unintentional misuse or overdose:

▶ Read the product information and use products only as directed.
▶ Ask your physician or pharmacist about the intended use and side effects of prescription and over-the-counter medications. If you are taking more than one medication, check for possible interaction effects.
▶ Never use another person's prescribed medications; what is right for one person is seldom right for another.
▶ Always keep medications in their appropriate, marked containers.
▶ Destroy all out-of-date medications. Time can alter the chemical composition of medications, causing them to be less effective and possibly even toxic.
▶ Always keep medications out of the reach of children.

SUMMARY

There are six major categories of substances that, when abused or misused, can produce a variety of signals, some of which are indistinguishable from those of other medical emergencies. Remember, you do not have to diagnose the condition to give care. If you suspect that the victim's condition is caused by substance misuse or abuse, give care for a poisoning emergency. Call 9-1-1 or the local emergency number or poison control center personnel and follow their directions. Also call the police if necessary. If the victim becomes violent or threatening, go to a safe place and wait for EMS personnel and police to arrive.

APPLICATION QUESTIONS

1. What are the signals of Susan's condition?

3. Should Susan's friends call 9-1-1 or the local emergency number? Why or why not?

2. What do you think is the cause of Susan's condition? Can you be sure?

STUDY QUESTIONS

1. Match each term with the correct definition.

   a. Addiction
   b. Dependency
   c. Medication
   d. Drug

   e. Overdose
   f. Substance abuse
   g. Tolerance
   h. Withdrawal

   _____ Deliberate, persistent, excessive use of a substance.

   _____ A drug given to prevent or treat a disease, or otherwise enhance mental or physical well-being.

   _____ Any substance other than food intended to affect the functions of the body.

   _____ An excess use of a drug, resulting in adverse reactions ranging from mania and hysteria to coma and death; specific reactions include changes in blood pressure and heartbeat, sweating, vomiting and liver failure.

   _____ The compulsive desire or need to use a substance.

   _____ The condition produced when a person stops using or abusing a substance to which he or she is addicted.

   _____ A desire to continually use a substance, out of a feeling that it is needed to function normally.

   _____ A condition that occurs when a substance user has to increase the dose and frequency of use of a substance to obtain the desired effect.

2. List four signals that might indicate substance abuse or misuse.

3. List four commonly misused or abused legal substances.

4. List four things you can do to prevent unintentional substance misuse.

5. Describe the care for a victim of suspected substance misuse or abuse.

6. Match each type of substance with the effects it has on the body.

a. Depressants
b. Hallucinogens
c. Inhalants
d. Stimulants
e. Narcotics
f. Cannabis products

_____ Affect mood, sensation, thought, emotion and self-awareness; alter perception of time and space; and produce hallucinations and delusions.

_____ Produce mood-altering effects similar to those of alcohol. Found in glues and solvents.

_____ Slow down the physical activities of the brain, producing temporary feelings of relaxation.

_____ Speed up the physical and mental activity of the brain, producing temporary feelings of alertness and improved task performance.

_____ Relieve pain.

_____ Produce feelings of elation, disoriented perceptions of time and space and impaired judgment.

In questions 7 through 9, circle the letter of the correct answer.

7. Which of the following is true of substance abuse?

a. It occurs only among the elderly who are forgetful and may have poor eyesight.
b. It is the use of a substance for intended purposes but in improper amounts or doses.
c. It is the use of a substance without regard to health concerns or accepted medical practices.
d. Its effects are minor and rarely result in medical complications.

8. The effects of designer drugs are—

a. Well-known.
b. Unpredictable.
c. Harmless.
d. Easily controlled.

9. Which of the following guidelines can help prevent unintentional substance misuse?

a. Read the product information and use only as directed.
b. Check for possible interaction effects if you are taking more than one medication.
c. Destroy all out-of-date medications.
d. All of the above.

Answers are listed in Appendix A.

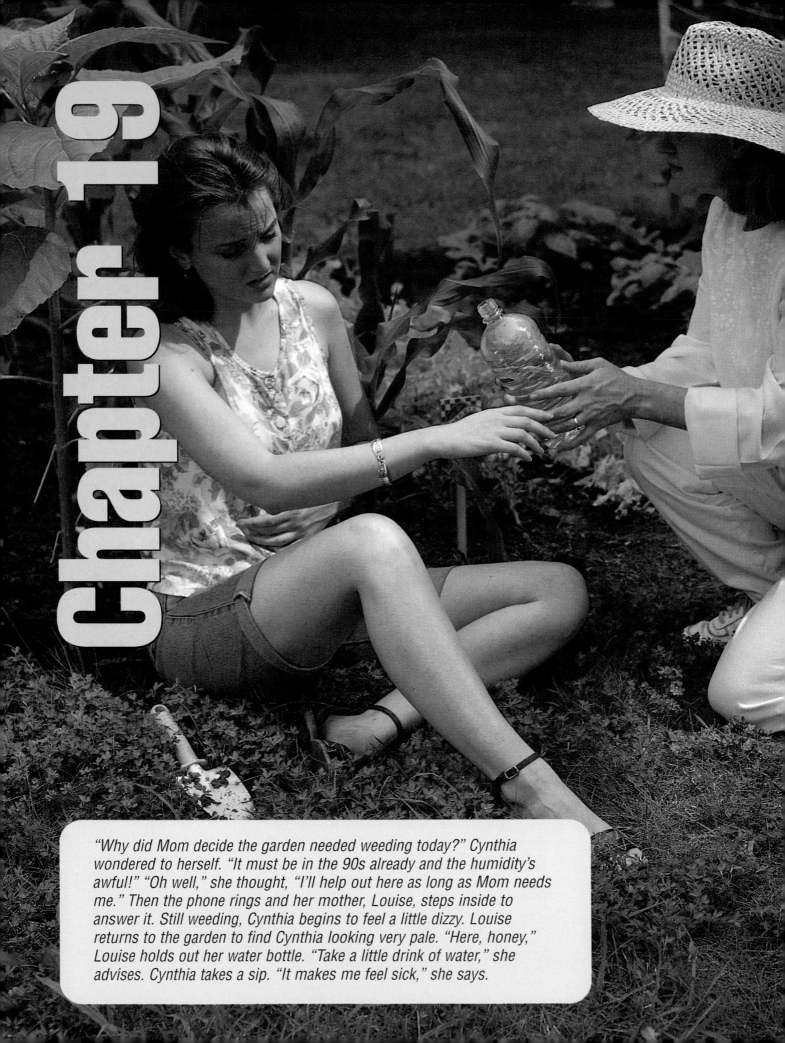

Chapter 19

"Why did Mom decide the garden needed weeding today?" Cynthia wondered to herself. "It must be in the 90s already and the humidity's awful!" "Oh well," she thought, "I'll help out here as long as Mom needs me." Then the phone rings and her mother, Louise, steps inside to answer it. Still weeding, Cynthia begins to feel a little dizzy. Louise returns to the garden to find Cynthia looking very pale. "Here, honey," Louise holds out her water bottle. "Take a little drink of water," she advises. Cynthia takes a sip. "It makes me feel sick," she says.

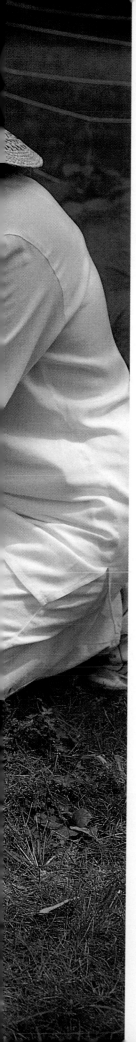

Heat- and Cold-Related Emergencies

Objectives

After reading this chapter, you should be able to—

■ *Describe how body temperature is controlled.*

■ *Identify three main factors that influence how well the body maintains its temperature.*

■ *Identify seven risk factors that increase a person's susceptibility to a heat- or cold-related emergency.*

■ *List the signals of heat cramps, heat exhaustion and heat stroke.*

■ *Describe the care for heat cramps, heat exhaustion and heat stroke.*

■ *List the signals of frostbite and hypothermia.*

■ *Describe the care for frostbite and hypothermia.*

■ *Describe five ways to help prevent heat- and cold-related emergencies.*

Introduction

The human body is equipped to withstand extremes in temperature. Under normal circumstances, its mechanisms for regulating body temperature work very well. However, when the body is overwhelmed, a heat- or cold-related emergency can occur. A heat- or cold-related emergency can happen anywhere—indoors or outdoors and under a variety of conditions. The signals of a heat- or cold-related emergency are progressive and can quickly become life threatening. A person can develop a heat- or cold-related emergency even when temperatures are not extreme. The effects of humidity, wind, clothing, living and working environments; physical activity; age; and health all play a role in determining an individual's susceptibility. In this chapter, you will learn how to recognize and give care for a victim of a heat- or cold-related emergency.

HOW BODY TEMPERATURE IS CONTROLLED

In order to work efficiently, the human body must maintain a constant temperature. Normal body temperature is 98.6° F (37° C). The body maintains its temperature by balancing heat loss with heat production. The amount of heat exchanged between the environment and the body is determined by the difference in temperature between the body and the environment.

Body heat is generated primarily through the conversion of food to energy. Heat is also produced by muscle contractions, as in exercise or shivering. Because the body is usually warmer than the surrounding air, it tends to lose heat to the air (**Fig. 19-1**). The heat produced in routine activities is usually enough to compensate for normal heat loss.

In a warm environment, a part of the brain called the *hypothalmus* detects an increase in blood temperature and sets a series of events in motion. Blood vessels near the skin dilate, or widen, to bring more blood to the surface, which allows heat to escape (**Fig. 19-2, A**). The body can also be cooled by sweat evaporating or by air moving over the skin.

When the body reacts to cold, blood vessels near the skin constrict (narrow) and move warm blood to the center of the body. Thus, less heat escapes through the skin, and the body stays warm (**Fig. 19-2, B**). When constriction of blood vessels fails to keep the body warm, the body shivers to produce heat through muscle action.

Factors Affecting Body Temperature Regulation

Three main factors affect how well the body maintains its temperature:

▸ Air temperature.
▸ Humidity.
▸ Wind.

KEY TERMS

Frostbite: A condition in which body tissues freeze; most commonly occurs in the fingers, toes, ears and nose.

Heat cramps: Painful spasms of skeletal muscles after exercise or work in warm or moderate temperatures; usually involve the calf and abdominal muscles.

Heat exhaustion: The early stage and most common form of heat-related illness; often results from strenuous work or exercise in a hot environment.

Heat stroke: A life-threatening condition that develops when the body's cooling mechanisms are overwhelmed and body systems begin to fail.

Hypothalmus: Part of the brain that is responsible for regulating body temperature.

Hypothermia: A life-threatening condition in which the body's warming mechanisms fail to maintain normal body temperature and the entire body cools.

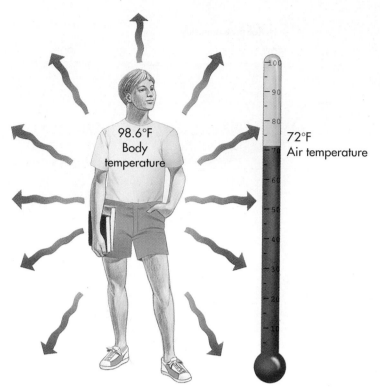

Figure 19-1   Because the body is usually warmer than the surrounding air, it tends to lose heat to the air.

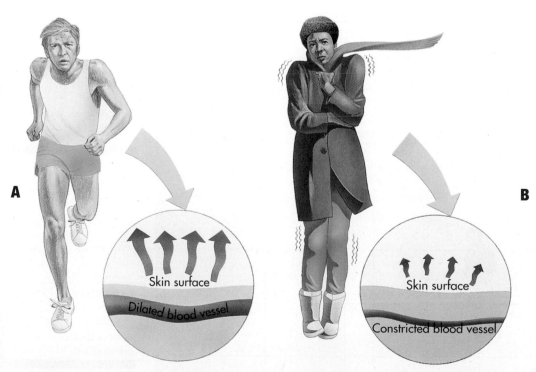

Figure 19-2   **A,** Your body removes heat by dilating the blood vessels near the skin's surface. **B,** The body conserves heat by constricting the blood vessels near the skin.

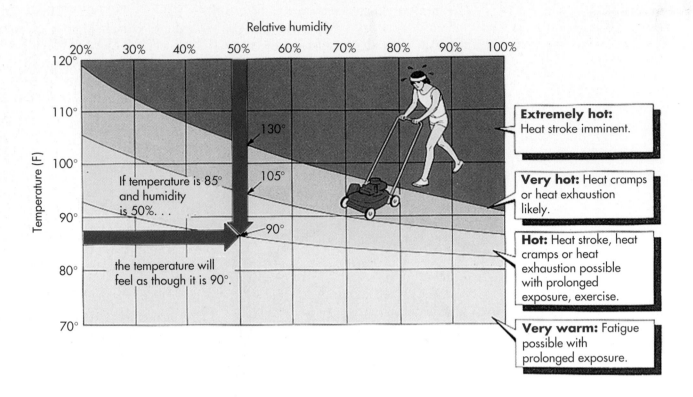

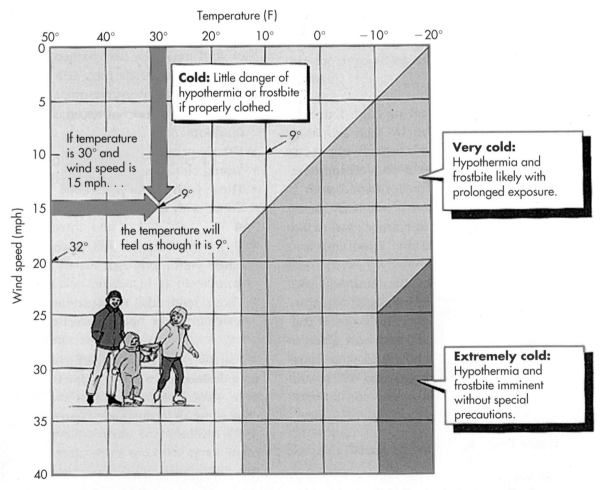

Figure 19-3 Temperature, humidity and wind are the three main factors affecting body temperature.

Extreme heat or cold accompanied by high humidity or wind speed reduces the body's ability to maintain temperature effectively (**Fig. 19-3**).

Other factors, such as the clothing you wear, how often you take breaks from exposure to extreme temperature, how much and how often you drink water and how intense your activity is, also affect how well the body manages temperature extremes. These are all factors you can control to prevent heat- or cold-related emergencies.

People at Increased Risk

Although anyone can be at risk for heat- and cold-related illness, some people are at greater risk than others. People more susceptible to a heat- or cold-related emergency include—

▶ Those who work or exercise strenuously in a warm or cold environment.
▶ Elderly people.
▶ Young children.
▶ Those with predisposing health problems, such as diabetes or heart disease.
▶ Those who have had a previous heat- or cold-related emergency.
▶ Those who have cardiovascular disease or other conditions that cause poor circulation.
▶ Those who take medications to eliminate water from the body (diuretics).

Usually people seek relief from an extreme temperature before they begin to feel ill. However, some people do not or cannot easily escape these extremes (**Fig. 19-4**). Athletes and those who work outdoors often keep working even after they de-velop the first indications of illness. Many times, they may not even recognize the signals.

Heat- or cold-related emergencies occur more frequently among the elderly, especially those living in poorly ventilated or poorly insulated buildings or buildings with poor heating or cooling systems. Young children and people with health problems are also at risk because their bodies do not respond as effectively to temperature extremes.

TYPES OF HEAT-RELATED EMERGENCIES

Heat cramps, *heat exhaustion* and *heat stroke* are conditions caused by overexposure to heat. Heat cramps are the least severe but, if not cared for, may be followed by heat exhaustion and heat stroke.

Heat Cramps

Heat cramps are painful spasms of skeletal muscles. Heat cramps usually affect the legs and the abdomen but they can occur in any voluntary muscle. The exact cause of heat cramps is not known, although it is believed to be a combination of loss of fluid and salt from heavy sweating. Heat cramps develop fairly rapidly and usually occur after heavy exercise or work in warm or even moderate temperatures. The victim's body temperature is usually normal and the skin moist. However, heat cramps may also indicate that a person is in the early stages of a more severe heat-related emergency.

To care for heat cramps, have the victim rest comfortably in a cool place. Lightly stretch the muscle, then gently massage it (**Fig. 19-5**). Provide cool

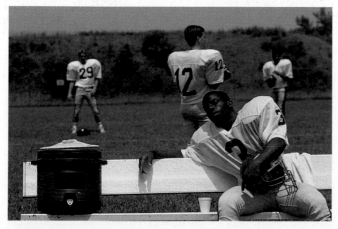

Figure 19-4   In certain situations, it is difficult to escape temperature extremes.

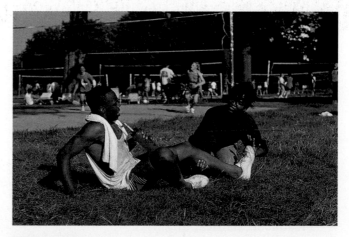

Figure 19-5   Resting, lightly stretching and massaging the affected muscle and replenishing fluids are usually enough for the body to recover from heat cramps.

water or a commercial sports drink that contains nutrients, such as carbohydrates, electrolytes and simple sugars, to replace those lost through heavy sweating. Usually, rest and fluids are all the body needs to recover. The victim should not take salt tablets or salt water. Ingesting high concentrations of salt, whether in tablet or liquid form, can hasten the onset of heat-related illness.

When the cramps stop and no other signals of illness are present, the person can usually resume activity. The person should be watched carefully, however, for signals of developing heat-related illness. He or she should continue to drink plenty of fluids during and after activity.

Heat-Related Illness

Heat-related illness, if not cared for promptly, can get progressively worse in a very short period of time. By recognizing the signals of the early stages of heat-related illness and responding appropriately, you may be able to prevent the condition from becoming life threatening.

Early Stages of Heat-Related Illness

Heat exhaustion is the early stage and the most common form of heat-related illness. It typically occurs after long periods of strenuous exercise or work in a hot environment. Although heat exhaustion is commonly associated with athletes, it also affects firefighters, construction workers, factory workers and others who are very active and wear heavy clothing in a hot, humid environment. However, strenuous activity is not a prerequisite for heat exhaustion—it can happen when a person is relaxing or standing still in the heat.

Heat exhaustion is an early indication that the body's temperature-regulating mechanism is becoming overtaxed. It is not always preceded by heat cramps. Over time, the victim loses fluid through sweating, which decreases the blood volume. Blood flow to the skin increases, reducing blood flow to the vital organs. The circulatory system is affected, and the person goes into a form of shock (see Chapter 9).

The signals of heat exhaustion include—

▶ Cool, moist, pale, ashen or flushed skin.
▶ Headache, nausea, dizziness.
▶ Weakness, exhaustion.
▶ Heavy sweating.

Heat exhaustion in its early stage can usually be reversed with prompt care.

Late Stages of Heat-Related Illness

Heat stroke is the least common and most severe heat-related emergency. Heat stroke most often occurs when people ignore the signals of heat exhaustion or do not act quickly enough to give care. Heat stroke develops when the body systems are so overtaxed by heat that they begin to stop functioning. Sweating often stops because body fluid levels are low. When sweating stops, the body cannot cool itself effectively through evaporation. Body temperature rises quickly, soon reaching a level at which the brain and other vital organs, such as the heart and kidneys, begin to fail. If the body is not cooled, convulsions, coma and death will result. Heat stroke is a serious medical emergency. You must recognize the signals of heat stroke and give care immediately.

The signals of heat stroke include—

▶ Red, hot, dry or moist skin.
▶ Changes in level of consciousness.
▶ Vomiting.

Care for Heat-Related Illness

Time is of the essence when caring for heat-related illness. The longer a heat-related illness goes untreated, the worse the condition becomes. Specific steps for care depend on whether you find a victim in the early or late stages of a heat-related illness.

Care in Early Stages

If you recognize heat-related illness in its early stages, you can usually reverse it. Follow these general steps:

▶ Cool the body.
▶ Give fluids if the victim is conscious.
▶ Take steps to minimize shock.

Remove the victim from the hot environment and give him or her cool water to drink. Moving the victim out of the sun or away from the heat allows the body's own temperature-regulating mechanisms to recover, cooling the body more quickly. Loosen any tight clothing and remove clothing soaked with perspiration. Apply cool, wet cloths, such as towels or sheets, to the wrists, ankles, armpits, groin and

TOO MUCH OF A GOOD THING

Although brief exposure to the sun stimulates the skin to produce the vitamin D necessary for the healthy formation of bones, prolonged exposure can cause problems such as skin cancer and premature aging—a classic case of too much of a good thing being bad.

There are two kinds of ultraviolet (UV) light rays to be concerned about. Ultraviolet beta rays (UVB) are the burn-producing rays that more commonly cause skin cancer. These are the rays that damage the skin's surface and cause blistering and perhaps peeling. The other rays, ultraviolet alpha rays (UVA), have been heralded by tanning salons as "safe rays." Tanning salons claim to use lights that only emit UVA rays. Although UVA rays may not appear as harmful as UVB rays to the skin's surface, they more readily penetrate the deeper layers of the skin. This increases the risk of skin cancer, skin aging, eye damage and genetic changes that may alter the skin's ability to fight disease.

To avoid getting too much sun, avoid exposure to the sun between 10:00 A.M. and 4:00 P.M. UV rays are most harmful during this period. Wear proper clothing to prevent overexposure. Also, take care to protect the skin and eyes whenever exposure to the sun is expected.

Commercial sunscreens come in various strengths. The American Academy of Dermatology recommends year-round sun protection, including use of a high sun protection factor (SPF) sunscreen, for all individuals, but particularly for those who are fair-skinned and sunburn easily. The Food and Drug Administration (FDA) has evaluated SPF readings and recognizes values between 2 and 15. The American Cancer Society recommends an SPF containing a rating of 15 or higher. To get a sense of the effectiveness of SPF, an SPF 4 blocks out 75 percent of the sun's burning UV rays, an SPF 15 blocks out 93 percent and an SPF 30 blocks out 97 percent of the burning UV rays.

For maximum effect, sunscreen should be applied 20 to 30 minutes before exposure to the sun and reapplied frequently. Swimmers should use sunscreens labeled as water resistant and reapply them as described in the labeling. Remember also to use lip balm with an SPF of 15 or higher.

Choose sunscreen that claims to be broad spectrum—protecting against both UVB and UVA rays. Carefully check the label to determine the protection a product offers. Some products only offer protection against UVB rays.

It is equally important to protect the eyes from sun damage. Wear polarized sunglasses that absorb at least 90 percent of UV sunlight. Polarized sunglasses are like sunscreen for the eyes and protect against damage that can occur from UV rays.

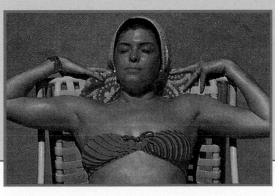

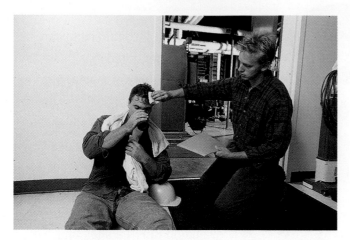

Figure 19-6 For early stages of heat-related illness, apply cool, wet cloths and fan the victim to increase evaporation. Give cool water to drink.

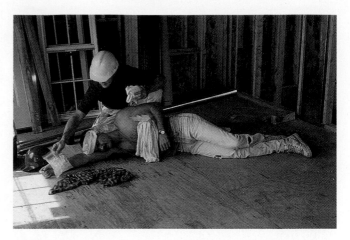

Figure 19-7 To cool the body of the victim of heat-related illness, cover the body with cool, wet towels and apply ice packs.

back of the neck, and fan the victim to increase evaporation.

If the victim is conscious, slowly drinking cool water will help replenish the vital fluids lost through sweating (**Fig. 19-6**). The victim is likely to be nauseated. Water is less likely than other fluids to cause vomiting and is more quickly absorbed into the body from the stomach. Do not let the victim drink too quickly. Let the victim rest in a comfortable position, and watch carefully for changes in his or her condition. A victim of heat-related illness should not resume normal activities the same day.

Care in Late Stages

If you observe changes in the victim's level of consciousness, call 9-1-1 or the local emergency number and cool the body quickly by any means available. Soak towels or sheets in cool water and apply them to the victim's body. Use a water hose, if one is available, to cool the victim. If you have ice or cold packs, wrap them in a cloth and place them on each of the victim's wrists and ankles, on the groin, in each armpit and on the neck to cool the large blood vessels (**Fig. 19-7**). A person in heat stroke may experience respiratory or cardiac arrest. Be prepared to perform rescue breathing or CPR, if needed.

COLD-RELATED EMERGENCIES

Frostbite and *hypothermia* are two types of cold-related emergencies. Frostbite occurs in body parts exposed to the cold. Hypothermia develops when the body can no longer generate sufficient heat to maintain normal body temperature.

Frostbite

Frostbite is the freezing of body tissues. It usually occurs in exposed areas of the body, depending on the air temperature, length of exposure and the wind. Frostbite can be superficial or deep. In superficial frostbite, the skin is frozen but the tissues below are not. In deep frostbite, both the skin and underlying tissues are frozen. Both types of frostbite are serious. The water in and between the body's cells freezes and swells. The ice crystals and swelling damage or destroy the cells. Frostbite can cause the eventual loss of fingers, hands, arms, toes, feet and legs.

The signals of frostbite include—

▸ Lack of feeling in the affected area.
▸ Skin that appears waxy.
▸ Skin that is cold to the touch.
▸ Skin that is discolored (flushed, white, yellow or blue).

Care

▸ Get the person out of the cold.
▸ Do not attempt to rewarm the frostbitten area if there is a chance that it might refreeze or if you are close to a medical facility.
▸ Handle the area gently; never rub the affected area.
▸ Warm gently by soaking the affected area in warm water (100-105° F) until normal color returns and feels warm (**Fig. 19-8, A**).
▸ Loosely bandage the area with dry, sterile dressings (**Fig. 19-8, B**).

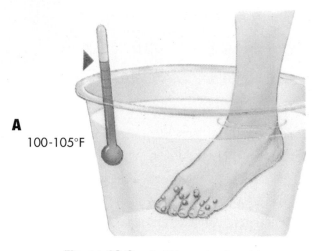
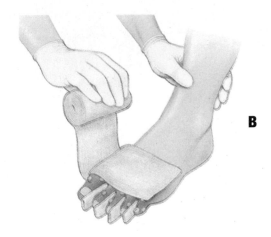

A
100-105°F
B

Figure 19-8   A, Warm the frostbitten area gently by soaking it in water. Do not allow the frostbitten area to touch the container. **B,** After rewarming, bandage the area with a dry, sterile dressing. If fingers or toes are frostbitten, place gauze between them.

▶ If the person's fingers or toes are frostbitten, place dry, sterile gauze between them to keep them separated.
▶ Avoid breaking any blisters.
▶ Take precautions to prevent hypothermia.
▶ Call 9-1-1 or seek emergency medical care as soon as possible.

Hypothermia

Hypothermia is the general cooling of the entire body. In hypothermia, body temperature drops below 95° F (35° C). As the body cools, an abnormal heart rhythm (ventricular fibrillation) may develop and the heart eventually stops. The victim will die if not given care.

The signals of hypothermia include—

▶ Shivering (may be absent in later stages of hypothermia).
▶ Numbness.
▶ Glassy stare.
▶ Apathy or decreasing level of consciousness.
▶ Weakness.
▶ Impaired judgment.

In cases of severe hypothermia, the victim may be unconscious. Breathing may have slowed or stopped. The body may feel stiff as the muscles become rigid.

The air temperature does not have to be below freezing for people to develop hypothermia. Elderly people in poorly heated homes, particularly those who suffer from poor nutrition and who get little exercise, can develop hypothermia at higher temperatures. Certain substances, such as alcohol and barbiturates, can also interfere with the body's normal response to cold, causing hypothermia to occur more easily. Medical conditions, such as infection, insulin reaction, stroke and a brain tumor also make a person more susceptible to hypothermia. Anyone remaining in cold water or wet clothing for a prolonged time may also easily develop hypothermia.

Care

▶ Gently move the person to a warm place.
▶ Care for life-threatening conditions.
▶ Call 9-1-1 or the local emergency number.
▶ Remove any wet clothing and dry the person.
▶ Warm the person by wrapping in blankets or by putting dry clothing on the person (passive re-warming) (**Fig. 19-9**).
▶ If available, apply heat pads or other heat sources to the body. Hot water bottles and chemical hot packs may be used when first wrapped in a towel or blanket before applying.
▶ Do not warm the person too quickly, such as by immersing him or her in warm water. Rapid warming may cause dangerous heart rhythms.
▶ If person is alert, give warm liquids that do not contain alcohol or caffeine.

Monitor ABCs and continue to warm the victim until EMS personnel arrive. Be prepared to perform CPR if necessary.

High-Tech War Against Cold

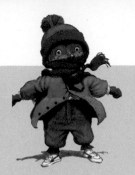

In the past, humans depended entirely on nature for clothing. Animal skins, furs and feathers protected us from freezing temperatures. As long as seasonal changes and cold climates exist, preventing cold-related illness, such as hypothermia, remains important when we work or play outside. Although natural fibers like wool and down are still practical, synthetic fibers are now used in clothing to make being outdoors a lot more comfortable than in the past.

The best way to use outdoor fabrics is to layer them. Layering creates warmth by trapping warm air between the layers to insulate the body. Layering is an old concept. It enables you to regulate your body temperature and deal with changes in the environment. By wearing several layers of clothing, you can take clothes off when you become too warm and put them back on if you get cold.

Start off with an underwear layer. Commonly called long underwear, it includes thin, snug-fitting pants and a long-sleeved shirt. Underwear should supply you with basic insulation and pull moisture away from your skin—damp, sweaty skin can chill you when you slow down or stop moving. Natural fibers, such as wool and silk, can be quite warm and are sufficient for light activity. For heavier exercise, however, synthetic fabrics absorb less moisture and actually carry water droplets away from your skin. Polypropylene and Capalene are two popular synthetic fabrics for underwear.

Next, to provide additional warmth, add one or more insulating layers. The weight of insulating clothing should be considered in relation to planned activities, weather conditions and how efficiently the garment compresses to pack. Depending on the temperature, a wool sweater or a down jacket may provide an insulating layer for the upper body. But do not forget your legs. Wool pants are a better choice than jeans or corduroys. Synthetic materials used in jackets and pants include Thinsulate™, Quallofil®, Polartec® and pile (a plush, nonpiling polyester fiber). Although down is an excellent lightweight insulator, it becomes useless when wet, so a water-repellent or quick-drying fabric like pile may keep you warmer in a damp climate.

Finish with a windproof, and preferably waterproof, shell layer. Synthetic, high-tech fabrics make a strong showing here. Windproof fabrics have names like Supplex, Silmond, Captiva or rip-stop nylon. Coatings, such as Hypalon, applied to jackets and pants are completely water repellent. However, most waterproof fabrics are "breathable." They repel wind and rain but allow your perspiration to pass through the fabric so that you stay dry and warmer. Gore-Tex®, Thintech, Ultrex, and Super Microft are some of the names given to these fabrics. Pay close attention to vents and closures in garments; they should seal tightly and open freely to adapt to changing activities and weather conditions. It is also important to make sure your outer garments are big enough to fit over several layers of clothing.

A hat is vital to staying truly warm. Gloves, insulating socks, neck "gaiters" and headbands all protect you from the cold. Visit your local outdoor store for more information about the best clothing for your specific work or recreational activities.

SOURCES
National Ski Patrol,
   www.nsp.org/nsp2002/safety_info_template.asp?mode=dress. Accessed 10/29/04.
Recreation Equipment Incorporated: *Layering for comfort: FYI, an informational brochure from REI*, Seattle, 1991.
Recreation Equipment Incorporated: *Understanding outdoor fabrics: FYI, An informational brochure from REI*, Seattle, 1991.
Recreation Equipment Incorporated: *Outerwear product information guide*, Seattle, 1995.

Care for Heat- and Cold-Related Emergencies

HEAT EMERGENCIES

HEAT CRAMPS
▸ Have the victim rest in a cool place.
▸ Give cool water to drink.
▸ Lightly stretch and gently massage the muscle.
▸ DO NOT GIVE SALT TABLETS.
▸ Watch for signals of heat illness.

HEAT-RELATED ILLNESS
▸ Move the victim to a cool place.
▸ Loosen tight or remove perspiration-soaked clothing.
▸ Apply cool, wet cloths to the skin or mist with cool water and fan the victim.
▸ If conscious, give cool water to drink.
▸ If the victim refuses water, vomits or loses consciousness:
  • Send someone to CALL 9-1-1 or the local emergency number and place the victim on his or her side.
  • Continue to cool by placing ice packs or cold packs on the victim's wrists, ankles, groin, neck and in the armpits.
  • If the victim becomes unconscious, give rescue breathing or CPR if needed.

COLD EMERGENCIES

FROSTBITE
▸ Get the person out of the cold.
▸ Do not attempt to rewarm the frostbitten area if there is a chance that it might refreeze or if you are close to a medical facility.
▸ Handle the area gently; never rub the affected area.
▸ Warm gently by soaking the affected area in warm water (100-105° F) until normal color returns and feels warm.
▸ Loosely bandage the area with dry, sterile dressings.
▸ If the person's fingers or toes are frostbitten, place dry, sterile gauze between them to keep them separated.
▸ Avoid breaking any blisters.
▸ Take precautions to prevent hypothermia.
▸ Call 9-1-1 or seek emergency medical care as soon as possible.

HYPOTHERMIA
▸ Gently move the person to a warm place.
▸ Care for life-threatening conditions.
▸ Call 9-1-1 or the local emergency number.
▸ Monitor ABCs.
▸ Give rescue breathing or CPR if needed.
▸ Remove any wet clothing and dry the person.
▸ Warm the person by wrapping in blankets or by putting dry clothing on the person (passive rewarming).
▸ Hot water bottles and chemical hot packs may be used when first wrapped in a towel or blanket before applying.
▸ Do not warm the person too quickly, such as by immersing him or her in warm water. Rapid warming may cause dangerous heart rhythms.

An Icy Rescue

Rescuers who pulled Michelle Funk from an icy creek near her home thought she was dead. The child's eyes stared dully ahead, her body was chilled and blue and her heart had stopped beating. The 2½ year-old had been under the icy water for more than an hour. By all basic measurements of life, she was dead.

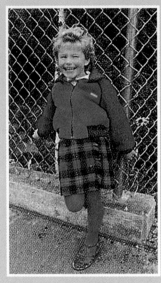

Years ago, Michelle's family would have prepared for her funeral. Instead, paramedics performed CPR on Michelle's still body as they rushed her to a children's medical center, where Dr. Robert G. Bolte took over care. Bolte had been reading about a rewarming technique used on adult hypothermia victims and thought it would work on Michelle. Surgeons sometimes intentionally cool a patient when preparing for surgery and use heart-lung machines to rewarm the patient's blood after surgery. This cooling helps keep oxygen in the blood longer. Bolte attached Michelle to the heart-lung machine, which provided oxygen and removed carbon dioxide in addition to warming the blood. When Michelle's temperature reached 77° F (25° C), the unconscious child gasped. Soon her heart was pumping on its own.

Doctors once believed the brain could not survive more than 5 to 7 minutes without oxygen, but survivals like Michelle's have changed opinions. Ironically, freezing water actually helps to protect the body from drowning.

In icy water, a person's body temperature begins to drop almost as soon as the body hits the water. The body loses heat in water 25 to 30 times faster than it does in the air. As the body's core temperature drops, the metabolic rate drops. Activity in the cells comes almost to a standstill, and the cells require very little oxygen. Any oxygen left in the blood is diverted from other parts of the body to the brain and heart.

This state of suspended animation allows humans to survive underwater at least four times as long as physicians once believed possible. Nearly 20 cases of miraculous survivals have been documented in medical journals, although unsuccessful cases are rarely described. Most cases involve children who spent 15 minutes or longer in water temperatures of 41° F (5° C) or lower. Children survive better because their bodies cool faster than an adult's.

Researchers once theorized that the physiological responses were caused by a "mammalian dive reflex" similar to a response found in whales and seals. They believed the same dive mechanism that allowed whales and seals to stay underwater for long periods of time was triggered in drowning humans. Experiments have failed to support the idea. Many researchers now say the best explanation for the slowdown is simply the body's response to extreme cold.

After being attached to the heart-lung machine for nearly an hour, Michelle was moved into an intensive care unit. She stayed in a coma for more than a week. She was blind for a short period, and doctors were not sure she would recover. But slowly she began to respond. First she smiled when her parents came into the room, and soon she was talking like a 2½ year-old again. After she left the hospital, she suffered a tremor from nerve damage. But Michelle was one of the lucky ones—eventually she regained her full sight, balance and coordination.

Although breakthroughs have saved many lives, parents still must be vigilant when their children and others are near water. Most near-drowning victims are not as lucky as Michelle. One out of every three survivors suffers neurological damage. There is no substitute for close supervision.

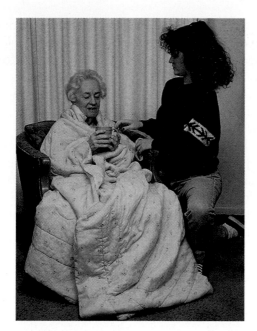

Figure 19-9 For a hypothermia victim, rewarm the body gradually.

PREVENTING HEAT- AND COLD-RELATED EMERGENCIES

Generally, illnesses caused by overexposure to extreme temperatures are preventable. To prevent heat- or cold-related emergencies from happening to you or anyone you know, follow these guidelines:

▶ Avoid being outdoors in the hottest or coldest part of the day.
▶ Dress appropriately for the environment.
▶ Change your activity level according to the temperature.
▶ Take frequent breaks by removing yourself from the environment.
▶ Drink large amounts of nonalcoholic or decaffeinated fluids before, during and after activity.

The easiest way to prevent illness caused by temperature extremes is to avoid being outside during the parts of the day when temperatures are most extreme. For instance, if you plan to work outdoors in hot weather, plan your activity for the early morning and evening hours when the sun is not as strong. Likewise, if you must be outdoors on cold days, plan your activities for the warmest part of the day.

Always wear clothing appropriate to the environmental conditions and your activity level. When possible, wear light-colored clothing in the heat. Light-colored clothing reflects the sun's rays.

When you are in the cold, wear layers of clothing made of tightly woven fibers, such as wool, that trap warm air against your body. Wear a head covering in both heat and cold. A hat protects the head from the sun's rays in the summer and prevents heat from escaping in the winter. Also, protect other areas of the body, such as the fingers, toes, ears and nose, from cold exposure by wearing protective coverings.

You can take additional precautions, such as changing your activity level and taking frequent breaks. For instance, in very hot conditions, exercise only for brief periods, then rest in a cool, shaded area. Frequent breaks allow your body to readjust to normal body temperature, enabling it to better withstand brief periods of exposure to temperature extremes (**Fig. 19-10**). Avoid heavy exercise during the hottest or coldest part of the day. Extremes of temperature promote fatigue, which hampers the body's ability to adjust to changes in the environment.

Whether in heat or cold, be sure to drink enough fluids. Drinking at least six 8-ounce (236.6 milliliters) glasses of fluids is the most important way to prevent heat- or cold-related illness. Plan to drink fluids when you take a break. Just as you would drink cool fluids in the summer, drink warm fluids in the winter. Cool and warm fluids help the body maintain a normal temperature. If cold or hot drinks are not available, drink plenty of plain water. Do not drink beverages containing caffeine

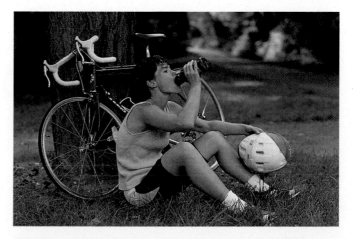

Figure 19-10 Taking frequent breaks when exercising in extreme temperatures allows your body to readjust to normal body temperature.

or alcohol. Caffeine and alcohol hinder the body's temperature-regulating mechanism.

SUMMARY

Overexposure to extreme heat or cold may cause a person to become ill. The likelihood of illness also depends on factors such as physical activity, clothing, wind, humidity, working and living conditions, and a person's age and physical condition. Heat cramps are an early indication that the body's normal temperature-regulating mechanism is not working efficiently. They may signal that the person is in the early stage of a heat-related illness. For heat-related illness, it is important for the victim to stop physical activity. Cool the victim and call 9-1-1 or the local emergency number. Heat stroke can rapidly lead to death if it is left untreated.

Both hypothermia and frostbite are serious cold-related conditions, and their victims need professional medical care. Hypothermia can be life threatening. For both hypothermia and frostbite, it is important to warm the victim gradually and handle him or her with care.

APPLICATION QUESTIONS

1. Why does Cynthia feel dizzy?

2. What can Louise do to help Cynthia's condition improve?

3. What could Cynthia have done to prevent heat exhaustion?

STUDY QUESTIONS

1. Match each term with the correct definition.
   a. Frostbite
   b. Heat cramps
   c. Heat exhaustion
   d. Heat stroke
   e. Hypothermia

   _____ The early stage and most common form of heat-related illness.

   _____ A life-threatening condition that develops when the body's warming mechanisms fail to maintain normal body temperature.

   _____ A life-threatening condition that develops when the body's cooling mechanism fails.

   _____ The freezing of body tissues caused by overexposure to the cold.

   _____ Painful spasms of skeletal muscles that develop after heavy exercise or work outdoors in warm or moderate temperatures.

2. List four factors that affect body temperature.

3. List three conditions that can result from overexposure to heat.

4. List four signals of heat-related illness.

5. List two signals of a heat-related illness for which EMS personnel should be called.

6. List two ways to cool a victim of a suspected heat-related illness.

7. List two conditions that result from overexposure to the cold.

8. List four ways to prevent heat and cold emergencies.

In questions 9 and 10, circle the letter of the correct answer.

9. To care for heat cramps—

   a. Have the victim rest comfortably in a cool place.
   b. Call 9-1-1 or the local emergency number.
   c. Give salt tablets.
   d. All of the above.

10. What should you do if the victim of a suspected heat-related illness begins to lose consciousness?

    a. Cool the body using wet sheets and towels or cold packs.
    b. Cool the body by applying rubbing alcohol.
    c. Call 9-1-1 or the local emergency number.
    d. a and c.

Use the following scenario to answer questions 11 and 12.

You and a friend have been skiing all morning. The snow is great, but it is really cold. Your buddy has complained for the last half hour or so that his hands and feet are freezing. Now he says he can't feel his fingers and toes. You decide to return to the ski lodge. Once inside, your friend has trouble removing his mittens and ski boots. You help him take them off and notice that his fingers look waxy and white and feel cold. Your friend says he still can't feel them.

11. Circle the signals of frostbite you find in the scenario above.

12. How would you care for your friend's hands and feet?

Use the following scenario to answer questions 13 and 14.

You are working on a community service project delivering meals to elderly, homebound individuals. It is a blustery winter day that has you running from the van to each front door. As you enter the last home, you notice that it is not much warmer inside the house than it is outside. An elderly woman, bundled in blankets, is sitting as close as possible to a small space heater. You speak to her, introducing yourself and asking how things are, but you get no response. The woman's eyes are glassy as she makes an effort to look at you. She seems weak and exhausted, barely able to keep her head up. You touch her arm, but she does not seem to feel it.

13. Circle the signals in the scenario above that would lead you to suspect a cold-related illness.

14. Describe the actions you would take to care for the woman in the scenario.

Answers are listed in Appendix A.

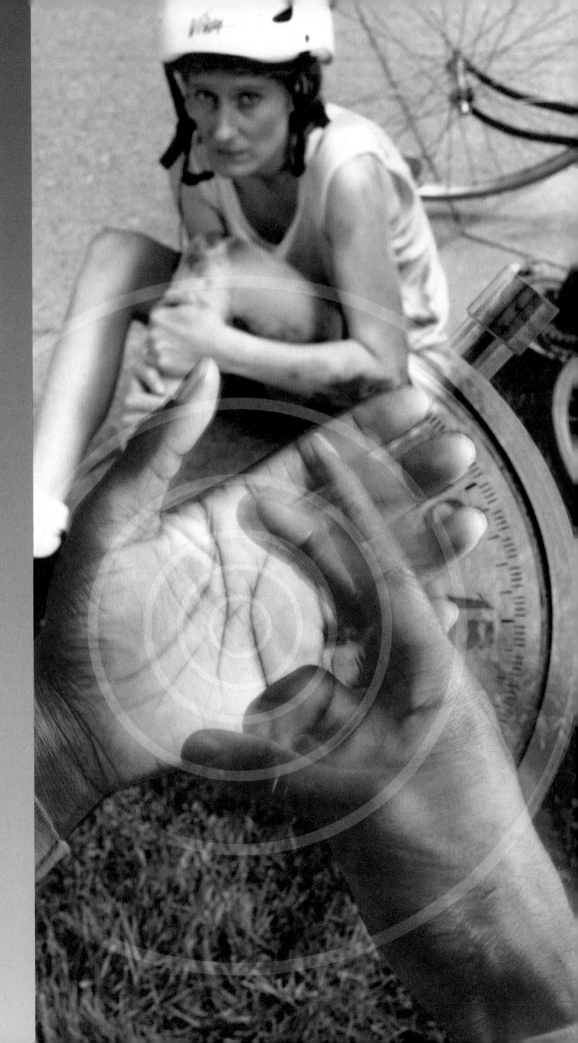

Part SIX

SPECIAL SITUATIONS

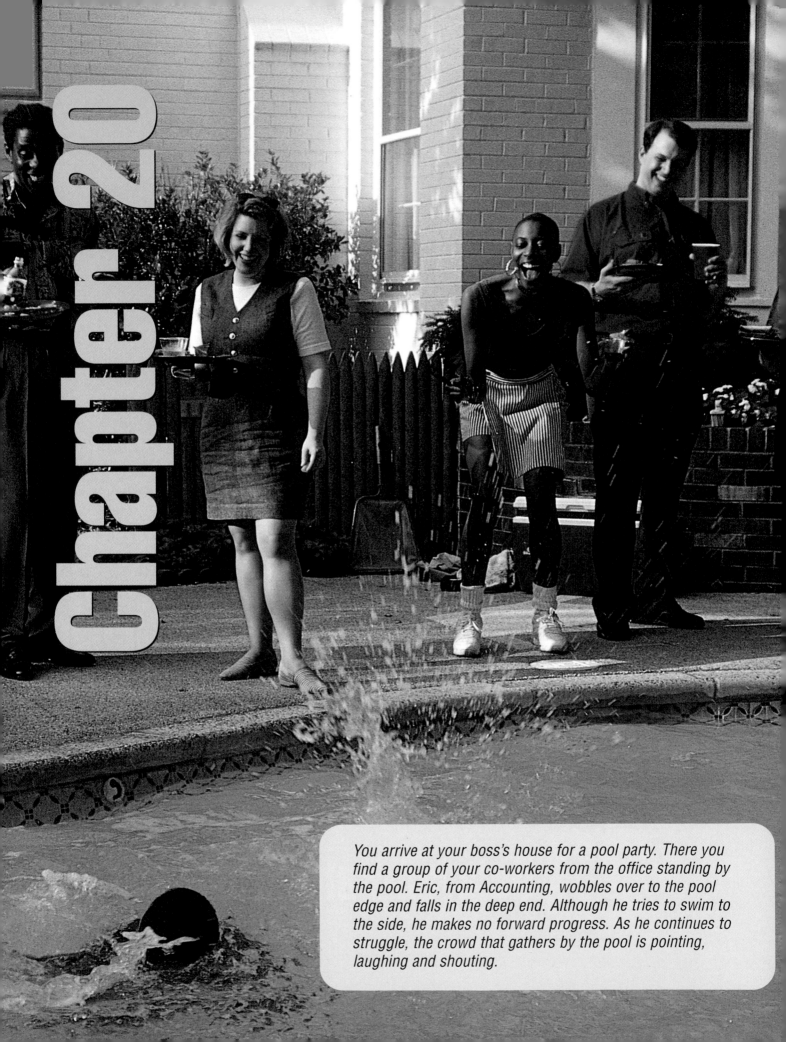

Chapter 20

You arrive at your boss's house for a pool party. There you find a group of your co-workers from the office standing by the pool. Eric, from Accounting, wobbles over to the pool edge and falls in the deep end. Although he tries to swim to the side, he makes no forward progress. As he continues to struggle, the crowd that gathers by the pool is pointing, laughing and shouting.

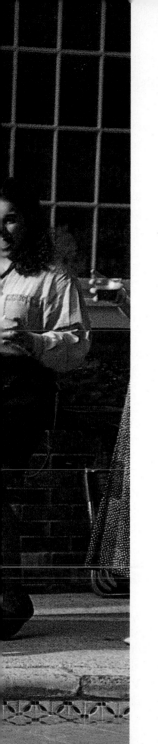

Reaching and Moving Victims in the Water

Objectives

After reading this chapter, you should be able to—

■ Describe two out-of-water assists that you can use to help someone who is in trouble in the water.

■ Describe how to perform an in-water assist that you can use to help someone who is in trouble in the water.

■ List the general guidelines for caring for someone who you suspect may have a head, neck or back injury and is in the water.

■ Describe two methods to support or stabilize a victim's head, neck and back in the water.

Introduction

Water provides people with some of the most enjoyable recreational activities, but water can be dangerous. **Drowning** *is death by suffocation in water. Drownings may occur during swimming, boating, hunting, fishing or while taking a bath. Everyone should learn how to swim well. Everyone should know basic water rescue methods to help themselves or someone else in an emergency. In this chapter, you will learn how to safely reach and assist victims in water without endangering or injuring yourself.*

THE RISK OF DROWNING

Children younger than age 5 and young adults ages 15 to 24 have the highest rates of drowning. As frightening as the risk of drowning is, it can usually be prevented. Regardless of where you are swimming and what activities you may be involved in, you can follow simple guidelines to reduce the risk of drowning.

PREVENTING AQUATIC EMERGENCIES

The best thing anyone can do to stay safe in, on and around the water is to learn to swim. The American Red Cross has swimming courses for people of any age and swimming ability. To enroll in a swimming course, contact a local Red Cross chapter. Follow these general guidelines whenever you are swimming in any body of water (pools, lakes, ponds, quarries, canals, rivers or oceans):

▸ Always swim with a buddy; never swim alone.
▸ Read and obey all rules and posted signs (**Fig. 20-1**).
▸ Swim in areas supervised by a lifeguard.
▸ Children or inexperienced swimmers should take extra precautions, such as wearing a U.S. Coast Guard-approved life jacket when around the water.
▸ Watch out for the "dangerous too's"—too tired, too cold, too far away from safety, too much sun, too much strenuous activity.
▸ Be knowledgeable of the water environment and the potential hazards (deep and shallow areas, currents, depth changes, obstructions and where the entry and exit points are located).
▸ Know how to prevent, recognize and respond to emergencies.
▸ Use a feet-first entry when entering the water.
▸ Enter head-first only when the area is clearly marked for diving and has no obstructions.
▸ Do not mix alcohol with swimming, diving or boating. Alcohol impairs judgment, balance and coordination; affects swimming and diving skills; and reduces the body's ability to stay warm.

RECOGNIZING AN AQUATIC EMERGENCY

An emergency can happen to anyone in, on or around the water, regardless of how good a swimmer the person is or what he or she is doing at the time. A strong swimmer can get into trouble in the water because of sudden illness or injury. A non-swimmer playing in shallow water can be knocked down by a wave or pulled into deeper water by a rip current. The key to recognizing an emergency is staying alert and knowing the signals that indicate an emergency is happening. Use all your senses when observing

KEY TERMS

Active drowning victim: A person exhibiting universal behavior that includes struggling at the surface for 20 to 60 seconds before submerging.

Distressed swimmer: A victim capable of staying afloat but likely to need assistance to get to safety.

Passive drowning victim: An unconscious victim face-down, submerged or near the surface of the water.

Reaching assist: A non-swimming rescue in which one extends an object, such as an arm, leg or tree branch to a victim.

Throwing assist: A non-swimming water rescue in which one throws a line with a floating object attached to a victim.

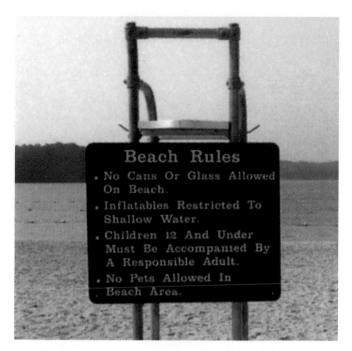

Figure 20-1   Read and obey all rules and posted signs.

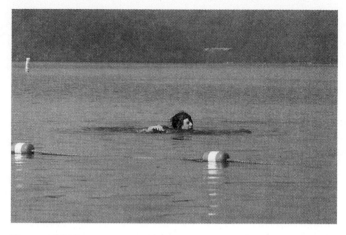

Figure 20-2   A distressed swimmer can stay afloat and usually call for help.

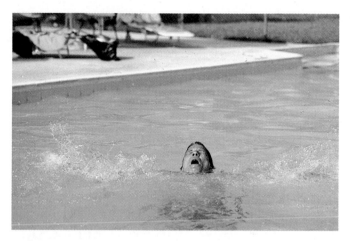

Figure 20-3   An active drowning victim struggles to stay afloat and is unable to call out for help.

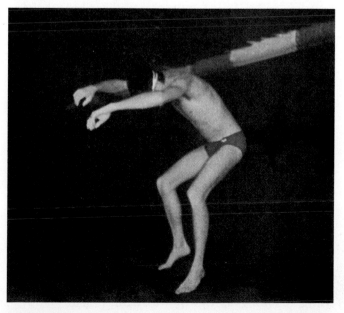

Figure 20-4   A passive drowning victim can be found floating near the surface or submerged on the bottom of the pool.

others in and around the water. A swimmer may be acting oddly, or you may hear a scream or sudden splash. Watch for anything that may seem unusual.

Being able to recognize a person who is having trouble in the water may help save that person's life. Most drowning people cannot or do not call out for help. They spend their energy just trying to keep their heads above water to get a breath. They may slip under water quickly and never resurface. There are two kinds of water emergency situations: a swimmer in distress and a drowning person. Each kind poses a different danger and can be recognized by different behaviors.

A *distressed swimmer* may be too tired to get to shore or to the side of the pool but is able to stay afloat and breathe and may be calling for help. The victim may be floating, treading water or clinging to a line for support (**Fig. 20-2**). Someone who is trying to swim but making little or no forward progress may be in distress. If not helped, a person in distress may lose the ability to float and become a drowning victim.

An *active drowning victim* is vertical in the water but unable to move forward or tread water. The victim's arms are at the side pressing down in an instinctive attempt to keep the head above water to breathe. All energy is going into the struggle to breathe, and the victim cannot call out for help (**Fig. 20-3**). A *passive drowning victim* is not moving and will be floating face-down on the bottom or near the surface of the water (**Fig. 20-4**). Table 20-1 compares the behaviors of distressed swimmers and drowning victims to those of swimmers.

Table 20-1 Behaviors of Distressed Swimmers and Drowning Victims Compared with Swimmers

BEHAVIORS	SWIMMER	DISTRESSED SWIMMER	ACTIVE DROWNING VICTIM	PASSIVE DROWNING VICTIM
Breathing	Rhythmic breathing	Can continue breathing and may call for help	Struggles to breathe; cannot call out for help	Not breathing
Arm and Leg Action	Relatively coordinated	Floating, sculling or treading water; may wave for help	Arms to sides alternately moving up and pressing down; no supporting kick	None
Body Position	Horizontal	Horizontal or diagonal, depending on means of support	Vertical	Horizontal or vertical; face-down, face-up or submerged
Locomotion	Recognizable	Little or no forward progress; less and less able to support self	None; has only 20-60 seconds before submerging	None

TAKING ACTION IN AN AQUATIC EMERGENCY

As in any emergency situation, follow the emergency action steps: **CHECK—CALL—CARE.** Make sure the scene is safe—do not rush into a dangerous situation where you too may become a victim. Always check first to see whether a lifeguard or other trained professional is present before helping someone who may be having trouble in the water. Do not swim out to a victim unless you have the proper training, skills and equipment. If the appropriate safety equipment is not available and there is a chance that you cannot safely help a person in trouble, call for help immediately. If you must assist someone who is having trouble in the water, you must have the appropriate equipment for your own safety and the victim's. Send someone else to call 9-1-1 or the local emergency number while you start the rescue.

Out-of-Water Assists

You can help a person in trouble in the water by using reaching assists or throwing assists. Out-of-water assists are safer for you. Whenever possible, start the rescue by talking to the victim. Let the vic-

tim know that help is coming. If it is too noisy or if the victim is too far away, use gestures. Tell the victim what he or she can do to help with the rescue, such as grasping the line, rescue buoy or any other floating device. Ask the victim to move toward safety by kicking or stroking his or her arms. Some victims have reached safety by themselves with the calm and encouraging assistance of someone calling to them.

Reaching Assists

If the victim is close enough, you can use a *reaching assist* to help him or her out of the water. If available, use any object that will extend your reach, such as a pole, an oar or paddle, a tree branch, a shirt, a belt or a towel (**Fig. 20-5**). Community pools and recreational areas, as well as hotel and motel pools, often have reaching equipment beside the water, such as a **shepherd's crook** (an aluminum or fiberglass pole with a large hook on one end) (**Fig. 20-6**). If using a rigid object, such as a pole or oar, sweep it toward the victim until it makes contact with an arm or hand. If using a shirt or towel, lie down and flip it into the victim's hands.

If there is equipment available:

1. Brace yourself on a pool deck, pier surface or shoreline.

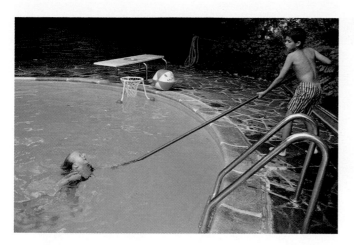

Figure 20-5   With a reaching assist, you remain safe while reaching out to the victim.

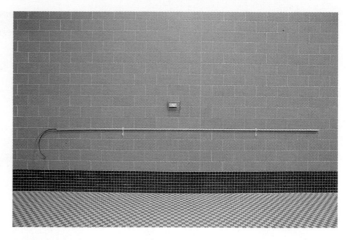

Figure 20-6   A shepherd's crook can be found at most public swimming facilities.

2. Extend the object to the victim.

3. When the victim grasps the object, slowly and carefully pull him or her to safety. Keep your body low and lean back to avoid being pulled into the water.

If there is no equipment available to perform a reaching assist, you should:

1. Brace yourself on the pool deck or pier surface.

2. Reach with one arm and grasp the victim.

3. Pull the victim to safety.

If you are already in the water:

1. Hold onto the pool ladder, overflow trough (gutter), piling or another secure object with one hand.

2. Extend your free hand or one leg to the victim (**Fig. 20-7, A** and **B**). Do not let go of the secure object or swim out into the water.

3. Pull the victim to safety.

Throwing Assists

You can rescue a conscious victim out of reach by using a ***throwing assist.*** Use anything that will provide the victim support. A floating object with a line attached is best. The victim can grasp the object and then be pulled to safety. However, lines and floats can also be used alone. Suitable throwing objects include a heaving line, ring buoy, throw bag, **rescue tube** or homemade device (**Fig. 20-8**). You can use any object at hand that will float, such as a picnic jug or life jacket. A throwing object

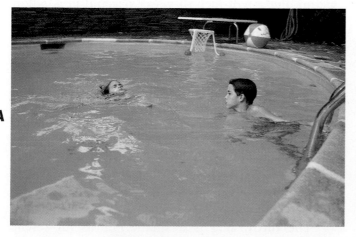

A

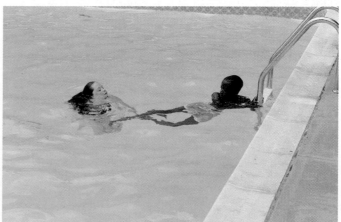

B

Figure 20-7   When no object is available to extend to the victim, try to extend your **A,** hand or **B,** foot to the victim.

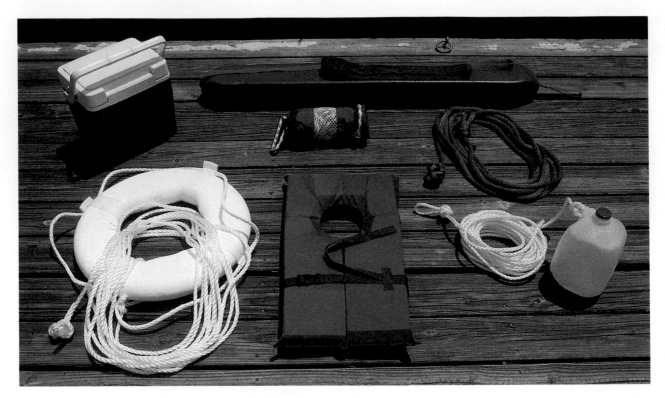

Figure 20-8 Throwing devices.

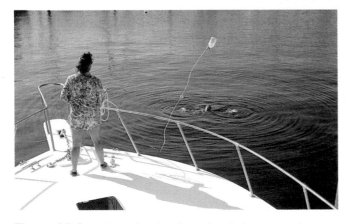

Figure 20-9 A heaving jug is a simple homemade device that can be thrown to a victim.

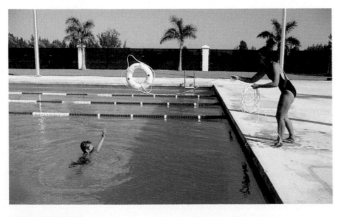

Figure 20-10 A ring buoy is another piece of rescue equipment that is commonly found at public swimming facilities.

with a coiled line should be kept in a prominent location that is accessible to the water so that anyone can quickly grasp it to throw to someone in trouble.

A **heaving line** should float. It should be white, yellow or some other highly visible color. Tying a buoyant, weighted object on the end will make throwing easier and more accurate. Hang about half the coiled line on the open palm of your non-throwing hand, and throw the other half underhand to the victim.

A homemade **heaving jug** can be thrown to a victim. Put a half-inch of water or sand in a gallon plastic container, seal it and attach 50 to 75 feet of floating line to the handle. Throw it by holding the handle and using an underhand swinging motion. The weight of the water in the jug helps direct the throw (**Fig. 20-9**).

A **ring buoy** is made of buoyant material and weighs about 2 pounds. It should have a towline or lightweight line with something at the end to keep the line from slipping out from under your foot when you throw it. Hold the underside of the ring with your fingers, and throw it underhand (**Fig. 20-10**).

The **throw bag** is a small, but useful rescue device. It is a nylon bag containing 50 to 75 feet of coiled floating line. A foam disk in the bag gives it shape and keeps it from sinking. Throw bags are

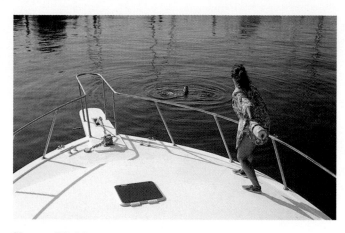

Figure 20-11 A throw bag is a compact rescue device that can be thrown to a victim.

often used in canoes and other boats. Hold the end of the line with one hand and throw the bag with your other hand, using an underhand swing (**Fig. 20-11**).

To perform a throwing assist, follow these guidelines:

1. Get into a stride position: the leg opposite your throwing arm is forward. This helps to keep your balance when you throw the object.
2. Step on the end of the line with your forward foot. Avoid stepping on the coiled line with your other foot.
3. Shout to get the victim's attention. Make eye contact and say that you are going to throw the object now. Tell the victim to grab it.
4. Bend your knees, and throw the object to the victim. Try to throw the object upwind or up current, just over the victim's head, so that the line drops within reach.

5. When the victim has grasped the object or the line, slowly pull him or her to safety. Keep your weight low and lean back. Lean away from the water as you bring the victim to safety.
6. If the object does not reach the victim, quickly pull the line back in and throw it again. Try to keep the line from tangling, but do not waste time trying to coil it. If using a throw bag, partially fill the bag with some water and throw it again.

If the throwing assist does not work and the water is shallow enough for wading, try a wading assist with equipment.

In-Water Assists

Wading Assist with Equipment

If the water is shallow enough that you can stand with your chest out of the water, wade into the water to assist the victim using a rescue tube, ring buoy, kickboard or a life jacket.

A tree branch, pole, air mattress or paddle can also be used (**Fig. 20-12, A** and **B**). If a current or soft bottom makes wading dangerous, do not enter the water. If possible, wear a life jacket when attempting a wading assist with equipment.

To perform a wading assist—

1. Take a buoyant object to extend out to the victim.
2. Wade into the water and extend the object to the victim.
3. When the victim grasps the object, tell him or her to hold onto the object tightly for support and pull him or her to safety. Keep the object

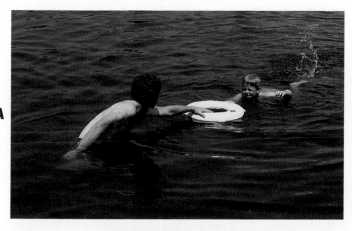
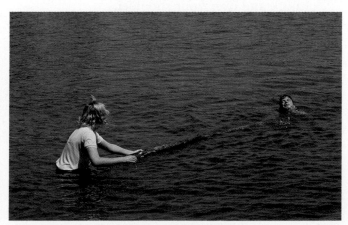

A

B

Figure 20-12 If you can enter the water without endangering yourself, wade in and reach to the victim. If possible, extend your reach with a **A,** ring buoy, **B,** tree branch or similar object.

between you and the victim to help prevent the victim from grasping you.

A victim who has been lying motionless and face-down in the water for several seconds is probably unconscious.

1. If the water is not over one's chest, wade into the water carefully with some kind of flotation equipment and turn the person face-up.
2. Bring him or her to the side of the pool or shoreline.
3. Remove the victim from the water.
4. Give care if needed.

Submerged Victim

If a victim is discovered on or near the bottom of the pool in deep water, call for trained help immediately. If in shallow water less than chest deep and a head, neck or back injury is not suspected—

1. Reach down and grasp the victim.
2. Pull the victim to the surface.
3. Turn the victim face-up and bring him or her to safety.
4. Remove the victim from the water.
5. Give care if needed.

Helping Victims from the Water

Walking Assist

If the victim is in shallow water where he or she can stand, he or she may be able to walk out of the water with some support. To perform a walking assist, follow these guidelines:

1. Place one of the victim's arms around your neck and over your shoulder.
2. Grasp the wrist of the arm that is over your shoulder, and wrap your free arm around the victim's back or waist.
3. Maintain a firm grasp, and help the victim walk out of the water (**Fig. 20-13**).

Beach Drag

You may use the beach drag with a victim in shallow water on a sloping shore or beach. This method works well with a heavy or unconscious victim. To perform the beach drag—

1. Stand behind the victim, and grasp him or her under the armpits, supporting the victim's head, when possible, with your forearms.

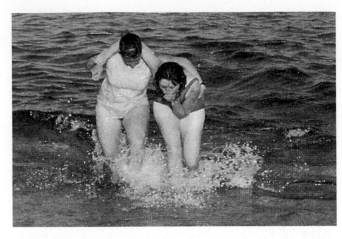

Figure 20-13 When performing a walking assist, maintain a firm grasp on the victim while walking out of the water.

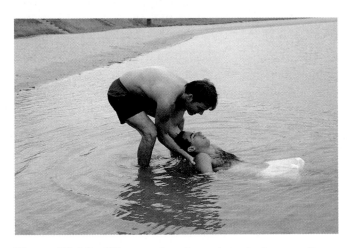

Figure 20-14 When performing a beach drag, walk backward slowly while dragging the victim toward shore.

2. While walking backward slowly, drag the victim toward the shore (**Fig. 20-14**).
3. Remove the victim completely from the water or at least to a point where the victim's head and shoulders are out of the water.

You may also use a two-person beach drag if another person is available to help (**Fig. 20-15**).

Two-Person Lift

The two-person lift can be used for removing a person from the water if there is no slope for you to easily remove the victim. **Do not use the two-person lift if you suspect the victim has a head, neck or back injury.** To perform the two-person lift—

1. Place the victim's hands, one on top of the other, on the deck or overflow trough (gutter).

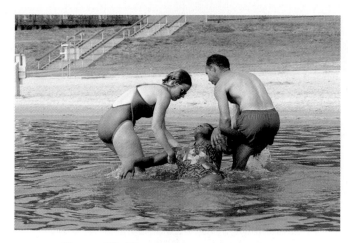

Figure 20-15   Two-person beach drag.

5. If necessary, pull the victim's legs out of the water, taking care not to twist the victim's back. Roll the victim onto his or her back. Support the victim's head and take care not to twist the victim's body as it is rolled.

Head, Neck or Back Injury

Most injuries to the head, neck or back occur in shallow water. Many involve the use of alcohol or other drugs. Diving into shallow water, diving from the deck into the shallow end of a pool, diving into above-ground pools and unsupervised diving from **starting blocks** cause most diving accidents. Injuries can also result from head-first entry into the surf at a beach, off a pier at a lake, from a cliff into a water-filled **quarry** or from falling while surfing or boogie boarding.

Recognizing a Head, Neck or Back Injury

2. Take the victim's hands and pull the victim up slightly to keep the head above the water. Be sure the victim's head is supported so that it does not fall forward and strike the deck (**Fig. 20-16, A**). Note: If in the water, climb out to help the second person.
3. Each person grasps one of the victim's wrists and upper arms (**Fig. 20-16, B**). Lift together until the victim's hips or thighs are at deck level.
4. Step backward and lower the victim to the deck. Be sure to protect the victim's head from striking the deck (**Fig. 20-16, C**).

Usually a head, neck or back injury is caused by hitting the bottom or an object in the water. Your major concern is to keep the victim's face out of the water to let him or her breathe and to prevent the victim's head and back from moving further. Movement can cause more injury and increase the risk of the victim's being paralyzed.

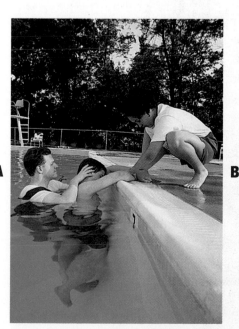

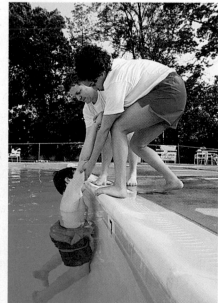

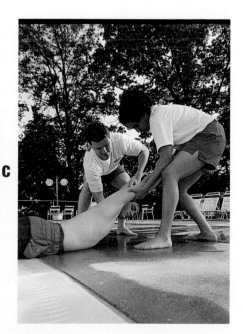

Figure 20-16   Two-person lift, **A,** One rescuer in the water supports the victim while one rescuer grasps the victim's hands. **B,** Both rescuers grasp the victim's arms and begin to lift. **C,** Rescuers removing the victim from the water.

Preventing Head, Neck and Back Injuries in Water

Every year, there are approximately 11,000 spinal cord injuries in the United States. About 9 percent of these injuries occur during sports and recreation.[1] Along with the risk of drowning, some water activities also involve the risk of head, neck or back injury. When the injury damages the spinal cord, severe disability is likely, including permanent paralysis. This means the person may never be able to move his or her arms or legs again.

Like drowning, head, neck or back injuries can be prevented by following basic guidelines such as these:

- ▶ Learn how to dive safely from a qualified instructor.
- ▶ Follow safety rules at all times.
- ▶ Obey "No Diving" signs. They are there for safety.
- ▶ Be sure of the water depth and ensure that the water is free from obstructions. The first time in the water, ease in or walk in; do not jump or dive.
- ▶ Never dive into an above-ground pool, the shallow end of any in-ground pool or at the beach.
- ▶ Never dive into cloudy or murky water.
- ▶ In open water, always check first for objects under the surface, such as logs, stumps, boulders and pilings.
- ▶ At lakes or rivers, enter head-first only when the area is clearly marked for diving.
- ▶ Check the shape of the pool bottom to be sure the diving area is large enough and deep enough for the intended dive.

- ▶ The presence of a diving board does not necessarily mean it is safe to dive. Pools at homes, motels and hotels might not have a safe diving envelope.
- ▶ When diving from a deck, the area of entry should be free of obstructions (such as lane lines and kickboards) for at least 4 feet on both sides. For dives from a 1-meter diving board, 10 feet of clearance is needed on both sides.
- ▶ For springboard diving, use equipment that meets standards for competition.
- ▶ Dive only from the end of a diving board. Diving off the side of a diving board might result in striking the side of the pool or entering water that is not deep enough.
- ▶ Do not bounce more than once on the end of a diving board to avoid missing the edge or slipping off the diving board.
- ▶ Do not run on a diving board or attempt to dive a long way through the air. The water might not be deep enough at the point of entry.
- ▶ Swim away from the diving board after entering the water. Do not be a hazard for the next diver.
- ▶ Do not dive from a height greater than 1 meter unless trained in elevated entry.
- ▶ Starting blocks should be used only by trained swimmers under the supervision of a qualified coach.
- ▶ Running into the water and then diving head-first into breaking waves is dangerous.
- ▶ If you are bodysurfing, always keep your arms out in front of you to protect your head and neck.
- ▶ Never use alcohol or other drugs when diving and swimming.

[1] Spinal Cord Injury Information Network. *Spinal Cord Injury, Facts and Figures at a Glance.* August 2004. *http://www.spinalcord.uab.edu/.* Accessed 11/01/04.

If you suspect a head, neck or back injury and the victim is in the water, your goal is to prevent any further movement of the head, neck or back and move the victim to safety. *Always check first whether a lifeguard or other trained professional is present before touching or moving a victim who may have a head, neck or back injury.*

General Guidelines for Care

A victim's head, neck or back can be stabilized in several ways while the victim is still in the water. These methods are described in the next section. Follow these general guidelines for a victim with a suspected head, neck or back injury in shallow water:

1. Be sure someone has called 9-1-1 or the local emergency number. If others are present, ask someone to help you.
2. Minimize movement of the victim's head, neck and back. Gently hold the victim's head in the position in which you found it and support it in that position until EMS arrives.
3. Position the victim face-up at the surface of the water. Keep the victim's face out of the water to let the victim breathe.
4. Check for consciousness and breathing once you have stabilized the victim's head, neck and back. A victim who can talk or is gasping for air is conscious and breathing.
5. Support the victim with his or her head, neck and back immobilized until help arrives. If the head is sharply turned to one side, DO NOT move it. Support it in the position found.

Specific Immobilization Techniques

The following sections describe two methods for stabilizing the victim's head, neck and back in the water. These methods will allow you to care for the victim whether he or she is face-up or face-down.

Hip and Shoulder Support

This method helps limit movement to the head, neck and back. Use it for a victim who is face-up. Support the victim at the hips and shoulders to keep the face out of the water. To perform the hip and shoulder support—

1. Approach the victim from the side, and lower yourself to chest depth.
2. Slide one arm under the victim's shoulders and the other arm under the hip bones. Support the victim's body horizontally, keeping the face clear of the water (**Fig. 20-17**).
3. Do not lift the victim, but support him or her in the water until help arrives.

Head Splint

This method provides better stabilization than the hip and shoulder support. Use it for a victim who is face-down at or near the surface of the water. To perform the head splint technique—

1. Approach the victim from the side.
2. Gently move the victim's arms up alongside the head by grasping the victim's arms midway between the shoulder and elbow. Grasp the victim's right arm with your right hand.

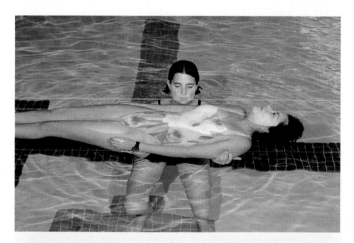
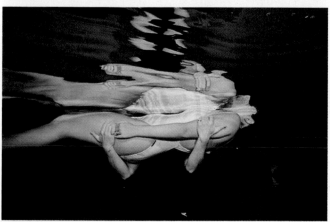

Figure 20-17 The hip and shoulder support helps limit movement of the head, neck or back, while keeping the victim's face clear of water.

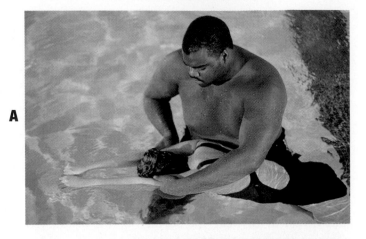

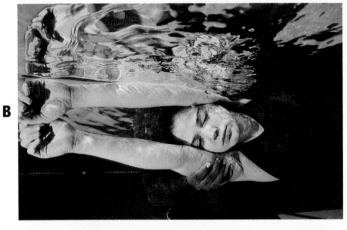

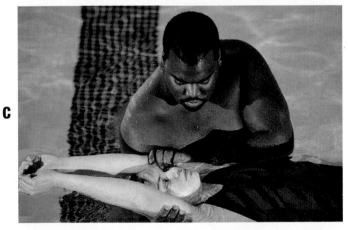

Figure 20-18 When performing the head splint technique, **A,** Squeeze the victim's arms against her head, **B,** Move the victim slowly forward and rotate the victim toward you until she is face-up, and **C,** Position the victim's head in the crook of your arm with the head in line with the body.

Grasp the victim's left arm with your left hand.

3. Squeeze the victim's arms against his or her head. This helps keep the head in line with the body (**Fig. 20-18, A**).
4. With your body at shoulder depth in the water, glide the victim slowly forward.
5. Continue moving slowly, and rotate the victim until he or she is face-up. This is done by pushing the victim's arm that is closest to you under water, while pulling the victim's other arm across the surface (**Fig. 20-18, B**).
6. Position the victim's head in the crook of your arm with the head in line with the body (**Fig. 20-18, C**).
7. Maintain this position in the water until help arrives.

Helping Someone Who Has Fallen Through Ice

If a person falls through ice, never go out onto the ice yourself to attempt a rescue. This is a very dangerous situation, and you are likely to become a victim too. Instead, follow these guidelines:

1. Send someone to call 9-1-1 or the local emergency number immediately. Trained rescuers may be needed to get the victim out of the ice, and even if you succeed in rescuing the victim, he or she will probably need medical care.
2. From a secure place on land, try a reaching or throwing assist. Use anything at hand that the victim can grasp for support, such as a tree branch, pole, life jacket or weighted rope (**Fig. 20-19**). Act quickly, because the victim's hands may become too numb to grasp the object.
3. If it is possible to do so safely, pull the victim to shore. If it is not, talk to the victim and make sure he or she is secure as possible with the object until help arrives.

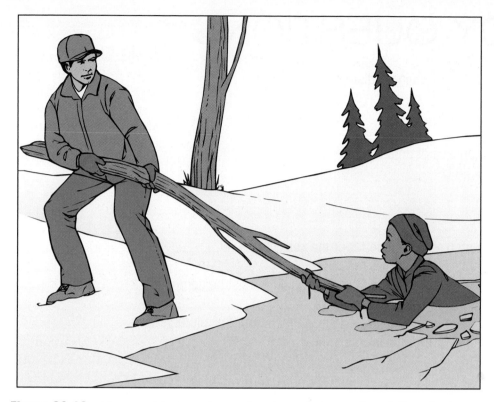

Figure 20-19   Use an object, such as a tree branch, to reach a victim who has fallen through the ice.

SUMMARY

Many drownings can be prevented by following simple precautions when in, on or around water. Use the basic methods of reaching, throwing or wading to reach or assist a victim in the water without endangering yourself. Always remember to stay safe. If there is any chance that you cannot safely and easily help the victim in trouble, call for professional assistance. Further training in water safety and lifeguarding is available through the local Red Cross chapter.

APPLICATION QUESTION

1. What can you do to help Eric once he has fallen into your boss's pool?

STUDY QUESTIONS

1. List three methods of rescuing a distressed swimmer.

2. List four characteristics of an active drowning victim.

In questions 3 through 6, circle the letter of the correct answer.

3. In which of the following situations would a wading assist be appropriate?

    a. You can reach the victim by extending a branch from the shore.
    b. You suspect or see strong currents.
    c. The bottom is not firm.
    d. The water is shallow, and you can stand with your head out of the water.

4. You see a man struggling in the rushing waters of a flooded creek. Which is the best way to try to rescue him without endangering yourself?

    a. Dive into the water and grab him.
    b. Wade in and reach out to him with an object.
    c. From the shoreline, extend an object for him to reach.
    d. Yell to him to kick forcefully.

5. If a victim is unconscious and too heavy for you to carry, which method could you use to get the victim out of the water?

    a. A walking assist
    b. A wading assist
    c. The two-victim seat carry
    d. The beach drag

6. Which two techniques can be used for stabilizing the head, neck and back of a victim with a suspected head, neck or back injury?

    a. Head and back support and head splint
    b. Hip/shoulder support and head splint
    c. Head splint and head/back immobilization technique
    d. Head and chin support and head and back support

Answers are listed in Appendix A.

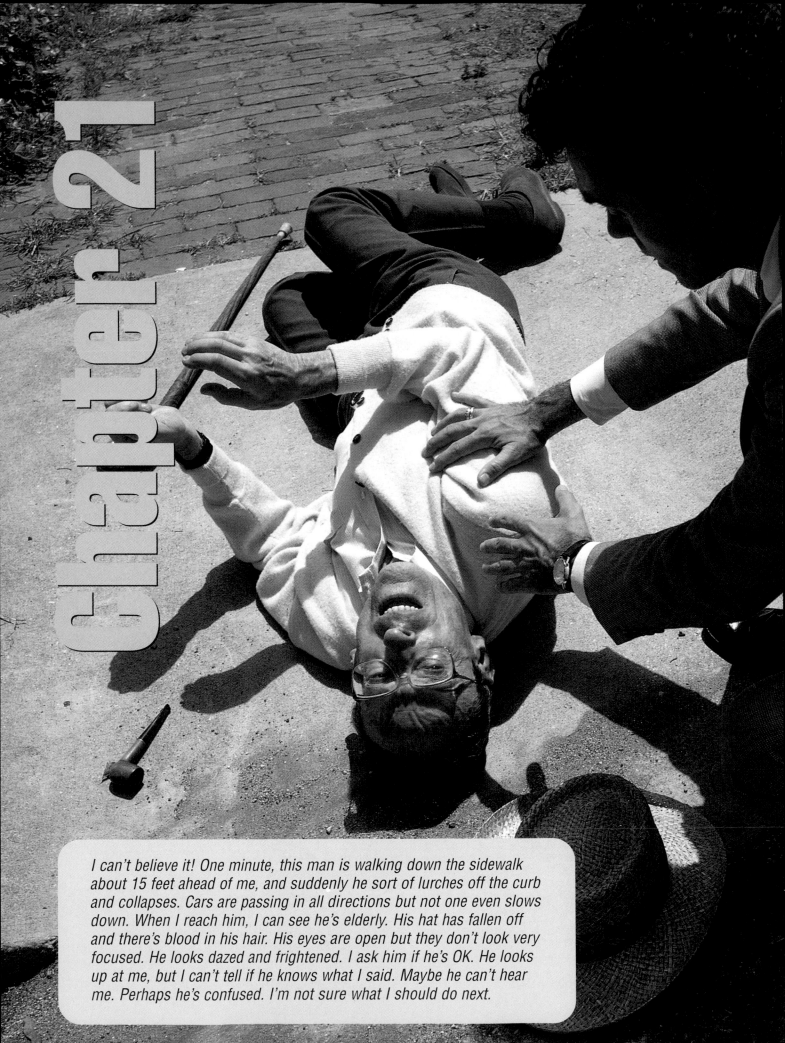

I can't believe it! One minute, this man is walking down the sidewalk about 15 feet ahead of me, and suddenly he sort of lurches off the curb and collapses. Cars are passing in all directions but not one even slows down. When I reach him, I can see he's elderly. His hat has fallen off and there's blood in his hair. His eyes are open but they don't look very focused. He looks dazed and frightened. I ask him if he's OK. He looks up at me, but I can't tell if he knows what I said. Maybe he can't hear me. Perhaps he's confused. I'm not sure what I should do next.

People with Special Needs

Objectives

After reading this chapter, you should be able to—

- Describe considerations for checking an infant, a toddler, a preschooler, a school-age child and an adolescent.

- Explain how to observe an ill or injured child and how to communicate with the parents or guardian.

- Describe how to check an older adult.

- Describe four problems that can affect older adults and their implications for care.

- Explain ways of communicating with victims who have hearing loss.

- Explain options available when trying to communicate with a victim and there is a language barrier.

- Explain what you should do if you encounter a crime scene or hostile victim.

Introduction

In an emergency, you should be aware of the special needs and considerations of children, older adults, people with disabilities and people who do not speak the same language you speak. Knowing these needs and considerations will help you better understand the nature of the emergency and give appropriate care. A young child may be terrified. An elderly adult may be confused. A person with a disability may be unable to hear or see you. A victim may not speak the language(s) you speak. Being able to communicate with and reassure people with special needs will help you to care for them effectively.

INFANTS AND CHILDREN

Infants and children have unique needs and require special care. Assessing a conscious infant's or child's condition can be difficult, especially if he or she does not know you. At certain ages, infants and children do not readily accept strangers. Infants and very young children cannot tell you what is wrong.

Communicating with an Ill or Injured Child

We tend to react more strongly and emotionally to a child who is in pain or terror. You will need to try exceptionally hard to control your emotions and your facial expressions. Doing so will be helpful to both the child and any concerned adults. To help an ill or injured child, you also need to try to imagine how the child feels. A child is afraid of the unknown. He or she is afraid of being ill or hurt, being touched by strangers and being separated from his or her parents or guardian.

How you interact with an ill or injured infant or child is very important. You need to reduce the child's anxiety and panic and gain the child's trust and cooperation if possible. Move in slowly. The sudden appearance of a stranger may upset the child. Get as close to the infant's or child's eye level as you can, and keep your voice calm (**Fig. 21-1**). Smile at the child. Ask the child's name, and use it when you talk with him or her. Talk slowly and distinctly, and use words the child will easily understand. Ask questions the child will be able to answer easily. Explain to the child and the parents or guardian what you are going to do. Reassure the child that you are there to help and will not leave him or her.

Checking Infants and Children

To be able to effectively check infants and children, it is helpful to be aware of certain characteristics of children in specific age groups.

KEY TERMS

Alzheimer's disease: A progressive, degenerative disease that affects the brain, resulting in impaired memory, thinking and behavior.

Child abuse: The physical, psychological or sexual assault of a child, resulting in injury and emotional trauma.

Disability: The absence or impairment of motor, sensory or mental function.

Hearing loss: Partial or total loss of hearing.

Impairment: Damage or reduction in quality, quantity, value or strength of a function.

Mental (cognitive) function: The brain's capacity to reason and to process information.

Motor function: The ability to move the body or a body part.

Motor impairment: The total or partial inability to move or to use a body part.

Sensory function: The ability to see, hear, touch, taste and smell.

Sudden infant death syndrome (SIDS): The sudden death of a seemingly normal, healthy infant; occurs during the infant's sleep without evidence of disease; sometimes called crib death.

Vision loss: Partial or total loss of sight.

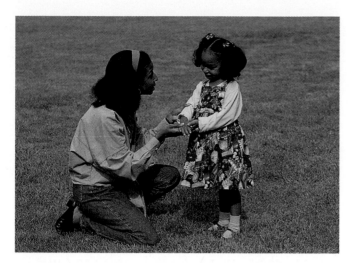

Figure 21-1 To communicate with a child, get as close to eye level as you can.

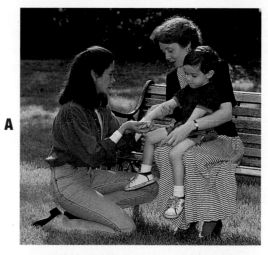

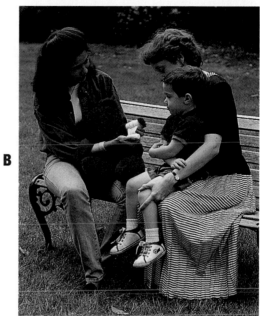

Figure 21-2 **A,** Allow a parent to hold the child while you check him or her. **B,** Demonstrating first aid steps on a stuffed animal or doll helps a toddler understand how you will care for him or her.

Characteristics of Infants and Children

Children up to 1 year of age are commonly referred to as infants. Infants less than 6 months old are relatively easy to approach and are unlikely to be afraid of you. Older infants, however, often show "stranger anxiety." They may turn away from you and cry and cling to their parent or guardian. If a parent or the guardian is calm and cooperative, ask him or her to help you. Try to check the infant in the parent's or guardian's lap or arms.

Children ages 1 and 2 years are often referred to as toddlers. Toddlers may not cooperate with your attempts to check them. They are usually very concerned about being separated from a parent or guardian. If you reassure the toddler that he or she will not be separated from a parent or guardian, the toddler may be comforted. If possible, give the toddler a few minutes to get used to you before attempting to check him or her and check the toddler in the parent's or guardian's lap (**Fig. 21-2, A**). A toddler may also respond to praise or be comforted by holding a special toy or blanket.

Children ages 3, 4, and 5 are commonly referred to as preschoolers. Children in this age group are usually easy to check if you use their natural curiosity. Allow them to inspect items such as bandages. Opportunities to explore can reduce many fears and provide distraction. Reassure the child that you are going to help and will not leave him or her. Sometimes you can show what you are going to do on a stuffed animal or doll (**Fig. 21-2, B**). The child may be upset by seeing his or her cut or other injury, so cover it with a dressing as soon as possible.

School-age children are between 6 and 12 years of age. They are usually cooperative and can be a good source of information about what happened. You can usually talk readily with school-age children. Do not let the child's chronological age influence you to expect an injured or ill child to behave in a way consistent with that age. An injured 11-year-old, for example, may behave more like a 7-year-old. Be especially careful not to talk down to these children. Let them know if you are going to do anything that may be painful. Children in this age group are becoming conscious of their bodies and may not like exposure. Respect their modesty.

Adolescents are between 13 and 18 years of age and are typically more adult than child. Direct your questions to an adolescent victim rather than to a parent or guardian. Allow input from a parent or guardian, however. Occasionally, if a parent or guardian is present, you may not be able to get an accurate idea of what happened or what is wrong. Adolescents are modest and often respond better to a responder of the same gender.

Interacting with Parents and Caregivers

If the family is excited or agitated, the child is likely to be too. When you can calm the family, the child will often calm down as well. Remember to get consent to give care from any adult responsible for the child when possible. Any concerned adults need your support, so behave as calmly as possible.

Observing an Infant or Child

You can obtain a lot of information by observing the infant or child before actually touching him or her. Look for signals that indicate changes in the level of consciousness, any trouble breathing and any apparent injuries and conditions. Realize that the situation may change as soon as you touch the child because he or she may become anxious or upset. Do not separate the infant or child from loved ones. Often a parent or guardian will be holding a crying infant or child. In this case, you can check the child while the adult continues to hold him or her. Unlike some ill or injured adults, an infant or child is unlikely to try to cover up or deny how he or she feels. An infant or child in pain, for example, will generally let you know that he or she hurts and the source of the pain as well as he or she can.

Whenever possible, begin your check of a conscious child at the toe rather than the head. Checking this way is less threatening to the child and allows him or her to watch what is going on and take part in it. Ask a young child to point to any place that hurts. An older child can tell you the location of painful areas. If you need to hold an infant, always support the head when you pick him or her up.

Special Problems

Certain problems are unique to children, such as specific kinds of injury and illness. The following sections discuss some of these concerns.

Injury

Injury is the number one cause of death for children in the United States. Many of these deaths are the result of motor vehicle crashes. The greatest dangers to a child involved in a motor vehicle incident are airway obstruction and bleeding. Severe bleeding must be controlled as quickly as possible. A relatively small amount of blood lost by an adult is a large amount for an infant or child. Because a child's head is large and heavy in proportion to the rest of the body, the head is the most often injured area. A child injured as the result of force or a blow may also have damage to the organs in the abdominal and chest cavities. Such damage can cause severe internal bleeding. A child secured only by a lap belt may have serious abdominal or spinal injuries in a car crash. Try to find out what happened, because a severely injured child may not immediately show signals of injury.

To avoid some of the needless deaths of children involved in motor vehicle crashes, laws have been enacted requiring that children ride in safety seats or wear safety belts. As a result, more children's lives are saved. You may have to check and care for an injured child while he or she is in a safety seat. A safety seat does not normally pose any problems while you are checking a child. Leave the child in the seat if the seat has not been damaged. If the child is to be transported to a medical facility for examination, he or she can often be safely secured in the safety seat for transport.

Illness

Certain signals in an infant or child can indicate specific illnesses. Often these illnesses are not life threatening, but some can be. A high fever in a child often indicates some form of infection. In a young child, even a minor infection can result in a rather high fever, which is often defined as a temperature above 103° F (40° C). Prolonged or excessively high fever can result in seizures (see Chapter 15). Your initial care for a child with a high fever is to gently cool the child. Remove excessive clothing or blankets and sponge the child with lukewarm water. Call a physician at once. *Do not give the child aspirin.* For a child, taking aspirin can result in an extremely serious medical condition called Reye's syndrome. See Chapter 6 for details on breathing emergencies in infants and children.

Sudden Infant Death Syndrome (SIDS)

"For the first few months, I would lie awake in bed at night and wonder if she was still breathing. I mean you just never know. I couldn't get to sleep until I checked on her at least once." This is how one mother described her first experience with parenting.

Sudden infant death syndrome (SIDS) is the sudden, unexpected and unexplained death of apparently healthy babies. It is the leading cause of death for infants between the ages of 1 month and 1 year, with the greatest number of deaths occurring in infants younger than age 6 months. In the United States, SIDS, sometimes called crib death, is responsible for the death of about 7000 infants each year.

Because it cannot be predicted or prevented, SIDS causes many new parents to feel anxious. However there are several things you can do to lower the risk of SIDS. These include—

- Placing an infant on his or her back while he or she is asleep.
- Placing an infant on a firm mattress. Placing an infant to sleep on soft mattresses, sofas, sofa cushions, waterbeds, sheepskins or other soft surfaces greatly increases the risk of SIDS.
- Removing all soft, fluffy and loose bedding and stuffed toys from the infant's sleeping area.
- Keeping blankets and other coverings away from an infant's mouth and nose. The best way to do this is to dress the baby in nightclothes so you will not have to use any other covering. If you do use a blanket or other covers, make sure that the baby's feet are at the bottom of the crib, the blanket is no higher than the baby's chest and the blanket is tucked in around the bottom of the crib mattress.
- Not allowing people to smoke around your baby.
- Preventing an infant from getting too warm during sleep. An infant's room should be at a temperature that is comfortable for an adult. Too many layers of clothing or blankets can overheat your baby.

The best prevention for SIDS, as well as many other infant diseases, is for women to practice healthy behaviors while pregnant. They should get proper prenatal care, eat a balanced diet, not smoke, not drink alcoholic beverages and get adequate rest and exercise.

For more information on sleep position for babies and reducing the risk of SIDS, visit the National Institute of Child Health & Human Development Web site at *www.nichd.nih.gov.*

SOURCES
National Institute of Health Web site, *www.nichd.nih.gov/sids/reduce_infant_risk.htm#WhatCan.* Accessed 10/8/04.

Poisoning

Poisoning is the fifth-largest cause of unintentional death in the United States for people ages 1 to 24. For the youngest of these victims, mainly children under 5 years of age, poisoning often occurs from ingesting household products or medications. Care for poisoning is discussed in Chapter 16, and how to help prevent poisoning of children in the home is discussed in Chapters 16 and 24.

Child Abuse

At some point, you may encounter a situation involving an injured child in which you have reason to suspect child abuse. *Child abuse* is the physical, psychological or sexual assault of a child resulting in injury and emotional trauma. Child abuse involves an injury or a pattern of injuries that do not result from an accident. Suspect child abuse if the child's injuries cannot be logically explained, or a parent or guardian gives an inconsistent or suspicious account of how the injuries occurred.

The signals of child abuse include—

▶ An injury that does not fit the parent or guardian's description of what caused the injury.
▶ Obvious or suspected fractures in a child younger than 2 years of age; any unexplained fractures.
▶ Injuries in various stages of healing, especially bruises and burns.
▶ Bruises and burns in unusual shapes, such as bruises shaped like belt buckles or burns the size of a cigarette tip.
▶ Unexplained lacerations or abrasions, especially to the mouth, lips and eyes.
▶ Injuries to the genitalia; pain when the child sits down.
▶ More injuries than are common for a child of the same age.

When caring for a child who may have been abused, your first priority is to care for the child's illness or injuries. An abused child may be frightened, hysterical or withdrawn. He or she may be unwilling to talk about the incident in an attempt to protect the abuser. If you suspect abuse, explain your concerns to responding police officers or EMS personnel if possible.

If you think you have reasonable cause to believe that abuse has occurred, report your suspicions to a community or state agency, such as the Department of Social Services, the Department of Child and Family Services or Child Protective Services. You may be afraid to report suspected child abuse because you do not wish to get involved or are afraid of getting sued. However, in most states, when you make a report in good faith, you are immune from any civil or criminal liability or penalty, even if you made a mistake. In this instance, "good faith" means that you honestly believe that abuse has occurred or the potential for abuse exists and a prudent and reasonable person in the same position would also honestly believe abuse has occurred or the potential for abuse exists. You do not need to identify yourself when you report child abuse, although your report will have more credibility if you do.

Sudden Infant Death Syndrome

Sudden infant death syndrome (SIDS) is a disorder that causes seemingly healthy infants to stop breathing while they sleep. SIDS is a leading cause of death for infants between 1 month and 1 year of age. By the time the infant's condition has been discovered, he or she will be in cardiac arrest. Make sure someone has called 9-1-1 or the local emergency number or call yourself. Perform CPR on the infant until EMS personnel arrive.

An incident involving a severely injured or ill infant or child or one who has died can be emotionally upsetting. After such an episode, find someone you trust with whom you can talk about the experience and express your feelings. If you continue to be distressed, seek some professional counseling. The feelings engendered by such incidents need to be dealt with and understood or they can result in serious stress reactions. For more information on stress, see Chapter 24.

Older Adults

Older adults, or the elderly, are generally considered those people over 65 years of age. They are quickly becoming the fastest growing age group in the United States. A major reason is an increase in life expectancy because of medical advancements and improvements in health care and knowledge. Since 1900, life expectancy has increased by 57 percent. For example, in 1900, the average life expectancy was 49 years. Today, the average life expectancy is over 75 years.

Normal aging brings about changes. People age at different rates, however, and so do their organs and body parts. A person may have a "young" heart but "old" skin, for example, and someone with wrinkled, fragile skin may have strong bones or excellent respiratory function.

Overall, however, body function generally declines as we age, with some changes beginning as early as age 30. The lungs become less efficient, so older people are at higher risk of developing pneumonia and other lung diseases. The amount of blood pumped by the heart with each beat decreases, and the heart rate slows. The blood vessels harden, causing increased work for the heart. Hearing and vision usually decline, often causing some degree of sight and hearing loss. Reflexes become slower, and arthritis may affect joints, causing movement to become painful. Four out of five older adults develop some sort of chronic condition or disease.

Checking an Older Adult

To check an injured or ill older adult, attempt to learn the person's name and use it when you speak to him or her. Consider using Mrs., Mr. or Ms. as a sign of respect. Get at the person's eye level so that he or she can see and hear you more clearly (**Fig. 21-3**). If the person seems confused at first, the confusion may be the result of impaired vision or hearing. If he or she usually wears eyeglasses and cannot find them, try to locate them. Speak slowly and clearly, and look at the person's face while you talk. Notice if he or she has a hearing aid. Someone who needs glasses to see or a hearing aid to hear is likely to be very anxious without them. If the person is truly confused, try to find out if the confusion is the result of the injury or a condition he or she already has. Information from family members or bystanders is frequently helpful. The person may be afraid of falling, so if he or she is standing, offer an arm or hand. Remember that an older person may need to move very slowly.

Try to find out what medications the person is taking and if he or she has any medical conditions so that you can tell EMS personnel. Look for a medical ID tag or bracelet that will give you the victim's name and address and information about any specific condition the victim has. Be aware that an elderly person may not recognize the signals of a serious condition. An elderly person may also minimize any signals for fear of losing his or her independence or being placed in a nursing home.

Special Situations

Physical and mental changes can occur as a result of aging. As a result of these changes, many older adults are particularly susceptible to certain problems. These problems may require you to adapt your way of communicating and to be aware of certain potential age-related conditions.

Falls

Falls are the sixth-leading cause of death for people over 65 years of age. As a result of slower reflexes, failing eyesight and hearing, arthritis and problems such as unsteady balance and movement, older adults are at increased risk of falls. Falls frequently result in fractures because the bones become weaker and more brittle with age.

Head Injuries

An older adult is also at greater risk of serious head injuries. As we age, the size of the brain decreases. This decrease results in more space between the surface of the brain and the inside of the skull. This space allows more movement of the brain within the skull, which can increase the likelihood of serious head injury. Occasionally, an older adult may not develop the signals of a head injury until days after a fall. Therefore, unless you know the cause of a behavior change, you should always suspect a head injury as a possible cause of unusual behavior in an elderly person, especially if the victim has had a fall or a blow to the head.

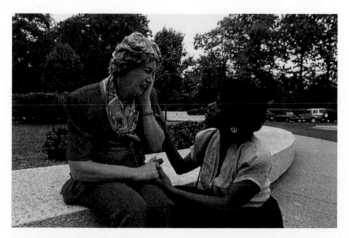

Figure 21-3   Speak to an elderly victim at eye level so that he or she can see or hear you more clearly.

Memories Memories Memories

Alzheimer's disease affects an estimated 4 million American adults and results in 100,000 deaths annually. Most victims are older than 65; however, Alzheimer's disease can strike people in their 40s and 50s. Men and women are affected almost equally. At this time, scientists are still looking for the cause of Alzheimer's disease. A confirmed diagnosis of the disease can only be made by examining the victim's brain tissue after death. While there are no treatments to stop or reverse a person's mental decline from Alzheimer's disease, several drugs are available now to help manage some of its signals.

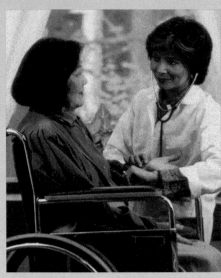

Signals of Alzheimer's disease develop gradually. They include confusion; progressive memory loss; and changes in personality, behavior and the ability to think and communicate. Eventually, victims of Alzheimer's disease become totally unable to care for themselves.

A number of disorders have signals similar to those of Alzheimer's disease. Some of them can be treated. Therefore, it is very important for anyone who is experiencing memory loss or confusion to have a thorough medical examination.

Most people with illnesses such as Alzheimer's disease are cared for by their families for much of their illness. Giving care at home requires careful planning. The home has to be made safe, and routines must be set up for daily activities, such as mealtimes, personal care and leisure.

Services That Help

It is important for anyone caring for a person with Alzheimer's disease or a related problem to realize that he or she is not alone. There are people and organizations that can help both you and the person with Alzheimer's disease. For health-care services, a physician—perhaps your family physician—or a specialist can give you medical advice, including help with difficult behavior and personality changes.

If you are caring for an Alzheimer's disease victim living at home, you may need help with basic services such as nutrition and transportation. A visiting nurse or nutritionist can help you, and a volunteer program like Meals-on-Wheels may be helpful. Volunteer or paid transportation services may also be available to take Alzheimer's disease victims to and from health-care facilities, adult day care and other programs.

Visiting nurses, home health aides and homemakers can come to your home and give help with health care, bathing, dressing, shopping and cooking. Many adult day-care centers provide recreational activities designed for people with Alzheimer's disease. Some hospitals, nursing homes and other facilities may take in Alzheimer's disease victims for short stays. For Alzheimer's disease victims who can no longer live at home, group homes or foster homes may be available. Nursing homes offer more skilled nursing, and some specialize in the care of victims of Alzheimer's disease or similar diseases. A few hospice programs accept Alzheimer's disease victims who are nearing the end of their lives. Search to find out which, if any, services are covered by Medicare, Medicaid, Social Security, disability or veterans benefits in your state. A lawyer or a social worker may be able to help you.

To locate services that can help you, the Alzheimer's disease victim and other family members, check the yellow pages under Social Service Organizations and state and local government listings in the phone directory. You can also contact your local health department, area office on aging, and department of social services or senior citizens' services. Churches, synagogues and other religious institutions may also have information and programs; so may senior centers and nursing home staffs, hospital geriatric departments, physicians, nurses, social workers and counselors. You may have a nearby chapter of the Alzheimer's Association. To locate a chapter near you, call the association's 24-hour, toll-free number: 1-800-272-3900 or log onto *www.alz.org/overview.asp*.

SOURCES
American Red Cross, *Caring for a Loved One with Alzheimer's Disease or Dementia*, StayWell, Yardley, PA. 2004.

Confusion

The elderly are at increased risk of altered thinking patterns and confusion. Some of this change is the result of aging. Certain diseases, such as *Alzheimer's disease,* affect the brain, resulting in impaired memory and thinking and altered behavior. Confusion that comes on suddenly, however, may be the result of medication, even a medication the person has been taking regularly. An ill or injured person who has problems seeing or hearing may also become confused when ill or injured. This problem increases when the person is in an unfamiliar environment. A head injury can also result in confusion.

Confusion can be a signal of a medical emergency. An elderly person with pneumonia, for example, may not run a fever, have chest pain or be coughing, but because sufficient oxygen is not reaching the brain, the person may be confused. An elderly person can have a serious infection without fever, pain or nausea. An elderly person having a heart attack may not have chest pain, pale or ashen skin or other classic signals, but may be restless, short of breath and confused.

Depression is common in older adults. A depressed older adult may seem confused at first. A depressed person may also have signals, such as sudden shortness of breath or chest pains, with no apparent cause. Whatever the reason for any confusion, do not talk down to the victim or treat the victim like a child.

Problems with Heat and Cold

An elderly person is more susceptible to extremes in temperature. The person may be unable to feel temperature extremes because his or her body may no longer regulate temperature effectively. Body temperature may change rapidly to a dangerously high or low level.

The body of an elderly person retains heat because of a decreased ability to sweat and the reduced ability of the circulatory system to adjust to heat. If an elderly person shows signals of heat-related illness, take his or her temperature, and if it is above normal, call 9-1-1 or the local emergency number. Slowly cool the person off with a lukewarm sponge bath, and give care as described in Chapter 19. If you find an elderly person hot to the touch, unable to speak and unconscious or semiconscious, call 9-1-1 or the local emergency number immediately. Put the person in a cooler location if possible, but do not try to quickly cool the person with cold water or put him or her in front of a fan or air conditioner.

An elderly person may become chilled and suffer hypothermia simply by sitting in a draft or in front of a fan or air conditioner. Hypothermia can occur at any time of the year in temperature that is 65° F (18° C) or less. People can go on for several days suffering from mild hypothermia that they do not recognize. The older person with mild hypothermia will want to lie down frequently, which will lower the body temperature even further. If you suspect hypothermia, feel the person's skin to see if it is cold. Take the person's temperature. If his or her temperature is below 98.6° F (37° C), put the person in a warm room; wrap him or her in one or two blankets; give the person warm, decaffeinated and nonalcoholic liquid to drink; and call a physician for advice. However, if the body temperature is below 95° F (35° C), call 9-1-1 or the local emergency number immediately. This condition is life threatening. Do not apply any direct heat, such as a heating pad, electric blanket turned high or a hot bath. Doing so will cause blood flow to increase to the area being heated and take blood away from the vital organs.

PEOPLE WITH DISABILITIES

The absence or loss of motor, sensory or mental function is called a *disability. Impairment* is damage or reduction in quality, quantity, value or strength of the function. People who have a disability may be impaired in one or more functions. The Centers for Disease Control and Prevention estimates that over 33 million people in the United States have disabilities. With many disabled people, communication can be a major challenge in finding out what has happened and what might be wrong in an emergency situation.

Physical Disability

Physical disability includes impairment of *motor function,* or movement, and of *sensory function,* impairment of one or more of the senses—including sight, hearing, taste, smell and touch. People may be impaired in one or both of these functions.

General hints for approaching an injured or ill person who you have reason to believe is in some way disabled include the following:

▶ Speak to the person before touching him or her.

▶ Ask "How can I help?" or "Do you need help?"

▶ Ask for assistance and information from the person who has the disability—he or she has been living with the disability and best understands it. If the person is not able to communicate, ask any of his or her family members, friends or companions who are available.

▶ Do not remove any braces, canes, other physical support, eyeglasses or hearing aids. Removal of these items puts the person at a disadvantage of losing necessary physical support for the body.

▶ Look for a medical ID tag at the person's wrist or neck.

▶ A person with a disability may have an animal assistant, such as a guide dog or hearing dog. Be aware that this animal may be protective of the person in an emergency situation. Someone may need to calm and restrain the animal. Allow the animal to stay with the person if possible, which will help reassure them both.

Hearing Loss

Hearing loss is a partial or total loss of hearing. Some people are born with a hearing loss. Hearing loss can also result from an injury or illness affecting the ear, the nerves leading from the brain to the ear or the brain itself. You may not initially be aware that the injured or ill person has a hearing loss. Often the victim will tell you, either in speech or by pointing to the ear and shaking the head no. Some people carry a card stating that they have a hearing loss. You may see a hearing aid in a person's ear.

The biggest obstacle you must overcome in caring for a person with a hearing loss is communication. You will need to figure out how to get that person's consent to give care, and you need to find out what the problem may be. Often the injured or ill person can read lips. Position yourself where the victim can see your face clearly. Look straight at the victim while you speak, and speak slowly. Do not exaggerate the way you form words. Do not turn your face away while you speak. Many people with a hearing impairment, however, do not read lips. Using gestures and writing messages on paper may be the most effective way you can communicate in an emergency. If you and the victim know sign language, use it. Some people who are hearing impaired have a machine called a telecommunications device for the deaf (TDD). You can use this device to type messages and questions to the victim, and the victim can type replies to you (**Fig. 21-4, *A-D***). Many people who have hearing impairments can speak, some distinctly, some not

so clearly. If you have trouble understanding, ask the person to repeat what he or she said. Do not pretend to understand. If the person cannot speak, use written messages.

Vision Loss

Vision loss is a partial or total loss of sight. Vision loss can have many causes. Some people are born with vision loss. Others lose vision as a result of disease or injury. Vision loss is not necessarily a problem with the eyes. It can result from problems with the vision centers in the brain.

People with vision loss are generally not embarrassed by their condition. It is no more difficult to communicate orally with a person who has a partial or total loss of sight than with someone who can see. You do not need to speak loudly or in overly simple terms. Checking a person who has a vision loss is like checking a victim who has good vision. The victim may not be able to tell you certain things about how an injury occurred but can usually give you a generally accurate account based on his or her interpretation of sound and touch.

When caring for a person with vision loss, help to reassure him or her by explaining what is going on and what you are doing. If you must move a visually impaired person who can walk, stand beside the person and have him or her hold onto your arm (**Fig. 21-5**). Walk at a normal pace, alert the person to any obstacles in the way such as stairs and identify whether to step up or down. If the person has a seeing eye dog, try to keep them together. Ask the person to tell you how to handle the dog or ask him or her to do it.

Motor Impairment

The person with ***motor impairment*** is unable to move normally. He or she may be missing a body part or have a problem with the bones or muscles or the nerves controlling them. Causes of motor impairment include stroke, **muscular dystrophy, multiple sclerosis,** paralysis, **cerebral palsy** or loss of a limb. In caring for an injured or ill person with motor impairment, be aware that the person may view accepting help as failure and may refuse your help to prove that he or she does not need it.

Determining which problems are pre-existing and which are the result of immediate injury or illness can be difficult. If you care for all problems you detect as if they are new, you can hardly go wrong. Be aware that checking one side of the body against

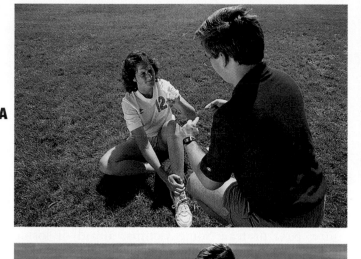
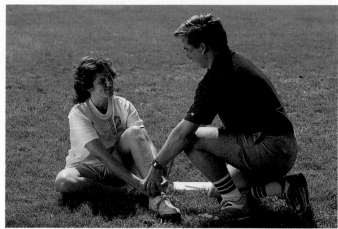
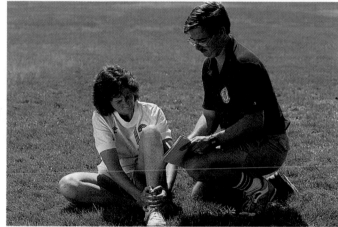
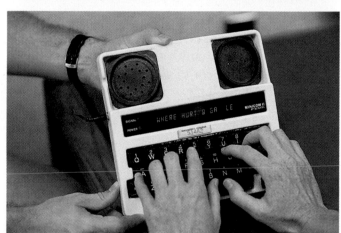

Figure 21-4 Communicate with a victim of hearing loss in the best way possible:
A, signing; **B,** lip reading; **C,** writing; **D,** TDD.

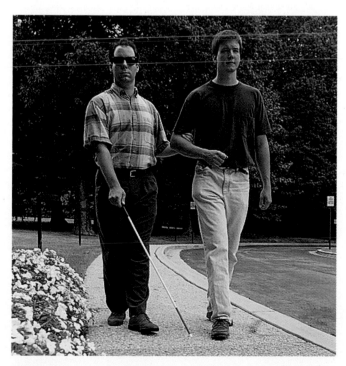

Figure 21-5 If a victim with a vision loss can walk, stand beside him or her and have the person hold your arm.

the other in your check for non-life-threatening conditions may not be effective with a person with motor impairment, since body parts may not look normal as a result of a specific condition.

Mental Impairment

Mental, or *cognitive, function* includes the brain's capacity to reason and to process information. A person with mental impairment has problems performing these operations. Some types of mental impairment are genetic, or, such as **Down syndrome,** are genetic alterations. Others result from injuries or infections that occur during pregnancy, shortly after birth or later in life. Some causes are never determined.

You may not be able to determine if a victim is mentally impaired, or it may be obvious. Approach the victim as you would any other person in his or her age group. When you speak, try to determine the person's level of understanding. If the person appears not to understand you, rephrase what you were saying in simpler terms. Listen carefully to what the person says. People who are mentally impaired often lead very orderly and structured lives. A sudden illness or injury can disrupt the order in a person's life and cause a great deal of anxiety and fear. Take time to explain who you are and what you are going to do. Offer reassurance. Try to gain the victim's trust. If a parent, guardian or caregiver is present, ask that person to help you care for the person.

LANGUAGE BARRIERS

Another reason for an uncomprehending look when you speak to a victim is that the person may not understand English or any other language you may speak. Getting consent to give care to a victim with whom you have a language barrier can be a problem. Find out if any bystanders speak the victim's language and can help translate. Do your best to communicate nonverbally. Use gestures and facial expressions. If the person is in pain, he or she will probably be anxious to let you know where that pain is. Watch his or her gestures and facial expressions carefully. When you speak to the victim, speak slowly and in a normal tone. The victim probably has no trouble hearing you. When you call 9-1-1 or the local emergency number, explain that you are having difficulty communicating with the victim and say what nationality you believe the victim is or what language you believe the victim speaks. The EMS system may have someone available, such as a call taker, who can help with communication. If the victim has a life-threatening condition, such as severe bleeding, consent is implied. The victim will most likely be willing for you to give care in such a case anyhow.

SPECIAL SITUATIONS

Special situations such as a crime scene or a hostile victim may arise that you should handle with extreme caution. In certain instances, your first reaction may be to go to the aid of a victim. Instead, call 9-1-1 and stay at a safe distance until the scene is secured. Do not enter the scene of a suicide. If you happen to be on the scene when an unarmed person threatens suicide, call 9-1-1 or the local emergency number and the police. If the scene is safe, listen to the person and try to keep him or her talking until help arrives. Do not argue with the person. Leave or do not enter any scene where there is a weapon or where a crime has been committed. Do not approach the scene of a physical or sexual assault. These are crime scenes. Call 9-1-1 or the local emergency number and stay at a safe distance.

Sometimes a victim may be hostile or angry. A victim's rage or hostility may be caused by the injury, pain or fear. Some victims, afraid of losing control, will act resentful and suspicious. Hostile behavior may also result from the use of alcohol or other drugs, lack of oxygen or a medical condition. Once a victim realizes that you are there to help and are not a threat, the hostility usually goes away. If a victim refuses your care or threatens you, withdraw. Never try to argue with or restrain a victim. Call 9-1-1 or the local emergency number if someone has not already done so.

Uninjured family members may also display anger. They may pressure you to do something immediately. Often this anger stems from panic, anxiety or guilt. Try to remain calm, and be sympathetic but firm. Explain what you are going to do. If possible, find a way that family members can help, such as by comforting the victim.

SUMMARY

No two emergency situations are alike. Situations involving people with special needs, problems and characteristics require your awareness and understanding. To give effective care to an older adult, an infant or child; a person with a disability; or anyone with whom communication is a challenge, you may need to adapt your approach and your attitude. Situations may also occur in which you should not intervene. If a situation is in any way unsafe, do not approach the victim and if you have already approached, withdraw. If the situation is a crime scene, keep your distance and stay away and call for appropriate help.

APPLICATION QUESTIONS

1. What steps should you take when you see the man fall?

2. What factors could have been responsible for the man's collapse and behavior?

STUDY QUESTIONS

1. Match each term with the correct definition.

   a. Sensory function   d. Disability
   b. Child abuse   e. Impairment
   c. Alzheimer's disease   f. Motor impairment

   _____ The absence or impairment of motor, sensory or mental function.

   _____ A progressive, degenerative disease that affects the brain, resulting in impaired memory, thinking and behavior.

   _____ The total or partial inability to move or to use a body part.

   _____ The physical, psychological or sexual assault of a child, resulting in injury and emotional trauma.

   _____ Damage or reduction in quality, quantity, value or strength of a function.

   _____ The ability to see, hear, touch, taste and smell.

2. You are walking to the mailbox. A child on a skateboard suddenly rolls into the street from between two parked cars. A car, fortunately moving very slowly, strikes the child, knocking him to the pavement. Three people in the vicinity run to the scene. The driver gets out of the car, looking shocked and stunned.
   Describe in order the steps you should take.

3. A neighbor phones saying her grandmother has fallen and is lying on the bathroom floor. She asks you to come help. When you get there, the grandmother is conscious but unable to get up. She does not recognize her granddaughter. She says her left leg and hip hurt. What steps should you take?

In questions 4 through 8, circle the letter of the correct answer.

4. In which of the following ways should you move a victim with vision loss who can walk?

   a. Grasp the victim's arm or belt, and support the victim as you walk.
   b. Walk in front of the victim, and have him or her keep a hand on your shoulder.
   c. Walk behind the victim with a hand on the person's back.
   d. Walk beside the victim, and let him or her grasp your arm while you are walking.

5. The best position you can take in talking to an ill or injured young child is—

   a. Holding the child in your arms or lap.
   b. Being at eye level with the child.
   c. Standing up, looking down at the child.
   d. Behind the child, out of direct sight.

6. Which should you do if an ill or injured elderly person appears to be confused?

   a. Assume the person is in a permanent state of confusion.
   b. Inquire about any medications the person is taking.
   c. Assume the person has fallen and injured his or her head.
   d. All of the above.

7. What should you do if you become aware that a physical assault has taken place?

   a. Call 9-1-1 or the local emergency number and then approach the victim.
   b. Call 9-1-1 or the local emergency number and do not enter the scene.
   c. Approach the victim and have someone call 9-1-1 or the local emergency number.
   d. Assess the victim for life-threatening conditions.

8. A small child in a car seat is in an automobile collision. How would you check the child?

   a. Remove the child from the car seat.
   b. Ask any relative of the child who is on the scene to remove the child from the seat.
   c. Check the child while the child is in the car seat.
   d. Wait until EMS personnel arrive.

In questions 9 through 11, write the correct answer on the line.

9. You enter the apartment of an elderly person and find him lying down and semi-conscious. His skin is hot to the touch. The room is very warm and stuffy. This person could be suffering from
   _____.

10. If an elderly person's body temperature is below 95° F (35° C), you should immediately
    _____.

11. A conscious person who does not appear to hear or understand what you say may be
    _____, _____ or may _____.

12. List four possible causes of confusion in an elderly person.

Answers are listed in Appendix A.

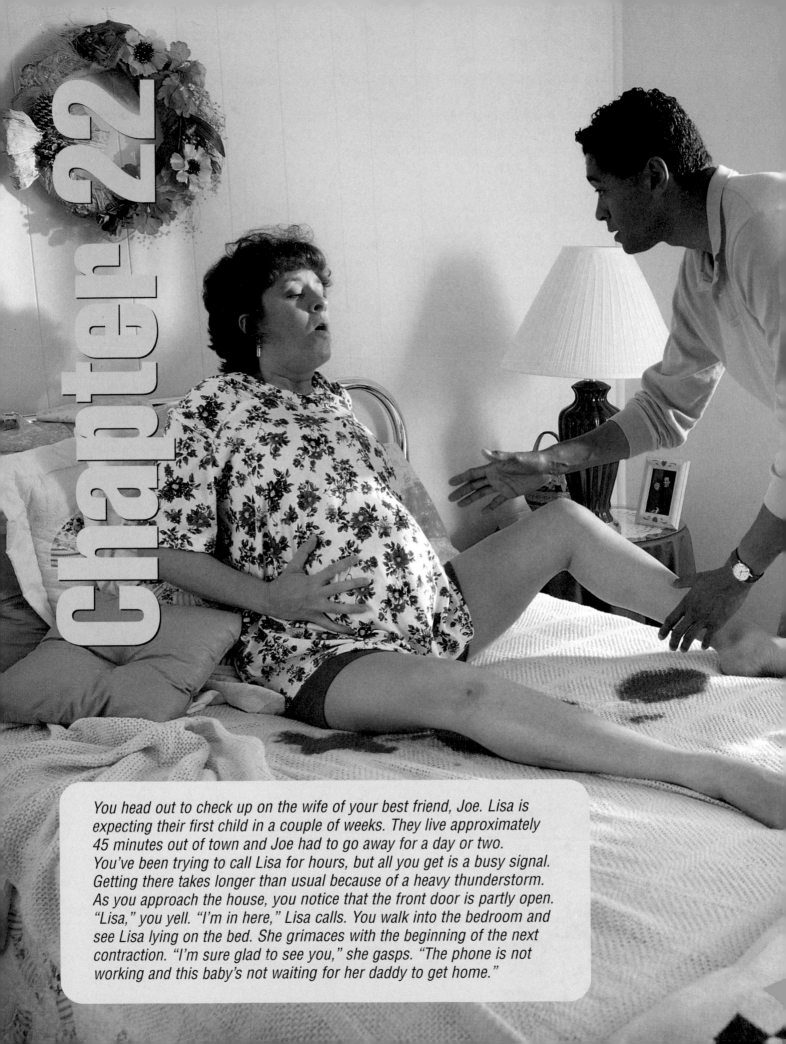

You head out to check up on the wife of your best friend, Joe. Lisa is expecting their first child in a couple of weeks. They live approximately 45 minutes out of town and Joe had to go away for a day or two. You've been trying to call Lisa for hours, but all you get is a busy signal. Getting there takes longer than usual because of a heavy thunderstorm. As you approach the house, you notice that the front door is partly open. "Lisa," you yell. "I'm in here," Lisa calls. You walk into the bedroom and see Lisa lying on the bed. She grimaces with the beginning of the next contraction. "I'm sure glad to see you," she gasps. "The phone is not working and this baby's not waiting for her daddy to get home."

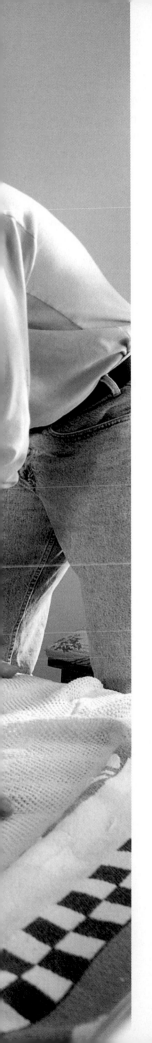

Childbirth

Objectives

After reading this chapter, you should be able to—

■ *Describe the three stages of labor.*

■ *Identify six factors you need to know to determine the mother's condition before the birth.*

■ *Describe two techniques the expectant mother can use to cope with labor pain and discomfort.*

■ *Identify equipment and supplies needed to assist with the delivery of a newborn.*

■ *Describe how to assist with the delivery of a newborn.*

■ *Identify the two priorities of care for a newborn.*

■ *Describe three steps to take in caring for the mother after delivery.*

■ *Identify four possible complications during childbirth that require immediate medical care.*

Introduction

Words such as exhausting, stressful, exciting, fulfilling, painful and scary are sometimes used to describe a planned childbirth: one that occurs in the hospital or at home under the supervision of a health-care provider. If you find yourself assisting with the delivery of a newborn, however, it is probably not happening in a planned situation. Therefore, your feelings, as well as those of the expectant mother, may be intensified by fear of the unexpected or the possibility that something might go wrong.

Take comfort in knowing that things rarely go wrong. Childbirth is a natural process. Thousands of children all over the world are born each day, without complications, in areas where no medical care is available.

By following a few simple steps, you can effectively assist in the birth process. This chapter will help you better understand the birth process and includes instruction on how to assist with the delivery of a newborn, how to give care for both the mother and newborn after the delivery and how to recognize complications requiring care from EMS personnel.

PREGNANCY

Pregnancy begins when an egg (ovum) is fertilized by a sperm, forming an **embryo**. The embryo implants itself within the lining of the mother's *uterus,* a pear-shaped organ that lies at the top center of the pelvis. The embryo is surrounded by the *amniotic sac.* This fluid-filled sac is also called the "bag of waters." The fluid helps protect the newborn from injury and infection.

As the embryo grows, its organs and body parts develop. After about 8 weeks, the embryo is called a **fetus.** To continue to develop properly, the fetus must receive nutrients. The fetus receives these nutrients from the mother through a specialized organ called the *placenta,* which is attached to the lining of the uterus. The placenta is attached to the fetus by a flexible structure called the **umbilical cord.** The fetus will continue to develop for approximately 40 weeks, at which time the birth process will begin (**Fig. 22-1**).

THE BIRTH PROCESS

The birth process begins with the onset of labor. *Labor* is the final phase of pregnancy. It is a process in which many systems work together to bring about birth. Labor begins with a rhythmic contraction of the uterus. As these contractions continue, they dilate the *cervix*—a short tube at the upper end of the *birth canal,* or *vagina.* The birth canal is the passageway from the uterus to the vaginal opening.

KEY TERMS

Amniotic sac: A fluid-filled sac that encloses, bathes and protects the developing newborn; commonly called the bag of waters.

Birth canal: The passageway from the uterus to the vaginal opening through which a newborn passes during birth.

Cervix: A short tube at the upper end of the birth canal; the opening of the uterus.

Contraction: The rhythmic tightening of muscles in the uterus during labor.

Crowning: The point in labor when the newborn's head is visible at the opening of the vagina.

Labor: The birth process, beginning with the contraction of the uterus and dilation of the cervix and ending with the stabilization and recovery of the mother.

Placenta: An organ attached to the uterus and unborn child through which nutrients are delivered to the newborn; expelled after the newborn is delivered.

Pregnancy: Begins when an egg (ovum) is fertilized by a sperm, forming an embryo.

Umbilical cord: A flexible structure that attaches the placenta to the unborn child, allowing for the passage of blood, nutrients and waste.

Uterus: A pear-shaped organ in a woman's pelvis in which an embryo forms and develops into a newborn.

Vagina: *See* birth canal.

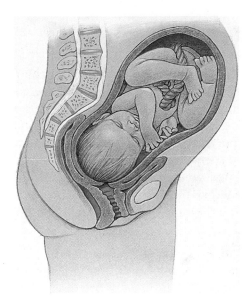

Figure 22-1   Mother and fetus at 40 weeks.

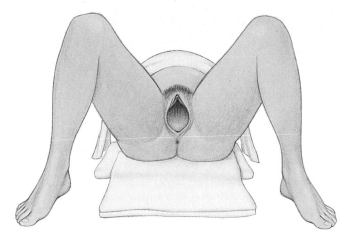

Figure 22-2   When crowning begins, birth is imminent.

As soon as the cervix is sufficiently dilated, the newborn travels from the uterus through the birth canal. The newborn emerges from the vaginal opening at the lower end of the canal. For first-time mothers, this process normally takes between 12 and 24 hours. Subsequent births are usually quicker.

Labor

Labor has three distinct stages. The length and intensity of each stage vary.

Stage One—Preparation

In the first stage, the mother's body prepares for the birth. This stage covers the period of time from the first contraction until the cervix is fully dilated. Most of the hours of labor are spent in stage one. A *contraction* is a rhythmic tightening of the muscles in the uterus. It is like a wave. It begins gently, rises to a peak of intensity, then drops off and subsides. The muscles then relax, and there is a break before the next contraction starts. As the time for delivery approaches, the contractions become closer together, last longer and feel stronger. Normally, when contractions are less than 3 minutes apart, childbirth is near.

Stage Two—Delivery of the Newborn

The second stage of labor involves the delivery of the newborn. It begins when the cervix is completely dilated and ends with the newborn's birth and occurs 15 minutes to 3 hours after the newborn moves into the birth canal. The mother makes pushing efforts by tightening the muscles to assist the newborn's progress. The newborn's head becomes visible as it emerges from the vagina. The moment during labor when the top of the head begins to emerge is called *crowning* (**Fig. 22-2**). When crowning occurs, birth is imminent and you must be prepared to receive the newborn. Stage two ends with the birth of the baby.

Stage Three—Delivery of the Placenta

The third stage of labor begins after the newborn's body emerges. During this stage, the placenta usually separates from the wall of the uterus and is expelled from the birth canal. This process normally occurs within 30 minutes of the delivery of the newborn.

After the placenta is delivered, the uterus contracts to control bleeding and the mother begins to recover from the physical and emotional stresses that occurred during childbirth.

Assessing Labor

If you must care for a pregnant woman, you will want to determine whether she is in labor. If she is in labor, you should determine in what stage of labor she may be and whether she expects any complications. You should find out if anyone has called 9-1-1 or the local emergency number; if not, immediately call. You can determine these and other factors by asking a few key questions and making some observations.

Ask the following questions:

▸ Has 9-1-1 or the local emergency number been called? If so, how long ago and what was the response?

▸ Is this the first pregnancy? The first stage of labor normally takes longer with first pregnancies than with subsequent ones.

▸ Does the mother expect any complications?

▸ Is there a bloody discharge? This pink or light red, thick discharge from the vagina is the mucous plug that falls from the cervix as it begins to dilate, also signaling the onset of labor.

▸ Has the amniotic sac ruptured (or water broken)? When the sac ruptures, fluid flows from the vagina in a sudden gush or a trickle. Some women think they have lost control of their bladder. The breaking of the sac usually signals the beginning of labor, but not always. People often describe the rupture of the sac as "the water breaking."

▸ What are the contractions like? Are they very close together? Are they strong? The length and intensity of the contractions will give you valuable information about the progress of labor. As labor progresses, contractions become stronger, last longer and are closer together. When contractions are 2 to 5 minutes apart and 45 to 60 seconds long, the newborn is beginning to pass out of the uterus and into the birth canal. Labor may continue from 15 minutes to 3 hours.

▸ Does she have the urge to bear down, or push? If the expectant mother expresses a strong urge to push, this signals that labor is far along.

▸ Is the newborn's head visible? If so, begin preparing for the delivery—the newborn is about to be born.

PREPARING FOR DELIVERY

Although childbirth can be exciting, it can also be frightening to witness. Remember that you are only assisting in the process; the expectant mother is doing all the work. Therefore, it is important that you remain calm. Try not to be alarmed at the loss of blood. It is a normal part of the birth process. Take a deep breath and try to relax. Prepare the scene by gathering your supplies and putting them where they are easily accessible.

Preparing the Mother

Explain to the expectant mother that the newborn is about to be born. Be calm and reassuring. A woman having her first child often feels fear and apprehension about the pain and the condition of the newborn. Labor pain ranges from discomfort, similar to menstrual cramps, to intense pressure or pain. Many women experience something in between. Factors that can increase pain and discomfort during the first stage of labor include—

▸ Irregular breathing.
▸ Tensing up because of fear.
▸ Not knowing what to expect.
▸ Feeling alone and unsupported.

You can help the expectant mother cope with the discomfort and pain of labor. Begin by reassuring her that you are there to help. If necessary and possible, explain what to expect as labor progresses. Suggest specific physical activities that she can do to relax, such as regulating her breathing. Ask her to breathe in slowly and deeply in through the nose and out through the mouth. Ask her to try to focus on one object in the room while regulating her breathing. By staying calm, firm and confident and offering encouragement, you can help reduce fear and apprehension. Reducing fear will aid in relieving pain and discomfort.

Breathing slowly and deeply in through the nose and out through the mouth during labor can help the expectant mother in several ways:

▸ It aids muscle relaxation.
▸ It offers a distraction from the pain of strong contractions as labor progresses.
▸ It ensures adequate oxygen to both the mother and the newborn during labor.

Taking childbirth classes, such as those offered at local hospitals, helps people become more competent in techniques used to help an expectant mother relax. Many expectant mothers also participate in such training, which could greatly simplify your role while assisting with the birth process. Many books and videos on the subject of childbirth are available.

ASSISTING WITH DELIVERY

It is difficult to predict how much time you have before the newborn is delivered. However, if the expectant mother says that she feels the need to push or feels as if she has to have a bowel movement, delivery is near.

You should time the expectant mother's contractions from the beginning of one contraction to the beginning of the next. If they are less than 3 minutes apart and last for 45 to 60 seconds, prepare to assist with the delivery of the newborn.

Assisting with the delivery of the newborn is often a simple process. The expectant mother is doing all the work. She will be pushing down, using certain muscles. Your job is to create a clean environment and to help guide the newborn from the birth canal, minimizing injury to the mother and newborn. Begin by positioning the mother. She should be lying on her back, with her head and upper back raised, not lying flat. Her legs should be bent, with the knees drawn up and apart (**Fig. 22-3, A**). Positioning the mother in this way will make her more comfortable.

Next, establish a clean environment for delivery. Because it is unlikely that you will have sterile supplies, use items such as clean sheets, blankets, towels or even clothes. Newspapers, which are very absorbent, can be used if nothing else is available. To make the area around the mother as sanitary as possible, place these items over the mother's abdomen and under her buttocks and legs (**Fig. 22-3, B**). Keep a clean, warm towel or blanket handy to wrap the newborn. Because you will be coming in contact with the mother's and newborn's body fluids, be sure to wear disposable gloves. If gloves are not available, try to find some other item to use as a barrier. For example, a plastic bag or plastic wrap may be secured around your hands. Put something on over your clothing, if possible, to protect yourself from splashing fluids.

Other items that can be helpful include a bulb syringe to suction secretions from the infant's nose and mouth immediately after birth, gauze pads or sanitary pads to help absorb secretions and vaginal bleeding, and a large plastic bag or towel to hold the placenta after delivery.

As crowning begins, place a hand on the top of the newborn's head and apply light pressure

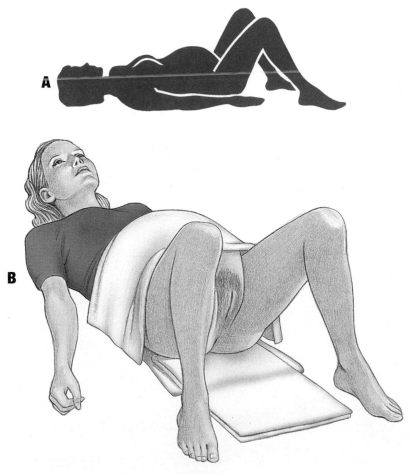

Figure 22-3   **A,** Position the mother with her legs bent and knees drawn up and apart. **B,** Place clean sheets, blankets, towels or even clothes under the mother.

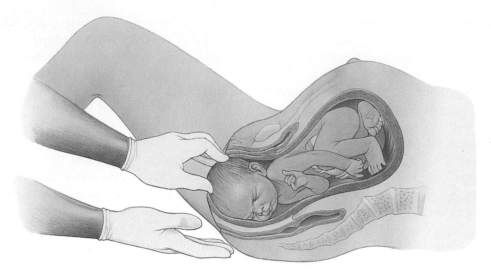

Figure 22-4   Place your hand on top of the newborn's head and apply light pressure.

(**Fig. 22-4**). In this way, you allow the head to emerge slowly, not forcefully. This will help prevent tearing of the vagina and avoid injury to the newborn. At this point, the expectant mother should stop pushing. Instruct the mother to concentrate on her breathing techniques. Ask her to pant. This technique will help her stop pushing and help prevent a forceful birth.

Once the head is out, the newborn's shoulders should rotate with another push. Support the head (**Fig. 22-5**). This will enable the shoulders and the rest of the body to pass through the birth canal. Slide your forefinger along the newborn's neck to see if the umbilical cord is looped around it. If the umbilical cord is around the neck, gently slip it over the newborn's head. If this cannot be done, slip it over the newborn's shoulders as they emerge. The newborn can slide through the loop.

Guide one shoulder out at a time. Do not pull the newborn. As the newborn emerges, he or she will be wet and slippery. Use a clean towel to catch the newborn. Place the newborn on his or her side, between the mother and you so that you can give care without fear of dropping the newborn. If possible, note the time the newborn was born.

CARING FOR THE NEWBORN AND MOTHER

Your first priority of care when the newborn arrives is to take some initial steps of care for him or her. Once these steps are accomplished, you can care for the mother.

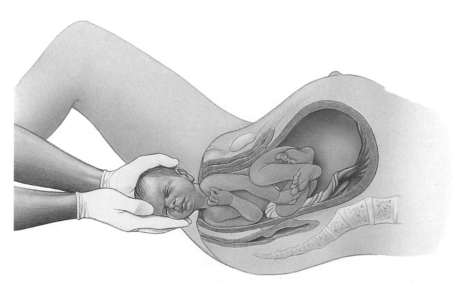

Figure 22-5   As the infant emerges, support the head.

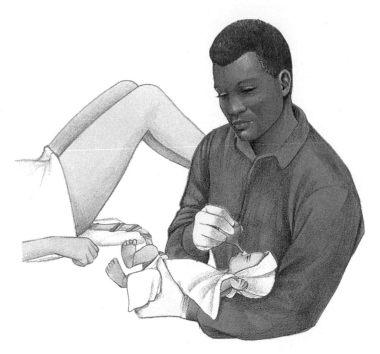

Figure 22-6   A bulb syringe can be used to clear a newborn's mouth and nose of any secretions.

Caring for the Newborn

The first few minutes of the newborn's life are a difficult transition from life inside the mother's uterus to life outside. You have two priorities at this point. Your first is to see that the newborn's airway is open and clear. Because a newborn breathes primarily through the nose, it is important to immediately clear the nasal passages and mouth thoroughly. You can do this by using your finger, a gauze pad or a bulb syringe (**Fig. 22-6**). When using a bulb syringe, make sure you compress the bulb before you place it in the newborn's mouth. Place the bulb syringe in and clean the mouth first, then in each nostril. The tip of the syringe should not be placed more than 1 to 1½ inches into the newborn's mouth and no more than ½ inch into the newborn's nostril.

Most babies begin crying and breathing spontaneously. If the newborn does not make any sound, stimulate the newborn to elicit the crying response by flicking your fingers on the soles of the newborn's feet. Crying helps clear the newborn's airway of fluids and promotes breathing. If the newborn does not begin breathing on his or her own within the first minute after birth, begin rescue breathing. If the newborn does not have signs of life and a pulse, begin CPR. You can review these techniques in Chapters 6 and 7.

Your second responsibility to the newborn is to maintain normal body temperature. Newborns lose heat quickly; therefore, it is important to keep him or her warm. Dry the newborn and wrap him or her in a clean, warm towel or blanket. Continue to monitor breathing, circulation and skin color. You may place the baby on the mother's abdomen.

Caring for the Mother

You can continue to meet the needs of the newborn while caring for the mother. Help the mother to begin nursing the newborn if possible. This will stimulate the uterus to contract and help slow bleeding. The placenta will still be in the uterus, attached to the newborn by the umbilical cord. Contractions of the uterus will usually expel the placenta within 30 minutes. Do not pull on the umbilical cord. Catch the placenta in a clean towel or container. It is not necessary to separate the placenta from the newborn. In the event that you or another citizen responder must transport the mother and child to the hospital, leave the placenta attached to the newborn and place the placenta in a plastic bag or wrap it in a towel.

Expect some additional vaginal bleeding when the placenta is delivered. Gently clean the mother using gauze pads or clean towels. Place a sanitary pad or a towel over the vagina. Do not insert anything inside the vagina. Have the mother place her legs together. Feel for a grapefruit-sized mass in the lower abdomen. This is the uterus. Gently massage the lower portion of the mother's abdomen. Massage will cause the uterus to contract and slow bleeding.

Many new mothers experience shock-like signals, such as cool, pale, moist skin; shivering; and slight dizziness. Keep the mother positioned on her back. Keep her from getting chilled or overheated, and continue to monitor her condition.

SPECIAL CONSIDERATIONS

Most deliveries are fairly routine, with few if any surprises or problems. However, you should be aware of certain complications or special situations that can occur.

Complications During Pregnancy

Complications during pregnancy are rare; however, they do occur. One such complication is a **miscarriage**, also called a **spontaneous abortion**. Because the nature and extent of most complications can only be determined by medical professionals during or following a more complete examination, you should not be concerned with trying to diagnose a particular problem. Instead, concern yourself with recognizing signals that suggest a serious complication during pregnancy. Two important signals you should be concerned about are vaginal bleeding and abdominal pain. Any persistent or profuse vaginal bleeding, or bleeding in which tissue passes through the vagina during pregnancy, is abnormal, as is any abdominal pain.

An expectant mother showing these signals needs to receive advanced medical care quickly. While waiting for EMS personnel, place a pad or other absorbent material between the mother's legs. Also, take steps to minimize shock. These include—

▶ Helping the mother into the most comfortable position.
▶ Keeping the mother from becoming chilled or overheated.

Complications During Childbirth

The vast majority of all births occur without complication. However, this fact is reassuring only if the birth you are assisting with is not complicated. For the few that do have complications, delivery can be stressful and even life threatening for the expectant mother and the newborn. More common complications include persistent vaginal bleeding, prolapsed umbilical cord, breech birth and multiple births. Learn to recognize the signals of a complicated birth and give the appropriate care. Call 9-1-1 or the local emergency number immediately if you have not already done so. All of these conditions require the help of more advanced medical care.

Persistent Bleeding

The most common complication of childbirth is persistent vaginal bleeding. While waiting for the ambulance to arrive, you should take steps to absorb the blood. Do not pack the vagina with dressings. Try to keep the mother calm and take steps to minimize shock, as explained in Chapter 9.

Prolapsed Umbilical Cord

A **prolapsed umbilical cord** occurs when a loop of the umbilical cord protrudes from the vagina while the unborn baby is still in the birth canal (**Fig. 22-7**). This condition can threaten the unborn baby's life. As the unborn baby moves through the birth canal, the cord will be compressed between the unborn baby and the birth canal, and blood flow to the unborn baby will stop. Without this blood flow, the unborn baby will die within a few minutes because of lack of oxygen. If you notice a prolapsed cord, have the expectant mother assume a knee-chest position (**Fig. 22-8**). This will help take pressure off the cord.

Breech Birth

Most babies are born head-first. However, on rare occasions, the newborn is delivered feet- or buttocks-first. This condition is commonly called a **breech birth.** If you encounter a breech delivery, support the newborn's body as it leaves the birth canal while you are waiting for the head to deliver. Do not pull on the newborn's body. Pulling will not help deliver the head.

Because the weight of the unborn baby's head lodged in the birth canal will reduce or stop blood flow by compressing the umbilical cord, the unborn baby will be unable to get any oxygen. Should the unborn baby try to take a spontaneous breath, he or she will also be unable to breathe because the face is pressed against the wall of the birth canal. When the unborn baby's head is deliv-

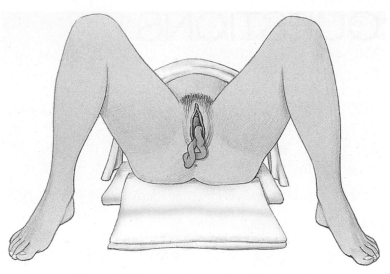

Figure 22-7   A prolapsed umbilical cord.

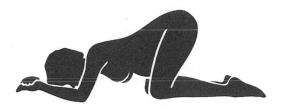

Figure 22-8   The knee-chest position will take pressure off the cord.

ered, check the infant for breathing and signs of life, including a pulse. Be prepared to give rescue breathing or CPR as necessary.

Multiple Births

Although most births involve only a single newborn, a few will involve delivery of more than one newborn. If the mother has had proper prenatal care, she will probably be aware that she is going to have more than one newborn. Multiple births should be handled in the same manner as single births. The mother will have a separate set of contractions for each baby being born. There may also be a separate placenta for each baby, although this is not always the case.

SUMMARY

Ideally, childbirth should occur in a controlled environment under the guidance of health-care professionals trained in labor and delivery. In this way, the necessary medical care is immediately available for mother and newborn should any problem arise. However, unexpected deliveries may occur outside of the controlled environment and may require your assistance. To assess the mother's condition before delivery and to assist in the delivery, be familiar with the three stages of labor and understand the birth process. By knowing how to prepare the expectant mother for delivery, assist with the delivery and give proper care for the mother and newborn, you can help bring a new child into the world.

APPLICATION QUESTIONS

1. Which stage of labor is Lisa in? Why do you think so?

2. What information can Lisa give that will help you to assist with the delivery?

STUDY QUESTIONS

1. Match each term with the correct definition.

   a. Amniotic sac   e. Crowning
   b. Birth canal   f. Cervix
   c. Placenta   g. Contraction
   d. Umbilical cord   h. Uterus

   _____ A pear-shaped organ in a woman's pelvis in which a fertilized egg develops into a newborn.

   _____ A rhythmic tightening of certain muscles during delivery.

   _____ An organ attached to the uterus that supplies nutrients to the fetus.

   _____ The appearance of the newborn's head at the vaginal opening.

   _____ The upper part of the birth canal.

   _____ A fluid-filled structure that protects the developing fetus.

   _____ A flexible structure that attaches the placenta to the fetus; it carries blood, nutrients and waste.

   _____ The passageway from the uterus to the vaginal opening through which the newborn passes during birth.

2. Name and briefly describe the three stages of labor.

3. List the two priorities of care for a newborn.

4. List six factors in determining a mother's condition before the birth.

Base your answers for questions 5 through 10 on the scenario below.

You happen upon a small gathering of people only to discover a woman has gone into labor. The woman is lying on the floor in pain. She says this is her first child. She tells you that her labor pains started about an hour ago, but she thought it was only gas. She also says that the newborn is not due for another 3 weeks.

5. You are reassured that there is enough time for the ambulance to arrive because labor for a first newborn usually lasts—

   a. 4 to 8 hours.
   b. 8 to 12 hours.
   c. 12 to 24 hours.
   d. 24 to 36 hours.

6. When the newborn's head is crowning at the vaginal opening, you should—

   a. Maintain firm finger pressure against the center of the skull.
   b. Place your hand lightly on the top of the newborn's head.
   c. Place the palm of your hand firmly against the newborn's skull.
   d. Place one hand on either side of the newborn's head.

7. If the mother has a breech delivery, what part of the newborn will be seen first?

   a. Head
   b. Arms
   c. Foot (feet) or buttocks
   d. b and c

8. If the newborn is not crying or does not appear to be breathing, you should first—

   a. Hold the newborn up by its ankles and spank its buttocks.
   b. Suction the newborn's throat with the bulb syringe.
   c. Flick the soles of the newborn's feet with your fingers.
   d. Begin rescue breathing.

9. To assist with delivery of the newborn, what preparations should you make?

   a. Have someone start a large pan of water boiling on the stove.
   b. Place clean sheets, blankets or towels under the mother's buttocks.
   c. Have the mother lie flat on her back with legs extended.
   d. All of the above.

10. What can the woman do to help cope with the pain and discomfort of labor?

   a. Focus on an object in the room while regulating her breathing.
   b. Assume a knee-chest position.
   c. Hold her breath then suddenly release it.
   d. Alternately tense and relax all muscles in her body.

Answers are listed in Appendix A.

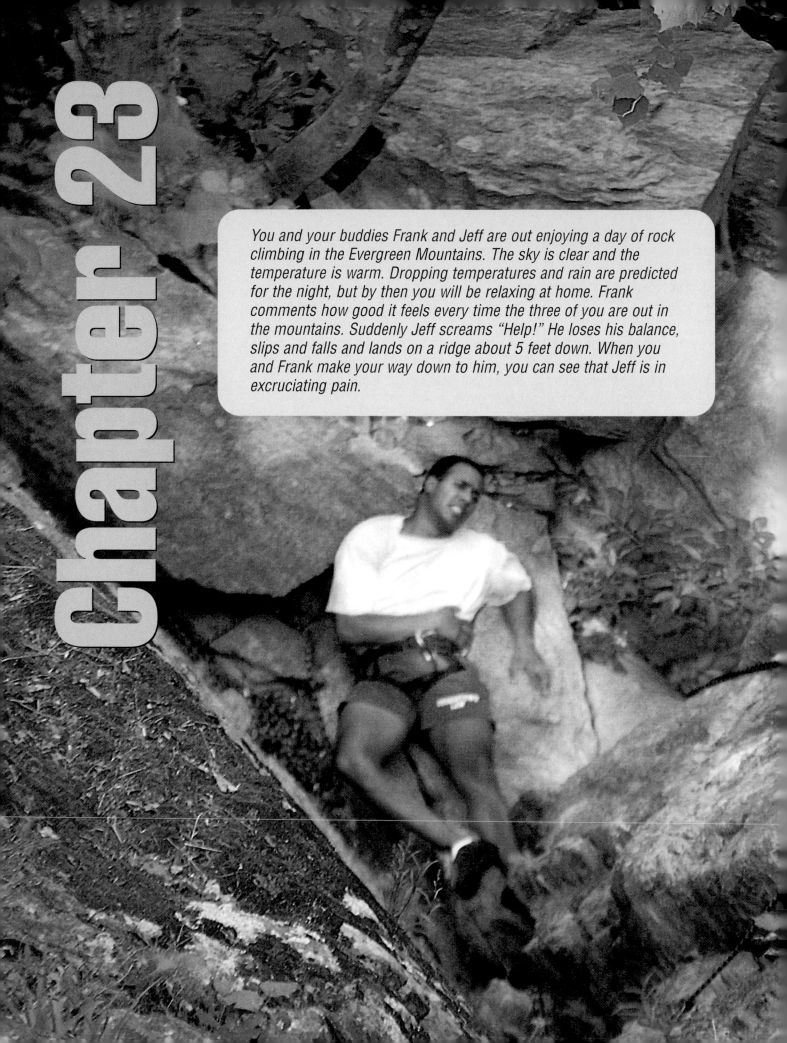

Chapter 23

You and your buddies Frank and Jeff are out enjoying a day of rock climbing in the Evergreen Mountains. The sky is clear and the temperature is warm. Dropping temperatures and rain are predicted for the night, but by then you will be relaxing at home. Frank comments how good it feels every time the three of you are out in the mountains. Suddenly Jeff screams "Help!" He loses his balance, slips and falls and lands on a ridge about 5 feet down. When you and Frank make your way down to him, you can see that Jeff is in excruciating pain.

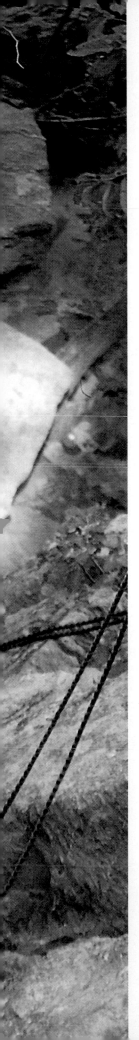

Delayed-Help Situations

Objectives

After reading this chapter, you should be able to—

■ *List three types of environments that could create a delayed-help situation.*

■ *Describe the information you should gather in a delayed-help situation before making a plan to get help.*

■ *List four ways to get help in a delayed-help situation.*

■ *Describe four of the options to consider in getting help in a delayed-help situation.*

■ *List the steps to take before leaving a victim alone for an extended period of time.*

■ *Describe how to protect a victim from heat or cold.*

■ *Describe four types of shelters you can use or construct.*

■ *List three general types of preparation for venturing into an environment where help may be delayed.*

Introduction

In previous chapters, you learned how to apply the emergency action steps: CHECK—CALL—CARE. In some situations, however, advanced medical care is not easy to contact or is not nearby. Situations in which medical care is delayed for 30 minutes or more are called delayed-help situations.

This chapter provides information to help you use the emergency action steps: CHECK—CALL—CARE in delayed-help situations. You will also learn how to prepare for such emergencies.

TYPES OF DELAYED-HELP SITUATIONS

Rural Areas

Rural areas include country and farm areas, which are less settled and populated than cities and where neighbors often live far away. Although it is usually easy to communicate with emergency medical personnel, response time is often delayed because of long distances and adverse road conditions. Temporary events, such as power outages and rising water, may cut off communication and access to EMS personnel.

Emergencies that occur in a rural environment usually involve equipment, animals, electricity, falls, fires, overturned vehicles, chemicals or pesticides and agricultural machinery mishaps, such as those resulting from tractors, combines and augurs. It is important to be aware of situations and circumstances that may put you or someone else in danger.

In rural areas, people are usually aware that help may be delayed. If telephone or mobile phone service is available, it may be possible to communicate with an emergency call taker who can tell you how to care for the victim until more advanced care arrives.

Wilderness Areas

A *wilderness* is an area that is not settled, is uncultivated and has been left in its natural condition. A phone and emergency personnel may be miles away. Some people work in wilderness areas. Others are drawn to wilderness activities because of the challenge, the adventure and the opportunity to discover the unknown. However, those same features that attract people to the wilderness often present barriers to getting help in an emergency.

If an emergency occurs in the wilderness, you need to consider how you are going to get help and what care you will give. If the victim cannot move and you have no means of transport, you may need to send someone to get help or go yourself. If the victim is able to move or be moved, you need to decide how to safely transport him or her. If he or she cannot be moved, you will have to shelter the victim from the elements to prevent his or her condition from deteriorating until you return.

Disaster Situations

Disasters, such as hurricanes, earthquakes or mass trauma (for example, explosions, acts of terror) are likely to create delayed-help situations. Phone and electrical services may be cut off or restricted; roads may be damaged; and medical facilities may be crowded or destroyed. It is important to plan ahead if you live, work or plan to travel in an area in which such disasters may occur.

KEY TERMS

Delayed-help situation: A situation in which emergency assistance is delayed for more than 30 minutes.

Tourniquet: A wide band of cloth or other material that is wrapped tightly around an extremity to control severe bleeding; used as a last resort measure.

Wilderness: An area that is uninhabited by human beings, is uncultivated and has been left in its natural condition.

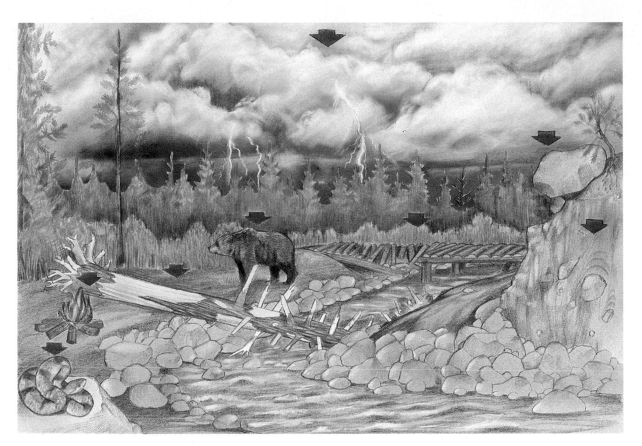

Figure 23-1   Check the scene for dangers that could threaten your safety or the safety of the victim.

Boating activities may also involve delayed-help situations. On the water, communication with medical personnel may be possible, but transportation to a medical facility may be limited or delayed.

TAKING ACTION IN A DELAYED-HELP SITUATION

In a delayed-help situation, you may have to modify the emergency action steps: CHECK—CALL—CARE to meet the specific needs of your situation.

Check the Scene

Check the entire scene to get a general impression of what happened. Look for dangers that could threaten your safety or the victim's safety, such as falling rocks or tree limbs (**Fig. 23-1**). If you see any dangers, do not approach the victim until you have carefully planned how you will avoid or eliminate the danger. Note any impending problems, such as a threatening storm.

Check the Victim

When you are sure it is safe, approach the victim carefully and check for life-threatening conditions.

Check for loss of consciousness, signs of life and severe bleeding (**Fig. 23-2**). If the victim has fallen

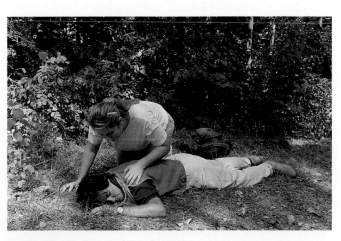

Figure 23-2   Check the victim for life-threatening conditions.

or if you do not know how the injury occurred, assume that he or she has a head, neck or back injury. Give care for the conditions you find.

Next, check the victim for any other problems that are not life threatening but may become so over time. In delayed-help situations, this check may need to occur before getting help. This ensures that you have all the information about the victim's condition that you need to make a plan for getting help. Whenever possible, perform a head-to-toe check even if the victim is unconscious or has life-threatening conditions. Write down the information that you gather so that you remember it (**Fig. 23-3**). Make a mental note of the most important or unusual observations if you do not have anything to write with.

The Unreckoned Cost

Rippling grain, cattle grazing by a stream, apple orchards in the spring, dark green fields of soy beans stretching as far as the eye can see—to many, a farm or ranch may not seem a particularly dangerous place. Yet historically, farming has been one of the most hazardous occupations in the United States. The death rate for agricultural workers is five times the national average for all industries.

The very nature of farming puts workers at risk. Crops must be planted and harvested under pressure from weather and time. Money is not always available to make needed equipment repairs or hire necessary labor. Equipment tends to be large and heavy, and much farm machinery is designed to chop, crush, cut or compress. Although newer equipment usually includes some safety features, such as rollover protection structures on tractors, older equipment provides little, if any, built-in safety protection.

There are many possibilities for injury. Equipment turns over, crushing the driver or passenger. Machinery traps arms and legs, mangling or amputating them. Gas generated by stored grain causes serious lung damage or death. Shifting grain buries people alive. The list goes on and on. The greatest number of deaths are caused by tractor overturns and runovers, followed by other machinery injuries, drowning, firearms, falls, fires, electric current, animals, poisoning, suffocation and lightning.

Children up to age 16 make up a disproportionate number of these farm fatalities and injuries. Nationally, one in five agricultural fatality victims is under age 18. Each year, approximately 33,000 children under 20 years of age are injured on farms and over 100 are killed. Too often, these children lack adequate supervision or are doing a task beyond their capabilities. Farm children tend to take on adult work at an early age. Children only 8 years old drive tractors. Five-year-olds feed farm animals, including animals with young who therefore may be extremely aggressive and protective. Children also play around machinery, tools, wire, gasoline pumps and other potential hazards in barns and other areas.

Nowhere is the need for training to deal with delayed-help emergency situations greater than in farming communities. Farms are often isolated, far from neighbors, towns or easily traveled roads. Many roads have no identifying signs. Injuries may occur in isolated areas of the farm where vehicle access is problematic. Weather may make reaching the injured person difficult or even immediately impossible. Emergency medical service is generally more limited than in urban areas. Responders are often volunteers who have other duties and may be far from the scene of the emergency. The first person on the scene, often a family member, is generally the person who gives the initial care and whose actions often determine whether the victim lives or dies.

Check for Resources

Check the scene for resources. Resources include people available to help, communication or signaling devices, food and water, shelter, first aid supplies and means of transportation. Check the surrounding environment for conditions or developing conditions that could endanger you or the victim during the time it will take to get help. Also, note any conditions that would make it difficult for you to go get help. Consider whether you may have to move the victim.

Call

In a delayed-help situation, the Call step can be divided into two phases: making a plan for getting help and executing the plan.

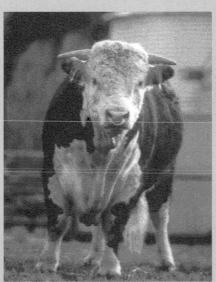

Various individuals, groups and organizations have developed resources to address the farm injury situation. First Care is a program developed by Allen L. Van Beek, M.D., a microsurgeon and plastic surgeon. Raised on a farm, at age 13, he had a firsthand experience with farm injuries when a tractor ran over both his legs. In 1968, as an army flight surgeon stationed in Vietnam, he worked with Col. George Omer, M.D., a hand surgeon who told him about microsurgery, a new form of surgery that had the potential to save severed limbs. After Vietnam, Dr. Van Beek studied reconstructive and plastic surgery. Performing surgery with the aid of a microscope and microscopic needles, he has repaired or reattached countless fingers, hands, arms and legs mangled or severed in farm injuries. Many of the victims are children.

Dr. Van Beek developed First Care to fill what he felt was a huge void in the rural health-care system. First Care is designed to teach the person who first comes upon a victim how to cope in those first minutes after an emergency and give care until advanced medical help can arrive. The program is sponsored by the Minnesota Farm Bureau Federation and The North Memorial Medical Center. For more information about this program, visit the Minnesota Farm Bureau Federation Web site at *www.minnesotafarmbureau.org*.

Other organizations include Farm Safety 4 Just Kids, an organization located in Earlham, Iowa, that works to prevent farm-related childhood injuries, health risks and fatalities. It puts out a variety of resource materials and activity ideas, including a catalogue of items to teach farm safety. One of its efforts is to raise the awareness of farm families about the developmental stages of children and how parents can apply that knowledge to tailor farm tasks to a child's skills, judgment and maturity. To learn more about this program visit the Farm Safety 4 Just Kids Web site: *www.fs4jk.org*.

FARMEDIC Training, Inc. is a nonprofit corporation that has been training EMS personnel in responding to farm emergencies. FARMEDIC is currently working also to train farm families and workers who are the first people on the scene of an emergency to respond appropriately. FARMEDIC has developed a program called "First on The Scene." This program is for farm family members, farm workers, agricultural business people and agricultural students. For more information visit the FARMEDIC Web site at: *www.farmedic.com*.

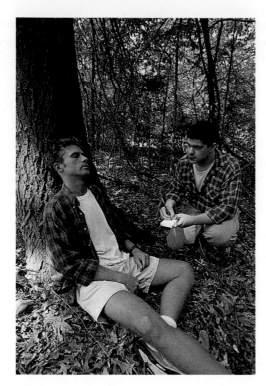

Figure 23-3 Write down the information you gather while interviewing the victim.

Making a Plan

In a delayed-help situation, you have four options for getting help:

▶ Stay where you are and call, radio or signal for help.
▶ Send someone to go get help or leave the victim alone to get help.
▶ Transport the victim to help.
▶ Care for the victim where you are until the victim has recovered enough to travel on his or her own.

Consider all the information you have gathered during the Check step about the conditions at the scene, the victim's condition, the resources available where you are and the available means for summoning help. Discuss your options with others, including the victim, if appropriate. To help decide on the best approach, ask yourself and others these questions:

▶ **Is advanced medical care needed and if so, how soon?** If you discovered any conditions for which you would normally call 9-1-1 or if these conditions seem likely to develop, you should plan to get help immediately.
▶ **Is there a way to call from the scene for help or advice?** If communication is possible, call

9-1-1 or the local emergency number as soon as you have enough information about the victim's condition and he or she is safe from dangers at the scene. Emergency medical personnel can tell you how to care for the victim and advise you about getting help.

▶ **If phone or radio communication is not possible, is there a way to signal for help?** The advantages of signaling are that it is faster and safer than going for help. The disadvantages include not knowing if your signal has been received and not being able to communicate to the receiver the type of help you need.
▶ **If there is no way to call for help, is it possible to go get help?** Consider whether you can get help safely while not jeopardizing the victim's safety. Carefully weigh the decision if going to get help means leaving the victim alone.
▶ **Is there a way to transport the victim to help?** Consider whether you have a safe and practical way to transport the victim. Ask whether the victim's injuries allow for safe transport. If the victim cannot walk, it will be extremely difficult to carry him or her any distance, even if you have a large number of people to assist. Unless a vehicle or other means of transportation is available, you probably will not be able to transport the victim to help without great difficulty.
▶ **Is it possible to give care where you are until the victim can travel?** Think about the risks of caring for the victim without medical assistance and the possibility that serious complications may develop. On the other hand, consider how quickly the victim may be able to recover, allowing you to safely transport him or her to medical care.
▶ **Is it safe to wait for help where you are?** Environmental hazards, such as a threatening storm or falling temperatures, may make it unsafe to wait for help.

You may discover that there is no "best" plan for getting help. You may have to compromise, reducing overall risk by accepting certain risks. For example, you are hiking in a remote area late in the afternoon on a cold, sunny day. One of your companions injures an ankle. Generally, the safest thing to do for the victim would be to immobilize the ankle, send someone for help and wait with the victim until emergency transportation arrives. However, if you know that it will take until nightfall for someone to summon help and no one in your party is dressed to survive the low temperatures overnight,

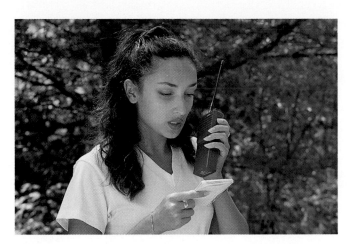

Figure 23-4 When calling for help, describe all important aspects of the victim's condition, your location and other information responders will need.

you may decide to immobilize the ankle and assist the victim in walking to shelter, even though following this plan may cause further injury to the ankle.

Getting Help

Once you have a plan, you need to execute it. Getting help may mean calling or signaling for help, sending for help, taking the victim to help or even going without additional help until the victim has recovered enough to travel.

Calling for Help

If you have some means of quickly calling for help, such as a mobile phone or two-way radio, make sure you have gathered all the necessary information about the victim's condition and your location so that EMS or rescue personnel will be able to plan their response (**Fig. 23-4**). Having essential information when you call reduces confusion and improves the likelihood that the right type of help will be sent to the right location. In addition, if you include all essential information in your first communication, emergency personnel will be able to respond even if later communication attempts fail.

Make sure you give the rescuers specific information about your location. Identifying prominent landmarks and marking your area can help rescuers find your location. Consider that some landmarks are clearly visible during the day but are not visible at night. Flares are one way of marking your location. Do not use flares in heavily wooded or dry areas that could ignite. You may need to send someone to meet EMS personnel at a main road or easy-to-identify location and have him or her guide

EMS personnel to the victim. Do not give mileage approximations to the EMS call taker unless you are sure of the distance.

Improvised Distress Signals

If you have no way to call for help and it is dangerous or impractical to use flares or send someone for help, you may have to improvise. Two of the most widely used general distress signals are—

▶ **Signals in Threes.** A series or set of three signals can be used to signal "Help!" Three shots, three flashes of light, three shouts, three whistles or three smoky fires are all examples (**Fig. 23-5**). Use extreme caution when building fires. Always remain near the fire and have water or dirt close by to extinguish sparks. Do not use fires in dry areas. A small fire can easily get out of control. Build your fires in a triangle at least 50 yards (45 meters) apart so that they are visible as separate fires.

▶ **Ground-to-Air Signals.** To signal an aircraft, use either signals in threes (three fires or three flashes of light) or else mark a large "X" on the ground. The X ground-to-air signal is a general distress signal meaning "unable to proceed" or "need immediate help." If constructing an X signal, make sure that you choose a large, open area and that the X you construct stands out against its background. The X signal should be at least 20 feet (6 meters) across.

In addition, smoke, mirrors, flare guns and whistles create visual or auditory signals to attract responders (**Fig. 23-6**). Smoke signals can be effective because they can be seen for many miles. If you are on a boat, making an urgent call over marine radio indicates that you have an emergency. You should be familiar with various ways of signaling that are appropriate for your location and environment.

Sending for Help

When you send someone to get help, he or she should carry the following information:

▶ A note indicating the victim's medical condition.
▶ A map indicating the location of the victim.
▶ A list of other members in the group.
▶ A list of available resources.
▶ A description of the weather, terrain and access routes if known.

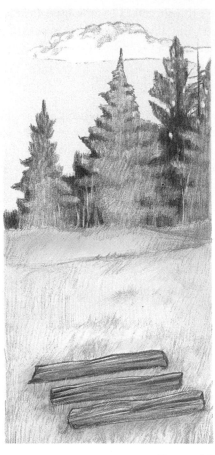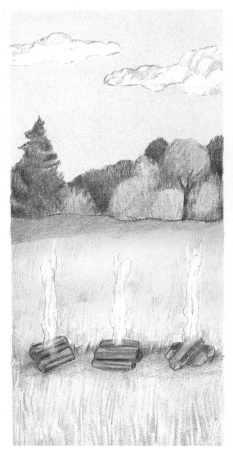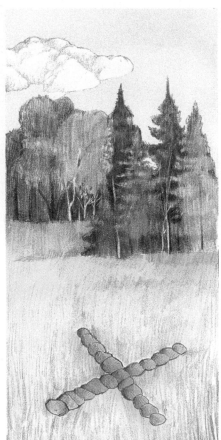

Figure 23-5 A set of three or an "X" is used to signal "Help."

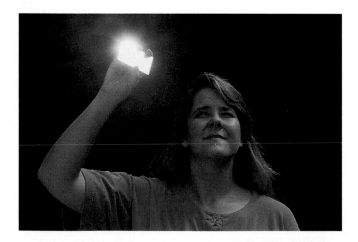

Figure 23-6 A mirror can be used to summon help.

This information will help emergency personnel determine their needs for the rescue. The information should be carried in writing in the event that the person becomes lost or something happens to him or her.

The safety of the messenger seeking help is extremely important. Make sure you send enough people to ensure the messenger's safety and success in delivering the message. If going for help involves hazards or challenges, do not send people who are not prepared to overcome these problems.

Another consideration in going for help is making sure you can lead rescuers back to the victim. When in the wilderness or on the water, the most accurate way to describe your location is to use compass readings. You should be trained in map and chart reading and the use of a compass if you travel or work in delayed-help environments.

Always mark your way so that you can find your way back. Regularly look back at the area you just traveled, which can assist you on your return trip. What you see behind you may look different from the area you are facing.

When sending someone for help, make sure that you leave enough people to care for the victim while waiting for help. Those remaining with the victim should be those equipped to care for the victim.

Finally, before sending anyone for help, consider whether tasks at the scene require everyone's help. For instance, moving a victim a short distance to a shelter is easier to do when everyone helps.

Leaving a Victim Alone

Generally, it is not a good idea to leave a victim alone. However, if you are alone with the victim, have no way to call or signal for help and are reasonably sure that no one will happen by, then you may decide that it is best to leave the victim and go get help.

Plan the route you will follow to go for help. Make sure you know how to lead rescuers back to the victim. Write down the route, the time you are leaving and when you expect to arrive. Leave this information with the victim.

Be sure to provide for the victim's needs while you are gone. Ensure that the victim has food, water and a container to use as a urinal or bedpan. If the victim cannot move, make sure that these things are within reach.

Make certain that the victim has adequate clothing and shelter and that he or she is protected from the ground. See "Protection from the Elements" in this chapter for more information. Recheck any splints or bandages, and adjust them if necessary so that they are not too tight. If the victim is unconscious or completely unable to move, place him or her in the recovery position, lying on one side with the face angled toward the ground, to protect the airway in case of vomiting (**Fig. 23-7**). Be careful to keep the head and spine as straight as possible.

Before you go, make sure that a conscious victim understands that you are going to get help. Give the victim an idea of when to expect a response. Be as reassuring and positive as the situation allows.

Transporting a Victim to Help

In situations involving injury or sudden illness, it is usually best to have help come to you. Consider transporting a victim to help only if a vehicle or other means of transportation is available rather than simply carrying the victim. Carrying a victim is very difficult and can be hazardous, especially if the terrain is not smooth and flat.

Factors to consider when deciding to move the victim include the extent of the injuries, distance to be traveled and available help at the scene. Remember that excessive movement may aggravate or worsen the victim's condition. You should not attempt to move or transport a victim with a suspected head, neck or back injury unless the scene is not safe or a potential for danger exists.

If you decide to transport a victim to help, plan the route you will follow. Remember that you may need to travel more slowly to avoid further injury to the victim. It is better to have a person besides the driver who will care for the victim during transport. If possible, inform someone else of your route and alternate plans.

Plan and rehearse how you will move the victim into the vehicle. To minimize pain and injury during the move, immobilize any possible bone or joint injuries before moving the victim to the vehicle. Select a place in the vehicle for the victim that will be as comfortable as possible and that will allow you to give care during transport. Make sure he or she will fit in the location you have selected. Use an uninjured person as a "test victim" to make sure the space is adequate. Transport the victim at a safe speed following the route you have planned. Monitor the victim's condition and work with the driver to make any necessary changes in transport conditions.

Care

In a delayed-help situation, you may need to care for the victim for a long time. It is important that you remain calm so that you can give the best care possible, whether for a few minutes or a few hours. Provide support and reassurance to the victim until EMS personnel arrive and take over.

Monitoring the Victim

After you complete your initial check of the victim and give care for the conditions found, continue to monitor the victim's condition while waiting for help. Monitoring is especially important in a delayed-help situation because the longer help is delayed, the more time there is for the victim's condition to change.

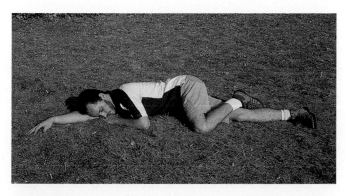

Figure 23-7   If you must leave an unconscious victim to go get help, position the person on one side in case he or she vomits while you are gone.

Continuously monitor the breathing of a victim who is unconscious or has an altered level of consciousness. Listen to and watch the victim's breathing. If the victim stops breathing or vomits, you will need to give care. Otherwise, the victim should be rechecked about every 15 minutes. If the victim can answer questions, ask the victim if his or her condition has changed. You should also watch for changes in skin appearance and temperature and level of consciousness. Changes in these conditions may indicate developing problems, such as heat- or cold-related emergencies and shock. Recheck any splints or bandages, and adjust them if they are too tight.

Keep a written record, noting any changes you find and the time the changes occur. Also note the care you give.

Fractures and Dislocations

In Chapters 11 and 12, you learned how to recognize and give care for musculoskeletal injuries. You should not attempt to move a person with a possible fracture unless it is absolutely necessary or the injury does not affect the person's ability to walk. Do not attempt to move a person or have the person move without first splinting the injured part. If you must move or transport the victim, splint the injured body part. Be sure to loosen the splint and recheck the limb about every 15 minutes.

Bleeding

In delayed-help situations, use the same principles that you learned to control severe bleeding in Chapter 8—apply direct pressure, first with your gloved hand after applying a dressing and then with a pressure bandage. Take steps to minimize shock and call 9-1-1.

Most external bleeding can be easily controlled. Direct pressure should be maintained for at least 10 minutes to allow a blood clot to form.

If bleeding cannot be controlled, consider applying a tourniquet in addition to maintaining direct pressure. A *tourniquet* is a wide band of cloth or other material placed tightly just above a wound to stop all flow of blood beyond the point of application. Do not use a narrow band, rope or wire. Application of a tourniquet can control severe bleeding from an open wound of the arm or leg, but it is rarely needed and should not be used except in situations where other measures fail. *Using a tourniquet is very dangerous.* When left in place for an extended period, uninjured tissues may die from lack of blood and oxygen. Releasing the tourniquet increases the danger of shock, and bleeding may resume. If a tourniquet is applied too loosely, it will not stop arterial blood flow to the affected limb and will only slow or stop venous blood flow from the limb. Applying a tourniquet means risking the loss of a limb in order to save a life.

To apply a tourniquet, place it just above the wound. Do not allow the tourniquet to touch the wound edges. If the wound is in a joint area or just below, place the tourniquet immediately above the joint.

▶ Wrap the tourniquet band twice tightly around the limb, and tie an overhand knot (**Fig. 23-8,** *A*).

▶ Place a short, strong stick or similar object that will not break on the overhand knot; tie two overhand knots on top of the stick (**Fig. 23-8,** *B*).

▶ Twist the stick to tighten the tourniquet until bleeding stops (**Fig. 23-8,** *C*).

▶ Secure the stick in place with the loose ends of the tourniquet, a strip of cloth or other material (**Fig. 23-8,** *D* and *E*).

▶ Make a written note of the location of the tourniquet and the time it was applied, and attach the note to the victim's clothing.

▶ Treat the victim for shock, and give first aid for other injuries.

▶ Do not cover a tourniquet.

Note the time the tourniquet was applied. Loosen it after 5 minutes to determine if bleeding has stopped. If bleeding continues, tighten the tourniquet for another 5-minute period. Then, loosen the tourniquet and recheck bleeding. If bleeding has stopped, leave the loosened tourniquet in place. Follow-up medical care is imperative.

Burns

General steps for caring for a burn in a delayed-help environment are the same as in any other situation:

▶ **Stop the burning by removing the victim from the source of the burn.** Smother flames with blankets or other material if water is not available.

▶ **Cool the burn.** Immerse the burned area in cold water until pain is relieved. However, using cold water on serious burns increases the possi-

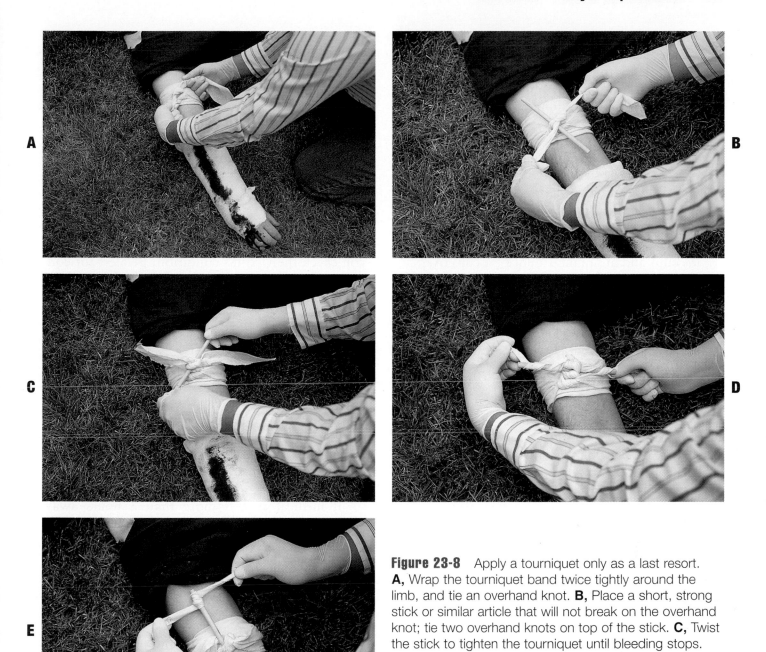

Figure 23-8   Apply a tourniquet only as a last resort. **A,** Wrap the tourniquet band twice tightly around the limb, and tie an overhand knot. **B,** Place a short, strong stick or similar article that will not break on the overhand knot; tie two overhand knots on top of the stick. **C,** Twist the stick to tighten the tourniquet until bleeding stops. **D,** Secure the stick in place with the loose ends of the tourniquet. **E,** A strip of cloth or other improvised material may also be used to secure the tightened tourniquet in place.

bility of hypothermia and shock, especially in a cold environment. Be careful not to use more water than necessary and to immerse only the burned area.

▶ **Cover the burned area.** Once the burn has been cooled, your main concern is keeping the area clean. Use a clean, dry cloth or a sterile burn dressing (such as one with a water-based gel coating) to cover the burn loosely. Be sure

that the gel on the dressing can easily be washed away with water.

▶ **Prevent infection.** Since the danger of infection is greater in delayed-help environments, apply a thin layer of triple antibiotic ointment to the cooled burn. Keep a dressing over the burn as mentioned. If an emergency facility is more than a day away, you must redress the burn daily. Redressing includes taking old dressings off, cleaning the burned area with sterile water and mild soap, reapplying a thin layer of triple antibiotic ointment and covering with a clean dressing. If none of these materials are available, leave the burn alone; it will form a scab.

▶ **Minimize shock.** Partial- and full-thickness burns, or burns covering more than one body part, can cause serious loss of body fluids. Give fully conscious victims water or clear juices to drink. Adults should receive 4 ounces (½ cup) over a 20-minute period, sipping slowly. A child should receive 2 ounces (¼ cup) and an infant 1 ounce (⅛ cup) over the 20-minute period. Elevate burned areas above the level of the heart and keep the burned victim from becoming chilled. Always monitor breathing and consciousness. The victim of serious burns requires transport to a medical facility as soon as possible.

Sudden Illness

When caring for a victim of sudden illness, such as someone experiencing a diabetic emergency or a seizure, follow the same procedures as if you were not in a delayed-help situation. However, there are additional factors to consider when you are far from help or transportation.

A victim recovering from an episode of low blood sugar should rest after eating or drinking something sweet. If he or she does not show signs of improvement within 5 minutes, you need to give the victim water in the amounts described in the following section on shock. Transport him or her to a medical facility. Some wilderness first aid experts recommend rubbing small amounts of a sugar and water mixture (or some other sweet liquid, such as fruit juice or a sports drink) on the gums of an unconscious person. Remember, victims of diabetic emergencies need to get a sugary substance into their system immediately. However, never give an unconscious victim anything to eat or drink.

To care for someone who has experienced a seizure in a delayed-help environment, do no further harm and complete a detailed check for injuries after the seizure is over. Maintain the victim's body temperature and help to prevent shock by putting some form of insulation between the victim and the ground. Cover the victim with a blanket or coat if necessary. Consider ending the trip if you suspect any injuries or possible recurrence of the seizure.

Shock

In a delayed-help situation, it is likely you will have to give care for shock. Although treatment for shock is carried out by advanced medical personnel, you can do your best to minimize or delay its onset.

Remember that shock does not always occur right away. It may develop while you are waiting for help. Check for signals of shock every time you check the victim's condition. Be alert for conditions that may cause shock to develop over time, such as slow bleeding, vomiting, diarrhea or heat loss.

If you or someone you are with is susceptible to a severe form of anaphylaxis or anaphylactic shock as a result of a bite or sting, be sure someone knows the location of necessary medication, such as oral antihistamines or injectable epinephrine, and knows how to use it. Anaphylactic shock can be life threatening if the victim does not receive care immediately. Quickly transport a person who shows signals of anaphylactic shock, such as swelling and trouble breathing, to a medical facility.

If medical care is more than 2 hours away, you may need to give preventive care for shock by giving a conscious victim cool water or clear juices. You can give an adult about 4 ounces (½ cup) or more of water to sip slowly over a 20-minute period. For a child, give 2 ounces (¼ cup) and for an infant, 1 ounce (⅛ cup) over the same 20-minute period. Giving frequent, small amounts, rather than fewer large amounts, reduces the chance of vomiting.

Even in a delayed-help situation, do not give fluids if the victim is unconscious; is having seizures; has a serious head or abdominal injury; or if vomiting is frequent and sustained. If you give fluids and the victim then starts to vomit, wait before giving the victim any more to drink. Remember to keep the victim from becoming chilled or overheated.

Head, Neck and Back Injuries

If you suspect a head, neck or back injury, the goal and the care are the same as in any other emergency: prevent further injury by providing manual stabilization (**Fig. 23-9**).

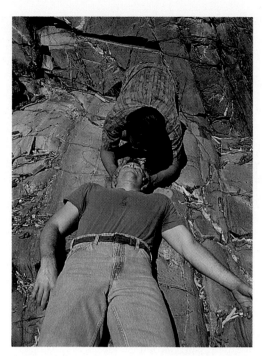

Figure 23-9 Provide manual stabilization if you suspect a head, neck or back injury.

Caring for a victim with a head, neck or back injury who will be outdoors for an extended period of time may be even more difficult. The victim will not be able to maintain normal body temperature without help. The person will need help with drinking, eating and going to the bathroom. If you are alone and need to free yourself from maintaining manual stabilization of the victim's head and neck, place two heavy objects wrapped in clothing next to each side of the head to hold it in line.

Help the victim maintain normal body temperature by placing insulation underneath him or her or by providing shelter from the weather. If two or more people are available, roll the victim onto one side to place insulation underneath the body, being careful not to twist the head, neck or back (**Fig. 23-10**).

DIFFICULT DECISIONS

One of the most stressful and emotionally draining situations you can be faced with is dealing with a life-threatening condition when advanced medical care is not easily obtainable. In a delayed-help situation, you may be faced with the difficult question of how long to continue resuscitation efforts if the victim's condition does not improve and advanced medical help is hours away. There is no

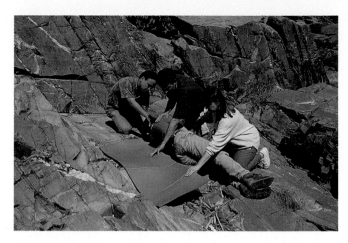

Figure 23-10 Place an insulating barrier between the victim and the ground.

simple answer to this question. In such a situation, you will ultimately need to make your own decision. However, some general principles can help you decide.

As you learned in Chapter 7, the purpose of CPR is to partially and temporarily substitute for the functions of the respiratory and circulatory systems. However, CPR is not designed for and is not capable of sustaining a victim's life indefinitely. Usually, the longer CPR is continued, the less likely the victim will survive.

The victim's survival depends largely on what caused the heart to stop in the first place. If the cause was a direct injury to the heart, such as from a heart attack or from crushing or penetrating trauma to the chest, little chance exists that the victim will survive in a delayed-help environment, whether or not CPR is performed. On the other hand, if the heart is not injured but stops as a result of hypothermia, lightning strike or drowning, the victim's heart has a better chance of starting. CPR can limit brain damage in case the heart starts and may even improve the chance that the heart will start. In such a case, CPR should be continued until the heart starts beating, you are relieved by another trained responder, EMS personnel arrive and take over, you are too exhausted to continue or the situation becomes unsafe.

PROTECTION FROM THE WEATHER

When caring for a victim in a delayed-help situation, it is critical to protect the victim from environmental conditions such as heat, cold, wind, rain, sleet or snow. You may need to construct a shelter for the victim using whatever materials you have on hand.

Protecting the Victim

A person who has an injury and is not able to move may develop a heat- or cold-related emergency. To keep the victim from getting chilled or overheated, provide some type of insulation to protect the victim. If the ground is dry, you can use cloth items such as towels, blankets, clothing or sleeping bags to insulate the victim from the ground. You can also improvise insulation from dry leaves or grass. In cold weather, lying on the ground draws heat away from the body and increases the chances of hypothermia. If the ground is too hot, the heat from the ground will travel to the body and raise the temperature. If the ground is wet, put a waterproof tarp, raincoat or poncho between the insulating material and the ground. If the victim is exposed to hot sun, rain, snow or chilling wind, provide an appropriate shelter.

Constructing Shelter

The following are four basic types of shelters:

▸ Natural shelters
▸ Artificial shelters
▸ Snow shelters
▸ Tents and bivouac bags

The type of shelter needed depends on where you are, the resources you have and whether you can move the victim safely into a shelter. It might be best to construct a shelter over the victim. Natural shelters are structures existing naturally in the environment, such as caves, overhangs and even large trees (**Fig. 23-11, A**). Artificial shelters are those you construct of materials, such as small trees or branches. An insulated tarp attached to branches makes a good temporary shelter (**Fig. 23-11, B**). You can make a snow shelter by digging out a snow cave, which is easy if it only has to hold one person (**Fig. 23-11, C**). Larger snow caves involve hard work and may take a while to dig. Snow cave shelters are also not advisable if the temperature is above freezing, because as the temperature rises, the strength and stability of a snow shelter weaken, making it unsafe. Many people carry a light tent, such as a pole tent or a bivouac bag, that can be

---

Vehicle Survival Kit

▸ Jumper cables
▸ Extra fuses
▸ Small tool kit
▸ Extra quart(s) of oil
▸ Gallon of antifreeze
▸ Tire inflator
▸ Tire pressure gauge
▸ Rags
▸ Spray bottle with washer fluid
▸ Tin can
▸ Help sign
▸ Reflective triangles
▸ Roadside flares
▸ Pocket knife
▸ Mobile phone
▸ Emergency preparedness kit
  • Battery powered flashlight and extra batteries
  • Battery powered radio and extra batteries
  • Emergency blanket
  • Emergency preparedness information card
  • Non perishable foods, such as granola or energy bars
  • Work gloves
  • Light sticks
  • Waterproof matches
  • Moist towelettes
  • Rain poncho
  • First aid kit (see Chapter 1 for a list of contents)
  • Roll of duct tape
  • Bottled water
  • Water container (2.5 gallon)
  • Toilet paper
  • Roll of paper towels
  • Pen and paper
▸ Additional items for winter travel
  • Sleeping bag(s)
  • Blankets
  • Extra winter clothing (gloves, socks, caps and scarves)
  • Chains
  • Sand or kitty litter
  • Small shovel
▸ Heavy-duty nylon bag to carry equipment

SOURCES:
www.redcross.org
www.creighton.edu/EHS/Newsletter/Wint3.htm. Accessed 01/20/05.
www.isu.edu/departments/pubsafe/industrial_safety/newsletters/
    June_2002.html. Accessed 01/20/05.

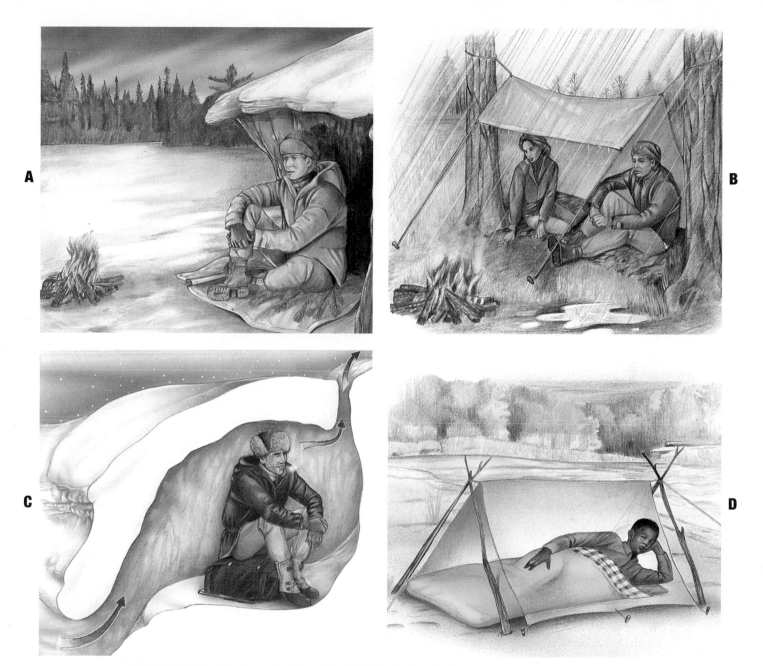

Figure 23-11   **A,** Natural shelter. **B,** Artificial shelter. **C,** Snow shelter. **D,** A pole tent.

easily assembled (**Fig. 23-11, D**). Although tents will keep you dry, they are usually not warm in extreme cold. Bivouac sacs made from Gore-Tex® are better at holding warmth.

A car can be an effective shelter. If you are stranded, it is better to stay in your car than to go find help. If you need heat, you can to keep the heater on for 15 to 20 minutes each hour. Make sure snow or ice does not block the exhaust pipe and cause carbon monoxide fumes to back up into the car. Leave the window opened a little to prevent carbon monoxide poisoning. You can also use candles as a source of heat. It is important,

especially in the winter months, that you keep your car in good working condition, filled with gasoline and carry a vehicle survival kit. Whether a shelter is natural or artificial, it should be well ventilated to prevent buildup of condensation or toxic fumes.

PREPARING FOR EMERGENCIES

If you live or work in a delayed-help environment or plan to be in one, develop a plan for how you will respond to emergencies that may arise.

Kit for Overnight Camping

CASE
Durable in temperature extremes
Water and dust tight
Sized to meet personal needs

CONTENTS
Scissors
Tweezers
Hypothermia thermometer (reads down to
   85° F (29.4° C)
Over-the-counter pain medication
Over-the-counter antihistamine
Antacids
Triple antibiotic ointment
Sunblock (SPF 15 or higher)
Sunburn lotion or cream
Lip protection, such as ointment or cream
Adhesive tape
Roller gauze, 2-inch, 4-inch
Sterile dressings, 4 x 4-inch squares
Nonstick dressings
Adhesive bandages

Sewing kit (safety pins, needle, thread)
Soap
Cotton swabs
Tongue depressors
Eye drops
Disposable gloves
Allergy kit
Water purification tablets or filter
Knife
Waterproof container of matches, with flint bar
   or lighter
Extra socks
Heliograph mirror, whistle
Flashlight and extra batteries
Foot powder
Magnifying glass
Sheet of aluminum foil
Nylon cord
Mosquito netting, emergency blanket
Compass
Insect repellent
Towel

Types of Preparation

There are three general types of preparation—knowledge, skills and equipment.

Knowledge includes learning about the emergency care resources available and how to access them. It also includes finding out the local geography, including landmarks and hazards. For instance, if you are going on a hiking trip, talk with park rangers or others who know the environment (**Fig. 23-12, A**). Plan your route and decide when and where you will check in (**Fig. 23-12, B**). If you are planning a boating expedition, consult the Coast Guard about possible weather hazards for that time of year. If you will be boating on inland waters, also consult with the local authority with control over dam water releases. People in rural areas should meet with local EMS personnel and ask what to do if an emergency occurs and estimated response time to their particular location.

Skills include proficiency in wilderness or survival techniques, and the technical skills necessary to safely engage in certain activities, such as scuba diving or rock climbing. For instance, if you plan to use a two-way radio, you need to know how to operate it and how to call for help. Rural inhabitants should know how to safely handle the hazards that they encounter on a regular basis, such as pesticides or farm machinery. Courses are available that address specific situations, such as wilderness first aid and farming emergencies.

Equipment includes appropriate clothing for your location and activities, first aid supplies suitable for your activities and expected hazards, as well as devices for signaling and communication. Basic first aid supplies are listed in Chapter 1. The contents of a first aid kit should be modified to suit your particular needs. For example, boaters should waterproof their kits by placing the contents in a waterproof container. People driving on long trips

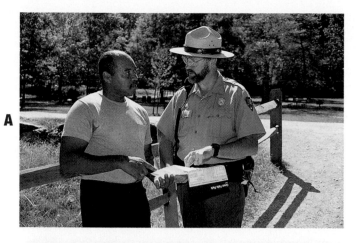

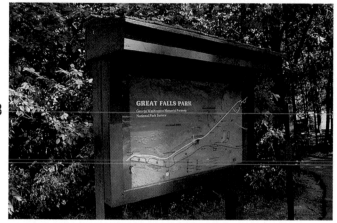

Figure 23-12   Appropriate preparation includes **A,** talking to a park ranger who knows the environment, and **B,** using a map to plan your route.

Being Prepared

When you are traveling in a wilderness or back-country area, the Boy Scouts of America recommend having the following with you at all times:

1. Map, preferably a **topographic map,** of the area in which you will be traveling.
2. **Compass**—and know how to use it before you leave.
3. **Matches** in a waterproof container.
4. 24 hours of **EXTRA high energy food.**
5. **Water,** 1-2 liters (2-3 quarts).
6. Extra **clothes,** such as socks and a sweater.
7. **Rain gear.**
8. A pocket **knife and whistle.**
9. **Sun protection** such as a wide-brimmed hat, sun glasses, and sun screen.
10. **First-aid kit with an emergency blanket.**

---

may want to add flares, a blanket and a flashlight to their kits.

Ensuring Adequate Preparation

Planning for emergencies is an important part of preparation for any trip or activity. Adequate preparation will not only reduce the risk of certain problems, but will also help make your trip more enjoyable. When planning a trip, several major considerations will help you determine special safety needs. These include—

▶ Level of first aid training among group members.
▶ Distance you will be from medical help.
▶ Duration of the trip or activity.
▶ Level of risk associated with the activity and environment.

▶ Group-related factors, such as pre-existing medical or physical conditions.
▶ Requirements for special equipment and supplies for high-risk or other specific activities.
▶ Group size. It is best to travel in a group larger than two so that at least one person is always available to stay with a victim.

The sooner you start to plan your trip, the more information you will be able to gather. You will also have more time to act.

Get trained. Take courses and talk to people with experience. Professionals, such as guides, park rangers and Coast Guard personnel, as well as enthusiasts of the activity you will be engaged in are good sources of information. You may find experienced people in clubs or in stores that sell equipment for the activity. Ask what preparations they recommend to make your experience safe and enjoyable. If possible, talk to more than one person to get a range of viewpoints.

Look for books, magazines and Web sites that include information on your intended destination and activity. Find more than one source of written information so that you get more than one author's point of view.

Find out about local weather conditions for the time you will be there. Make sure that you know the environmental conditions you need to be prepared for. An atlas or reference book and people knowledgeable about your destination may provide you with information about weather-related challenges for the area in which you will be traveling.

Find out about local emergency resources in the area you will be, including how to call for help. Find out if the emergency number is 9-1-1; if it is not, find out what the local emergency number is. Get other important phone numbers, such as hospitals, clinics and law enforcement agencies. If traveling to a foreign country, find out whatever details you can about the medical care that is available.

Plan your route and write it down. Let others know about your timing, routes, destination and companions. Letting others know your destination and estimated time of arrival may lessen the response time in the event of an emergency.

SUMMARY

Emergencies do not always happen where it is quick and easy for you to call 9-1-1 or the local emergency number, for advanced medical personnel to reach the victim or for the victim to be transported to a medical facility. In these delayed-help situations, you will need to give care for a much longer time than usual.

As with all other emergency situations, use the emergency action steps: **CHECK—CALL—CARE.** However, in a delayed-help situation, you will need to check the scene and the victim in greater detail before getting help. You may also need to develop a more detailed plan for getting help and caring for the victim. Getting help may involve calling for help, sending for help, leaving the victim alone and going for help, transporting the victim to help or allowing the victim to recover sufficiently so that he or she can walk to help.

In general, the care you give a victim in a delayed-help situation is no different from what you have learned in previous chapters. However, you will spend more time caring for the victim. Regularly checking the victim's condition while waiting for help and writing down any changes that you find are important in a delayed-help situation. You may also need to protect the victim from heat and cold or construct a shelter if help is delayed for an extended period of time.

If you are planning to venture into a delayed-help environment or if you live or work in one, think about how you can reduce the risk of emergencies. Adequately preparing yourself for a delayed-help environment includes early planning, talking to people with experience, reading, finding out about local weather conditions and emergency resources, planning your route and constructing plans to deal with emergencies should they arise.

APPLICATION QUESTIONS

1. Are you, Frank and Jeff in a delayed-help situation? If so, what factors make it a delayed-help situation?

2. What dangers should you look for at the scene of Jeff's fall? What life-threatening conditions might Jeff have, and what conditions might shortly become life threatening?

3. What do you think would be the best method for getting help in this situation? Why?

4. What should you do to care for Jeff while Frank goes for help?

STUDY QUESTIONS

1. Match each term with the correct definition.

   a. Tourniquet
   b. Bivouac sac
   c. Wilderness
   d. CHECK—CALL—CARE
   e. Delayed-help situation

   _____ Emergency Action Plan

   _____ A wide band of clothing placed above a wound to stop all blood flow as a last resort to control bleeding in a delayed-help situation

   _____ An emergency situation in which medical care is delayed for 30 minutes or more

   _____ A lightweight single person shelter made of waterproof and insulating materials

   _____ A delayed-help environment

2. List three types of problems that can create a delayed-help situation.

3. List two types of environments that can create a delayed-help situation.

4. List four options for getting help in a delayed-help situation.

In questions 5 through 9, circle the letter of the correct answer.

5. Periodically rechecking the victim's condition while giving care until help arrives is necessary because—

   a. It helps you remember changes in his or her condition.
   b. The victim may become hungry.
   c. The victim's condition may worsen.
   d. The victim needs to be comfortable.

6. The type of shelter that can be built from readily available materials, such as branches and trees, is called a(n)—

   a. Natural shelter.
   b. Artificial shelter.
   c. Snow shelter.
   d. Tent shelter.

7. Flare guns, whistles and mirrors are examples of—

   a. Hunting gear.
   b. First aid supplies.
   c. Signaling devices.
   d. Ground-to-air signals.

8. To prevent further injury to a person who may have a head, neck or back injury, you should provide—

   a. Manual immobilization.
   b. Manual traction.
   c. Manual stabilization.
   d. Manual reduction.

9. Which would you do if you would have to leave the victim alone for an extended period of time?

   a. Give the victim instructions to give the rescuers.
   b. Tighten any splints or bandages before you leave.
   c. Write down the route you are going to take and the time you are leaving.
   d. Do not leave any food within the victim's reach.

10. In the following scenario, circle the information you should consider before making a plan to get help.

    You are hiking with your hiking club in Greenleaf National Forest and are now on a trail about 5 miles from the main road. As you are crossing a stream, a group member slips and falls into the icy water. You all help him out and help him sit on the bank. He is shivering violently in the cool breeze. He says his right knee is very painful and feels as if it is swelling. The sky is overcast and the temperature is about 50° F (10° C). The sun will begin to set in about 4 hours. A group member gives you a sweater, which you substitute for the victim's soaked jacket. Other group members provide clothing.

11. To keep a victim from getting chilled or overheated, you would _____.

12. Three general types of preparation that can help you plan for going into a delayed-help environment are _____, _____ and _____.

Answers are listed in Appendix A.

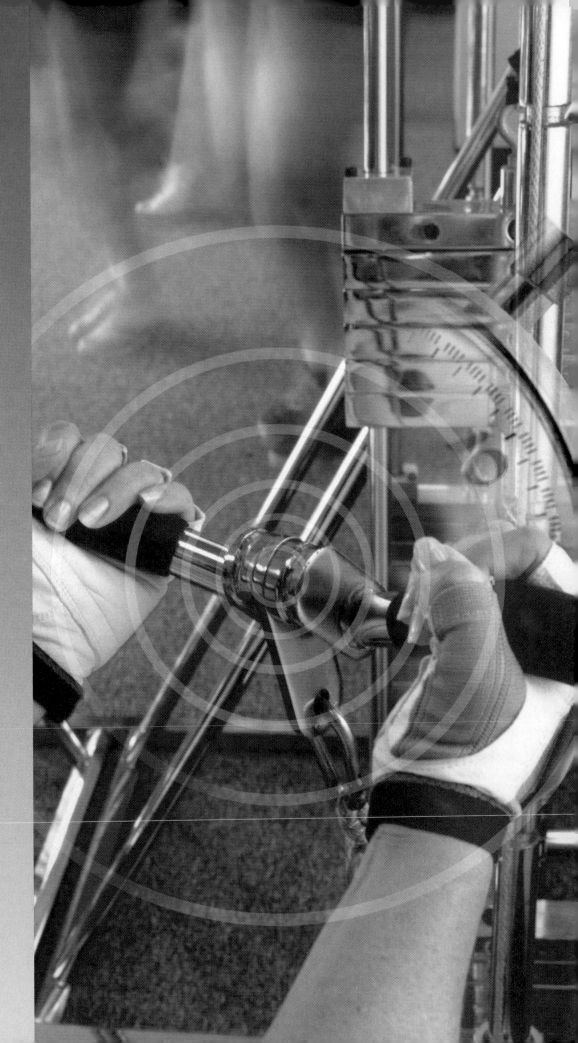

Part
SEVEN

HEALTHY LIFESTYLES

24 A Safer and Healthier Life

Rosanna was excited to be entering her first 10K of the season. At the registration tables, she was surprised to see a trim gray-haired woman signing up. "Mrs. Gallagher!" she gasped. "What are you doing here? I mean—well, I guess you're here for the walk..."Mrs. Gallagher smiled. "Why, Rosanna, I'm no older than your mother!" After warming up, they joined the crowd at the starting line. Bang! The sea of people began to move out. Rosanna managed to keep up for the first mile, but before long, Mrs. Gallagher had moved so far ahead she was almost out of sight.

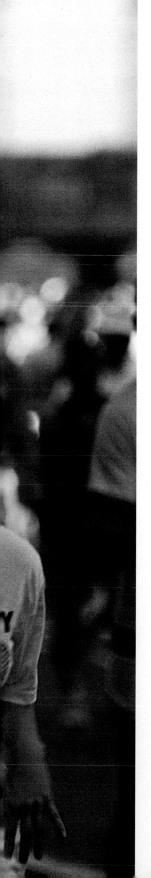

A Safer and Healthier Life

Objectives

After reading this chapter, you should be able to—

■ *List three general strategies for preventing injuries.*

■ *List four steps you can take to reduce your risk of personal injury.*

■ *List two steps you can take to help prevent personal injury from a motor vehicle accident.*

■ *List four elements of a fire escape plan.*

■ *Identify five ways to improve safety at home, work or at play.*

■ *Describe the contents of a food label.*

■ *Identify six physical indicators of negative stress.*

■ *List five risks of smoking.*

■ *Identify five ways to keep alcohol consumption under control.*

Introduction

Injuries and illness have a significant impact on our society. The costs in lost wages, medical expenses, insurance, property damage and other indirect costs are staggering—many billions of dollars a year. But illness and injury are not simply unpleasant facts of life to be shrugged off as inevitable. Often you can prevent them by taking safety precautions and choosing a lifestyle that promotes optimal health.

INJURY

Each year in the United States an estimated one in 12 people require medical treatment for an injury. An estimated 150,000 people die from the injuries they receive. Injury is the leading cause of death for people ages 1 to 39 years.

Factors Affecting Risk of Injury

A number of factors affect risk of injury—age, gender, geographic location, economic status and alcohol use and abuse. Technology also affects the type and frequency of injury. As certain activities, such as skateboarding and rollerblading, gain and lose popularity, the injury statistics reflect the changes.

▶ Injury rates are highest among people younger than age 39. People ages 65 and older and people ages 15 to 24 have the highest rate of deaths from injury.

▶ Gender is also a significant factor in risk of injury. Males are at greater risk than females for any type of injury. In general, men are about twice as likely to suffer a fatal injury as women.

▶ Many environmental factors influence injury statistics. Whether you live on a farm or in the city, whether your home is built out of wood or brick, the type of heat used in your home and the climate all affect your degree of risk. For instance, death rates from injury are higher in rural areas. The death rate from injuries is twice as high in low-income areas as in high-income areas.

▶ The use and abuse of alcohol is a significant factor in many injuries and fatalities, even in teenagers. In 2002, approximately 17,500 people in the United States died in alcohol-related motor vehicle crashes. This figure accounts for 41 percent of all traffic related deaths. It is also estimated that a significant number of victims who die as a result of falls, drownings, fires, assaults and suicides have blood alcohol concentrations over the legal limit.

Figure 24-1 shows the leading causes of deaths from injuries in 2003.

KEY TERMS

Aerobic: Requiring additional effort by the heart and lungs to meet the body's increased demand by the skeletal muscles for oxygen.

Calorie: A measure of the energy value of food.

Carbohydrates: Compounds that contain carbon, oxygen and hydrogen; the main source of energy for all body functions.

Cardiorespiratory endurance: The ability to take in, deliver and extract oxygen for physical work; the ability to persevere at a physical task.

Fat: A compound made up of carbon, hydrogen, oxygen and three fatty acids; a storage form of energy in the body; a type of body tissue composed of cells containing stored fat.

Nutrition: The science that deals with study of the food you eat and how your body uses it.

Obesity: A condition characterized by excess body fat.

Proteins: Compounds made up of amino acids necessary to build tissues.

Saturated fat: The fat in animal tissue and products.

Sodium: A mineral abundant in table salt; associated with high blood pressure.

Stress: A physiological or psychological response to real or imagined influences that alter an existing state of physical, mental or emotional balance.

Stressor: An event or condition that triggers the stress response.

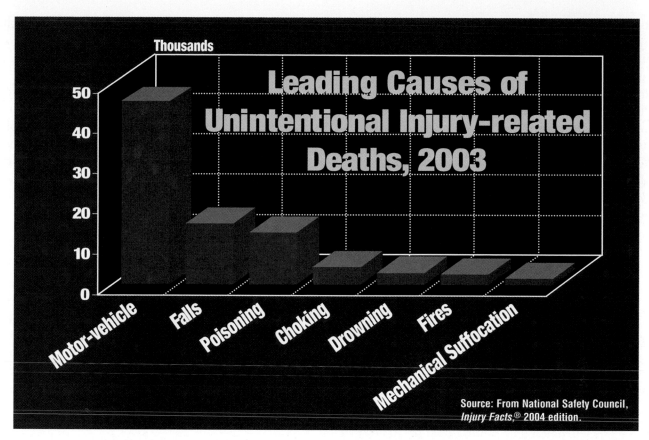

Figure 24-1 Leading causes of unintentional injury-related deaths, 2003.

Reducing Your Risk of Injury

Despite the statistics showing that people of certain ages and gender are injured more often than others, your chances of injury have more to do with what you do than who you are. Injuries do not just happen. Many injuries are preventable, predictable events resulting from the way people interact with the potential dangers in the environment.

The following are general strategies for preventing injuries:

▸ Encourage or persuade people at risk to change their behavior.
▸ Require people at risk to change their behavior, such as with laws requiring people to wear safety belts.
▸ Provide products that offer automatic protection, such as air bags, designed to reduce the risk of injury.

In addition, you can reduce your own risk of an injury by taking the following steps:

▸ Know your risk. Complete the Health Check Boxes in this chapter. Note the areas that indicate where you are at risk.

▸ Take measures that make a difference. Change behaviors that increase your risk of injury and risk injuring others.
▸ Think safety. Be alert for and avoid potentially harmful conditions or activities that increase your injury risk. Take precautions, such as wearing appropriate protective devices—helmets, padding and eyewear—and buckle up when driving or riding in motor vehicles. Let your state and congressional representatives know that you support legislation that ensures a safer environment for us all.
▸ Learn and use first aid skills. Despite dramatic improvements in the last decade in emergency medical systems nationwide, the person who can often make the difference between life and death is you, when you apply your first aid training.

Vehicle Safety

When riding in a motor vehicle, buckle up. Although more cars than ever are equipped with air bags, and many have air bags on the driver and passenger sides, wearing a safety belt is the easiest and best action you can take to prevent injury in a motor-vehicle collision. Always wear a safety belt, including a shoulder restraint when riding in the front or back seats. In all states, except for New Hampshire, wearing a safety belt is a law. In 2002 safety belts saved more than 14,000 lives. The economic cost of motor vehicle crashes (police-reported and nonreported crashes) that occurred in 2000 totaled $230.6 billion.

Infants and children should always ride in approved safety seats. Infants weighing less than 20 pounds should ride in a safety seat facing the rear of the vehicle to protect the infant's head and neck. For children, motor-vehicle crashes are the major cause of death as a result of injury. All 50 states and the District of Columbia require the use of child safety seats. Unsecured toys and other objects can turn into high-speed missiles in a vehicle crash. Do not leave objects loose in your vehicle.

Do not drink and drive. Plan ahead to find a ride or take a cab or public transportation if you are going to a party where you may drink alcohol. If you are with a group, have a designated driver who agrees not to drink on this occasion. Do not drink if you are in a boat. The U.S. Coast Guard reports that more than 50 percent of drownings from boating incidents involve alcohol.

Fire Safety

Between 1999 and 2001, an average of 4266 Americans lost their lives and approximately 25,000 were injured annually as the result of fire. Cooking is the leading cause of home fires in the United States. Fires are also caused by heating equipment, appliances, electrical wiring and careless smoking. Regardless of the cause of fires, everyone needs to

---

Vehicle Safety

The following statements represent an awareness of vehicle safety that can reduce your chances, and the chances of others, of injury in a vehicle crash. Check each statement that reflects your lifestyle.

☐ I put on a safety belt whenever I am a driver or passenger in a motor vehicle.

☐ My vehicle is equipped with an air bag.

☐ I am alert to the actions of other drivers, pedestrians, motorcyclists and bikers.

☐ I obey traffic rules.

☐ I use turn signals when turning or changing lanes, giving the driver behind me sufficient warning.

☐ I drive a safe distance behind the car in front of me (10 mph = 1 car's length).

☐ I keep my vehicle in good working order.

☐ I do not drink and drive.

☐ I am aware of environmental and weather conditions that increase driving risks.

If you only checked one or two statements, you should consider making changes in your lifestyle now.

Fire Safety

The following statement represents an awareness of fire safety that can reduce your chances, and the chances of others, of injury from a fire. Check each statement that reflects your lifestyle.

☐ I have a fire-escape plan for my home and I practice it.

☐ I have fire extinguishers in at least two rooms in my home, and the other occupants and I know how to use them.

☐ I have smoke detectors in my home, and I check the batteries every month and change them every 6 months.

☐ I keep irons and other heating appliances unplugged when not in use.

If you only checked one or two statements, you should consider making changes in your lifestyle now.

be aware of the danger fire presents and act accordingly. Install a smoke detector on every floor of your home. Check the batteries once a month, and change the batteries at least twice a year.

Plan and practice a fire escape route with your family or roommates (**Fig. 24-2**). Gather everyone together at a convenient time. Sketch a floor plan of all rooms, including doors, windows and hallways. Include all floors of the home.

Plan and draw the escape plan with arrows showing two ways, if possible, to get out of each room. Sleeping areas are most important, since many fires happen at night. Plan to use stairs only, never an elevator. Plan where everyone will meet after leaving the building.

Designate who should call the fire department and from which phone. Plan to leave the burning building first and then call from a phone nearby, if possible. Many, but not all, locations in the United States use 9-1-1 for the emergency number. When you travel, take a moment to find out and write down the local emergency number.

Remember and use the following guidelines to escape from fire:

▸ If smoke is present, crawl low to escape. Because smoke rises in a fire, breathable air is often close to the floor.
▸ Make sure children can open windows, go down a ladder and lower themselves to the ground. Practice with them. Always lower

children to the ground first before you go out a window.
▸ Get out quickly and do not, under any circumstances, return to a burning building.
▸ If you cannot escape, stay in the room and stuff door cracks and vents with wet towels, rags or clothing. If a phone is available, call the fire department—even if rescuers are already outside—and tell the call taker your location.

Contact your local fire department for additional safety guidelines.

Install a smoke detector on every floor of your home. Ninety percent of homes in the United States have smoke detectors, but half of them do not work because of old or missing batteries, according to the International Association of Fire Chiefs. A good way to remember the batteries is to change them twice a year when you reset your clocks for daylight savings time.

Knowing how to exit from a hotel in a fire could save your life. Locate the fire exits and fire extinguisher on your floor. If you hear an alarm while in your room, feel the door first and do not open it if it is hot (**Fig. 24-3**). Do not use the elevator. If the

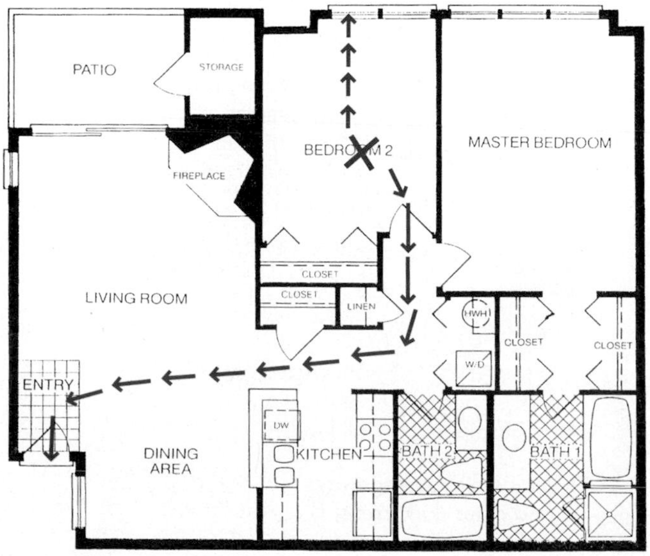

Figure 24-2 Plan a fire escape route for your home.

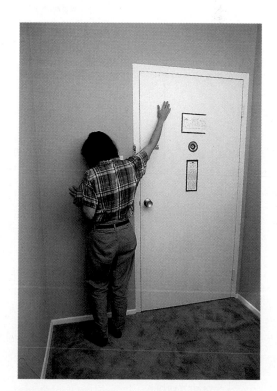

Figure 24-3 In a fire, do not open a door if it feels hot.

hall is relatively smoke free, use the stairs to exit. If the hall is filled with smoke, crawl to the exit. If you cannot get to the exit, return to your room. Turn off the ventilation system, stuff door cracks and vents with wet towels and call the front desk or the fire department to report the fire and your location.

Safety at Home

About 8 million disabling injuries occur in homes each year in the United States. The three leading causes of accidental death in the home are poisoning, falls and fire. Most falls occur around the home. Young children and the elderly are frequent victims of falls. Removing hazards and practicing good safety habits will make your home safer (**Fig. 24-4**). Make a list of needed improvements. Safety at home is relatively simple and relies largely on common sense. Taking the following steps will help make your home a safer place:

▶ Post emergency numbers—9-1-1 or the local emergency number, poison control center, physician, as well as other important numbers—near every phone.

▶ Make sure that stairways and hallways are well lit.

▶ Equip stairways with handrails, and use non-slip tread or securely fastened rugs.

▶ Secure rugs to the floor with double-sided tape.

▶ If moisture accumulates in damp spots, correct the cause of the problem. Clean up spills promptly.

▶ Keep medicines and poisonous substances separate from each other and from food. They should be out of reach of children and in secured cabinets.

▶ Keep medicines in their original containers, with safety caps.

▶ Keep your heating and cooling systems and all appliances in good working order. Check heating and cooling systems annually before use.

▶ Read and follow manufacturers' instructions for electrical tools, appliances and toys.

▶ Turn off the oven and other appliances when not using them. Unplug certain appliances, such as an iron, curling iron, coffee maker or portable heater, after use.

▶ Make sure that your home has at least one working, easily accessible fire extinguisher and everyone knows how to use it.

▶ Keep any firearms in a locked place, out of the reach of children and stored separately from ammunition.

PREVENT ACCIDENTS AT HOME

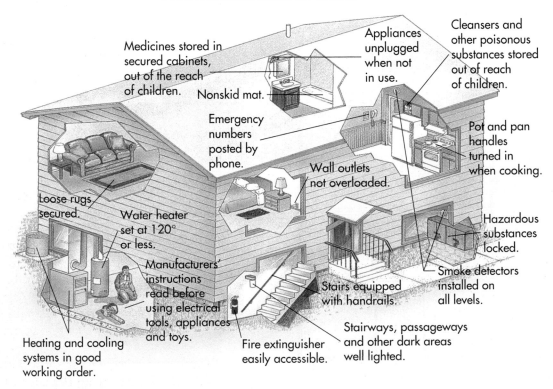

Figure 24-4 Follow home safety practices to prevent injuries at home.

▶ Have an emergency fire escape plan and practice it.

▶ Try crawling around your home to see it as an infant or young child sees it. You may become aware of unsuspected hazards.

▶ Turn pot handles toward the back of the stove.

▶ Ensure that cords for lamps and other items are not placed where someone can trip over them.

This list does not include all the safety measures you need to take in your home. If young children or elderly or ill individuals live with you, you will need to take additional steps, depending on the individual characteristics of your home.

For an elderly person, you may need to install handrails in the bathtub or shower and beside the toilet. You may need a bath chair or bench. Always have mat with a suction base if your tub does not have nonslip strips built in. A safe bath water temperature is 101° F (38° C).

If you have a residential pool, you will need to take additional steps:

▶ Learn to swim—and be sure everyone in the household knows how to swim.

▶ Never leave a child unattended who may gain access to any water. Even a small amount of water can be dangerous to young children.

▶ Teach your child not to go near the water without you; the pool area is off limits without adult supervision.

▶ Adult supervision is essential. Adult eyes must be on the child at all times.

▶ Enclose the pool completely with a fence with vertical bars (so that it is not easy to climb) that has a self-closing, self-latching gate. Openings in the fence should be no more than 4 inches wide. The house should not be part of the barrier. If the house is part of the barrier for an existing pool, an additional fence should be installed and the doors and windows leading from the house to the pool should remain locked and be protected with an alarm that produces sounds when the door is unexpectedly opened.

▶ Post the rules for your pool and enforce them without exception. For example, never allow anyone to swim alone, do not allow bottles or glass around the pool, do not allow running or pushing and do not allow diving unless your pool meets the safety standards.

▶ Post depth markers and "No Diving" signs, as appropriate. Use a buoyed line to show where the depth changes from shallow to deep. Limit nonswimmer activity to shallow water.

▶ Never leave furniture or toys near the fence that would enable a child to climb over the fence.

▶ Keep toys away from the pool and out of sight when it is not in use. Toys can attract young children into the pool.

▶ Pool covers should always be completely removed prior to pool use and completely secured when in place.

▶ Have an emergency action plan to address potential emergencies.

▶ Post CPR and first aid instructions.

▶ Post the emergency telephone number for the Emergency Medical Services (EMS) system by your telephone. Keep a telephone near the pool or bring a fully charged cordless or mobile phone poolside. Also post your address and the nearest cross streets so that anyone can read them to an emergency call taker.

▶ Always keep basic lifesaving equipment by the pool and know how to use it. A reaching pole, rope and flotation devices, such as ring buoys, rescue tubes and life jackets, are recommended. A well-stocked first aid kit should also be available. Store the safety gear in a consistent, prominent, easily accessed location. A "safety post" may be used.

▶ Learn Red Cross CPR and first aid. Insist that babysitters, grandparents and others who care for your children know these lifesaving skills.

▶ If a child is missing, check the pool first. Go to the edge of the pool and scan the entire pool, bottom surface, as well as the surrounding pool area.

▶ Keep the pool water clean and clear. Water should be chemically treated and tested regularly. If you cannot clearly see the bottom of the deep end, close the pool. Contact a local pool store or health department for information and instruction.

▶ Store pool chemicals—chlorine, soda ash, muriatic acid, test kits—in childproof containers and out of children's reach. Clearly label the chemicals. Follow manufacturer's directions and safety instructions.

▶ Consult the National Spa and Pool Institute, state law and local building codes for pool dimension guidelines to help you establish rules for your pool to ensure safe diving activities. For example:
   • Prohibit all dives into shallow water.
   • Only allow dives from the edge of the pool into deep water.

Make Your Home Safe for Kids

Use this checklist to spot dangers in your home. When you read each question, circle either the "Yes" box or the "No" box. Each "No" shows a possible danger for you and your family. Work with your family to remove dangers and make your home safer.

Storage Areas

YES | NO   Are pesticides, detergents and other household chemicals kept out of child's reach?

YES | NO   Are tools kept out of child's reach?

General Safety Precautions Inside the Home

YES | NO   Are stairways kept clear and uncluttered?

YES | NO   Are stairs and hallways well lit?

YES | NO   Are safety gates installed at tops and bottoms of stairways?

YES | NO   Are guards installed around fireplaces, radiators or hot pipes and wood-burning stoves?

YES | NO   Are sharp edges of furniture cushioned with corner guards or other material?

YES | NO   Are unused electric outlets covered with tape or safety covers?

YES | NO   Are curtain cords and shade pulls kept out of child's reach?

YES | NO   Are windows secured with window locks?

YES | NO   Are plastic bags kept out of child's reach?

YES | NO   Are fire extinguishers installed where they are most likely to be needed?

YES | NO   Are smoke detectors in working order?

YES | NO   Do you have an emergency plan to use in case of fire? Does your family practice this plan?

YES | NO   Is the water set at a safe temperature? (A setting of 120° F [49° C] or less prevents scalding from tap water in sinks and in tubs. Let the water run for 3 minutes before testing it.)

YES | NO   If you have a firearm, is it locked in a place where your child cannot get it? Is the ammunition stored separately from the firearm?

YES | NO   Are all purses, handbags, briefcases and other packages or bags, including those of visitors, kept out of child's reach?

YES | NO   Are all poisonous plants kept out of child's reach?

YES | NO   Is a list of emergency phone numbers posted near a telephone?

YES | NO   Is a list of instructions posted near a telephone for use by children and/or babysitters?

Bathroom

YES | NO   Are the toilet seat and lid kept down when the toilet is not in use?

YES | NO   Are cabinets equipped with safety latches and kept closed?

YES | NO   Are all medicines in child-resistant containers stored in a locked medicine cabinet?

YES | NO   Are shampoos and cosmetics stored out of child's reach?

YES | NO   Are razors, razor blades and other sharp objects kept out of child's reach?

YES | NO   Are hair dryers and other appliances stored away from sink, tub and toilet?

YES | NO   Does the bottom of tub or shower have rubber stickers or a rubber mat to prevent slipping?

YES | NO   Is the child always watched by an adult while in the tub?

Kitchen

YES NO Do you cook on back stove burners when possible and turn pot handles toward the back of the stove?

YES NO Are hot dishes kept away from the edges of tables and counters?

YES NO Are hot liquids and foods kept out of child's reach?

YES NO Are knives and other sharp items kept out of child's reach?

YES NO Is the child's highchair placed away from stove and other hot appliances?

YES NO Are matches and lighters kept out of child's reach?

YES NO Are all appliance cords kept out of child's reach?

YES NO Are cabinets equipped with safety latches?

YES NO Are cabinet doors kept closed when not in use?

YES NO Are cleaning products kept out of child's reach?

YES NO Do you test the temperature of heated food before feeding the child?

Child's Room

YES NO Is child's bed or crib placed away from radiators and other hot surfaces?

YES NO Are crib slats no more than $2\frac{3}{8}$ inches apart?

YES NO Does the mattress fit the sides of the crib snugly?

YES NO Is paint or finish on furniture and toys nontoxic?

YES NO Are electric cords kept out of child's reach?

YES NO Is the child's clothing, especially sleepwear, flame resistant?

YES NO Does the toy box have a secure lid and safe closing hinges?

YES NO Are the toys in good repair?

YES NO Are toys appropriate for the child's age?

Parents' Bedroom

YES NO Are space heaters kept away from curtains and flammable materials?

YES NO Are cosmetics, perfumes and breakable items stored out of child's reach?

YES NO Are small objects, such as jewelry, buttons and safety pins, kept out of child's reach?

Outside the Home/Play Areas

YES NO Is trash kept in tightly covered containers?

YES NO Are walkways, stairs and railings in good repair?

YES NO Are walkways and stairs free of toys, tools and other objects?

YES NO Are sandboxes and wading pools covered when not in use?

YES NO Are swimming pools nearby enclosed with a fence that your child cannot easily climb over?

YES NO Is playground equipment safe? Is it assembled according to the manufacturer's instructions and anchored over a level, soft surface such as sand or wood chips?

Child Safety

The following statements represent an awareness of child safety that can reduce the chances of injury to your child. Check each statement that reflects your lifestyle.

☐ I buckle my child into an approved automobile safety seat even when making short trips.

☐ I teach my child safety by behaving safely in my everyday activities.

☐ I supervise my child whenever he or she is around water and maintain fences and gates that act as barriers to water.

☐ I have checked my home for potential fire hazards and smoke detectors are installed and working.

☐ I have placed foods and small items that can choke my child out of his or her reach.

☐ I inspect my home, day-care center, school, babysitter's home or wherever my child spends time for potential safety and health hazards.

If you only checked one or two statements, you should consider making changes in your lifestyle now.

Home Safety

The following statements represent a safety-conscious lifestyle that can reduce your chances, and the chances of others, of injury in your home.

☐ The stairways and halls in my home are well lit.

☐ I have nonskid tread or securely fastened rugs on my stairs.

☐ I keep all medications out of reach of children and in a locked cabinet.

☐ I keep any poisonous materials out of the reach of children and in a locked cabinet.

☐ All rugs are firmly secured to the floor.

☐ I store all firearms, unloaded, in a locked place out of the reach of children, and ammunition is stored separately.

☐ I keep the handles of pots and pans on the stove turned inward when I am using them.

If you only checked one or two statements, you should consider making changes in your lifestyle now.

- Diving from a diving board should only occur if there is a safe diving envelope (the area of water in front of, below and to the sides of a diving board that is deep enough that a diver will not strike the bottom, regardless of the depth of the water or the design of the pool).

▶ Make sure your homeowner's insurance policy covers the pool.

Safety at Work

Most people spend approximately one-third of their day at work. To improve safety at work, you should be aware of the following:

▶ Fire evacuation procedures

▶ How to activate your emergency response team and how to call 9-1-1 or the local emergency number

▶ Location of the nearest fire extinguisher and first aid kit

If you work in an environment where hazards exist, wear recommended safety equipment and follow safety procedures (**Fig. 24-5**). Both employers and employees must follow safety rules issued by

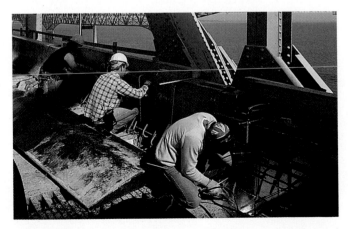

Figure 24-5   Safety clothing and/or equipment are required for some jobs.

Workplace Safety

The following statements represent a safety-conscious lifestyle that can reduce your chances, and the chances of others, of injury at your workplace. Check each statement that reflects your lifestyle.

- ☐ I know the fire evacuation procedures at my workplace.
- ☐ I know the location of first aid supplies and the nearest fire extinguisher at my workplace.
- ☐ I wear the recommended safety equipment and follow all recommended safety procedures.
- ☐ I know how to report an emergency at work.
- ☐ I know how to activate the workplace emergency response team.

If you only checked one or two statements, you should consider making changes in your lifestyle now.

Recreational Safety

The following statements represent a safety-conscious lifestyle that can reduce your chances, and the chances of others, of injury during recreational activity. Check each statement that reflects your lifestyle.

- ☐ I follow the rules established for any sport in which I participate.
- ☐ I wear the recommended safety gear, such as a helmet or goggles, for any sport or activity.
- ☐ I wear a life jacket when I am in a boat.
- ☐ I enter the water feet-first to check unknown water depths.
- ☐ I keep my recreational equipment in good condition.

If you only checked one or two statements, you should consider making changes in your lifestyle now.

the Occupational Safety and Health Administration (OSHA). Anytime you operate machinery or perform an activity that may involve flying particles, you should wear protective eyewear, such as goggles. Inspect mechanical equipment and ladders periodically to ensure good working order. Check for worn or loose parts that could break and cause a mishap. Before climbing a ladder, place its legs on a firm, flat surface and have someone anchor it while you climb. Take workplace safety training seriously. Ask your employer about first aid and CPR refresher courses.

Safety at Play

Make sports and other recreational activities safe by always following accepted guidelines for the activity (**Fig. 24-6**).

Each year, approximately 500,000 people are non-fatally injured while riding a bicycle. Ninety percent of bicyclists killed in 2000 reportedly were not wearing helmets. When cycling, always wear an approved helmet. The head or neck is the most seriously injured part of the body in most fatally in-

jured cyclists. Children should wear a helmet even if they are still riding along the sidewalk on training wheels. Some states have helmet laws that apply to young children. Look for a helmet approved by the Snell Memorial Foundation or the American National Standards Institute (ANSI), and make sure the helmet is the correct size and that it fits comfortably and securely. Keep off roads that are busy or have no shoulder. Wear reflective clothing, and make sure you have a headlight, taillight and reflectors on your bicycle wheels if you cycle at night. Make sure your bicycle and your child's bicycle are in good condition. Most bicycle mishaps happen within a mile of home.

With any activity in which eyes could be injured, such as racquetball, wear protective goggles. Appropriate footwear is also important in preventing injuries. For activities involving physical contact, wear properly fitted protective equipment to avoid serious injury. Above all, know and follow the rules of the sport.

If you do not know how to swim, learn how or always wear an appropriate flotation device if you are going to be in, on or around the water. Many

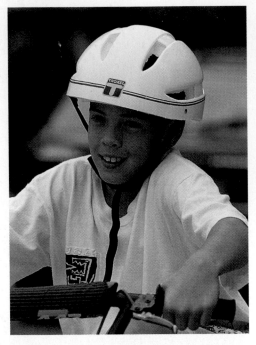

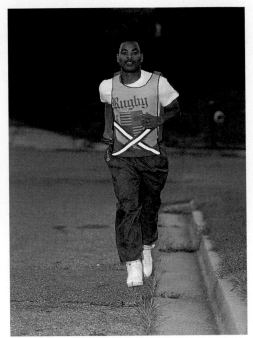

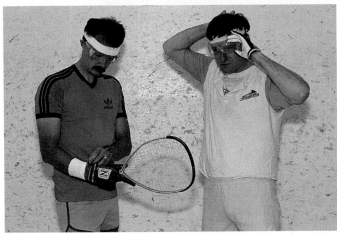

Figure 24-6 Wear proper safety equipment during recreational activities.

people who drown never intended to be in the water at all. Be careful when walking beside rivers, lakes and other bodies of water. Dangerous undercurrents in shallow water can catch even the best of swimmers.

If you are on a boat, always wear a flotation device. Never drink while you drive a boat and do not travel in a boat operated by a driver who has been drinking.

If you run, jog or walk, plan your route carefully. Exercise only in well-lit, well-populated areas, and consider exercising with another person. Keep off busy roads. If you must exercise outdoors after dark, wear reflective clothing and move facing traffic. Be alert for cars pulling out at intersections and driveways.

Whenever you start an activity unfamiliar to you, such as boating, skiing or motorcycle riding,

take lessons to learn how to do the sport safely. Many mishaps result from inexperience. Make sure your equipment is in good working order. Ski bindings, for instance, should be professionally inspected, adjusted and lubricated before each season. It is an added expense, yes, but far less than serious injuries.

REDUCING YOUR RISK OF ILLNESS

The choices you make about your lifestyle affect your health and general well-being. Informed choices can reduce or eliminate your risk of cancer, stroke, cardiovascular disease, pneumonia, diabetes, HIV infection and disease of the liver. These diseases are the leading causes of chronic illness and death in the United States.

Nutrition

Nutrition is the science that deals with the food you eat and how your body uses it. Studies indicate that poor diet is a contributing factor to many diseases. Therefore, changing your diet to make it healthier and more nutritious is one of the lifestyle decisions you may decide to make. This chapter touches on a few basic facts about nutrition; to understand this important subject in more detail, you should take a nutrition course, consult a nutritionist or at least read a book or visit a Web site recommended by a health-care professional or a nutritionist. However, learning to interpret the nutritional information on packaged food labels is a basic and important step you can take toward ensuring that you eat a proper diet.

Food Labels

Food labels describing a product's nutritional value are required by law on most packaged food and began appearing on many food products in 1993. The labels provide specific information about certain **nutrients,** substances found in foods that are required by the body because they are essential elements of a nutritious diet. Weights and percentages are provided so that consumers can evaluate the nutrients as to how they fit as part of a total daily diet.

Food is made up of six classes of nutrients—carbohydrates, fats, proteins, vitamins, minerals and water. Food labels are now required to list the amounts per serving of the following in a packaged product (**Fig. 24-7**):

▶ Calories—A *calorie* is a measure of the energy value of a food. On some labels, they are called kilocalories or kcalories (1000 calories of heat energy), the term used in nutritional science.

▶ Calories from fat—*Fat* is an important supplier of the body's heat and energy. However, the kind and amount of certain dietary fat increases the risk of some cancers, coronary heart disease, diabetes and obesity. Fat should provide no more than 25 to 30 percent of the daily calories in a well-balanced diet—approximately 65 grams per day for a 2000-calorie diet.

▶ Total fat—The **total fat** includes the amount of saturated and unsaturated fat. Overconsumption of foods high in fat, especially when they replace healthier foods, such as carbohydrates and fiber, is a major health concern for Americans.

▶ Saturated fat—*Saturated fat* is the fat in animal tissue and products. It should make up no more than 10 percent of daily calories. Saturated fat is solid at room temperature. Eating high levels of saturated fat contributes to high levels of cholesterol in the blood and therefore to coronary artery disease. Foods high in saturated fat include palm and coconut oil, butter, ice cream, milk chocolate, cheddar and American cheese and beef hot dogs.

▶ Trans fat—**Trans fats** are created when vegetable oil is heated in a process known as hydrogenation. The consumption of trans fats is linked to increasing the risk of heart disease. These types of fats can be found in commercially fried foods and baked goods.

▶ Cholesterol—**Cholesterol** is a waxy chemical substance found in animal tissue. It is not a fat, although it is chemically related to fat. High levels of cholesterol are considered to be a risk factor for cardiovascular disease. Foods high in cholesterol include eggs, shrimp, meat, fish, liver and kidneys.

▶ Sodium—**Sodium** is a mineral abundant in table salt. The main health problem associated with sodium is hypertension (high blood pressure). Use salt only in moderation, and check

Nutrition facts	Amount/Serving	% Daily value*	Amount/Serving	% Daily value*	*Percent Daily Values are based on a 2,000 calorie diet. Your daily values may be higher or lower depending on your calorie needs:		
	Total fat 7 g	11%	**Total Carbohydrate** 19 g	6%			
	Saturated fat 3 g	14%	Dietary Fiber 1 g	4%		Calories:	2,000	2,500
Serving size 7 slices (28g) Servings per Container 5	**Cholesterol** 0 mg	0%	Sugars 8g		Total Fat Less than 65g 80g		
					Sat Fat Less than 20g 25g		
	Sodium 360 mg	15%	**Protein** 2 g		Cholesterol Less than 300mg 300mg		
Calories 141 Calories from Fat 57	Vitamin A 21%	Vitamin C 27%	Calcium 1%	Iron 9%	Sodium Less than 2,400mg 2,400mg Total Carbohydrate 300g 375g Dietary Fiber 25g 30g Calories per gram: Fat 9 Carbohydrate 4 Protein 4		

Figure 24-7   Food label.

the sodium content of packaged food carefully. Many foods contain surprisingly large amounts of sodium. High sodium content is found in smoked meat and fish, many canned and instant soups, many frozen dinners and some canned or bottled sauces.

▶ **Total carbohydrate**—*Carbohydrates* are compounds that contain carbon, hydrogen and oxygen. In the body, they are easily converted to energy and are the main source of energy for all body functions. Sources of carbohydrates include grain and grain products, such as cereal, rice, pasta, baked goods, potatoes, beans and peas, seeds, nuts, fruits, vegetables and sugars.

▶ **Dietary fiber**—**Dietary fiber** consists of the carbohydrates that are not broken down by the human digestive process. Soluble fiber, fiber that dissolves in hot water, lowers blood cholesterol levels and has other beneficial effects. Fruit, vegetables and grains are good sources of soluble fiber. Insoluble fiber adds bulk to the contents of the intestine and speeds the transit time of undigested food through the intestines. Wheat bran, other whole grains, dried beans and peas and most fruits and vegetables are good sources of insoluble fiber.

▶ **Sugars**—**Sugars** are forms of carbohydrates. Sugar should be used in moderation—no more than 10 percent of daily calories. Sugar contributes to tooth decay, and high sugar consumption is considered by some to be a contributing factor to obesity, diabetes, heart disease and malnutrition. On lists of ingredients, sugar is often hidden by being listed as corn syrup, fructose or sucrose.

▶ **Protein**—*Proteins* are compounds made up of amino acids and contain the form of nitrogen most easily used by the human body. Protein contains the basic material for cell growth and repair, but if you take in more than the 15 percent of daily calories the body requires from proteins, the excess amount is converted to energy or stored as fat. Sources of protein include milk products, meat and fish.

▶ **Vitamin A**—**Vitamin A** is essential for the growth of the cells of skin, hair and mucous membranes. It contributes to bone and tooth development and increases resistance to infection. Sources include milk, cheese, butter, eggs, liver, carrots, cantaloupe, yellow squash and sweet potatoes.

▶ **Vitamin C**—**Vitamin C** aids in protection against infection and in the absorption of iron

and calcium. It contributes to the formation of bones and teeth and aids in wound healing. Sources include citrus fruits, melons, broccoli, green peppers, spinach and strawberries.

▶ **Calcium**—**Calcium** contributes to tooth and bone formation and general body growth. It helps maintain nerve function, good muscle tone and the regulation of normal heartbeat. Sources include dairy products, dried beans, dark green vegetables and shellfish.

▶ **Iron**—**Iron** aids in the formation of red blood cells, the production of antibodies and the use of energy. It facilitates the transportation of carbon dioxide and oxygen. Sources include lean red meat, seafood, eggs, dried beans, nuts, grains and green leafy vegetables.

The label information also shows the size of a serving, given as a household measure, such as a piece or cup, followed by the metric weight in parentheses and the total number of servings per container. The term "Daily Value" relates the total nutritional value of the product to a 2000-calorie daily diet and to a 2500-calorie daily diet. For example, using the label in **Figure 24-7**, a person on a 2000-calorie daily diet consuming one serving of that product would take in 19 grams of carbohydrates. This amount is 6 percent of 300 grams, which is the largest recommended daily amount. The person would also consume 7 grams, or 11 percent of the largest recommended daily amount of fat (65 grams or less).

Next to oxygen, water is the substance we need most to survive. Water regulates the body temperature through perspiration and carries oxygen and nutrients to the cells as part of the blood. Water lubricates the joints, removes wastes and aids in respiration by moistening the lungs, which facilitates the intake of oxygen and the removal of carbon dioxide. Most health-care professionals advise drinking six to eight 8-ounce glasses of water a day and more if you exercise regularly or drink alcohol or caffeine.

A Healthy Diet

One size doesn't fit all

USDA's new MyPyramid (**Fig. 24-8**) symbolizes a personalized approach to healthy eating and physical activity. The symbol has been designed to be simple. It has been developed to remind consumers to make healthy food choices and to be active every day. The different parts of the symbol are described below.

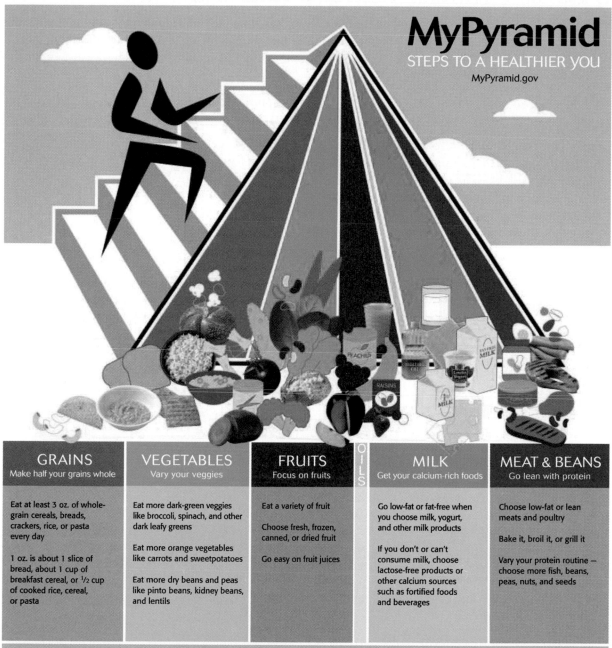

Figure 24-8 MyPyramid. (U.S. Department of Agriculture. [on-line]. http://www.mypyramid.gov)

Activity

Activity is represented by the steps and the person climbing them, as a reminder of the importance of daily physical activity.

Moderation

Moderation is represented by the narrowing of each food group from bottom to top. The wider base stands for foods with little or no solid fats or added sugars. These should be selected more often. The narrower top area stands for foods containing more added sugars and solid fats. The more active you are, the more of these foods can fit into your diet.

Personalization

Personalization is shown by the person on the steps, the slogan and the URL. Find the kinds and amounts of food to eat each day at MyPyramid.gov.

Proportionality

Proportionality is shown by the different widths of the food group bands. The widths suggest how much food a person should choose from each group. The widths are just a general guide, not exact proportions. Check the Web site for how much is right for you.

Variety

Variety is symbolized by the 6 color bands representing the 5 food groups of the Pyramid and oils. This illustrates that foods from all groups are needed each day for good health.

Weight-Loss Strategies

Use some of the following strategies to help you lose weight—

- Keep a log of the times, settings, reasons and feelings associated with your eating.
- Set realistic, long-term goals (for example, losing one pound per week instead of five pounds per week).
- Occasionally reward yourself with small amounts of food you enjoy.
- Eat slowly, and take time to enjoy the taste of the food.
- Be more physically active (take stairs instead of elevators, or park in the distant part of the parking lot).
- Reward yourself when you reach your goals (for example, with new clothes, sporting equipment).
- Share your commitment to losing weight with your family and friends who will support you.
- Keep a record of the food you eat each day.
- Weigh yourself once a week at the same time of day and record your weight.
- Be prepared to deal with occasional plateaus as you lose weight.

Nutrition and Weight

The following statements represent a healthy lifestyle that can reduce your chance of disease. Check each statement that reflects your lifestyle.

- ☐ I eat a balanced diet.
- ☐ I read the nutrition labels on food products to help me eat a balanced diet.
- ☐ I monitor my intake of foods high in fats.
- ☐ I monitor my intake of sodium and sugars.
- ☐ I do not fry foods.
- ☐ I maintain an appropriate weight.
- ☐ If I need to lose weight, I use medically approved diet techniques.
- ☐ For snacks, I eat fruit, vegetables and other healthy food rather than "junk foods."
- ☐ I drink 6 to 8 glasses of water daily.

If you only checked one or two statements, you should consider making changes in your lifestyle now.

Gradual Improvement

Gradual improvement is encouraged by the slogan. It suggests that individuals can benefit from taking small steps to improve their diet and lifestyle each day.

Weight

Many adults are overweight. Some are overweight to the point of obesity. *Obesity,* defined as a condition characterized by excess body fat, contributes to heart disease, high blood pressure, diabetes and gallbladder disease. For males, obesity is defined as body fat equal to or greater than 25 percent of the total body weight of the body and for females, it is equal to or greater than 32 percent of total body weight. See your physician or health-care professional for help if you want to have your body fat measured.

Losing weight, especially fat, is no easy task. Calories that are not used as energy are stored as fat. Weight loss and gain depend on the balance of caloric intake and energy output. If you take in more calories than you use, you gain weight. If you use more calories than take in, you lose weight. There are several guides to weight control.

Day-to-day fluctuations in weight reflect changes in the level of fluids in your body. So, if you are watching your weight, pick one day and time per week as weigh-in time. Track your weight loss based on this weekly amount, not on day-to-day differences. Even better, have a body fat analysis done. The term "overweight" does not take body composition into account. **Body composition** is the ratio of fat to all the tissues, such as muscles, that are fat free. One person may weigh more than is termed desirable for his or her height, but the weight may be mainly in muscle rather than fat. Someone else may be within an acceptable weight range but have a large proportion of his or her weight in body fat, which is not healthy.

Weight loss or gain should always be combined with regular exercise—another part of a healthy lifestyle. Any activity—walking to the bus, climbing the stairs, cleaning house—uses calories. You even burn off a few while you sleep. The more active you are, the more calories you use. Activity allows you to eat a few more calories and still maintain body weight.

Your eating habits should change as you grow older. A person who eats the same number of calories between the ages of 20 to 40 and maintains the same level of activity during this time will be con-siderably heavier at 40 than at 20. It is more important as you grow older to eat foods that provide your body with essential nutrients but are not high in calories.

Pregnant women should follow their physician's advice regarding diet. Severely limiting calories and fat can be detrimental to the developing fetus.

Fitness

Many of us would like to be fit. In general, fitness involves cardiorespiratory endurance, muscular strength, muscular endurance and flexibility. You do not need to take part in sports, such as tennis, basketball or soccer, to achieve fitness. You can become fit for health purposes by taking part in such activities as walking, jogging, swimming, cycling, hiking and weight training, among others.

Exercise

The "no pain, no gain" theory is not a good approach to exercise. In fact, experiencing pain usually means you are exercising improperly. You achieve the health benefits of exercise when it is somewhat uncomfortable, but not painful. Be sure to warm up to prepare the body before vigorous exercise and cool down afterwards. Make flexibility exercises part of the warm-up and cool-down process. When possible, add exercises or activities that strengthen the muscles to your fitness routine. Turn your daily activities into exercise (**Fig. 24-9**). Walk briskly instead of driving, whenever possible. Take the stairs instead of the elevator or the escala-

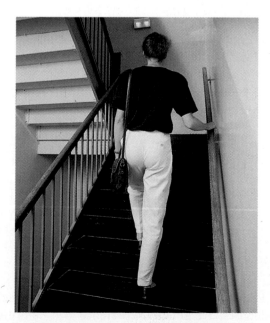

Figure 24-9 Build exercise into your daily activities.

Fitness

The following statements represent a healthy lifestyle that can reduce your chance of disease. Check each statement that reflects your lifestyle.

☐ I set realistic exercise goals and aim to achieve them.

☐ I exercise regularly for a minimum of 30 to 45 minutes at least three times a week.

☐ I warm up before exercise and cool down afterwards.

☐ I incorporate flexibility and muscle-strengthening activities into my fitness activities.

☐ I use aerobic exercise to build cardiorespiratory endurance.

☐ I know my target heart rate range and exercise within it.

☐ I walk or bike rather than drive whenever possible.

If you only checked one or two statements, you should consider making changes in your lifestyle now.

tor. Pedal an exercise bike while watching TV, listening to music or reading.

Many books and Web sites are available for those who want to improve their fitness and develop an exercise program. You can become physically fit, regardless of the condition you are in when you start. Set realistic goals and you will see regular progress. A variety of training programs are available. Make a commitment to exercise each week. Whatever activities you choose to achieve fitness, you must exercise regularly and maintain a level of activity to stay fit. You should exercise nonstop for a minimum of 30 to 45 minutes a day three to five times a week. The many benefits include loss of body fat, more resistance to disease, an ability to reduce the negative effects of stress and increased energy. If you have been sedentary or have health problems, see your physician before starting an exercise program. It is never too late to start exercising. People in nursing homes, many of them in wheelchairs, are able to experience and demonstrate the benefits of flexibility and strength training.

Cardiorespiratory Endurance

If you have limited time for limited exercise, it is best to build up *cardiorespiratory endurance,* the ability to take in, deliver and extract oxygen for physical work. Cardiorespiratory endurance is the foundation for total fitness. The best way to accomplish cardiorespiratory endurance is through aerobic exercise. The term *aerobic* refers to activities that require additional effort by the heart and lungs to meet the body's increased demand by the skeletal muscles for oxygen. **Aerobic exercise** is sustained, rhythmical exercise, using the large muscle groups, for at least 30 to 45 minutes within your target heart rate.

Taking part in aerobic exercise can—

▸ Reduce the risk of cardiovascular disease.
▸ Develop stronger bones that are less susceptible to injury.
▸ Promote joint stability.
▸ Contribute to fewer lower back problems.
▸ Improve self image.
▸ Help control diabetes.
▸ Stimulate other lifestyle changes.

Target Heart Rate Range

To achieve cardiorespiratory endurance, you must exercise your heart and lungs. To do this, you should exercise at least three to five times a week for a minimum of 30 to 45 minutes and at your appropriate target heart rate (THR) range. Your **target heart rate range** is 60 to 90 percent of your maximum heart rate. To find your maximum heart rate, subtract your age from 220. To find your target heart rate range, multiply that figure first by 0.60 and then by 0.90. For example, if you are 20 years old, 60 percent of your maximum heart rate would be 220 − 20 x 0.60 = 120 beats per minute (bpm). This figure is the lower limit of your target heart rate range. To find the upper limit, multiply 220 − 20 by 0.90, which is 180. Your target heart rate range is from 120 bpm to 180 bpm. You should get your pulse up to between 120 and 180 bpm and keep it there for 20 to 30 minutes. If you are age 20, with an average level of fitness, for example, aim for 150 to 160 bpm. Keep below the upper limit. In general, to improve cardiorespiratory endurance, a person must exercise at least 60 percent of his or her maximum heart rate.

As you exercise, take your pulse periodically at the wrist (radial artery) or neck (carotid artery) (**Fig. 24-10**). Your exercise must be continuous and vigorous to stay within your target heart rate range.

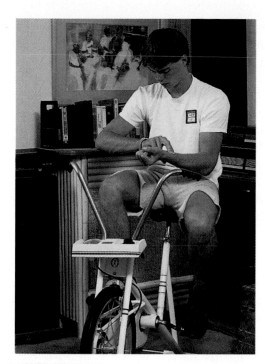

Figure 24-10 As you exercise, take your pulse periodically to see if you have reached your appropriate target heart rate.

As you build cardiorespiratory endurance, you will eventually be able to exercise for longer periods of time and at a higher THR.

Stress

Everyone experiences stress. Stress in itself is not harmful. How we deal with what we view as stress is what determines whether it has a positive or negative effect on our lives. *Stress* is a physiological or psychological response to real or imagined influences that alter an existing state of physical, mental or emotional balance. The reaction to stress can take such varied forms as muscle tension, dizziness, increased heart rate, acute anxiety, sleeplessness, anger, excitement, energy and even joy. A *stressor* is an event or condition that triggers the stress response. Stressors may be as varied as taking a test, speaking in public, poverty, loneliness, poor self-esteem, being stuck in traffic or winning a prize. A stressor for one person may not be a stressor for another, although some stressors, such as injury or loneliness, tend to stress everyone.

Positive, or "good," stress is productive. Good stress is the force that produces, for example, enhanced thinking ability, improved relationships with others and a greater sense of control. It can be part of the experience of being in a play, making a new friend or succeeding at a difficult task, for example. Good stress can help you perform better and be more efficient. Stress judged as "bad" (distress) can result in negative responses, such as sadness, fatigue, guilt and disease.

Most stressful situations involve harm and loss, threat or challenge. Harm and loss situations, for example, include the death or loss of a loved one, physical assault and physical injury. Threat situations, real or perceived, can be frightening or menacing and make it more difficult to deal with life. They can result in anger, anxiety or depression. Challenging situations often involve major life changes, such as moving, getting a new job, leaving home and forming or leaving a close relationship.

The Effects of Stress

Any stressful situation has an effect on the body. Because it affects the immune system, stress can be a major contributor to disease. The effects of stress on body systems can result in increased susceptibility to headaches, high blood pressure, clogging of the arteries, cancer and respiratory problems. When someone reacts to stress by over- or under-eating, overusing caffeine or alcohol, smoking or eating foods high in sugar and fat, for example, the physiological balance in the body is upset.

Stress

The following statements represent an awareness of stress that can reduce your chance of disease. Check each statement that reflects your lifestyle.

☐ I am aware of the physical and mental signals of stress.

☐ I know the effects stress has on my body.

☐ I would consult a professional counselor if necessary to help cope with stress.

☐ I am able to use several relaxation techniques to help manage stress.

If you only checked one or two statements, you should consider making changes in your lifestyle now.

The first step in learning to deal with stress is to become aware of the accompanying physical and mental signals. Some of the physical indicators of negative stress include severe headaches, sweating, lower back pain, weakness, sleep disturbance and shortness of breath. Other indicators, both emotional and mental, include depression, irritability, denial that a problem exists, increased incidences of illness, an inability to concentrate, feelings of unreality, inability to relax and becoming "accident prone." Becoming aware of how your body reacts to stress can help you recognize situations and conditions that are stressful for you.

Managing Stress

Stress management is a person's planned attempt to cope and deal with stress. Managing potentially harmful stress may require using a variety of techniques, including using time effectively, evaluating the activities that are important for you and establishing achievable goals. Perhaps the most difficult form of coping is change. It is especially hard to change an outlook or way of life, even if it has become unproductive and a source of negative stress. The advice and help of a professional counselor can be useful in such situations.

Relaxation techniques can also be helpful in reducing or avoiding the negative effects of stress. A few of these techniques are exercise, yoga, meditation, listening to quiet or soothing music and relaxation exercises, including deep breathing and muscle relaxation. **Biofeedback,** another technique, involves using instruments that measure bodily functions, such as heart rate and blood pressure. By receiving immediate feedback on responses such as muscle tension and skin temperature, the person can learn to consciously control these reactions. **Autogenics** uses self-suggestion to produce relaxation, using deep breathing, a conscious effort to relax and repeated phrases that carry a message of calming. **Imagery** involves using the imagination to create various scenes and wished-for situations. Commercial tapes of various relaxation exercises and books on stress management are available.

Smoking

Every year, close to 342,000 Americans die of lung disease. Smoking costs the United States over $150 billion each year in health-care costs. Cigarettes contain at least 69 distinct cancer-causing chemicals. During the past few decades, studies have made the negative effects of smoking clear. As a result, smoking has been banned or restricted in many work sites and public places around the nation. The nicotine in cigarettes is an addictive substance and a poison. The tars are carcinogenic (cancer causing). Nicotine, carbon monoxide and tars are all inhaled when you smoke.

Next time you are tempted to light up, consider that cigarette smoking is the single most preventable cause of heart and lung disease. Cigarette smoking is directly responsible for 87 percent of lung cancer cases and causes most cases of emphysema and chronic bronchitis. Cigarette smoking severely narrows the coronary arteries, giving the cigarette smoker an increased risk of heart attack and sudden cardiac arrest over the nonsmoker. Smokers are at risk for cancer of the esophagus, pancreas, bladder and larynx. A pregnant woman who smokes harms herself and her unborn baby. The carbon monoxide in cigarettes travels to the fetus through the umbilical cord and into the fetus's circulatory system. Smoking mothers have more stillbirths and babies with low birth weight and respiratory problems than nonsmokers. Inhaling the smoke generated by smokers is a health risk for nonsmokers, including infants and children.

Those who use smokeless tobacco also face serious risks. Nicotine is absorbed through the membranes of the mouth and cheeks. Chewing tobacco and snuff cause cancer of the mouth and tongue, so these products should also be avoided.

Sources of Help to Quit Smoking

American Heart Association
www.americanheart.org

American Lung Association
www.lungusa.org

American Cancer Society
www.cancer.org

National Cancer Institute
www.nci.nih.gov

Lungline National Jewish Center for Immunology and Respiratory Medicine
www.njc.org

Your risk of developing a disease or other conditions starts to go down as soon as you stop smoking and eventually decreases to that of any non-smoker. Stopping smoking or stopping the use of smokeless tobacco can be difficult, but most ex-smokers and former users say they feel better physically and emotionally. Many programs designed to help the smoker break the habit are available. If you want to quit smoking or know someone who does, the agencies listed in the *Sources of Help to Quit Smoking* box below may be able to help you.

Alcohol

Alcohol is the most popular drug in Western society. In addition to the hazardous relationship between drinking alcohol and driving, consuming alcohol in large amounts has other unhealthy effects on the body.

A blood alcohol concentration (BAC) of 0.05 percent or higher impairs judgment and reflexes and makes activities like driving unsafe (**Fig. 24-11**). How much drinking leads to this blood alcohol level? On an empty stomach, an average 160-pound person can reach this level after just two ordinary-size drinks in an hour or less—2 bottles of beer, 10 ounces of wine or 2 drinks with 1 ounce of alcohol in each. The faster alcohol enters the bloodstream, the faster the BAC increases. A small amount of alcohol enters the body quickly from the stomach, where food slows alcohol absorption. The major portion passes into the bloodstream from the small intestine, where food does not affect absorption. From the bloodstream, alcohol goes directly to the brain and to other parts of the body, such as the liver. Because of the time it takes for the body to process alcohol, you should always limit yourself to one drink per hour.

Only time can make a person sober after having too much to drink. Black coffee and a cold shower may make a person feel more alert, but the body must process the alcohol over time for the impairment of judgment and coordination to pass. Therefore, any group driving to a party should always have a designated, nondrinking driver for the return trip.

Whether hosting a party or participating in one, you can act responsibly by keeping alcohol consumption under control. To do this, remember these general principles:

▶ Drink slowly. Have no more than one drink per hour.

▶ As a host, have nonalcoholic beverages available.
▶ Do not drink before a party.
▶ Avoid drinking when angry or depressed.
▶ Eat plenty of food before and while drinking.
▶ Avoid salty foods—they may make you thirsty and cause you to drink more. As a host, do not provide foods that are high in salt.
▶ Do not play or promote drinking games.
▶ When mixing drinks, always measure the amount of alcohol. Do not just pour. As a host, hire a bartender and give clear instructions about measuring drinks or mix all the drinks yourself.
▶ As a host, do not have an open bar or serve someone who has had too much to drink.
▶ Stop drinking alcohol 1 hour before the party is over. If you are a host, stop serving alcohol.
▶ Do not drink and drive. Have a designated nondrinking driver or call a cab.

Smoking and Alcohol Use

The following statements represent an awareness of smoking and alcohol that can reduce your chance of disease. Check each statement that reflects your lifestyle.

☐ I am aware of the risks and negative effects of smoking.

☐ To prevent inhaling secondhand smoke as much as possible, I avoid being around people who are smoking.

☐ I do not use tobacco products.

☐ I drink alcohol in moderation or not at all.

☐ Whenever I am in a group driving to a party where alcohol will be served, I make sure the group has a designated driver.

☐ I am aware of the rate at which alcohol passes into the bloodstream.

☐ I do not drink more than one alcoholic drink per hour.

If you only checked one or two statements, you should consider making changes in your lifestyle now.

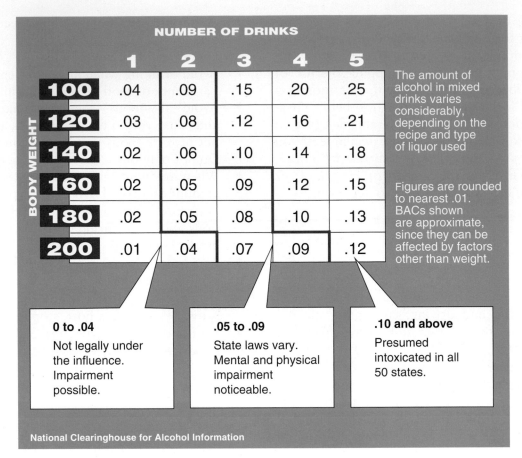

NUMBER OF DRINKS

BODY WEIGHT	1	2	3	4	5
100	.04	.09	.15	.20	.25
120	.03	.08	.12	.16	.21
140	.02	.06	.10	.14	.18
160	.02	.05	.09	.12	.15
180	.02	.05	.08	.10	.13
200	.01	.04	.07	.09	.12

The amount of alcohol in mixed drinks varies considerably, depending on the recipe and type of liquor used

Figures are rounded to nearest .01. BACs shown are approximate, since they can be affected by factors other than weight.

0 to .04
Not legally under the influence. Impairment possible.

.05 to .09
State laws vary. Mental and physical impairment noticeable.

.10 and above
Presumed intoxicated in all 50 states.

National Clearinghouse for Alcohol Information

Figure 24-11   BAC chart.

For help with an alcohol problem, refer to Chapter 18 for a list of organizations that provide help and support for substance abuse problems.

SUMMARY

You can help prevent injury and disease by taking safety precautions and making lifestyle choices that promote health. To reduce your risk of injury, it is important to take safety precautions in vehicles, at work, at play and in your home. To reduce your risk of illness, you need to make choices about your lifestyle. Making healthy choices will reduce your chances of cancer, stroke, heart attack, cardiovascular disease and other diseases that are the leading causes of chronic illness and death. Eating a healthy diet, exercising regularly, avoiding harmful substances and managing stress all contribute to a person's health and well-being.

APPLICATION QUESTION

1. What might Mrs. Gallagher have done to achieve her current state of fitness?

STUDY QUESTIONS

1. Match each term with the correct definition.

   a. Carbohydrates
   b. Obesity
   c. Stress
   d. Cardiorespiratory
      endurance

   e. Aerobic exercise
   f. Saturated fat
   g. Calorie

   _____ A measure of the energy value of food.

   _____ A physiological or psychological response to real or imagined influences that alter an existing state of physical, mental or emotional balance.

   _____ The ability to take in, deliver and extract oxygen for physical work.

   _____ The fat in animal tissues and products.

   _____ Activities that require additional effort by the heart and lungs to meet the increased demand by the skeletal muscles for oxygen.

   _____ A condition characterized by excess of stored body fat.

   _____ Compounds that contain carbon, oxygen and hydrogen; the main source of energy for all body functions.

2. Fill in the blanks with the correct word or words.

   The leading cause of death in the United States is _____. The disease that is the leading cause

   of death is _____. The leading cause of death for people ages 1 to 39 is _____.

3. List three ways to reduce your risk of personal injury.

4. List two motor-vehicle safety guidelines.

5. List four guidelines for what to do in case the building you are in catches fire.

6. When Jake learned that his grandmother had fallen in the upstairs hall, he went to her house to see what he could do to make it safer for her. What hazards might he have discovered in the hall? What could he do to make the hall safer?

7. Your 2-year-old nephew is coming to visit. What can you do to make your kitchen safe?

In questions 8 through 16, circle the letter of the correct answer.

8. Which best describes the purpose of the current food labels?

   a. They compare the beneficial effects of the nutrients listed.
   b. They point out the dangers of fat and sugar.
   c. They provide a way to evaluate the nutritional value of the food product.
   d. All of the above.

9. From which of these food groups should you get the majority of your daily nutrients?

   a. Fruits and vegetables
   b. Milk and cheese
   c. Fats, oils and sweets
   d. Bread, cereal, rice and pasta

10. Which of these statements is correct?

   a. You can eat as much fat as you wish as long as it is not saturated fat.
   b. Excess protein is always stored in the body as muscle.
   c. Carbohydrates are the body's main source of energy.
   d. Dietary fiber has no value for the body, since it is not digested.

11. Which of these statements is correct?

   a. To be beneficial, exercise must cause pain.
   b. Only vigorous activities burn off calories.
   c. If you take in more calories than you use, you will not gain weight.
   d. Too much body fat contributes to disease.

12. To improve cardiorespiratory endurance, which form of exercise is most effective?

   a. Strength training
   b. Flexibility training
   c. Aerobic exercise
   d. Vigorous walking

13. Which of these statements is correct?

   a. Stress can be positive as well as negative.
   b. Receiving an unexpected award can cause stress.
   c. Not all people are stressed by the same events.
   d. All of the above.

14. Which is the addictive substance in cigarettes?

   a. Tar
   b. Nicotine
   c. Carbon monoxide
   d. All of the above

15. Which of these statements is correct?

    a. Cigarette smoking contributes heavily to lung cancer.
    b. If you stop smoking, you remain at the same risk of heart attack as while you were smoking.
    c. The tars and carbon monoxide in cigarettes are harmless.
    d. Chewing tobacco and snuff are safe because you do not inhale smoke when you use them.

16. Which is the most effective way to sober up a person who has had too much to drink?

    a. Give the person a lot of black coffee.
    b. Put the person in a cold shower.
    c. Have the person eat a lot of food.
    d. None of the above.

17. List four ways in which you can be a responsible host.

Answers are listed in Appendix A.

Appendix A

CHAPTER 1

Answers to Application Questions

1. One person can find a phone and call EMS personnel; another can look around for a nearby citizen responder. Someone can begin to give first aid.
2. Although you may feel ill and be incapacitated by the sight of blood or cries of pain, you can still help. If possible, turn away for a moment and try to control your feelings. If you are still unable to proceed, make sure EMS personnel have been called. Then find other ways to help, such as asking bystanders to assist you or helping to keep the area safe.
3. People delayed calling EMS personnel; the caller gave an incorrect location of the crash; the ambulance was held up in traffic. EMS personnel may have had to cut the victim out of the car; the location of the car was hazardous; they had to use special equipment; a helicopter may have had to be called and would have had to land safely nearby; the hospital was far away.

Answers to Study Questions

1 a. I was fixing sandwiches and talking with my next-door neighbor, Mrs. Roberts, who had come by to borrow a book. My 3-year-old, Jenny, was in the next room playing with some puzzles. As Mrs. Roberts got up to leave, **I heard a loud thump and a shriek from upstairs.**

  b. I was on the bus headed for work. A man from the back of the bus came down the aisle, and **I noticed that he was moving unsteadily. I noticed he was sweating and looked very pale. "I don't know where I am," I heard him mumble to himself.**

  c. On my way into the grocery store from the parking lot, **I heard the loud screech of tires and the crash of metal. I saw that a car had struck a telephone pole, causing the telephone pole to lean at an odd angle. Wires are hanging down from the pole.** It was very frightening.

2. Five common barriers to taking action at the scene of an emergency are: the presence of bystanders; uncertainty about the victim; nature of the injury or illness; fear of disease transmission; and the fear of doing something wrong.
3. A citizen responder can overcome these barriers to action by thinking about these barriers and mentally preparing himself or herself to face these challenges ahead of time.
4. c, e, a, d, b, f
5. Bystanders can help at the scene of an emergency by calling, meeting and directing the ambulance; keeping the area free of unnecessary traffic; or giving first aid. Bystanders can go for additional supplies or give comfort to others on the scene. Finally, bystanders may be able to give you important information about the victim or what happened.

CHAPTER 2

Answers to Application Questions

1. The main danger in the garage could be the presence of carbon monoxide. Another danger could be fumes from a spilled toxic substance or an electrical hazard.
2. The presence of poisonous fumes would be the major factor that could cause you to decide to move your Dad immediately. Avoid breathing in poisonous fumes as you execute the move.
3. You would shout for help. If no one came, you would go to the phone and call 9-1-1 or the

local emergency number. If the car is running, you would suspect carbon monoxide, so you would turn off the engine and move your Dad from the garage.

Answers to Study Questions

1. Downed power lines; traffic; fire; dangerous fumes; freezing rain; broken glass; metal shards; spilled fuel.
2. Do not approach the victim. Go to a safe place and call 9-1-1 or the local emergency number.
3. Unconsciousness; trouble breathing; no signs of life (movement or breathing); severe bleeding.
4. The victim's condition, the care being given, the location and type of emergency (auto accident). Tell him or her to report back to you after making the call and tell you what the call taker said.
5. *Call First*, that is, call 9-1-1 or the local emergency number before giving care.

CHAPTER 3

Answers to Application Questions

1. The lifeguard should take steps to prevent disease transmission, such as wearing gloves to avoid contact with the victim's blood.
2. The lifeguard should immediately wash his hands and check for any open sores or cuts in his skin.

Answers to Study Questions

1. a. The victim may or may not be infected with the disease.
2. d. Indirect contact.
3. b. Using personal protective equipment such as disposable gloves.
4. a. Your level of training.
5. c. Clothes drag.
6. Fire; presence of toxic gas; risk of drowning; risk of explosion.
7. Dangerous conditions at the scene; the size of the victim; your physical ability; the victim's condition.
8. Only attempt to move a person you are sure you can comfortably handle; bend your body at the knees and hips; lift with your legs, not your back; walk carefully, using short steps.

9. Walking assist; pack-strap carry; two-person seat carry; clothes drag.

CHAPTER 4

Answers to Application Questions

1. His brain may have been injured by the blow to the head, and this damage to the nervous system could affect breathing and perhaps cause it to stop.
2. Respiratory—his breathing is changing, becoming faster, then slower. Nervous—he is unconscious. Integumentary—he has a cut on his head.
3. Jim may have sustained damage to other systems, but these injuries are the most obvious.

Answers to Study Questions

1. (a) Respiratory (b) airway, lungs (c) circulatory (d) transports oxygen and other nutrients to cells and removes wastes (e) skin, hair, nails (f) helps keep fluids in, prevents infection, sweat glands and pores in skin help regulate temperature, helps make vitamin D, stores minerals (g) bones, ligaments, muscles, tendons (h) supports body, allows movement, protects internal organs and structures, produces blood cells, stores minerals, produces heat (i) nervous (j) brain, spinal cord, nerves.
2. g, f, e, d, c, a, h, b
3. a
4. c
5. c
6. c
7. b
8. b
9. d

CHAPTER 5

Answers to Application Questions

1. In this particular emergency, you may not be able to do much to ensure scene safety, beyond guarding against the possibility that another biker might round the curve and hit you or the victim.
2. A head, neck or back injury is certainly a possibility, as well as a sudden illness, such as an allergic reaction or a heart attack.

3. Shout for help. If no one responds and the victim is unconscious, position the victim on one side (recovery position) and find a telephone or ask someone else to call 9-1-1 or the local emergency number. After calling 9-1-1 or the local emergency number, return to the victim as soon as possible. You may be asked to meet EMS personnel and take them to the victim. If you cannot find a phone or someone to place the call, go get help.

4. Ask the victim what happened. Check for non-life-threatening conditions to find out if the victim has any problems that require you to call 9-1-1 or the local emergency number. If you do not find life-threatening conditions, help the victim gradually to his or her feet.

Answers to Study Questions

1. (a) Look for bystanders who can help, look for victims, look for dangers, look for clues to determine what happened. (b) Open the airway, check for signs of life (movement and breathing), check for severe bleeding. (c) Call 9-1-1 or the local emergency number. (d) Interview the victim and bystanders, do a head-to-toe examination, obtain the victim's consent.

2. Unconsciousness; breathing in a strange way or trouble breathing; no signs of life (movement or breathing); severe bleeding.

3. There's a stopped car in the road and a mangled bicycle. You can use bystanders to direct traffic.

4. If the victim is conscious and has no life-threatening conditions, you can begin to check for other conditions that may need care. Checking a conscious victim with no immediate life-threatening conditions involves two basic steps: Interview the victim and bystanders and check the victim from head to toe.

5. 4, 1, 5, 2, 3
6. b
7. c
8. b
9. a

CHAPTER 6

Answers to Application Questions

1. Steve had signals of respiratory distress. Signals of Steve's emergency were holding his throat, pale skin and wheezing sounds when breathing.

2. No. The care for respiratory distress is basically the same, regardless of the condition that caused it.

3. Yes. If the passages narrow as a result of swelling, preventing air exchange, Steve may suffer respiratory arrest. The possibility of respiratory arrest is the reason to call 9-1-1 or the local emergency number right away.

4. Send Kevin to call 9-1-1 if someone has not already called. Your first step would be to open Steve's airway and check for signs of life (movement or breathing). If he is not breathing, give 2 rescue breaths. If he is breathing, maintain an open airway.

5. Yes, if Steve's condition is asthma or a severe allergic reaction, an airway obstruction could occur. Also, if Steve became unconscious, his tongue could fall to the back of his throat and block the airway. In Steve's case, airway obstruction could be a serious emergency, because abdominal thrusts would not relieve this obstruction caused by swelling. Make sure to call 9-1-1 or the local emergency number immediately.

Answers to Study Questions

1. c, d, a, f, h, b, g, e
2. High-pitched sounds; skin is unusually moist; fearful; skin has a flushed appearance; shortness of breath; pain in chest.
3. Trying to swallow large pieces of poorly chewed food; drinking alcohol before or during meals; wearing dentures; eating while talking excitedly or laughing or eating too fast; walking, playing or running with food or objects in the mouth.
4. c, a, b   13. a
5. d   14. b
6. b   15. b
7. a   16. c
8. a   17. 2, 3, 1, 4
9. c
10. b
11. d
12. a

CHAPTER 7

Answers to Application Questions

1. Yes. The exertion of mowing grass in the heat can add an extra burden on the body, increasing

its demand for oxygen. The heart works harder to keep up with the body's demand for oxygen, increasing its own oxygen needs. If the arteries are narrowed as a result of atherosclerosis, the delivery of oxygen-rich blood to the heart is severely restricted or completely cut off, causing the heart to beat irregularly or stop beating.

2. Resting reduces the heart's need for oxygen, allowing it to recover from the strain placed on it.

3. Yes. If Mr. Getz suffered a heart attack, he may go into cardiac arrest. A heart attack becomes cardiac arrest when so much of the heart muscle is destroyed that the heart is unable to contract regularly and subsequently stops beating. There is no way to predict the extent of the damage sustained by the heart during a heart attack or to predict when a heart attack might become cardiac arrest. Therefore, it is very important to recognize the signals of a heart attack and to call 9-1-1 quickly.

4. If Mr. Getz is suffering cardiac arrest, he needs defibrillation as quickly as possible. Someone must call 9-1-1 or the local emergency number immediately and CPR must be started immediately.

5. CPR—the combination of chest compressions and rescue breathing—sustains the vital organs, such as the brain, for a relatively short time. Prompt CPR, early defibrillation and other advanced cardiac life support measures in combination are needed to sustain life.

Answers to Study Questions

1. e, c, g, h, d, b, a, f
2. Absence of signs of life. The victim's skin may be pale, ashen or bluish, particularly around the face. The skin may also be moist from perspiration.
3. The scene becomes unsafe; the victim shows signs of life; an AED becomes available and is ready to use; another trained rescuer arrives and takes over; you are too exhausted to continue.
4. Motor vehicle crashes, drowning, smoke inhalation, poisoning, airway obstruction, firearm injuries and falls.
5. b
6. d
7. d
8. c
9. d
10. c
11. c
12. b
13. Persistent chest pain associated with shoulder pain; perspiring heavily; breathing fast; looking ill.
14. 2, 3, 1, 4, 5
15. 3, 4, 2, 1, 5

CHAPTER 8

Answers to Application Questions

1. The bleeding from Janelle's wound is probably from a vein. The blood is flowing rather than spurting. Spurting would indicate that the bleeding is from an artery.
2. Severe bleeding can reduce the blood volume in the body and become life threatening. An adequate amount of blood is needed to maintain the flow of oxygen-rich blood to the body, particularly to the vital organs.
3. Janelle's friend should first try to control the bleeding by applying direct pressure to the wound. She should then apply a pressure bandage and determine if the wound needs further medical attention.
4. Janelle's friend should use a barrier, such as disposable gloves or plastic wrap. If these items are not available, the friend could use a clean folded cloth or have Janelle use her hand to control the bleeding. The friend should wash her hands after giving care.

Answers to Study Questions

1. b, a, e, c, g, f, d
2. Blood spurts from the wound, making it difficult for clots to form; bleeding that fails to stop after all measures have been taken to control it.
3. Place direct pressure on the wound with a sterile gauze pad or any clean cloth, such as a washcloth, towel or handkerchief. Place your gloved hand over the pad and apply firm pressure. If you do not have disposable gloves or an appropriate barrier, have the injured person apply pressure with his or her hand. Apply a pressure bandage to hold the gauze pads or cloth in place. If blood soaks through the bandage, add more pads and bandages to help absorb the blood and continue to apply pressure. Do not remove any blood-soaked pads. If bleeding continues, call 9-1-1 or the local emergency number.

4. Soft tissues, such as those in the abdomen, that are tender, swollen or hard; swelling, tenderness or rigidity in the injured area; anxiety or restlessness; rapid, weak pulse; rapid breathing, shortness of breath; skin that feels cool or moist or looks pale, ashen or bluish; bruising in the injured area; nausea or vomiting; vomiting or coughing up blood; abdominal pain; excessive thirst; decreased level of consciousness; severe headache.

5. Apply an ice pack or a chemical cold pack to the injured area to help reduce pain and swelling. Place something, such as a gauze pad or a towel, between the source of cold and the skin to prevent damage to the skin.

6. Internal bleeding.

7. Get ice or a cold pack and apply it to the area. If the injury appears to be serious, call 9-1-1 or the local emergency number.

8. a

CHAPTER 9

Answers to Application Questions

1. Her body could not compensate for her significant injuries, which probably involved significant bleeding.

2. The man could minimize shock by keeping the woman from becoming chilled and by providing reassurance. He could also control any external bleeding and give any additional care that she needed.

Answers to Study Questions

1. f

2. Restlessness or irritability; altered consciousness; pale or ashen, bluish, cool or moist skin; rapid breathing, rapid and weak pulse; excessive thirst; nausea or vomiting.

3. Severe injury or sudden illness.

4. Care for life-threatening conditions. Make the victim as comfortable as possible. Keep the victim from getting chilled or overheated. Watch for changes in the victim's level of consciousness, breathing rate and skin appearance. Help the victim lie down on his or her back. Elevate the legs about 12 inches to help blood circulate to the vital organs. Do not elevate the legs if the victim is nauseated or having trouble breathing.

If you suspect head, neck or back injuries or possible broken bones involving the hips or legs, if moving causes more pain, if you are unsure of the victim's condition or if it is painful for him or her to move, leave the victim lying flat. Do not give the victim anything to eat or drink, even though he or she is likely to be thirsty.

5. d

6. b

7. d

8. d

9. b

10. Shock is life threatening because the circulatory system fails to circulate oxygen-rich blood to all parts of the body, causing vital organs to fail to function properly.

11. Elevating the legs helps to maintain blood flow to the vital organs.

CHAPTER 10

Answers to Application Questions

1. Joe's burn is probably a deep burn. The heat from steam and scalding fluid is likely to damage more than the first layer of skin.

2. Joe's burns will require medical attention. His burns cover more than one body part.

3. Call 9-1-1 or the local emergency number. Find a source of cool water and cool the burn. Remove any clothing from the burned areas. Cover the burned areas. Minimize shock by having Joe rest and keeping him from getting chilled or overheated. Consider the possibility of inhalation burns, and check for trouble breathing.

Answers to Study Questions

1. c, f, a, d, e, b

2. c, d, a, b

3. a, b, d, c

4. Swollen, red area around wound; area may be warm or painful, possible pus discharge; fever and feeling ill; red streaks from wound toward heart.

5. Hold dressings in place; to protect a wound from dirt and infection.

6. Laceration (cut); abrasion (scrape); puncture (penetrates—sharp object); avulsion; (torn tissue—may be torn completely away).

7. Heat; electricity; chemicals; radiation.

8. **a.** Involves only the top layer of the skin (first degree). Skin is red and dry, and the burn is usually painful. Heals in 5 to 6 days without permanent scarring.

   b. Involves the epidermis and dermis (second degree). May look red and have blisters. Blisters may open and weep clear fluid. Burned skin may look mottled. Burns are painful and often swell. Heals in 3 or 4 weeks. May scar.

   c. Destroys all layers of the skin and any or all of underlying structures (third degree). Burns look brown or charred (black). Tissues underneath may appear white. Burns can be extremely painful or painless if burn destroyed nerve endings. Burn is often life threatening, takes a long time to heal and results in scarring.

9.	a	17.	d
10.	b	18.	b
11.	d	19.	d
12.	b	20.	b
13.	d	21.	b
14.	a	22.	b
15.	b	23.	c
16.	b	24.	c

CHAPTER 11

Answers to Application Questions

1. Rita is obviously in pain—moaning and holding her shoulder. She seems unable to get up. She appears unable to move her left arm.

2. Rita could have a serious shoulder injury, possibly injuring the bones, muscles, ligaments and tendons. She might also have injured her neck or back.

3. Help her find the most comfortable position; keep from moving her head, neck and back as much as possible; immobilize her upper extremity and apply ice to the injured area; prevent her from becoming chilled or overheated to delay the onset of shock; and keep her comfortable until EMS personnel arrive.

4. Yes. Although the injury does not appear to be life threatening—the victim is conscious, breathing, has signs of life and is not bleeding severely—Rita is unable to get up and is in pain. She may have a fracture or dislocation and could also have injured her head, neck or back.

Answers to Study Questions

1. h, b, f, c, a, i, k, d, j, g, e
2. Pain; swelling; discoloration of the skin; inability to use the affected part normally; loss of sensation in the affected part.
3. Splint only if you have to move the injured person and you can do so without causing more pain and discomfort to the victim. Splint an injury in the position in which you find it. Do not move, straighten or bend the injured part. Splint the injured area and the joints or bones above and below the injury site. Check for proper circulation (feeling, warmth and color) before and after splinting.
4. c
5. b
6. b
7. a
8. b

CHAPTER 12

Answers to Application Questions

1. Yes; Sam's knee hurts, he cannot use it, and it is swelling.
2. He should make Sam as comfortable as possible and go find a phone to call 9-1-1 or the local emergency number. If he uses a phone in a home or business, he could ask for ice or a cold pack and a blanket or pillow to use to immobilize Sam's knee.

Answers to Study Questions

1. c, b, d, a
2. Falling on the hand of an outstretched arm.
3. A dislocation, separation, broken bone.
4. Unable to move the leg, which is beginning to swell; left arm looks deformed at the shoulder; no sensation in the fingers of that arm; arm is beginning to look bruised and is painful.
5. Call 9-1-1 or the local emergency number; immobilize the injured part; apply ice; elevate the injured extremity; place gauze or cloth between the source of cold and the skin. Help the victim rest in the most comfortable position; prevent him from becoming chilled or overheated; reassure him. Continue to monitor the victim's level of consciousness, breathing, skin color and temperature. Be alert for any signals, such as changes in breathing rate, skin color or level of

consciousness that may indicate the victim's condition is worsening. If needed, take steps to minimize shock.

6. Injured leg is noticeably shorter than the other leg; injured leg is turned outward; severe pain; inability to move the lower extremity.

7. Soft, rigid and anatomic.

8. b

9. c

10. Control any external bleeding. Wear disposable gloves or use a protective barrier. Call 9-1-1 or the local emergency number immediately. Immobilize the injured area and help the victim into the most comfortable position. If the victim's lower extremity is supported by the ground, do not move it. Rather, use rolled towels or blankets to support the leg in the position in which you found it. If one is available, place a pillow or rolled blanket between the lower extremities and bind them together above and below the site of the injury. Check for feeling, warmth and color before and after applying the splint. Apply ice or a cold pack. Take steps to minimize shock.

CHAPTER 13

Answers to Application Questions

No. Signals could develop later. He did strike his head and could have injured his neck or back in doing so.

Answers to Study Questions

1. b, a, c, e, d

2. A fall from a height greater than the victim's height; any diving mishap in which the person may have struck or otherwise injured the head, neck or back; a victim found unconscious for unknown reasons; any injury involving a severe blunt force to the head or trunk, such as being hit by a car or baseball bat; any injury that penetrates the head or trunk, such as a knife or gunshot wound; a motor vehicle crash involving a driver or passengers not wearing safety belts; any person thrown from a motor vehicle; any injury in which a victim's helmet is broken or cracked, including a bicycle, motorcycle, football or industrial helmet; anytime a victim is struck by lightning.

3. Changes in the level of consciousness; severe pain or pressure in the head, neck or back; tingling or loss of sensation in the extremities; partial or complete loss of movement of any body part; unusual bumps or depressions on the head or neck; sudden loss of memory; blood or other fluids in the ears or nose; profuse external bleeding of the head, neck or back; seizures in a person who does not have a seizure disorder; impaired breathing or impaired vision as a result of injury; nausea or vomiting; persistent headache; loss of balance; bruising of the head, especially around the eyes or behind the ears.

4. Wearing safety belts (lap and shoulder restraints) and placing children in car safety seats; when appropriate, wearing approved helmets, eyewear, faceguards and mouthguards; taking steps to prevent falls; obeying rules in sports and recreational activities; avoiding inappropriate use of alcohol and other drugs; inspecting work and recreational equipment periodically; thinking and talking about safety.

5. Place the victim on his or her back; do not attempt to remove any object embedded in the eye; wearing disposable gloves, place a sterile dressing around the object; stabilize any embedded object as best you can; you can stabilize the object by placing a paper cup around the object to support it; bandage loosely and do not put pressure on the injured eye/eyeball; seek immediate medical attention.

6. a

7. d

8. c

9. c

10. a

11. b

12. d

13. d

14. Do not put direct pressure on the wound; attempt to control bleeding with pressure on the area around the wound; secure the dressings with a roller bandage or triangular bandage; call 9-1-1 if you are unsure about the extent of the injury.

15. Minimize movement of the head, neck and back; keep the victim as still as possible until EMS personnel arrive; use a technique called in-line stabilization to minimize movement of the head and neck; check for life-threatening conditions; maintain an open airway; monitor consciousness and breathing; control any external bleeding with direct pressure unless the bleeding is located directly over a suspected fracture; wear disposable gloves or use another barrier; maintain normal body temperature.

CHAPTER 14

Answers to Application Questions

She should have Mr. McGuffy lie down, and she should call or have a bystander call 9-1-1 or the local emergency number. She should keep Mr. McGuffy as still as possible. Because the injury was the result of trauma, she should apply manual stabilization, watch for changes in his breathing and level of consciousness while waiting for EMS personnel to arrive. She should also keep Mr. McGuffy from getting chilled or overheated.

Answers to Study Questions

1. c, a, b, e, d
2. Calling 9-1-1 or the local emergency number; limiting movement; monitoring signs of life; controlling bleeding; minimizing shock.
3. Trouble breathing; severe pain at the site of the injury; flushed, pale, ashen or bluish skin; obvious deformity, such as that caused by a fracture; coughing up blood (may be bright red or dark like coffee grounds); bruising at the site of a blunt injury, such as that caused by a seat belt; a "sucking" noise or distinct sound when the victim breathes
4. Rib fracture. Have the victim rest in a position that will make breathing easier. Do not move the victim if you suspect a head, neck or back injury. Call 9-1-1 or the local emergency number. Bind the victim's upper arm to the chest on the injured side to help support the injured area and make breathing more comfortable. Use an object such as a pillow or rolled blanket to support and immobilize the area. Monitor breathing and skin condition, and take steps to minimize shock.
5. A sucking sound coming from the wound with each breath the victim takes
6. Severe pain; bruising; external bleeding: nausea; vomiting (sometimes containing blood); weakness; thirst; pain, tenderness or a tight feeling in the area; protruding organs; rigid abdominal muscles; other signals of shock.
7. a
8. A sucking chest wound.
9. Trouble breathing; severe pain at the site of the injury; hear a sucking sound when victim breathes.

CHAPTER 15

Answers to Application Questions

1. The signals of Julio's illness include his body collapsing to the ground and becoming rigid, his eyes rolling back and his arms and legs jerking uncontrollably.
2. During the seizure, Michelle could protect Julio's head, loosen any clothing that might restrict breathing and move any nearby objects that could cause injury. After the seizure, Michelle could ensure that Julio's airway is open, position Julio on his side so that any fluids could drain, look and care for non-life-threatening conditions that may have occurred during the seizure, provide reassurance, maintain crowd control or find Julio a more secluded place to rest, stay with Julio until he is fully conscious and aware of his surroundings and call 9-1-1 or the local emergency number, if necessary.
3. Michelle should call 9-1-1 or the local emergency number if Julio was injured when he fell or during the seizure, another seizure immediately follows the end of the first one, the seizure lasted more than 5 minutes, Julio is not known to have epilepsy, Julio is a known diabetic or Julio fails to regain consciousness after the seizure.

Answers to Study Questions

1. f, c, h, g, e, d, b, i, a
2. A victim of sudden illness may faint or complain of feeling lightheaded, dizzy or weak. He or she may feel nauseated or may vomit. Breathing, pulse, body temperature and skin color may change. A person who looks or feels ill generally is ill.
3. Do no further harm; monitor breathing and consciousness; help the victim rest in the most comfortable position; keep the victim from getting chilled or overheated; reassure the victim; give any specific care needed.
4. The seizure lasts more than five minutes; the victim has repeated seizures, one after another, without regaining consciousness in between; the victim appears to be injured; the victim is not known to have a predisposing condition, such as epilepsy, that could have brought on the seizure; the victim is pregnant; the victim is an

infant or child who is experiencing an initial febrile seizure; the victim is known to have diabetes; the seizure takes place in water; the victim fails to regain consciousness after the seizure.

5. Control your blood pressure; do not smoke; eat a healthy diet; exercise regularly; control diabetes.

6. Look for non-life-threatening conditions, checking to see if the victim was injured during the seizure; be reassuring and comforting; if the seizure occurred in public, try to provide a measure of privacy for the person; ask bystanders not to crowd around the person; if possible, take the victim to a nearby place, away from bystanders, to rest; if moving the victim to a more secluded location is not possible, use your body or an object, such as a blanket, to shield the victim from onlookers. Stay with the victim until he or she is fully conscious and aware of his or her surroundings.

7. Confusion; profuse sweating; pupils of unequal sizes; speech difficulty; weakness or fatigue.

8. Call 9-1-1 or the local emergency number. Allow the victim to rest in a comfortable position. Do not give her anything to eat or drink. Stay with her and offer comfort and reassurance until EMS personnel arrive.

9. a
10. c
11. c
12. a
13. b
14. a
15. c
16. d

CHAPTER 16

Answers to Application Questions

1. Ashley sees the chair used to climb up to the table and an empty vitamin container on the table next to Kristen.

2. Ashley should take the empty container to the phone, call the local poison control center and follow their directions.

Answers to Study Questions

1. e, b, f, c, a, d
2. Nausea; vomiting; diarrhea; chest or abdominal pain; trouble breathing; sweating; changes in consciousness; seizures; headache; dizziness; weakness; irregular pupil size; burning or tearing eyes; abnormal skin color; burn injuries around the lips or tongue or on the skin.

3. Depends on the type and amount of the substance; how and where it entered the body; the time elapsed since the poison entered the body; and the victim's size, weight, medical condition and age.

4. Immediately rinse the affected area thoroughly with water. Using soap cannot hurt, but soap may not do much to remove the poisonous plant oil that causes the allergic reaction. If the victim is wearing any jewelry that is contaminated or restricting circulation, ask him or her to remove it. If a rash or weeping lesion (an oozing sore) develops, seek advice from a pharmacist or physician about possible treatment. If the condition worsens and large areas of the body or the face are affected, the victim should see a physician, who may administer anti-inflammatory drugs, such as corticosteroids, or other medications to relieve discomfort. If other poisons, such as dry or wet chemicals, contact the skin, flush the affected area continuously with large amounts of water. Garden hoses and showers suit this purpose well. Call 9-1-1 or the local emergency number immediately, then continue to flush the area until EMS personnel arrive. If running water is not available, brush off dry chemicals, such as lime, with a gloved hand. Take care not to inhale any of the chemical or get any of the dry chemicals in your eyes or the eyes of the victim or any bystanders.

5. Keep all medications and household products well out of the reach of children. Special latches and clamps are available to keep children from opening cabinets. Consider all household or drugstore products to be potentially harmful. Use childproof safety caps on containers of medication and other potentially dangerous products. Keep products in their original containers, with the labels in place. Use poison symbols to identify dangerous substances, and teach children what the symbols mean. Dispose of outdated medications and household products properly and in a timely manner. Use potentially dangerous chemicals only in well-ventilated areas. Wear proper clothing when work or recreation may put you in contact with a poisonous substance. Immediately wash those areas of the body that you suspect may have come into contact with a poisonous plant.

6. Itching and burning hand; swollen fingers; red bumps all over her forearm.

7. Rinse the affected area thoroughly with water, and consult a doctor or pharmacist about possible treatments.
8. Wear protective clothing.
9. c
10. a

CHAPTER 17

Answers to Application Questions

1. The sounds of hissing and dry leaves crackling, as well as pain and bleeding at or near Tonya's ankle, indicate that she was probably bitten by a snake.
2. Darrell should use his mobile phone or contact a park ranger to call 9-1-1 or the local emergency number immediately. Then, if possible, Darrell should wash the wound, immobilize Tonya's leg, keep her leg lower than her heart and minimize her movement.
3. Darrell should consider the distance to professional help, whether he can get Tonya to help before help can get to her and whether he has a way to transport her to a medical facility.
4. To prevent her injury, Tonya could have made noise to scare away the snake, kept her socks and boots on and not used the log as a footrest.

Answers to Study Questions

1. b, a, c, e, d
2. With a gloved hand, grasp the tick with fine-tipped pointed, non-etched, non-rasped tweezers as close to the skin as possible and pull slowly and upwards. Do not burn the tick off, do not apply petroleum jelly or nail polish to the tick. These remedies are not always effective in removing the tick and can cause further harm to the victim. If you cannot remove the tick, or if its mouth parts remain embedded, get medical care. Place the tick in a sealable container for analysis. Wash the bite area with soap and warm water. Apply antiseptic or triple antibiotic ointment to help prevent infection. If rash, flu-like signals or joint pain appears, seek medical attention. Wash your hands thoroughly. If you do not have tweezers, use a glove, plastic wrap, a piece of paper or a leaf to protect your fingers.
3. Apply insect or tick repellent according to label instructions. Wear sturdy hiking boots. Wear long-sleeved shirts and long pants. Tuck your pant legs into your socks or boots. Tuck your shirt into your pants. Wear light-colored clothing to make it easier to see tiny insects or ticks. Use a rubber band or tape the area where pants and socks meet to prevent ticks or other insects from getting under clothing. Inspect yourself carefully for insects or ticks after being outdoors or have someone else do it. If you are outdoors for a long period of time, check yourself several times during the day. Check especially in moist, hairy areas of the body (including the back of the neck and the scalp line). Shower immediately after coming indoors, using a washcloth to scrub off any insects or ticks. Carefully inspect yourself for embedded ticks and remove them appropriately. Keep an eye out for and avoid the nests of wasps, bees and hornets. If you have pets that go outdoors, spray them with repellent made for your type of pet. Apply the repellent according to the label, and check your pet for ticks often. When hiking in woods and fields, stay in the middle of trails. Avoid underbrush, fallen trees and tall grass. Avoid walking in areas known to be populated with snakes. Make noise as you walk through areas that may be populated with snakes, because many snakes will retreat if they detect your movement. If you encounter a snake, look around, because other snakes may be nearby. Turn around and walk away, back on the same path you were just on. To prevent stings from marine animals, you might consider wearing a wet suit or dry suit or protective footwear in the water. To prevent dog bites: do not run past a dog. Avoid eye contact, try to remain motionless until the dog leaves, then back away slowly until the dog is out of sight. Do not approach a strange dog, especially one that is tied or confined. Always let a dog see and sniff you before you pet the animal.
4. A bite or sting mark at the point of injection (entry site). A stinger, tentacle or venom sac remaining in or near the entry site. Redness at or around the entry site. Swelling at or around the entry site. Pain or tenderness at or around the entry site.
5. Call 9-1-1 or the local emergency number. Wash the wound, if possible. Immobilize the affected part. Keep the affected area lower than the heart, if possible. Minimize the victim's movement. If possible, carry a victim who must be transported or have him or her walk slowly. If you know the victim cannot receive medical care within 30 minutes, consider suctioning the wound using a snakebite kit.

6. Try to get your sister away from the dog without endangering yourself. Do not try to capture the animal. Control the bleeding and apply a dressing. Do not clean the wound. Call 9-1-1 or the local emergency number. In case animal control personnel need to be summoned, try to describe what the dog looked like and the area in which it was last seen.

7. a	10. d
8. d	11. d
9. b	12. d

CHAPTER 18

Answers to Application Questions

1. The signals of Susan's condition are dizziness, nausea, vomiting, unconsciousness and unusually pale skin.
2. The signals of Susan's condition, along with the fact that she has been drinking, seem to indicate a case of alcohol poisoning. Although you cannot be sure of the cause of Susan's condition, the fact that she is unconscious means that she needs immediate care.
3. Yes, Susan's friends must call 9-1-1 or the local emergency number because EMS personnel should always be called in cases of unconsciousness.

Answers to Study Questions

1. f, c, d, e a, h, b, g
2. Trouble breathing; chest pain; altered level of consciousness; moist or flushed skin; mood changes; nausea; vomiting; sweating; chills; fever; headache; dizziness; rapid pulse; rapid breathing; restlessness; excitement; irritability; talkativeness; hallucinations; confusion; slurred speech; poor coordination; trembling.
3. Stimulants; depressants; hallucinogens; narcotics; inhalants; cannabis products.
4. Read the product information and use products only as directed. Ask your physician or pharmacist about the intended use and side effects of prescription and over-the-counter medication. If you are taking more than one medication, check for possible interaction effects. Never use another person's prescribed medications; what is right for one person is seldom right for another. Always keep medications in their appropriate, marked containers. Destroy all out-of-date medications. Time can alter the chemical composition of medications, causing them to be less effective and possibly even toxic. Always keep medications out of the reach of children.
5. Check the scene to be sure it is safe to help the person. Do not approach the victim if he or she is behaving in a threatening manner. Call 9-1-1, the local emergency number or the poison control center. Check for any life-threatening conditions. Care for any conditions you find.
6. b, c, a, d, e, f
7. c
8. b
9. d

CHAPTER 19

Answers to Application Questions

1. Cynthia feels dizzy because, in an effort to cool the body, blood flow to the skin is increased, bringing warm blood to the surface and allowing heat to escape. As more blood flows to the skin, blood flow to vital organs like the brain is reduced. This reduction of blood flow causes a lack of oxygen-rich blood in the brain, creating a temporary decline in the level of consciousness and making the person feel weak and dizzy or faint.
2. Louise should get Cynthia out of the sun immediately, then make sure that she rests in a cool place and sips cool water.
3. Cynthia could have worn a hat, taken frequent breaks and kept drinking liquids throughout her activity.

Answers to Study Questions

1. c, e, d, a, b
2. Air temperature; humidity; wind; clothing you wear; how often you take breaks from exposure to extreme temperature; how much and how often you drink water; how intense your activity is; how well your body manages temperature extremes.
3. Heat cramps; heat exhaustion; heat stroke.
4. Changes in body temperature; changes in skin temperature, color and moisture; headache; nausea; dizziness and weakness; exhaustion; progressive loss of consciousness; rapid, weak pulse; rapid, shallow pulse.

5. Changes in the victim's level of consciousness.

6. Move the victim away from the heat source. Have the victim rest in a cool place and drink cool water slowly. Loosen tight clothing. Remove clothing soaked with perspiration. Apply wet towels or sheets to the victim's body. Fan the victim. Apply ice and cold packs to the wrists, ankles, armpits, neck and groin.

7. Frostbite; hypothermia.

8. Avoid being outdoors in the hottest or coldest part of the day. Dress appropriately for the environment. Change your activity level according to the temperature. Take frequent breaks, by removing yourself from the environment. Drink large amounts of nonalcoholic or decaffeinated fluids before, during and after activity.

9. a

10. d

11. Lack of feeling in fingers; fingers look waxy and white; fingers feel cold.

12. Call 9-1-1 or the local emergency number. Attempt to remove jewelry or restrictive clothing. Handle the affected area gently; never rub the affected area. Rubbing causes further damage. If there is no chance that the frostbitten part will refreeze, you may begin rewarming the affected area gently by soaking the affected part in water (100° F to 105° F) until it appears red and feels warm. Loosely bandage area with a dry, sterile dressing. If fingers or toes are frostbitten, place dry, sterile gauze between them to keep them separated. Avoid breaking any blisters.

13. No response to your questions; glassy eyes; seems weak and exhausted; does not feel your touch.

14. Call 9-1-1 or the local emergency number. Carefully remove any wet clothing and dry the victim. Warm the body gradually by wrapping the victim in blankets or putting on dry clothing and moving him or her to a warm environment. If they are available, apply hot water bottles, chemical heat packs or other heat sources to the body. Keep a barrier, such as a blanket, towel or clothing, between the heat source and the victim to avoid burning him or her. If the victim is alert, give him or her warm nonalcoholic and decaffeinated liquids to drink. Do not warm the victim too quickly. Rapid rewarming can cause dangerous heart rhythms. Be extremely gentle in handling the victim. Monitor signs of life, give rescue breathing or CPR if necessary and continue to warm the victim until EMS personnel arrive.

CHAPTER 20

Answers to Application Questions

1. You can make a reaching assist by using rescue equipment that should be near the pool, such as a shepherd's crook. Other equipment available may include a leaf skimmer attached to a pole or a pole used to vacuum the pool. You may also firmly brace yourself on the pool deck and reach out to Eric, or you can extend your reach by using a towel or a shirt. You can also throw items that float out to him, such as a picnic jug, an air mattress or an inflatable toy. Remember that your first priority is to stay safe. Rushing into the water to help a victim may cause you to become a victim too.

Answers to Study Questions

1. Reaching assist; throwing assist; wading assist.

2. Struggles to breathe; cannot call out for help; arms to the sides pressing down; has no supporting kick; body position is vertical in the water; unable to move forward in the water.

3. d

4. c

5. d

6. b

CHAPTER 21

Answers to Application Questions

1. Check the scene for safety. If traffic is heavy or otherwise threatening, you might have to help the man move onto the sidewalk. Ask a bystander to call 9-1-1 or the local emergency number. Try to reassure the man and try to control the bleeding if it is severe, keeping a barrier between yourself and the victim's blood if possible. Try to keep the man from moving.

2. Depending on the weather, he could have been affected by heat or cold. He could have a sudden illness, such as a heart attack, stroke or seizure. He could have fainted. He could be confused, mentally impaired, unable to hear or have poor vision.

Answers to Study Questions

1. d, c, f, b, e, a
2. Check the scene for safety. Have a bystander call 9-1-1 or the local emergency number. Introduce yourself as someone who knows first aid. Find out if anyone on the scene is a parent or guardian of the child and, if so, ask permission to give care. Check the child for life-threatening conditions. If the child is conscious, try to reassure and comfort the child and ask the child's name and address. Have someone try to locate the parents if they are not present.
3. Introduce yourself and explain that you are there to help. Ask the woman her name and use it when you speak to her. Tell her to lie still; try to find out from the neighbor if the woman is generally confused or is taking any medication, if you haven't done so already. Have the neighbor call 9-1-1 or the local emergency number. Reassure and comfort the victim. Support and immobilize the injured area, probably using blankets and pillows.
4. d
5. b
6. b
7. b
8. c
9. Heat-related illness.
10. Call 9-1-1 or the local emergency number.
11. Hearing loss; confused or mentally impaired; not speak the same language you speak.
12. Medication; infection; vision or hearing problems; depression; Alzheimer's disease; mental impairment; shock.

CHAPTER 22

Answers to Application Questions

1. Because this is Lisa's first pregnancy, she is probably still in stage one, but getting close to stage two. The bloody fluid on the bed is probably the mucous plug, and possibly the amniotic sac has broken.
2. Lisa can tell you how close the contractions are, when she began to have them, if the water broke, where the clean sheets and towels are and where to find gloves.

Answers to Study Questions

1. h, g, c, e, f, a, d, b

2. Stage 1: Preparation—the mother's body prepares for birth; from the first contraction until the cervix is completely dilated.
   Stage 2: Delivery—Begins when the cervix is completely dilated and ends with the birth of a baby.
   Stage 3: Delivery of the Placenta—The placenta separates from the wall of the uterus and is expelled from the birth canal.
3. See that the airway is open and clear; keep the newborn from getting chilled.
4. a. Has 9-1-1 or your local emergency number been called? If so, how long ago and what was the response?
   b. Is this the first pregnancy?
   c. Does she expect any complications?
   d. Is there a bloody discharge?
   e. Has the amniotic sac ruptured (or water broken)?
   f. What are the contractions like? Are they very close together? Are they strong?
   g. Does she have the urge to bear down, or push?
   h. Is the newborn's head visible? If so, begin preparing for the delivery—the newborn is about to be born.
5. c
6. b
7. c
8. c
9. c
10. a

CHAPTER 23

Answers to Application Questions

1. The mountains where you, Frank and Jeff are located create a delayed-help situation. It will take more than 30 minutes for you and Frank to get help to Jeff. The mountain environment will also require specially trained rescue personnel to remove Jeff.
2. When checking the scene, you should check for dangerous conditions, such as loose or slippery rocks. You should be sure the area Jeff is lying on is safe and stable. It appears that Jeff is conscious; however, if his injuries are not cared for, he may develop shock, a life-threatening condition.
3. Jeff slipped and fell. He may have a head, neck or back injury, and you should not attempt to move him unless necessary. In this situation, because you are trained in first aid, you should stay with Jeff and Frank should go for help.

4. After checking for non-life-threatening conditions, you should give care and continue to check Jeff. You should prevent Jeff from getting dehydrated, chilled or overheated.

Answers to Study Questions

1. d, a, e, b, c
2. Hurricanes; earthquakes; mass trauma.
3. Wilderness; rural.
4. Stay where you are and call, radio or signal for help. Send someone to go get help or leave the victim alone to get help. Transport the victim to help. Care for the victim where you are until the victim has recovered enough to travel on his or her own.
5. c
6. b
7. c
8. c
9. c
10. He is shivering violently. His knee is very painful and feels as if it is swelling. The sky is overcast. The temperature is about 50° F. The sun will begin to set in 4 hours. Group members provide various dry items of clothing.
11. Provide some type of insulation.
12. Knowledge; skills; equipment.

CHAPTER 24

Answers to Application Questions

1. To have achieved her current state of fitness, Mrs. Gallagher would probably have eaten a healthy diet, exercised regularly, not smoked and drank alcohol only in moderation or not at all.

Answers to Study Questions

1. g, c, d, f, e, b, a
2. Disease, heart disease, injury.
3. Know your risk; change risky behaviors; think about safety; take precautions; wear protective devices; wear a safety belt; learn first aid.
4. Wear a safety belt including shoulder restraint; do not drink and drive.
5. Crawl low to escape smoke. Make sure children can open windows. If you cannot escape down a ladder, be prepared to lower children. Get out quickly and do not return to the building. If you cannot escape, stuff wet towels, rags or clothing into door cracks and vents. If a phone is available, call the fire department.
6. Poor lighting; rugs that are not fastened down. He could install bright lights, fasten down rugs, place handrails if necessary.
7. Turn pot handles toward the back of the stove; turn off the oven and other appliances when they are not in use; lock up all cleaning products and other poisonous items; clean up any spills promptly; fasten down any rugs.
8. c
9. d
10. c
11. d
12. c
13. d
14. b
15. a
16. d
17. Stop serving alcohol an hour before the party is to end. Have nonalcoholic beverages available. Do not promote or play drinking games. Do not have salty foods available. Do not have an open bar or serve anyone who has had too much to drink. Measure drinks if you are serving.

Glossary

PRONUNCIATION GUIDE

The accented syllable in a word is shown in capital letters.

River = RIV er

An unmarked vowel that ends a syllable or comprises a syllable has a long sound, such as the *o* in *open* and the *i* in *silent*.

O pen   SI lent

A long vowel in a syllable ending in a consonant is marked ⁻.

Snowflake = SNO flāk

An unmarked vowel in a syllable that ends with a consonant has a short sound, such as the *i* in *sister* and the *e* in *reset*.

SIS ter   re SET

A short vowel that comprises a syllable is marked ˘.

Decimal = DES ĭ mal

The sound of an unstressed vowel, such as the *a* in *ago* and the *o* in *connect*, is spelled.

Ahead = ə HED

Abdomen: The middle part of the trunk, containing the stomach, liver, intestines and spleen.

Abdominal cavity: An area in the body that contains many organs, including the liver, pancreas, intestines, stomach, kidneys and spleen.

Abrasion (ah BRA zhun): A wound characterized by skin that has been scraped or rubbed away.

Absorbed poison: A poison that enters the body after it comes in contact with the skin.

Active drowning victim: A person exhibiting universal behavior that includes struggling at the surface for 20 to 60 seconds before submerging.

Acute: Having a rapid and severe onset, then quickly subsiding.

Addiction: The compulsive need to use a substance. Stopping use would cause the user to suffer mental, physical and emotional distress.

Adhesive compress: A small pad of nonstick gauze on a strip of adhesive tape, applied directly to small injuries.

Advanced cardiac life support (ACLS): Techniques and treatments designed for use with victims of cardiac emergencies.

Aerobic: Requiring additional effort by the heart and lungs to meet the increased demand by the skeletal muscles for oxygen.

Aerobic exercise: Sustained, rhythmical exercise, using the large muscle groups, for at least 20-30 minutes within one's target heart rate range.

Airway: The pathway for air from the mouth and nose to the lungs.

Airway obstruction: Complete or partial blockage of the airway, which prevents air from reaching a person's lungs; the most common cause of respiratory emergencies.

Allergens: Substances that induce allergies.

Alveoli (al VE o li): Microscopic air sacs in the lungs where gases and wastes are exchanged between the lungs and the blood.

Alzheimer's disease: A progressive, degenerative disease that affects the brain, resulting in impaired memory, thinking and behavior.

Amnesia: Loss of memory.

Amniotic sac: A fluid-filled sac that encloses, bathes and protects the developing baby; commonly called the bag of waters.

Amputation: A type of avulsion injury in which a body part is severed.

Anaphylactic shock (an əfiiLAK tik) shock: A severe allergic reaction in which air passages may swell and restrict breathing; a form of shock.

Anaphylaxis (an əfii LAK sis): A severe allergic reaction; a form of shock.

Anaphylaxis kit: A container that holds the medication and any necessary equipment used to present or counteract anaphylactic shock.

Anatomical airway obstruction: Complete or partial blockage of the airway by the tongue or swollen tissues of the mouth or throat.

Aneurysm (AN u rizm): A condition in which the wall of an artery or vein weakens, balloons out and may rupture; usually caused by disease, trauma or a natural weakness in the vessel wall.

Angina (an JI nə) pectoris (PEK t əris): Chest pain that comes and goes at different times; commonly associated with cardiovascular disease.

Anorexia nervosa: An eating disorder characterized by a long-term refusal to eat food with sufficient nutrients and calories.

Antibiotic: A medicine used to help the body fight bacterial infection.

Antihistamines (an te HIS t əmenz): Drugs used to treat the signals of allergic reactions.

Anti-inflammatory (an te in FLAM ətor e) drug: A substance used to reduce heat, swelling, redness and pain in a body area.

Antiseptic: A substance that inhibits the growth and reproduction of microorganisms or germs.

Antitoxins: Antibodies capable of neutralizing specific disease-producing poisonous substances.

Antivenin: A substance used to counteract the poisonous effects of snake, spider or insect venom.

Arm: The part of the upper extremity from the shoulder to the hand.

Arteries: Large blood vessels that carry oxygenated blood away from the heart to the rest of the body.

Ashen: A grayish color; darker skin often looks ashen instead of pale.

Aspirate: Inhalation of blood, vomit or other foreign material into the lungs.

Asthma: A condition that narrows the air passages and makes breathing difficult.

Asystole: A condition where the heart has stopped generating electrical activity.

Atherosclerosis (ath er o skle RO sis): A condition in which fatty deposits build up on the walls of the arteries.

Aura (AW rah): An unusual sensation or feeling a person may experience before an epileptic seizure; it may be a visual hallucination; a strange sound, taste or smell; or an urgent need to get to safety.

Autogenics: A relaxation technique that uses self-suggestion to produce relaxation.

Auto-injector: A spring-loaded needle and syringe system with a single dose of epinephrine.

Automated external defibrillator (AED): An automatic device used to recognize a heart rhythm that requires an electric shock and either delivers the shock or prompts the rescuer to deliver it.

Avulsion: A wound in which a portion of the skin and sometimes other soft tissue is partially or completely torn away.

Bacteria: Microorganisms capable of causing infection.

Bandage: Material used to wrap or cover a part of the body; commonly used to hold a dressing or splint in place.

Bandage compress: A thick gauze dressing attached to a gauze bandage.

Barriers to action: Reasons for not acting or for hesitating to act in an emergency situation.

Biofeedback: A relaxation technique that uses instruments to measure bodily functions, such as heart rate and blood pressure.

Biological death: The irreversible damage caused by the death of brain cells.

Birth canal: The passageway from the uterus to the vaginal opening through which a baby passes during birth.

Bivouac: A temporary shelter.

Bladder: An organ in the pelvis in which urine is stored until it is released from the body.

Blood volume: The total amount of blood circulating within the body.

Body composition: The ratio of fat to all the tissues, such as muscles, that are fat free.

Body system: A group of organs and other structures that work together to carry out specific functions.

Bone: A dense, hard tissue that forms the skeleton.

Brachial (BRA ke əl) pulse: The pulse felt at the brachial artery on the inside of the upper arm.

Brain: The center of the nervous system; controls all body functions.

Breathing emergency: An emergency in which breathing is so impaired that life is threatened.

Breech birth: The delivery of a baby feet or buttocks first.

Bronchi (BRONG ki): The air passages that lead from the trachea to the alveoli.

Bronchioles: The air passage from the bronchi to the lungs.

Bronchitis: A disease resulting in inflammation of the lining of the trachea, bronchi and bronchioles.

Bronchodilator: A drug that widens the air passages that lead from the trachea to the alveoli. It most commonly is used for the treatment of asthma.

Bulimia: An eating disorder characterized by eating excessively then purging unwanted calories by vomiting or using laxatives.

Burn: An injury to the skin or other body tissues caused by heat, chemicals, electricity or radiation.

Calorie: A measure of the energy value of food.

Cannabis products: Substances, such as marijuana and hashish, that are derived from the *Cannabis sativa* plant; can produce feelings of elation, distorted perceptions of time and space and impaired motor coordination and judgment.

Capillaries (KAP i ler ez): Microscopic blood vessels linking arteries and veins; they transfer oxygen and other nutrients from the blood to all body cells and remove waste products.

Carbohydrates: Compounds that contain oxygen, carbon and hydrogen; the main source of energy for all body functions.

Carbon dioxide: A colorless, odorless gas; a waste product of respiration.

Carbon monoxide (CO): A clear, odorless, poisonous gas produced when carbon or other fuel is burned, as in gasoline engines.

Cardiac (KAR de ak) arrest: A condition in which the heart has stopped or beats too ineffectively to generate a pulse.

Cardiac emergency: Sudden illness involving the heart.

Cardiopulmonary (kar de o PUL mo ner e) resuscitation (re sus i TA shun) (CPR): A technique that combines chest compressions and rescue breathing for a victim whose heart and breathing have stopped.

Cardiorespiratory endurance: The ability to take in, deliver and extract oxygen for physical work; the ability to persevere in a physical task.

Cardiovascular (kar de o VAS ku lar) disease: Disease of the heart and blood vessels.

Carotid (kəROT id) arteries: Major blood vessels that supply blood to the head and neck.

Carpals: The bones of the wrist.

Cells: The basic unit of all living tissue.

Cerebral palsy: A dysfunction of the central nervous system in which a person has little or no control of the muscles.

Cervix (SERV ix): A short tube at the upper end of the birth canal; the opening of the uterus.

Chest: The upper part of the trunk, containing the heart, major blood vessels and lungs.

Child abuse: The physical, psychological or sexual assault of a child, resulting in injury or emotional trauma.

Cholesterol (ko LES ter ol): A fatty substance made by the body and found in certain foods; too much in the blood can cause fatty deposits on artery walls that may restrict or block blood flow.

Chronic: Persistent over a long period of time.

Circulatory (SER ku lə tor e) cycle: The flow of blood in the body.

Circulatory system: A group of organs and other structures that carries oxygen-rich blood and other nutrients throughout the body, removes wastes and returns oxygen-poor blood to the lungs.

Citizen responder: A layperson who recognizes an emergency and decides to act.

Clavicle: The collarbone; the slender, curved bone that extends from the sternum to the scapula (shoulder blade).

Clinically dead: The condition in which the heart stops beating and breathing stops.

Closed fracture: A fracture that leaves the skin unbroken.

Closed wound: An injury that does not break the skin and in which soft tissue damage occurs beneath the skin.

Clotting: The process by which blood thickens at a wound site to seal a hole or tear in a blood vessel and stops bleeding.

Concussion (kon CUSH ən): An injury to the brain caused by a violent blow to the head, followed by a temporary impairment of brain function, usually without permanent damage to the brain.

Consciousness: The state of being aware of one's self and one's surroundings.

Consent: Permission to give care, given by the victim to the rescuer.

Contraction: The pumping action of the heart; the rhythmic tightening of muscles in the uterus during labor.

Contusion: A bruise.

Coronary (KOR əner e) arteries: Blood vessels that supply the heart muscle with oxygen-rich blood.

Coronary heart disease (Also called coronary artery disease): Occurs when the coronary arteries that supply oxygen-rich blood to the heart muscle become hardened or narrowed from the build-up of fatty deposits.

Corticosteroid (KOR ti ko STIR oyd): A hormone, made synthetically or in the body, that is used in antiinflammatory medications.

Cranial cavity: An area in the body that contains the brain and is protected by the skull.

Cravats: Folded triangular bandages used to hold dressings or splints in place.

Critical burn: Any burn that is potentially life threatening, disabling or disfiguring.

Croup: An infection that causes swelling of the throat around the vocal cords.

Crowning: The point in labor when the baby's head is visible at the opening of the vagina.

Cyanosis (si əNO sis): A blue discoloration of the skin around the mouth and fingertips resulting from a lack of oxygen in the blood.

Cyanotic: Bluish discoloration of the skin around the mouth or the fingertips resulting from a lack of oxygen in the blood.

Deep burn: A burn that involves the epidermis and the two lower layers of skin, the dermis and the hypodermis, and may destroy underlying structures; it can be life threatening.

Defibrillation (de fib ri LA shun): An electrical shock that disrupts the electrical activity of the heart long enough to allow the heart to spontaneously develop an effective rhythm on its own.

Defibrillator (de FIB ri la tor): A device that sends an electric shock through the chest to the heart.

Delayed-help situation: A situation in which emergency assistance is delayed for more than 30 minutes.

Dependency: When one using a drug becomes physically and psychologically addicted to the drug.

Depressants: Substances that affect the central nervous system and decrease physical and mental activity, such as tranquilizers and sleeping pills.

Dermis: The deeper layer of skin; contains the nerves, hair roots, sweat and oil glands and blood vessels.

Designer drugs: Drugs that are chemically modified from medically prescribed substances to make them more potent or alter their effects.

Diabetes (di əBE tez): A condition in which the body does not produce enough insulin or does not use insulin effectively enough to regulate the amount of sugar (glucose) in the bloodstream.

Diabetes mellitus (mel I tus): *See* Diabetes.

Diabetic coma: A life-threatening emergency in which the body needs insulin.

Diabetic emergency: A situation in which a person becomes ill because of an imbalance of sugar (glucose) and insulin in the bloodstream.

Diabetic ketoacidosis (KE to a si DO sis): A life-threatening complication of uncontrolled diabetes mellitus.

Diaphragm: A dome-shaped muscle that aids in breathing and separates the chest from the abdomen.

Dietary fiber: The carbohydrates that are not broken down by the human digestive process.

Digestive system: A group of organs and other structures that digests food and eliminates wastes.

Direct contact transmission: Occurs when infected blood or body fluids from one person enter another person's body at a correct entry site.

Direct pressure: The pressure applied on a wound to control bleeding, for example, by one's gloved hand.

Disability: The absence or impairment of motor, sensory or mental function.

Disease transmission: The passage of a disease from one person to another.

Dislocation: The displacement of a bone from its normal position at a joint.

Distressed swimmer: A victim capable of staying afloat but likely to need assistance to get to shore.

Down syndrome: A condition caused by a genetic accident and characterized by varying degrees of mental retardation and physical defects.

Dressing: A pad placed directly over a wound to absorb blood and other body fluids and to prevent infection.

Drowning: Death by suffocation when submerged in water.

Drug: Any substance, other than food, intended to affect the functions of the body.

Drug paraphernalia (PAR əfer NAL yə): Devices used to contain or administer various kinds of drugs, such as needles and syringes for drugs that are injected.

Elapid snake: Family of venomous snakes that include coral snakes, cobras, mambas and others, such as the Australian brown snake or death adder.

Elastic roller bandage: A bandage designed to keep continuous pressure on a body part; the fabric is made of a yarn containing rubber.

Electrolyte (e LEK tro LIT): A substance that, in a solution or in liquid form, is capable of conducting an electric current.

Embedded object: An object that remains embedded in an open wound.

Embolus (EM bo lus): A sudden blockage of a blood vessel by a traveling clot or other material, such as fat or air, that circulates in the bloodstream until it becomes lodged in a blood vessel.

Embryo (EM bre o): The early stages of a developing baby in the uterus; characterized by the rapid growth and development of body systems.

Emergency: A situation requiring immediate action.

Emergency action steps: Three basic steps you should take in any emergency: CHECK—CALL—CARE.

Emergency medical services (EMS) personnel: Trained and equipped community-based personnel who provide emergency care for ill or injured victims and who are often dispatched through a local emergency number.

Emergency medical services (EMS) system: A network of community resources and medical personnel that provides emergency care to victims of injury or sudden illness.

Emergency medical technician (EMT): A person who has successfully completed a state-approved emergency medical technician training program. The levels of EMTs are the EMT-Basic, EMT-Intermediate and EMT-Paramedic.

Emphysema (em fəSE mə): A disease in which the lungs lose their ability to exchange carbon dioxide and oxygen effectively.

Endocrine (EN dəcrin) system: A group of organs and other structures that regulates and coordinates the activities of other systems by producing chemicals and hormones that influence the activity of tissues.

Epidermis: The outer layer of skin.

Epiglottis (ep i GLOT is): The flap of tissue that covers the trachea during swallowing to keep food and liquid out of the lungs.

Epiglottitis (ep i glot I tis): An infection that causes severe inflammation and potentially life-threatening swelling of the epiglottis.

Epilepsy (EP i lep se): A chronic condition characterized by seizures that may vary in type and duration; can usually be controlled by medication.

Esophagus (e SOF əgus): The tube leading from the mouth to the stomach.

Exhale: To breathe air out of the lungs.

External bleeding: Bleeding that can be seen coming from a wound.

Extremity: The shoulder to the fingers; the hip to the toes.

Fainting: A partial or complete loss of consciousness resulting from a temporary reduction of blood flow to the brain.

Fat: A compound made up of carbon, hydrogen, oxygen and three fatty acids, a storage form of energy for the body; a type of body tissue composed of cells containing stored fat.

Febrile (FEB ril) seizure (SE zhur): A seizure caused by a sudden change in body temperature.

Femoral arteries: The arteries that supply blood to the lower extremities.

Femur: The bone of the thigh.

Fetus (FE tus): The developing unborn offspring after the embryo stage.

Fibula: One of the two bones of the leg.

First aid: Immediate care given to a victim of injury or sudden illness until more advanced care can be obtained.

First responder: A person trained in emergency care that may be called on to give such care as a routine part of his or her job.

Food Guide Pyramid: A pictorial guide to the current five basic food groups.

Forearm: The part of the upper extremity from the elbow to the wrist.

Fracture: A break or disruption in bone tissue.

Frostbite: A condition in which body tissues freeze; most commonly occurs in the fingers, toes, ears and nose.

Gastric distention: A condition in which the abdomen becomes swollen with air.

Genitals: The external reproductive organs.

Genitourinary (jen i to UR ri nary) system: A group of organs and other structures that eliminates wastes and enables sexual reproduction.

Glands: Organs that release fluid and other substances into the blood or onto the skin.

Glucose: A simple sugar found in certain foods, especially fruits, and a major source of energy for all living organisms.

Good Samaritan laws: Laws that protect people who willingly give first aid without accepting anything in return.

Hallucinogens (həLOO sin ə jenz): Substances that affect mood, sensation, thought, emotion and self-awareness; alter perceptions of time and space; and produce hallucinations and delusions. Also known as psychedelics.

Head-tilt/chin-lift technique: A technique used to open a victim's airway by pushing down on the forehead while pulling up on the bony part of the jaw.

Hearing loss: Partial or total loss of hearing.

Heart: A muscular organ that circulates blood throughout the body.

Heart attack: A sudden illness involving the death of heart muscle tissue when it does not receive oxygen-rich blood; also known as myocardial infarction.

Heat cramps: Painful spasms of skeletal muscles after exercise or work in warm or moderate temperatures; usually involve the calf and abdominal muscles.

Heat exhaustion: The early stage and most common form of heat-related illness; often results from strenuous work or exercise in a hot environment.

Heat stroke: A life-threatening condition that develops when the body's cooling mechanisms are overwhelmed and body systems begin to fail.

Heaving jug: A homemade piece of rescue equipment for throwing to a victim, composed of a 1-gallon plastic container containing some water, with 50 to 75 feet of floating line attached.

Heaving line: Floating rope, white, yellow or some other highly visible color, used for water rescue.

Hemorrhage (HEM ə rij): A loss of a large amount of blood in a short period of time.

High blood pressure: A condition, often without any signals, of elevated blood pressure; also referred to as hypertension.

Hormone: A substance that circulates in body fluids and has a specific effect on cell activity.

Humerus: The bone of the arm.

Hyperglycemia (hi per gli SE me ə): A condition in which too much sugar (glucose) is in the bloodstream, and the insulin level in the body is too low.

Hyperventilation: Breathing that is faster than normal.

Hypodermis: A layer of skin located beneath the dermis and epidermis; contains fat, blood vessels and connective tissues.

Hypoglycemia (hi po gli SE me ə): A condition in which too little sugar (glucose) is in the bloodstream, and the insulin level in the body is too high.

Hypothalmus: Part of the brain that is responsible for regulating body temperature.

Hypothermia: A life-threatening condition in which the body's warming mechanisms fail to maintain normal body temperature and the entire body cools.

Imagery: A relaxation technique that involves using the imagination to create various scenes and wished-for situations.

Immobilize: Keep an injured body part from moving by using a splint or other method.

Impairment: Damage or reduction in quality, quantity, value or strength of a function.

Implied consent: Legal concept that assumes a person would consent to receive emergency care if he or she were physically able to do so.

Indirect contact transmission: Occurs when a person touches objects that have the blood or body fluid of an infected person, and that infected blood or body fluid enters the body through a correct entry site.

Infection: The growth of disease-producing microorganisms in the body.

Inhalants: Substances such as glue or paint thinners inhaled to produce mood-altering effect.

Inhale: To breathe air into the lungs.

Ingested poison: A poison that is swallowed.

Inhaled poison: A poison breathed into the lungs.

Injected poison: A poison that enters the body through the skin through a bite or sting, or as drugs or medications through a hypodermic needle.

Injury: Damage that occurs when the body is subjected to an external force, such as a blow, a fall, a collision, an electric current or extremes of temperatures.

Insulin (IN su lin): A hormone produced in the pancreas that enables the body to use sugar (glucose) for energy; frequently used to treat diabetes.

Insulin shock: A life-threatening condition in which too much insulin is in the bloodstream.

Integumentary (in teg YU men tәre) system: The skin, hair and nails; protects the body, retains fluid and helps prevent infection.

Internal bleeding: Bleeding inside the body.

Joint: A structure where two or more bones are joined.

Kidney: An organ that filters waste from the blood to form urine.

Labor: The birth process, beginning with the contraction of the uterus and dilation of the cervix and ending with the stabilization and recovery of the mother.

Laceration (las әRA shun): A cut, usually from a sharp object; may have jagged or smooth edges.

Larynx (LAR ingks): A part of the airway connecting the pharynx with the trachea; commonly called the voice box.

Layperson: Someone who does not have special or advanced first aid training or skills (also known as a citizen responder).

Leg: The part of the lower extremity from the pelvis to the ankle.

Life-threatening emergency: An illness or injury that impairs a victim's ability to circulate oxygenated blood to all the parts of his or her body.

Ligament: A fibrous band that holds bones together at a joint.

Lower extremity: The parts of the body from the hip to the toes.

Lower leg: The part of the lower extremity from the knee to the ankle.

Lungs: A pair of light, spongy organs in the chest that provide the mechanism for taking oxygen in and removing carbon dioxide during breathing.

Lyme disease: An illness transmitted by a certain kind of infected tick; victims may or may not develop a rash.

Manual stabilization: A technique used to minimize movement of a victim's head and neck and keep them in line with the body to protect the spine while giving care.

Mechanical airway obstruction: Complete or partial blockage of the airway by a foreign object, such as a piece of food or a small toy, or by fluids, such as vomit or blood.

Medical emergency: A sudden illness requiring immediate medical attention

Medication: A drug given therapeutically to prevent or treat the effects of a disease or condition or otherwise enhance mental or physical well-being.

Membrane: A thin layer of tissue that covers a surface, lines a cavity or divides a space.

Mental (cognitive) function: The brain's capacity to reason and process information.

Metabolism: The process by which cells convert nutrients to energy.

Metacarpals: The bones of the hand.

Metatarsals: The bones of the foot.

Microorganism (mi kro OOR gә nizm): A bacteria, virus or other microscopic structure that may enter the body. Those that cause an infection or disease are called pathogens.

Miscarriage: A spontaneous end to pregnancy before the twentieth week; usually because of defects of the fetus or womb.

Motor function: The ability to move the body or a body part.

Motor impairment: The total or partial inability to move or to use a body part.

Mucous membranes: A thin sheet of body tissue that covers parts of the body.

Multiple sclerosis: A progressive disease characterized by nerve degeneration and patches of hardened tissue in the brain or spinal cord.

Muscle: A soft tissue that contracts and relaxes to create movement.

Muscular dystrophy: A hereditary disease characterized by progressive deterioration of muscles, leading to disability, deformity and loss of strength.

Musculoskeletal (mus ku lo SKEL ә tәl) system: A group of tissues and other structures that supports the body, protects internal organs, allows movement, stores minerals, manufactures blood cells and creates heat.

Narcotics: Drugs that dull the senses and are prescribed to relieve pain.

Nerve: A part of the nervous system that sends electrical impulses to and from the brain and all body areas.

Nervous system: A group of organs and other structures that regulates all body functions.

Nitroglycerin: A prescribed medication, often in tablet form, given for the prevention or relief of angina pectoris.

Non-life-threatening emergency: A situation that does not have an immediate impact on a victim's ability to circulate oxygenated blood, but still requires medical attention.

Nutrients: Substances found in food that are required by the body.

Nutrition: The science that deals with the study of food you eat and how the body uses it.

Obesity: A condition characterized by an excess of stored body fat.

Occlusive dressing: A type of dressing that does not allow air or moisture to pass through.

Open fracture: A fracture that involves an open wound.

Open wound: An injury resulting in a break in the skin's surface.

Organ: A collection of similar tissues acting together to perform specific body functions.

Osteoporosis (os te o pəRO sis): The gradual, progressive weakening of bone.

Overdose: An excess use of a drug, resulting in adverse reactions ranging from mania and hysteria to coma and death. Specific reactions to an overdose include changes in blood pressure and heartbeat, sweating, vomiting and liver failure.

Oxygen: A tasteless, colorless and odorless gas necessary to sustain life.

Paralysis: A loss of muscle control; a permanent loss of feeling and movement; the inability to move.

Paramedic: A highly specialized EMT.

Passive drowning victim: An unconscious victim face-down, submerged or near the surface of the water.

Patella: The kneecap.

Pathogen: A disease-causing agent; also called a microorganism.

Pelvic cavity: The lowest part of the trunk, containing the bladder, rectum and female reproductive organs.

Pelvis: The lower part of the trunk, containing the intestines, bladder and internal reproductive organs.

Personal protective equipment: The equipment and supplies that help prevent the responder from directly contacting infected materials.

Phalanges: The bones of the fingers.

Pharynx (FAR ingks): A part of the airway formed by the back of the nose and the throat.

Placenta (plə CENT ə): An organ attached to the uterus and unborn child through which nutrients are delivered to the baby; expelled after the baby is delivered.

Plasma: The liquid part of the blood.

Platelets: Disk-shaped structures in the blood that are made of cell fragments; help stop bleeding by forming blood clots at wound sites.

Poison: Any substance that can cause injury, illness or death when introduced into the body in relatively small amounts.

Poison Control Center (PCC): A specialized health-care center that provides information in cases of poisoning or suspected poisoning emergencies.

Pregnancy: Begins when an egg (ovum) is fertilized by a sperm, forming an embryo.

Pressure bandage: A bandage applied snugly to create pressure on a wound to aid in controlling bleeding.

Prolapsed umbilical cord: A complication of childbirth in which a loop of umbilical cord protrudes through the vagina prior to delivery of the baby.

Proteins: Compounds made up of amino acids necessary to build tissues.

Pulse: The beat you feel with each heart contraction.

Puncture wound: A wound that results when the skin is pierced with a pointed object, such as a nail, a piece of glass, a splinter or a knife.

Quarry: A deep pit where stone or gravel was once excavated; when no longer in use, it may become filled with water.

Rabies: A disease caused by a virus transmitted through the saliva of infected mammals.

Radius: One of the two bones of the forearm.

Reaching assist: A non-swimming rescue in which one extends an object, such as an arm, leg or tree branch to a victim.

Recovery position: The position of an unconscious victim on his or her side in case he or she vomits.

Reproductive system: A group of organs and other structures that enables sexual reproduction.

Rescue breathing: A technique of breathing for a nonbreathing child or infant.

Rescue tube: A vinyl, foam-filled, floating support used in making rescues.

Respiration (res pi RA shun): The breathing process in which the body takes in oxygen and eliminates carbon dioxide.

Respiratory (re SPI rə to re) or (RES pərə tor e) arrest: A condition in which breathing has stopped.

Respiratory distress: A condition in which breathing is difficult.

Respiratory system: A group of organs and other structures that brings air into the body and removes wastes through a process called breathing or respiration.

Reye's (raz) syndrome: An illness that affects the brain and other internal organs, usually found in people under the age of 18.

Rib cage: The cage of bones formed by the 12 pairs of ribs, the sternum and the spine.

Ribs: Bones that attach to the spine and to the breastbone, forming a protective shell for vital organs, such as the heart and lungs.

Ring buoy: A rescue device made of buoyant cork, kapok or plastic-covered material attached to a line with an object or knot at the end to keep the line from slipping out from under your foot when you throw it.

Risk factors: Conditions or behaviors that increase the chance that a person will develop a disease.

Rocky Mountain spotted fever (RMSF): A disease transmitted by a certain kind of infected tick; victims develop a spotted rash.

Roller bandage: A bandage made of gauze or gauze-like material; generally wrapped around a body part over a dressing.

Saturated fats: The fat in animal tissue and products.

Scapula: The shoulder blade.

Seizure (SE zhur): An irregularity in the brain's electrical activity, often marked by loss of consciousness and uncontrollable muscle movement; also called a convulsion.

Sensory function: The ability to see, hear, touch, taste and smell.

Shepherd's crook: A long pole with a hook on the end that can be used to either pull a conscious drowning person to safety or encircle a submerged drowning person and pull the person to safety.

Shock: The failure of the circulatory system to provide adequate oxygen-rich blood to all parts of the body.

Signals: Signs or indications of observable evidence of injury or illness.

Signs of life: Normal movement or breathing.

Skeletal muscles: Muscles that attach to the bones.

Skin: The tough, supple membrane that covers the surface of the body.

Sodium: A mineral abundant in table salt; associated with high blood pressure.

Soft tissues: Body structures that include the layers of skin, fat and muscles.

Spinal cavity: An area of the body that contains the spinal cord and is protected by the bones of the spine.

Spinal column: The spine.

Spinal cord: A bundle of nerves extending from the brain at the base of the skull to the lower back; protected by the spinal column.

Spine: A strong, flexible column of vertebrae, extending from the base of the skull to the tip of the tailbone (coccyx), that supports the head and the trunk and encases and protects the spinal cord; also called the spinal column or the vertebral column.

Splint: A device used to immobilize body parts; to immobilize body parts with such a device.

Spontaneous abortion: A spontaneous or unintentional ending of pregnancy before the fetus can be expected to live, which usually occurs before the twentieth week of pregnancy. Also known as a miscarriage.

Sprain: The stretching and tearing of ligaments and other tissue structures at a joint.

Starting block: Platforms competitive swimmers dive from to start a race.

Sternum: The long, flat bone in the middle of the front of the rib cage; also called the breastbone.

Standard precautions: Safety measures taken to prevent exposure to blood and body fluids when giving care to ill or injured persons.

Stimulants: Substances that affect the central nervous system and increase physical and mental activity.

Stoma: An opening in the front of the neck through which a person whose larynx has been removed breathes.

Strain: The stretching and tearing of muscle and tendons.

Stress: A physiological or psychological response to real or imagined influences that alter an existing state of physical, mental or emotional balance.

Stress management: A person's planned attempt to deal with stress.

Stressor: An event or condition that triggers the stress response.

Stroke: A disruption of blood flow to a part of the brain, which causes permanent damage to brain tissue; also called a cerebrovascular accident (CVA).

Substance abuse: The deliberate, persistent, excessive use of a substance without regard to health concerns or accepted medical practices.

Substance misuse: The use of a substance for unintended purposes or for intended purposes but in improper amounts or doses.

Sucking chest wound: A penetrating chest injury producing a sucking sound each time the victim breathes.

Sudden death: Death from cardiac arrest without any prior signals of a heart attack.

Sudden illness: A physical condition requiring immediate medical attention.

Sudden infant death syndrome (SIDS): The sudden death of a seemingly normal, healthy infant; occurs during the infant's sleep without evidence of disease; sometimes called crib death.

Superficial burn: A burn involving only the outer layer of skin, the epidermis, characterized by dry, red skin.

Syncope (sing kə p e): A brief lapse in consciousness; *see* Fainting.

Synergistic effect: The interaction of two or more drugs to produce a certain effect.

Target heart rate range: Sixty to ninety percent of your maximum heart rate.

Tarsals: The bones of the ankle.

Tendon: A cordlike, fibrous band that attaches muscle to bone.

Tetanus: An acute infectious disease caused by a bacteria that produces a powerful poison; can occur in puncture wounds, such as human and animal bites; also called lockjaw.

Thigh: The part of the lower extremity from the pelvis to the knee.

Thoracic (tho RAS ik) cavity: An area in the body that contains the heart and the lungs and is protected by the rib cage and upper portion of the spine.

Thrombus (THROM bus): A collection of blood components that forms in the heart or vessels, obstructing blood flow.

Throw bag: A nylon bag containing 50 to 75 feet of coiled floating line; used as a rescue device.

Throwing assist: A non-swimming water rescue in which one throws a line with a floating object attached to a victim.

Tibia: One of the two bones of the leg.

Tissue: A collection of similar cells that act together to perform specific body functions.

Tolerance: The body becomes resistant to a drug or other substance because of continued use.

Tourniquet (TUR ni kit): A wide band of cloth or other material that is wrapped tightly around an extremity to control severe bleeding; used as a last resort measure.

Toxin: A poisonous substance.

Trachea (TRA keə): A tube leading from the upper airway to the lungs; also called the windpipe.

Transient (TRANZ e ent) ischemic (is KE mik) attack (TIA): A temporary episode that, like a stroke, is caused by a disruption of blood flow to the brain; sometimes called a mini-stroke.

Trauma: The violent force or mechanism that can cause injury

Triangular bandage: A bandage in the shape of a triangle; used to hold a dressing or splint in place or as a sling.

Trunk: The part of the body containing the chest, abdomen and pelvis.

Ulna: One of the two bones of the forearm.

Umbilical cord: A flexible structure that attaches the placenta to the unborn child, allowing for the passage of blood, nutrients and waste.

Upper arm: The part of the upper extremity from the shoulder to the elbow.

Upper extremity: The parts of the body from the shoulder to the fingers.

Urinary system: A group of organs and other structures that eliminates waste products from the blood.

Uterus (U ter us): A pear-shaped organ in a woman's pelvis in which an embryo forms and develops into a baby.

Vagina: *See* birth canal.

Veins: Blood vessels that carry oxygenated blood from all parts of the body to the heart.

Ventricular fibrillation (V-fib): An abnormal heart rhythm characterized by disorganized electrical activity, which results in the quivering of the ventricles.

Ventricular tachycardia (V-tach): An abnormal heart rhythm characterized by rapid contractions of the ventricles.

Vertebrae (VER tə bra): The 33 bones of the spine.

Vertebral column: The spine.

Virus: A disease-causing microorganism that, unlike bacteria, requires another organism to live and reproduce.

Vision loss: Partial or total loss of sight.

Vital organs: Organs whose functions are essential for life, including the brain, heart and lungs.

Wheezing: Hoarse whistling sounds made during breathing.

Wilderness: An area that is uninhabited by human beings, is uncultivated and has been left in its natural condition.

Withdrawal: The condition produced when a person stops using or abusing a substance to which he or she is addicted.

Wound: An injury to the soft tissues.

Sources

Altman L: New breakfast of champions: a recipe for victory or disaster?, *The New York Times*, November 20, 1988.

American Academy of Orthopaedic Surgeons: *Basic rescue and emergency care*, Park Ridge, IL, 1990,

American Academy of Orthopaedic Surgeons.

American Academy of Orthopaedic Surgeons: *Rural rescue and emergency care*, Park Ridge, IL, 1990. American Academy of Orthopaedic Surgeons.

American Academy of Orthopaedic Surgeons: *Your first response in emergency care*, Park Ridge, IL, 1990, American Academy of Orthopaedic Surgeons.

American Association of Poison Control Centers, http://www.aapcc.org.

American Cancer Society: *Prevention and early detection—Cigarette smoking.* http://www.cancer.org/docroot/PED/content/PED_10_2X_Cigarette_Smoking.asp?sitearea=PED.

American Cancer Society: *Statistics—Statistics for 2004.* http://www.cancer.org/docroot/STT/stt_O.asp.

American Cancer Society: *Reference information—Overview: Lung cancer.* http://www.cancer.org/docroot/CRI/content/CRI_2_2_2X_What_causes_lung_cancer_26.asp?sitearea=.

American College of Emergency Physicians: *Dental emergencies.* http://www.acep.org. Accessed 10/25/04.

American Dental Association: *Dental emergencies and injuries.* http://www.ada.org/public/manage/emergencies.asp. Accessed 10/25/04.

American Diabetes Association. http://www.diabetes.org.

American Heart Association: *Heart disease and stroke statistics — 2004 update*, Dallas, TX, 2003. http://www.americanheart.org.

American Heart Association: *Heart and stroke facts*, 1992.

American Lyme Disease Foundation: *A quick guide to Lyme disease*, 1995.

American Lyme Disease Foundation: *A homeowner's guide to the ecology and environmental management of Lyme disease*, 1995.

American Red Cross: *Caring for a loved one with Alzheimer's disease or dementia*, Yardley, PA, 2004, StayWell.

American Red Cross Advisory Council on First Aid And Safety (ACFAS): *Statement on ephinephrine administration*, 2001.

American Stroke Association: http://www.strokeassociation.org.

Berkow R: *The Merck manual of diagnosis and therapy*, ed 17, Rahway, NJ, 1993, Regents/PrenticeHall.

Bogart J, DDS: Executive Director, American Academy of Pediatric Dentists. Interview, April 1990.

Breuss CE, Laing SJ: *Decisions for health*, Dubuque, IA, 1985, William C. Brown.

Canadian Red Cross Society: *The vital link*, St. Louis, 1994, Mosby.

Centers for Disease Control and Prevention: *Behavioral risk factor surveillance system survey data.* U.S. Department of Health and Human Services, 1999, http://www.cdc.gov/brfss. Accessed 8/31/04.

Centers for Disease Control and Prevention: *Carpal tunnel syndrome.* http://www.cdc.gov/niosh/ctsfs.html. Accessed 10/15/04.

Centers for Disease Control, http://www.cdc.gov/ncidod.op/food.htm.

Centers for Disease Control and Prevention: *Measures of alcohol consumption and alcohol-related health effects from excessive consumption*, U.S. Department of Health and Human Services, 5 August 2004. http://www.cdc.gov/alcohol/factsheets/general_information. Accessed 8/31/04.

Chaikin T, Telander R: The nightmare of steroids, *Sports Illustrated*, 69:18, 1988.

Cohn AH: *It shouldn't hurt to be a child*, Chicago, 1987, National Committee for Prevention of Child Abuse.

Coil SM: *Poisonous plants*, New York, 1991, Franklin Watts.

CTS: *Relief at hand*, The University of California Berkeley Wellness Letter, 11(4): 7, 1995.

DISPATCH Monthly Magazine, http://www.911.dispatch.com. Accessed 06/24/04.

Division of Medical Sciences, National Academy of Sciences. National Research Council: *Accidental death and disability: the neglected disease of modern society*, Washington, DC, 1966.

Dorsman J: *How to quit drinking without AA: A complete self-help guide*, ed 2, Rocklin, CA, 1994, Prima Pub.

Driesbach RH, Robertson WO: *Handbook of poisoning*, ed 12, East Norwalk, CT, 1987, Appleton & Lange.

FDA Consumer Drug Information. http://www.fda.gov/cder/consumerinfo/default.htm. Accessed 08/12/04.

Federal Communications Commission, http://www.fcc.gov/911/enhanced. Accessed 06/24/04.

Gabor A: On-the-job-straining: Repetitive motion is the Information Age's hottest hazard, *US News and World Report* 108(20): 51-53, 1990.

Getchell B, Pippin R, Barnes J: *Health*, Boston, 1989, Houghton Mifflin.

Green M, ed: *Bright futures: Guidelines for health supervision of infants, children, and adolescents*, Arlington, VA, 1994, National Center for Education in Maternal and Child Health.

Guthrie HA, Picciano MF: *Human nutrition*, St. Louis, 1995, Mosby.

Hafen BO, Karren KJ: *First aid for colleges and universities*, ed 5, Englewood Cliffs, NJ, 1993, Regents/Prentice Hall.

Hahn DB, Payne WA, *Focus on health*, ed 2, St. Louis, 1994, Mosby.

Hauser WA, Hesdorffer DC: *Facts about epilepsy*, 1994, Epilepsy Foundation of America.

Hospital Shared Services of Colorado: *Stockard inventory program: your right to make health care decisions*, Denver, 1991.2.

Instant health boost: stop smoking, *Glamour*, May 1995, p. 48.

Isaac J, Goth P: *Wilderness first aid handbook*, New York, 1991, Lyons & Burford.

Juvenile Diabetes Foundation International. http://www.jdrf.org.

Katz RT: *Carpal tunnel syndrome: A practical review*, American Family Physician 49(6): 1371-1382, 1994.

Kessler E: *The thunderstorm in human affairs*, Norman, OK, University of Oklahoma, 1983.

Lerner C: *Dumb cane and daffodils: Poisonous plants in the house and garden*, New York, 1990, William Morrow.

Major R, M.D.: *A history of medicine*, Springfield, IL. Charles C. Thomas, 1954.

Marnell T: *Drug identification bible*, ed 1, Denver, Drug Identification Bible, 1993.

Medford H, DDS: Acute care of an avulsed tooth, *Annals of Emergency Medicine* 11:559-61, 1982.

Merenstein GB, Kaplan DW, Rosenberg AA: *Handbook of pediatrics*, ed 17, East Norwalk, CT, 1994, Appleton & Lange.

National Center for Chronic Disease Prevention and Health Promotion Centers for Disease Control and Prevention. http://www.cdc.gov/nccdphp/bb_diabetes/index.htm.

National Center for Injury Prevention and Control: *Water related injuries fact sheet*, U.S. Department of Health and Human Services, 5 August 2004, http://www.cdc.gov/ncipc/factsheets/drown.htm. Accessed 8/31/04.

National Committee for Injury Prevention and Control: *Injury prevention: Meeting the challenge*, New York, 1989, Oxford University Press as a supplement to the *American Journal of Preventive Medicine*, 5:3, 1989.

National Diabetes Education Program. http://www.ndep.nih.gov.

National Diabetes Information Clearinghouse (NDIC). http://www.diabetes.niddk.nih.gov/dm/pubs/medicines_ez/specific.htm. Accessed 08/12/04.

National Diabetes Information Clearinghouse (NDIC). http://diabetes.niddk.nih.gov/dm/pubs/insulin/index.htm. Accessed 08/12/04.

National Diabetes Information Clearinghouse (NDIC). http://www.diabetes.niddk.nih.gov/dm/pubs/pancreati-cislet.htm. Accessed 08/12/04.

National Emergency Number Association. http://www.nena.org. Accessed 6/24/04.

National Fire Protection Association: *Play it safe, plan your escape*, 1987, Quincy, MA (Ch. 24, Escape Route).

National Institute of Diabetes and Digestive and Kidney Diseases of the National Institutes of Health. http://www.niddk.nih.gov/.

National Institute of Health, http://www.nichd.nih.gov/sids/reduce_infant_risk.htm#WhatCan. Accessed 10/08/04.

National Institute of Neurological Disorders and Stroke: *Stroke: Hope through research*, NINDS, July 2004. http://www.ninds.nih.gov.

National Institute on Drug Abuse: *Anabolic steroids: A threat to body and mind*. National Institutes of Health, No. 94-3721, 1991. Reprinted 1994, 1996. Revised April, 2000. http://www.drugabuse.gov/ResearchReports/Steroids/AnabolicSteroids.html. Accessed 9/1/04.

National Registry of Emergency Medical Technicians. http://www.nremt.org/about/ems_learn.asp. Accessed 7/22/04.

National Safety Council: *Injury facts*, 2004, Chicago, National Safety Council.

National Safety Council, Thygerson AL, eds: *First aid essentials*, Boston, 1989, Jones and Bartlett.

National Ski Patrol, http://www.nsp.org/nsp2002/safety_info_template.asp?mode=dress. Accessed 10/29/04.

National Weather Service. http://www.lightningsafety.noaa.gov/outdoors.htm. Accessed 10/25/04.

Patient Self-Determination Act, U.S. Code 42 (1990), § Section 1395 cc(a)(1)(Q)(A).

Payne WA, Hahn WB: *Understanding your health*, St. Louis, 1989, Mosby.

Randall T: 50 million volts may crash through a lightning victim, *The Chicago Tribune*, Section 2D, August 13, 1989, p. 1.

Recreation Equipment Incorporated: *Layering for comfort: FYI*, an informational brochure from REI, Seattle, 1991.

Recreation Equipment Incorporated: *Outerwear product information guide*, Seattle, 1995.

Recreation Equipment Incorporated: *Understanding outdoor fabrics: FYI*, an informational brochure from REI, Seattle, 1991.

Rice DP, MacKenzie EJ, and associates: *Cost of injury in the United States: A report to Congress 1989*, San Francisco, 1989, Institute for Health and Aging, University of California, and Injury Prevention Center, The Johns Hopkins University.

Rideing WH: Hospital Life in New York, *Harper's New Monthly Magazine* 57(171), 1878.

Rob C: *The caregiver's guide: Helping elderly relatives cope with health and safety problems*, Boston, 1991, Houghton Mifflin.

Rodwell SR: *Basic nutrition and diet therapy*, ed 10, St. Louis, 1995, Mosby.

Safety IQ: A quiz for the whole family, *Geico Direct*, pp. 7-10, Spring, 1995, K. L. Publications.

Sanford JP: Tetanus—Forgotton but not gone, *New England Journal of Medicine* 332(12): 812-813.

Schimelpfenig T, Lindsey I: *NOLS wilderness first aid*, Lander, WY, 1991, NOLS Publications.

Seeley RR, Stevens TD, Tate P: *Anatomy and physiology*, ed 3, St. Louis, 1995, Mosby.

Simon JE, Goldberg AT: *Prehospital pediatric life support*, St. Louis, 1989, Mosby.

Spence WR: *Substance abuse identification guide*, Waco, TX: HEALTH EDCO, 1991.

Spinal Cord Information Network; *Spinal injury, facts and figures at a glance*. August 2004. http://www.spinalcord.uab.edu/. Accessed 11/01/04.

The White House: *National drug control strategy*, September 1989.

Treating for carpal tunnel syndrome, *Lancet* 338(8765): 479-481, 1991.

Turkington C: *Poisons and antidotes,* New York, 1994, Facts on File.

USA Today, Vol. 121, No. 2573, February 1993.

United States Coast Guard: *Boating Statistics—2003,* U.S. Department of Homeland Security, 8 October 2004. http://www.uscgboating.org/statistics/Boating Statistics 2003.pdf. Accessed 12/14/04.

U.S. Department of Agriculture: *USDA's Food Guide Pyramid.* USDA Human Nutrition, Pub No. 249, Washington, DC 1992.

U.S. Department of Health and Human Services: Public Health Service; Alcohol, Drug Abuse, and Mental Health Administration; and National Institute on Alcohol Abuse and Alcoholism: *Seventh special report to the U.S. Congress on alcohol and health,* Alexandria, VA, January, 1990, Editorial Experts.

U.S. Department of Health and Human Services: *The health consequences of smoking: A report of the surgeon general.* U.S. Department of Health and Human Services, Centers for Disease Control and Prevention, National Center for Chronic Disease Prevention and Health Promotion, Office on Smoking and Health, 2004. http://www.cdc.gov/tobacco/sgr/sgr_2004/Factsheets/2.htm.

U.S. Food and Drug Administration FDA. http://www.fda.gov/diabetes/glucose.html. Accessed 08/15/04.

U.S. Food and Drug Administration FDA. http://www.fda.gov/diabetes/insulin.html. Accessed 08/12/04.

Ventura SJ, Mosher WD, Curtin SC, Abma JC, Henshaw S: *Trends in pregnancies and pregnancy rates by outcome: Estimates for the United States, 1976–96.* National Center for Health Statistics. Vital and Health Statistics 2000; 21(56).

Wardlaw GM, Insel PM: *Perspectives in nutrition,* St. Louis, 1990, Mosby.

Wardlaw GM, Insel PM, Seyler MF: *Contemporary nutrition: Issues and insights,* ed 2, St. Louis, 1994, Mosby.

Weil A, Rosen W: *From chocolate to morphine: Everything you need to know about mind-altering drugs,* ed 2, New York, 1993, Houghton-Mifflin.

Westbrooks RG, Preacher JW: *Poisonous plants of eastern North America,* Columbia, SC, 1986, University of South Carolina Press.

Wilderness Medical Society: *Practice guidelines for wilderness emergency care,* Forgey WW, ed, Merrillville, IN, 1995, ICS Books.

Williams SR: *Basic nutrition and diet therapy,* ed 10, St. Louis, 1995, Mosby.

Woodward L: *Poisonous plants: a colorful field guide,* New York, 1985, Hippocrene Books.

Wyllie I: *The treatment of epilepsy: Principles and practice,* Philadelphia, 1993, Lea & Febiger.

Index

MISSION OF THE AMERICAN RED CROSS

The American Red Cross, a humanitarian organization led by volunteers and guided by its Congressional Charter and the Fundamental Principles of the International Red Cross Movement, will provide relief to victims of disaster and help people prevent, prepare for, and respond to emergencies.

ABOUT THE AMERICAN RED CROSS

The American Red Cross has helped people mobilize to help their neighbors for 125 years. Last year, victims of a record 72,883 disasters, most of them fires, turned to the nearly 1 million volunteers and 35,000 employees of the Red Cross for help and hope. Through more than 800 locally supported chapters, more than 15 million people each year gain the skills they need to prepare for and respond to emergencies in their homes, communities and world. Almost 4 million people give blood—the gift of life—through the Red Cross, making it the largest supplier of blood and blood products in the United States. The Red Cross helps thousands of U.S. service members separated from their families by military duty stay connected. As part of the International Red Cross and Red Crescent Movement, a global network of more than 180 national societies, the Red Cross helps restore hope and dignity to the world's most vulnerable people. An average of 91 cents of every dollar the Red Cross spends is invested in humanitarian services and programs. The Red Cross is not a government agency; it relies on donations of time, money, and blood to do its work.

FUNDAMENTAL PRINCIPLES OF THE INTERNATIONAL RED CROSS AND RED CRESCENT MOVEMENT

HUMANITY
IMPARTIALITY
NEUTRALITY
INDEPENDENCE
VOLUNTARY SERVICE
UNITY
UNIVERSALITY